UNDERSTANDING PHARMACOLOGY
Essentials for Medication Safety

M. Linda Workman, PhD, RN, FAAN

Linda LaCharity, PhD, RN

ELSEVIER

Elsevier
3251 Riverport Lane
St. Louis, Missouri 63043

Notice

Practitioners and researchers must always rely on their own experience and knowledge in evaluating and
using any information, methods, compounds or experiments described herein. Because of rapid advances
in the medical sciences, in particular, independent verification of diagnoses and drug dosages should be
made. To the fullest extent of the law, no responsibility is assumed by Elsevier, authors, editors or con-
tributors for any injury and/or damage to persons or property as a matter of products liability, negligence
or otherwise, or from any use or operation of any methods, products, instructions, or ideas contained in
the material herein.

Senior Content Strategist: Brandi Graham
Content Development Manager: Danielle Frazier
Senior Content Development Specialist: Rae L. Robertson
Publishing Services Manager: Julie Eddy
Book Production Specialist: Clay S. Broeker
Design Direction: Renee Duenow

Printed in Canada

Last digit is the print number: 9   8   7   6   5   4   3   2   1

To David, Emmy, and Violet, who complete my rainbow.

M. Linda Workman

To Ralph, Thal, and Anne with all my heart.

Linda LaCharity

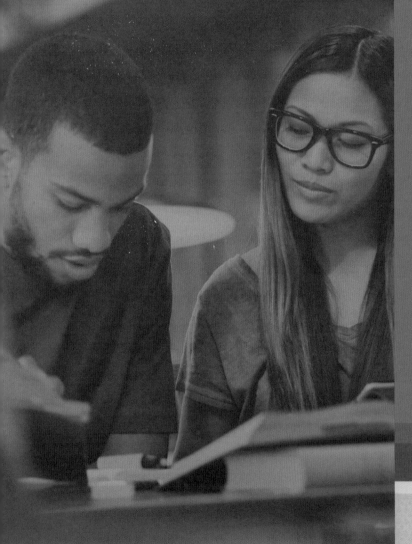

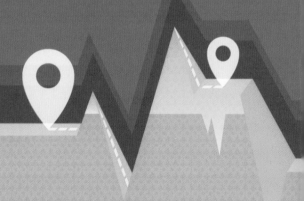

About the Authors

M. Linda Workman, a native of Canada, received her BSN from the University of Cincinnati College of Nursing and Health. She later earned her MSN and a PhD in Developmental Biology from the University of Cincinnati. Linda's more than 40 years of academic experience includes teaching at the diploma, associate degree, baccalaureate, and master's levels. Her areas of teaching expertise include medical-surgical nursing, pharmacology, physiology, and pathophysiology. Linda has been called the "Mr. Rogers" of nursing education for her ability to creatively present complex physiologic concepts in a manner that promotes student retention of the information. She has been recognized nationally for her teaching expertise and has received Excellence in Teaching awards from Raymond Walters College, the University of Cincinnati, and Case Western Reserve University. Currently she is a visiting professor at Case Western Reserve University, consults with a variety of nursing programs on teaching and curricular issues, and co-authors a genetics textbook.

Linda LaCharity received her BSN from Kent State University's College of Nursing. During her career in the U.S. Army Nurse Corps, she earned an MN from the University of Washington in Seattle. Linda earned her PhD from the University of Cincinnati. She worked as a staff nurse and nurse manager in adult medical-surgical and critical care settings supervising RNs, LPN/LVNs, and nursing assistant staff. Linda's academic experience includes teaching EMTs and critical care nurses for the military and across the curriculum at the University of Cincinnati (BSN, MSN, Accelerated BSN/MSN, and PhD). Her area of teaching expertise in both classroom and patient care settings is adult health. She was director of the Accelerated Program and an Assistant Professor in the College of Nursing at the University of Cincinnati in Cincinnati, Ohio. Retired in 2013, she continues to write textbooks, including *Prioritization, Delegation and Assignment, Practice Exercises for the NCLEX-RN Examination* and *Prioritization, Delegation, and Assignment, Practice Exercises for the NCLEX-PN Examination.*

Reviewers

Kimberly A. Amos, PhD, MSN, RN, CNE
Director
Foothills Nursing Consortium AND
Isothermal Community College
Spindale, North Carolina

Samantha Bonaduce, MSN, RN
Faculty
School of Nursing
Kent State University, Tuscarawas
New Philadelphia, Ohio

Laura Brennan, MS, RN
Assistant Professor
Director, Prelicensure Program
School of Nursing
Elmhurst University
Elmhurst, Illinois

Meera Brown, PharmD, MBA
Senior Manager
CVS Health
Woonsocket, Rhode Island

Heather Clark, DNP
LPN Program Director
Penn State University—Lehigh Valley
Allentown, Pennsylvania

Alice M. Hupp, BS, RN
Lead Instructor
North Central Texas College
Gainesville, Texas

Beth Kasprisin, RN, MSN
Associate Degree Director of Nursing
Texas Southmost College
Brownsville, Texas

Lorraine Kelley, DNP, RN
Faculty
Department of Nursing and Emergency Medical Services
Pensacola State College
Pensacola, Florida

Molly M. Showalter, MSN Ed, RN
Interim Vocational Nursing Program Director
Texas Southmost College
Brownsville, Texas

Cynthia Theys, MSN, RN, MSOLQ
Associate Dean
Health Sciences and Education
Northeast Wisconsin Technical College
Green Bay, Wisconsin

Brittany Williams, DNP, RN, CMSRN
Faculty
Central Texas College
Killeen, Texas

Jennifer J. Yeager, PhD, RN, APRN
Associate Professor
School of Nursing
Tarleton State University
Stephenville, Texas

Preface

We, the authors of this text, are pleased to announce that the third edition of this text represents much more than an update. With the addition of new content and revision of certain organizational elements while maintaining the text's essential and effective style, we hope to increase the ease with which students are able to assimilate and use the content. As nurses and educators with many decades of clinical and teaching experience and the understanding that increased scientific application now enhances drug therapy, we strive to prepare students to be aware of how genetics, biologics, and targeted therapies allow for more precise and individualized patient care. Incorporation of these concepts and applications complements our long-held views of what is needed in a pharmacology textbook to help students identify the most important content areas for safe drug administration and patient teaching. With this goal in mind, we continue to apply the unique format of our previous editions based on four focus areas:

- Why specific drugs are prescribed as therapy for common health problems
- How different drugs work to induce their intended responses
- What critical actions and assessments to perform before and after administering drugs
- Which points are most important to teach patients about their drug therapy

Using these focus areas, we present pharmacology content in a framework that promotes in-depth learning versus rote memorization, which is truly essential in understanding the principles of pharmacology and safe drug administration. It is our hope that this framework will provide students with the tools to continue their acquisition of the ever-changing pharmacology content throughout the years of their careers in nursing.

As in the second edition, interwoven within the textbook are areas that highlight specific safety issues with regard to medication administration. The impetus for this inclusion is the recommendations championed by the American Association of Colleges of Nursing, collectively known as the Quality and Safety Education for Nurses (QSEN) practice standards. Specific actions related to safety are noted with "QSEN" throughout the text.

CHAPTER ORGANIZATION

The text has been reorganized into 9 units totaling 29 chapters to streamline access to specific content areas. In addition, two chapters that are assigned less often by most instructors (Drug Therapy with Nutritional Supplements and Anticancer Therapy) have been revised, updated, and moved to the Evolve website. This change in actual text content allows the inclusion of the rationales for practice questions and clinical judgment activities within the text itself for ease of student assessment. Unit I provides an overview of general content important for safe medication administration. Unit II provides essential mathematical concepts and practice for safe dosage calculation. Unit III focuses on content that has application to many body systems, such as inflammation, infection, pain, and cancer. The remaining six units are divided by the body system most closely associated with the specific drug therapy. For example, Unit IV, Drug Therapy for Problems of the Circulatory and Cardiac Systems, is further divided into six chapters that include drug therapy affecting urine output, hypertension, heart failure, dysrhythmias, high blood lipids, and blood clotting. We believe this content arrangement synchronizes the information for students when they are studying specific health problems and issues. Although information regarding normal physiology and pathophysiology is still presented, this information has been streamlined to promote the pharmacology focus of the text.

Our presentation style for the content of this text is direct, active, and clear for the nursing student. Health care terms and related physiological mechanisms are explained in clear, straightforward, everyday language to promote better student understanding and application of the content in the clinical setting. Photographs and other illustrations have been selected and developed to better explain drug administration techniques, drug actions, and appropriate health care interventions.

Chapter **Objectives** presented at the beginning of each chapter focus the student on "need to know" information, clarifying which issues have the highest priority and relevance for safe drug administration. A list of **Key Terms** includes phonetic pronunciations, definitions, and page numbers where each term is first used.

The **mathematics review chapters** (Chapters 3, 4, and 5) are written in a self-paced, guided-study format and contain easy-to-understand explanations and examples. **Try This!** boxes provide more than 150 practice questions within these chapters, in addition to the end-of-chapter review material. Answers to these exercises are found at the end of the chapters.

In-text **drug tables** outline the most common drugs used to treat highlighted disorders and diseases. Although the number of tables has increased, the actual content has been revised by drug category and streamlined to reduce confusion. Generic and trade names as well as common dosage ranges and routes of administration for adults are included.

Discussion sections focus on essential nursing responsibilities in drug therapy. These headings have been revised with terminology consistent with the National Council to highlight important information and nursing actions. These headings now state **"Priority Actions to Take Before," "Priority Actions to Take After,"** and **"Teaching Priorities for Patients"** about each highlighted drug or drug category to emphasize the important aspects of drug administration, monitoring, follow-up, and patient teaching. Some of this content, especially in the "Teaching Priorities" sections, is now presented in a bullet point format suitable for sharing with patients and families during patient education sessions.

Life Span Considerations sections receive particular attention in most chapters. Differences in actions, the risks for side effects, precautions, or dosing for pediatric patients, pregnant or breastfeeding patients, or older adults are presented as appropriate for each drug class.

A **Get Ready for the NCLEX® Examination!** section at the end of each chapter features Key Points, Additional Learning Resources, Review Questions, and Clinical Judgment activities.

- **Key Points** emphasize selected need-to-know content from the chapter to help students study for tests and licensure exams.
- **Additional Learning Resources** sections refer students to related review material in the accompanying Study Guide and on the Evolve website at http://evolve.elsevier.com/Workman/pharmacology/.
- **Review Questions** have been completely revised for this edition. These self-assessment questions, expressed in an NCLEX Examination compatible style, correspond with the Objectives at the beginning of the chapter. Drug calculation questions are also included in this section. The majority of these questions were developed at the comprehension and application levels and focus on the student being able to determine the most relevant or important action to prevent harm in a given situation. Answers and rationales to the Review Questions are located in the appendix at the end of the book.
- **Clinical Judgment** activities are new true-to-practice case studies that present issues and problems requiring clinical judgment and decision-making related to individual patients receiving drug therapy. Answer guidelines to the questions also are available in the appendix at the end of the text.

LEARNER-FRIENDLY INSTRUCTIONAL DESIGN

One of the most innovative features of this text is its unique instructional design. A single column presents the narrative, and a wide margin is used to reinforce important concepts and prevent medication errors with special boxed features. This wide margin also allows generous space for note-taking. Examples of the special learning features found in the wide margin include the following:

 Drug Alert boxes help reinforce crucial actions or interventions, teaching, and drug administration information. Each of these boxes is classified into one of five categories: Teaching, Interaction, Administration, Dosage, or Action/Intervention.

 Memory Jogger boxes highlight and summarize essential information, including major categories of drugs and the diseases they are used to treat.

 Critical Point for Safety boxes focus on information vital for safe practice and medication administration.

 Common Side Effects boxes focus on individual drug groups and feature unique icons that promote rapid recognition. More than a dozen new icons for common side effects were developed specifically for this edition.

 Do Not Confuse boxes highlight look-alike/sound-alike drug names.

 Did You Know? boxes help students link pharmacology content to the world around them.

 Cultural Awareness boxes emphasize important cultural considerations related to pharmacology.

We believe you'll find that the authors and publisher have crafted a balance of these features to minimize wasted space and at the same time promote in-depth learning versus rote memorization.

TEACHING AND LEARNING PACKAGE

FOR STUDENTS

A companion **Study Guide**, available for purchase at elsevier.com, features a variety of engaging learning activities that complement those in the textbook. Clinically focused Medication Safety Practice questions and a Practice Quiz are provided in each chapter along with a variety of other Learning Activities that promote an understanding of pharmacology and safe drug administration. New Next-Generation NCLEX® Examination–Style Case Studies sections are included in drug-focused chapters.

The **Evolve website** at http://evolve.elsevier.com/Workman/pharmacology/ provides free student learning resources that include the following:

- New **Next-Generation NCLEX® Examination–Style Case Studies** sections for drug-focused chapters help students review important material in new test question formats. Separate **Answer Keys** are also provided.

- Over 450 **Interactive Review Questions** in multiple-choice and multiple response formats, with rationales for correct and incorrect answers, help students review important chapter material.
- **Video Clips** and **Animations** explain important concepts from anatomy and physiology to drug administration and are keyed to the text by distinctive icons.
- Supplemental **Appendices** on Medication Administration Skills, Anticancer Drugs, and Nutritional Therapy are provided as additional reference content for these key topics.
- Twelve interactive **Drug Dosage Calculators** offer a quick way to calculate IV dosages, body surface area, oral doses, and more.
- An extensive **Spanish/English Audio Glossary** provides a vast array of health care–related terms and their definitions (with audio) in both English and Spanish.
- A collection of **Essential Drug Patient Teaching Handouts** can be used to provide patients with information on almost any available drug in both English and Spanish.

FOR INSTRUCTORS

The comprehensive *Evolve Resources with TEACH Instructor Resource* provides everything a new or seasoned instructor will need to teach the content, including the following:

- **TEACH Lesson Plans,** based on textbook Objectives, tie together the text and all other learning resources in ready-to-use, customizable lessons.

- A high-quality **Test Bank,** delivered in ExamView, contains more than 760 test items created by the authors. Approximately 50% of these items are written at the Applying or higher cognitive level of Bloom's taxonomy. Each question includes the correct answer, rationale, and cognitive level.
- Additional **Next-Generation–Style Case Studies** are available to instructors for classroom discussion.
- A collection of **PowerPoint Lecture Slides** highlights key concepts and discussion in the text.
- **Answer Keys** are provided for the Study Guide questions.
- An **Image Collection** contains every reproducible image from the text. Images are suitable for incorporation into classroom lectures, PowerPoint presentations, or distance-learning applications.

Understanding Pharmacology: Essentials for Medication Safety, edition 3, together with its fully integrated multimedia ancillary package, provides the tools needed to fully understand pharmacology principles and how to apply them effectively and safely in today's health care environment. For more information on any of these innovative companion publications, or if you simply wish to provide us feedback, please contact your Elsevier sales representative, visit us at http://www.us.elsevierhealth.com/, or contact Elsevier Faculty Support at 1-800-222-9570 or sales.inquiry@elsevier.com.

Acknowledgments

Many talented people are needed to make any textbook a success. The authors wish to acknowledge the following individuals and groups for their guidance, dedication, hard work, constructive criticism, and creative input that were so important to this project: Nancy O'Brien, Brandi Graham, Rae Robertson, Julie Eddy, Abigail Bradberry, Clay Broeker, and Renee Duenow.

Special Features

Understanding Pharmacology: Essentials for Medication Safety, edition 3, focuses on an *understanding* of pharmacology principles and safety of drug administration by using clear, everyday language. Full-color illustrations and a unique, user-friendly design accompany practical, understandable discussions of important drugs and drug classes.

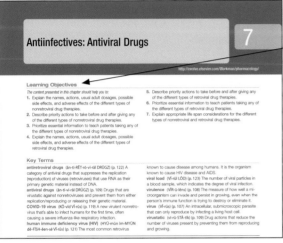

> Chapters open with **Objectives** and **Key Terms** with pronunciations and references to the pages where the terms are first used.

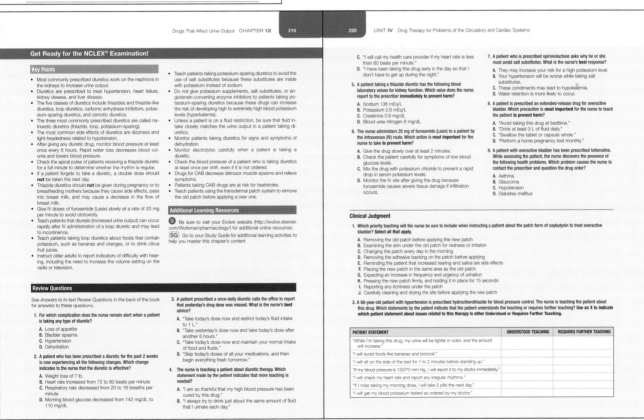

> **Get Ready for the NCLEX® Examination!** sections include **Key Points** and **Review Questions**, including **Clinical Judgment** assessments, to reinforce important concepts learned in the chapter.

Full-color illustrations explain key procedures, pathophysiology, and pharmacology concepts.

Try This! boxes in the math chapters let you practice math and dosage calculation concepts as you learn them. Answers are found at the end of the chapter.

Did You Know? boxes relate pharmacology content to everyday life.

Video clips illustrate medication administration procedures.

Do Not Confuse boxes highlight look-alike/sound-alike drugs to help you avoid drug errors.

Memory Jogger boxes summarize essential information, including major categories of drugs and the diseases they are used to treat.

Drug Alert boxes highlight important tips for safe medication administration.

Drug tables provide generic drug names, brand names, and typical dosage ranges. High-Alert drugs are noted with a special icon.

Common Side Effects boxes use memorable, easy-to-recognize icons to emphasize common side effects of drugs.

Critical Point for Safety boxes highlight critically important pharmacologic concepts to remember.

Priority icons emphasize content related to important aspects of drug administration, monitoring, follow-up, and patient teaching.

Animations supplement important concepts related to pharmacology.

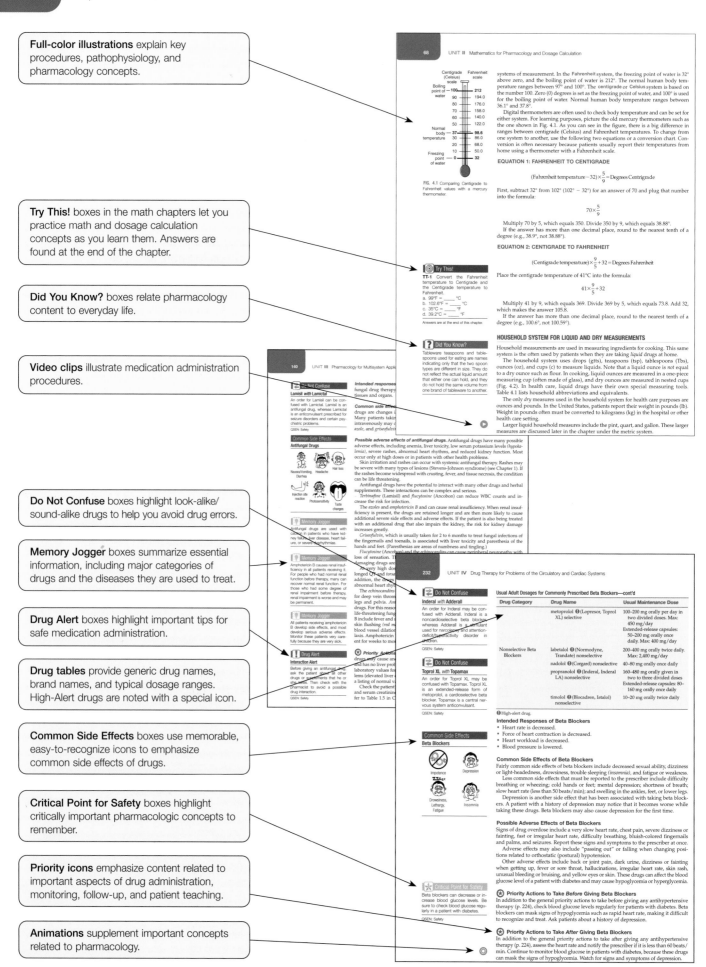

Contents

Animations and Videos (on Evolve)

Drug Therapy: Roles, Regulations, Actions, and Responses

1

http://evolve.elsevier.com/Workman/pharmacology/

Learning Objectives

The content presented in this chapter should help you to:

1. Understand the intended uses of drug therapy.
2. Explain the differences among a drug's therapeutic effects (intended actions), side effects, adverse effects, and unique or personal effects.
3. Compare the expected outcomes of agonist drug therapy with antagonist drug therapy.
4. Explain how genetic variation can be responsible for personal differences in expected responses to drugs, including allergic reactions.
5. Explain the purposes, advantages, and disadvantages of the different routes of drug administration.
6. Describe the processes and organs involved in drug metabolism and elimination.
7. Explain the influence of drug half-life, peak blood level, and trough of blood level on drug activity.
8. Describe the ways in which drug therapy for children and older adults differs from drug therapy for younger adults.
9. Explain how pregnancy and breastfeeding should be taken into consideration with drug therapy.

Key Terms

absorption (ăb-SŌRP-shŭn) (p. 12) Movement of a drug from the outside of the body into the bloodstream.

adverse drug reaction (ADR) (ĂD-vŭrs DRŬG rē-ĂK-shŭn) (p. 9) Same as adverse effect.

adverse effect (ĂD-vŭrs ĕf-FĔKT) (p. 9) A drug effect that is more severe than expected and has the potential to damage tissue or cause serious health problems. It may also be called a toxic effect or toxicity and usually requires intervention by the prescriber.

agonist (ĂG-ŏn-ĭst) (p. 7) An extrinsic drug that activates the receptor sites of a cell, which then mimics the actions of naturally occurring body substances (intrinsic drugs) and increases the cell's response.

allergic response (ă-LŬR-jĭk rē-SPŎNS) (p. 10) Type of adverse effect in which the presence of the drug stimulates the release of histamine and other body chemicals that cause inflammatory reactions. The response may be as mild as a rash or as severe and life threatening as anaphylaxis.

antagonist (ăn-TĂG-ŏn-ĭst) (p. 8) An extrinsic drug that blocks the receptor sites of a cell, which then prevents the naturally occurring body substance from binding to the receptor and decreases the cell's response.

bioavailability (bī-ō-ă-văl-ă-BĬL-ĭ-tē) (p. 12) The percentage of a drug dose that actually reaches the blood.

black box warning (BLĂK BŎKS WŌR-nĭng) (p. 10) A notice from the US Food and Drug Administration (FDA) that a drug may produce serious or even life-threatening effects in some people in addition to its beneficial effects.

brand name (BRĂND NĀM) (p. 4) A manufacturer-owned name of a generic drug; also called *trade name* or *proprietary name*.

contraindication (KŎN-tră-ĭn-dĭ-KĀ-shŭn) (p. 10) A personal or health-related reason for not administering a specific drug to an individual patient or group of patients.

cytotoxic (sī-tō-TŎKS-ĭk) (p. 9) Drug action that is intended to kill a cell or an organism.

distribution (dĭs-trĭ-BYŪ-shŭn) (p. 14) (drug distribution) The extent that a drug absorbed into the bloodstream spreads into the three body water compartments.

drug (DRŬG) (p. 2) Any small molecule that changes any body function by working at the chemical and cellular levels (same as medication).

drug therapy (DRŬG THĂR-ă-pē) (p. 2) A plan that uses a specific drug or drugs to prevent, reduce, improve, or correct a health problem.

duration of action (dū-RĀ-shŭn of ĂK-shŭn) (p. 11) The length of time a single drug dose is present in the blood at or greater than the level needed to produce an effect or response.

elimination (ē-lĭm-ĭ-NĀ-shŭn) (p. 17) The removal of drugs from the body accomplished by certain enzyme metabolizing systems and organs.

enteral route (ĔN-tĕr-ŭl ROWT) (p. 12) Movement of drugs from the outside of the body to the inside using the gastrointestinal tract.

first-pass loss (FŬRST PĂS LŎS) (p. 17) Rapid inactivation or elimination of oral drugs as a result of liver metabolism.

generic name (jĕn-ĂR-ĭk NĀM) (p. 4) National and international public drug name created by the United States Adopted Names Council to indicate the usual use or chemical composition of a drug.

half-life (HĂF LĪF) (p. 17) Time span needed for one half of a drug dose to be eliminated from the body.

1

high-alert drug (HĪ ă-LŮRT DRŬG) (p. 5) A specific drug or drug category that has an increased risk for causing patient harm if it is used in error (given at the wrong dose, wrong time, wrong patient, or not given).

intended action (ĭn-TĔN-dĕd ĂK-shŭn) (p. 3) Desired effect (main effect) of a drug on specific body cells or tissues; same as therapeutic response.

loading dose (LŌ-dĭng DŌS) (p. 18) The first dose of a drug that is larger than all subsequent doses of the same drug; used when it takes more drug to reach steady state than it does to maintain it.

mechanism of action (MĔK-ă-nĭz-ŭm of ĂK-shŭn) (p. 6) Exactly how, at the cellular level, a drug changes the activity of a cell.

metabolism (mĕ-TĂB-ō-lĭz-ĭm) (p. 15) (drug metabolism) Physiologic body actions by enzymes that change the chemical shape and content of a drug, most commonly preparing the drug for inactivation and elimination.

minimum effective concentration (MEC) (MĬN-ĭ-mŭm ĕf-FĔK-tĭiv kŏn-sĕn-TRĂ-shŭn) (p. 11) The smallest amount of drug necessary in the blood or target tissue to result in a measurable intended action.

over-the-counter (OTC) (Ō-vŭr THĒ KOWN-tŭr) (p. 4) Drugs that are approved for purchase without a prescription.

parenteral route (pă-RĔN-tĕr-ăl ROWT) (p. 12) Movement of a drug from the outside of the body to the inside of the body by injection (intra-arterial, intravenous, intramuscular, subcutaneous, intradermal, intracavitary, intraosseous, intrathecal).

peak (PĒK) (p. 18) The maximum or highest blood drug level that can be measured.

percutaneous route (pĕr-kū-TĂN-ē-ŭs ROWT) (p. 12) Movement of a drug from the outside of the body to the inside through the skin or mucous membranes.

pharmacodynamics (făr-mă-kō-dĭ-NĂM-ĭks) (p. 6) How drugs work to change cellular, tissue, organ, or whole-body function.

pharmacogenetics (făr-mă-kō-GĔN-ĔT-ĭks) (p. 16) How differences or variations in a person's genes affect the physiologic action of a drug.

pharmacogenomics (făr-mă-kō-GĔ-NōM-ĭks) (p. 15) How the general expression of all gene variations influences the effects of drug therapy.

pharmacokinetics (făr-mă-kō-kĭn-ĔT-ĭks) (p. 11) How the body changes drugs; drug metabolism.

pharmacology (făr-mă-KŎL-ō-jē) (p. 2) The science and study of drugs and their actions on living animals.

physiologic effect (fĭ-zē-ō-LŎ-jĭk ĕf-FĔKT) (p. 9) The change in action of cells, tissues, organs, or the whole body as a result of a drug's mechanism of action.

potency (PŌ-tĕn-sē) (p. 11) The strength of the intended action produced at a given drug dose.

prescription (prē-SKRĬP-shŭn) (p. 5) An order written or dictated by a state-approved prescriber for a specific drug therapy for a specific patient.

prescription drugs (prē-SKRĬP-shŭn DRŬGZ) (p. 4) The legal status of any drug that is considered unsafe for self-medication or has a potential for addiction and is only available by a prescription written by a state-approved health care professional.

receptors (rē-SĔP-TŮRZ) (p. 6) Physical places on or in a cell where a drug can attach itself (bind) and control cell activity.

side effect (SĪD ē-FĔKT) (p. 3) Any minor effect of a drug on body cells or tissues that is not the intended action of a drug.

steady state (STĔD-ē STĀT) (p. 11) Point at which drug elimination is balanced with drug entry, resulting in a constant effective blood level of the drug.

target tissue (TĂR-gĕt TĬ-shū´) (p. 6) The actual cells, tissues, or organs affected by the mechanism of action or intended actions of a specific drug.

transdermal (trănz-DŮR-mŭl) (p. 12) Type of percutaneous drug delivery in which the drug is applied to the skin or mucous membranes, passes through these tissues, and enters the bloodstream.

trough (TRŎF) (p. 18) The lowest or minimal blood drug level that can be measured.

vaporized (VĂ-pŭr-īzd) (p. 17) Changing of a drug from a liquid form to a gas or mist that can be absorbed into the body by inhalation.

INTRODUCTION TO DRUG THERAPY

OVERVIEW

Pharmacology is the science and study of drugs and how they work. A **drug** is any small molecule that changes a body function by working at the chemical and cell levels. Some people use the term *medication* for substances that are used to treat health problems and the term *drug* for substances that are harmful or can be misused. However, these terms mean the same thing, and any drug or medication can be misused. **Drug therapy** is a plan that uses one or more drugs to help prevent, reduce, improve, or correct a health problem. For example, a specific drug may be prescribed daily to help control high blood pressure *(hypertension)*. Some patients may require more than one drug type to keep blood pressure within normal levels.

Many everyday substances are actually drugs, including caffeine, alcohol, and nicotine. Some drugs are manufactured from chemicals, others are taken from plants, and still others are taken from a person or animal to be used by another person. For example, insulin can be made in a laboratory, or it can be taken from the pancreas of a cow or pig and given to humans. (There are no plant sources of insulin.)

Drug therapy includes these factors:

- Identifying the specific health problem
- Determining what drug or drugs would best help the problem
- Deciding the best delivery method and schedule
- Ensuring that the proper amount of the drug is given
- Helping the patient become an active participant in his or her drug therapy

The prescriber's primary role in drug therapy is to identify the health problem and, if needed, plan and select specific drug therapy. The authority to prescribe varies by state. State-approved prescribers may include physicians, dentists, podiatrists, advanced practice nurses, and physician's assistants, among other professionals. The pharmacist's primary role is to mix (*compound*) and dispense prescribed drugs. The nurse's primary role in drug therapy is to administer prescribed drugs directly to the patient and monitor him or her for outcomes related to the drug therapy. Nurses often are the last checkpoint for safe drug therapy, which makes understanding the purposes, actions, side effects, problems, delivery methods, usual dosages, and necessary follow-up care for different drugs a critical responsibility. Prescribers, pharmacists, and nurses all share responsibility for teaching patients about the drug therapies they have been prescribed.

Although drugs are prescribed or used to improve some condition or function, the body also makes some of its own drugs in the form of hormones, enzymes, growth factors, and other substances that change the activity of cells and tissues. The chemicals the body makes are called **intrinsic drugs**. The insulin made by the pancreas is one example of an intrinsic drug. Other drugs are made outside of the body and must be taken into the body to change cell, organ, or body action. These drugs are known as **extrinsic drugs**. The study of pharmacology is concerned mainly with extrinsic drugs. However, many effective extrinsic drugs are nearly identical to the drugs the body creates. For example, the body makes endorphin, which is very similar to the extrinsic drug morphine. Morphine is a very effective pain reliever because it has the same action as endorphin at the cell level.

Any drug affects some body tissues or organs. The reason a drug is prescribed is that it has at least one desired effect that improves body function, known as the **intended action** or the *therapeutic response*. Think about a drug that dilates blood vessels and thereby lowers blood pressure. The therapeutic response of such a drug is to lower blood pressure; thus it is classified as an antihypertensive drug. In addition to its intended action or therapeutic response, there may be many minor changes in body function that occur when the drug is taken. These minor effects of a drug on body cells or tissues that are not the intended actions are known as **side effects**. Side effects can be helpful or may cause problems. For example, a drug to treat hypertension that dilates blood vessels also may cause the side effects of dizziness and ankle swelling. All drugs have at least one intended action and at least one side effect. The safety of any drug is determined by balancing the seriousness of the side effects against the benefit of the therapeutic effect.

DRUG NAMES

Drugs usually have three names: the chemical name, generic name, and brand name (trade name). The chemical name of a drug is the exact chemical composition of atoms and molecules for the main ingredient of the drug. For example, the chemical name for furosemide is 4-chloro-2-(furan-2-ylmethylamino)-5-sulfamoylbenzoic acid. Chemical names are used only by the chemists who develop and manufacture the drug.

Memory Jogger

Any drug (medication) can be misused and harm a person.

Critical Point for Safety

Nurses who administer drugs to patients have responsibility for understanding the purposes, actions, side effects, problems, delivery methods, usual dosages, and necessary follow-up care for different drugs.

QSEN: Safety

Memory Jogger

All drugs have at least one intended action and at least one side effect.

Generic names are the shorter and simpler drug names used by clinical health care professionals such as pharmacists, physicians, and nurses. For example, furosemide is the generic name for Lasix and Furocot. The United States Adopted Names Council creates the generic names used for all drugs made in the United States. The rules used to name drugs help ensure that the generic name is relatively short, often give some clue as to its use or chemical composition, and does not sound too much like any other known drug name. Often some part of all generic names for drugs of one class (also known as a "drug family") will be the same. For example, most of the generic names for the type of blood pressure control drugs that are angiotensin II receptor antagonists (also known as angiotensin receptor blockers [ARBs]) end in "-sartan" (e.g., eprosartan, losartan, olmesartan, telmisartan). Most beta-blockers end in "-olol" or "-alol" (e.g., atenolol, metoprolol, propranolol, and sotalol). After the generic name is approved, it is public and not owned by any one drug company. When a generic drug name is written, the first letter is not capitalized.

Brand names are created by each drug company that makes and sells a specific drug. Other terms for brand name are *proprietary name* and *trade name*. Each company owns its brand names. For example, many drug companies make aspirin and each one has its own recognized brand name for it. St. Joseph Aspirin is the aspirin made by the McNeil Company; Bufferin is the aspirin made by Genomma Laboratories. The first letter of a brand name is always capitalized, and the name will often be followed by either the symbol ® (for registered trademark) or ™ (for trademark). Patients often only know their prescribed drugs by the brand name.

At one time, drugs were largely prescribed by brand name. Now most are prescribed by generic name unless the drug is a combination of two or more drugs. As a nurse, you are expected to know and refer to drugs by their generic names.

GENERAL DRUG GROUPS

Any drug has the potential to harm a person if it is taken improperly or in large quantities. Some drugs have more powerful and dangerous effects than others. The US government has divided drugs into two broad groupings based on their potential for harm. These groups are over-the-counter (OTC) drugs and prescription drugs. Drugs are also grouped by harm potential as high alert and whether they are considered a natural herbal substance. Most drugs fall into more than one group. For example, morphine is grouped as a prescription drug and as a high-alert drug.

Over-the-Counter Drugs

Drugs that are weaker at a lower dosage and have less potential for harmful side effects are available for purchase without a prescription. These drugs are called **over-the-counter (OTC)** drugs. OTC drugs are considered safe for self-medication when the package directions for dosage and schedule are followed. Examples of OTC drug types include aspirin and other nonsteroidal antiinflammatory drugs (NSAIDs), antacids, vitamin supplements, and antihistamines. Even when a prescriber recommends these drugs, they may be sold almost anywhere without a prescription.

OTC drugs are convenient and allow patients to control their own health care to some extent. However, some problems do exist with OTC drugs. Many patients do not consider them to be even slightly dangerous. *All drugs, even vitamins, can be misused and cause harmful side effects when taken too often or in high doses.* In addition, some people do not consider OTC drugs to be "real drugs" and may not mention them when they are asked what drugs they take on a daily basis. OTC drugs can cause health problems and may interact with prescription drugs.

Prescription Drugs

Prescription drugs are those with a legal status that has a greater potential for harm, strong sedating effects, or a potential for addiction and are considered too dangerous for self-medication. They are available only from a pharmacy with a drug order from a state-authorized prescriber. A **prescription** is an order written or dictated by a state-approved prescriber for a specific drug therapy for a specific patient.

High-Alert Drugs

A **high-alert drug** is one that has an increased risk for causing a patient harm if it is used in error. The error may be a dose that is too high, a dose that is too low, a dose given to a patient for whom it was not prescribed, and a dose not given to a patient for whom it was prescribed. One way to remember the more commonly prescribed high-alert drugs is with the term PINCH. In this term, *P* is for potassium, *I* is for insulin, *N* is for narcotics (more commonly called *opioids*), *C* is for cancer chemotherapy agents, and *H* is for heparin or any other drug that strongly affects blood clotting. Although calculating drug dosages and administering drugs always require care and concentration, extra care is needed when calculating and administering high-alert drugs. When possible, always check the order for a high-alert drug with another licensed health care professional or pharmacist. Specific high-alert drugs are highlighted throughout the clinical chapters of this textbook.

Herbal Products

Herbals are natural products made from plants that cause a physiologic response similar to that of a drug. Many herbal products, also called *botanicals,* have been used as drug therapy for centuries. This area of drug therapy is poorly understood and not regulated for consistent effectiveness, purity, or strength, because they are considered dietary supplements rather than conventional food or drugs. Such products are available for sale almost everywhere, and individuals may even grow, collect, or make their own. Use of these products with or without the supervision of a prescriber is often termed *herbal therapy, homeopathic therapy, natural therapy,* or *alternative therapy.*

Many people who use herbal preparations consider them to be "natural" and therefore safe. However, herbal products do have cellular effects that can be harmful or interact with other drugs. For example, both white willow bark products and gingko biloba reduce blood clotting. If either of these is taken by a person who is also taking a prescription drug to reduce clotting, such as warfarin, the risk for a brain hemorrhage is high. When asked what drugs he or she is taking, a patient may not even mention herbal preparations that are taken on a daily basis, increasing the risk for an interaction with a prescribed drug.

Because many people consider herbal products to be safe, they may take large quantities of the products, believing that if one dose is good, higher doses must be even better. For example, many people use the juice of the stinging nettle as a natural diuretic. It does increase urine output, but excessive doses cause dehydration and low blood potassium levels *(hypokalemia).*

DRUG REGULATION

The United States Pharmacopeia (USP) is a national group responsible for developing standards for drug manufacturing, including purity, strength, packaging, and labeling. The US Food and Drug Administration (FDA) is the US government agency that is responsible for enforcing the standards set by the USP. The FDA and the USP work together to ensure continuing public protection and drug safety.

The drug regulating body is the US Drug Enforcement Administration (DEA). All prescribers within the United States must register with the DEA and obtain a DEA number for full prescriptive authority. In addition, the DEA is responsible for enforcing all drug laws with regard to controlled substances and illegal drugs. The DEA has categorized drugs that have a potential for addiction or abuse as *"controlled substances."* These substances are further classified by the degree of their potential for addiction and abuse into one of five "schedules" that are regulated by the Federal Controlled Substances Act of 1970. Table 1.1 describes category differences and lists common examples for each schedule category.

 Memory Jogger

Use the term **PINCH** to remember common high-alert drugs: *P*otassium, *I*nsulin, *N*arcotics (opioids), *C*ancer chemotherapy agents, and *H*eparin or any drug that strongly affects blood clotting.

 Critical Point for Safety

Always check the order for a high-alert drug with another licensed health care professional or pharmacist.

QSEN: Safety

 Critical Point for Safety

Your responsibility with herbal therapy is to obtain correct information about what specific herbal products a patient is using and make sure that the prescriber is aware of this information.

QSEN: Safety

 Drug Alert

Interaction Alert

When taking a history, always ask what specific herbal products the patient uses daily, including the brand names and the amounts.

QSEN: Safety

Table 1.1	Classification of Controlled Substances (United States)	
SCHEDULE	**DESCRIPTION**	**EXAMPLES**
I	High potential for abuse No currently accepted medical use in treatment in United States. Lack of accepted safety for use of the drug or other substance under medical supervision.	More than 80 drugs or substances of which the following are the most well known: α-acetylmethadol, γ-hydroxybutyric acid, heroin, lysergic acid diethylamide, mescaline; peyote, methaqualone, methylenedioxymethamphetamine "ecstasy"
II	Currently accepted use for treatment in United States. Dangerous with high potential for abuse that may lead to severe psychological or physical dependence.	More than 30 drugs or substances of which the following are the most well known: Combination products with less than 15 mg of hydrocodone per dosage unit, cocaine, methamphetamine, methadone, morphine, hydromorphone, meperidine, oxycodone, fentanyl, Dexedrine, Adderall, and Ritalin
III	Currently accepted medical use for treatment in United States. Moderate to low potential for psychological or physical dependence. Potential for abuse is less than drugs/substances in schedules I and II.	Most drugs are compounds containing some small amounts of the drugs (less than 90 mg) from schedule II along with acetaminophen or aspirin. Other drugs include anabolic steroids such as testosterone preparations, ketamine.
IV	Currently accepted medical use for treatment in United States. Low potential for abuse or dependence relative to the drugs or substances in schedule III.	Include diet drugs with propionic acid Other well-known drugs include benzodiazepines (lorazepam, flurazepam, diazepam, midazolam, alprazolam; chloral hydrate; paraldehyde; pentazocine; tramadol; zolpidem
V	Currently accepted medical use in United States. Low potential for abuse relative to the drugs or substances in schedule IV consist of preparations containing limited quantities of certain narcotics.	Include cough preparations with small amounts of codeine, drugs for diarrhea, and drugs for analgesic purposes. Examples include diphenoxylate with atropine (Lomotil) (Robitussin AC), Motofen, Lyrica, Parepectolin.

Data from United States Department of Justice, Drug Enforcement Administration. (2020). Diversion Control Division: Controlled Substance Schedules, from: https://www.deadiversion.usdoj.gov/schedules/

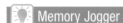 **Memory Jogger**

Drugs and drug products with the highest potential for addiction or abuse are classified as schedule I; those with the lowest potential for addiction or abuse are classified as schedule V.

The federal government requires that all schedule II and some schedule III drugs be carefully controlled. These drugs require a prescription written by a state-approved prescriber with a registered number from the DEA. These drugs are stored in a locked area of the facility and unit, and each drug dose is carefully tracked. On nursing units, these drugs are counted at the change of every shift, and the nurse must "sign out" each dose prescribed for a particular patient. States vary in whether or not licensed practical nurses (LPNs) or licensed vocational nurses (LVNs) are permitted to administer any or all schedule drugs.

HOW DRUGS AFFECT THE BODY: PHARMACODYNAMICS

MECHANISM OF ACTION

An important aspect of drug therapy is **pharmacodynamics**, or how drugs work to change cellular, tissue, organ, and body function. Think of this as what the drug does to the body. Drugs affect body function by changing the activity levels of individual cells. Remember that each body cell has at least one job that it must perform to make the whole body function correctly. The job that any cell performs can be slowed, stopped, or speeded up when that cell is exposed to a specific drug. Exactly how a drug changes the activity of a cell is its **mechanism of action**. Most cells have receptors that control their activity. The actual cells, tissues, and organs affected by the mechanism of action (intended action) of a drug are known as the **target tissues**.

Receptors

Receptors are places on or in a cell where a drug can attach itself (bind) and control cell activity. In this way, the receptor acts as an ignition slot for the cell's motor. When the right key (drug) is placed in the ignition (receptor) and turned, the cell motor starts, and the cell performs its special job better or faster. The right key for the ignition can be either an intrinsic drug such as the adrenaline made by the adrenal glands or an extrinsic drug such as epinephrine. (Chemically, epinephrine is almost identical to human adrenaline.) When the adrenal glands make and release adrenaline, one action it has is to bind to adrenaline receptor sites on the heart muscle cells and make those cells contract more strongly and rapidly. This action causes increased heart rate and higher blood pressure. When epinephrine is injected into a person, it binds to those same adrenaline receptor sites on the heart muscle cells and causes the same effects that adrenaline does. Fig. 1.1 and Animation 1.1 show how cell receptors are used in drug therapy to control cell activity.

A cell can have more than one type of receptor; thus different drugs can affect the same cell in different ways. Fig. 1.2 shows why a cell can respond to more than one drug. A cell can respond to a drug by changing its activity only when the proper drug fits into its receptor. If the wrong drug attempts to bind to a receptor, it will not activate that receptor—just as using the wrong key in a car's ignition will not start the motor.

Many types of drugs work through cell receptors. These receptors can be on the surface of a cell or actually inside the cell. A cell with a receptor for a specific drug is known as the target for that drug. For example, common targets of morphine are brain cells (neurons) that perceive pain. Drug types that work by affecting cell receptors include opioid pain drugs, drugs for high blood pressure, diuretics, insulin, antihistamines, antiinflammatory drugs, and antidiabetic drugs, to name only a few. For example, cells that are targets for antihistamines are those that have histamine receptors on their surfaces, such as mucous membrane cells, blood vessel cells, cells that line the airways, and stomach lining cells.

Receptor agonists. When an extrinsic drug binds to the receptor of a cell and causes the same response that an intrinsic drug does, the extrinsic drug is called a receptor *agonist* and it is the right key to turn on that cell's ignition. Thus an **agonist** is an extrinsic drug that activates the receptor site of a cell, which mimics the actions of naturally occurring body substances (intrinsic drugs) and increases the cell's response. Extrinsic drugs that are agonists have the same effects as the body's own hormones or natural substances (intrinsic drugs) that activate or turn on a specific receptor type in or on a cell (Fig. 1.3).

Agonist drugs must interact with the correct receptor for the drug to change the activity of the cell. Some agonist drugs change this activity to the same degree that intrinsic drugs do (see Fig. 1.3B). Other agonist drugs may work but not quite as well

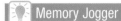

Memory Jogger

Receptors are physical places on or in cells that can bind with and respond to naturally occurring body chemicals. Their purpose is to control cell activity to meet the body's needs. A cell can respond to a drug by increasing its activity only when the drug fits properly into the receptor of the cell.

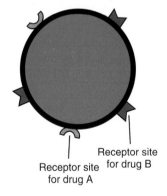

Cell with two different unbound receptors and two different free (loose) drugs

Receptor site for drug A

Receptor site for drug B

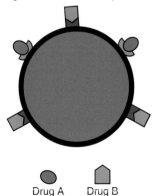

Cell with two different types of drugs bound to their receptor sites

Drug A   Drug B

FIG. 1.2 Cell with two types of receptors, unbound and bound.

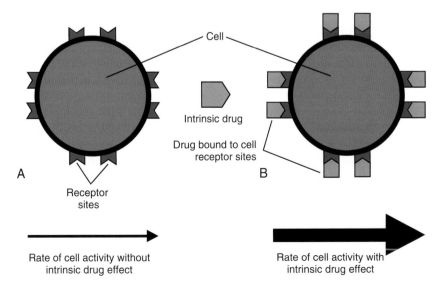

Cell

Intrinsic drug

Drug bound to cell receptor sites

A

Receptor sites

B

Rate of cell activity without intrinsic drug effect

Rate of cell activity with intrinsic drug effect

FIG. 1.1 Receptors controlling cell activity.

Intrinsic drug

Agonist drug

Powerful agonist drug

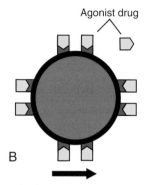

A

B

C

Rate of cell activity when each specific receptor is bound with the naturally occurring substance (intrinsic drug).

Rate of cell activity when each specific receptor is bound with an extrinsic drug that is nearly identical to the naturally occurring substance (drug is an agonist).

Rate of cell activity when each specific receptor is bound with an extrinsic drug that is even more powerful than the naturally occurring substance (drug is an agonist).

FIG. 1.3 Comparison of cell activity when receptor sites are bound with different substances.

 Memory Jogger

The effectiveness and "strength" of an agonist drug depend on how tightly and how long it remains bound to its receptor.

 Memory Jogger

Agonists are drugs that act like naturally occurring drugs and "turn on" receptors when they bind, speeding up cell action. Antagonists bind to receptors but "block" them, slowing cell action.

as the intrinsic drug. Still other agonist drugs work more powerfully than intrinsic drugs (see Fig. 1.3C). Agonist drug strength is determined by how tightly the drug binds to the receptor and how long it stays bound. The more tightly bound a drug is to its receptor and the longer it stays attached, the stronger the effect of the drug on the activity of the cell. For example, hydromorphone is an opioid agonist that binds to the opioid receptor better than morphine does. As a result, hydromorphone provides longer pain relief at lower doses than morphine.

Receptor antagonists. Sometimes the goal of drug therapy is to slow the activity of a cell. One way drugs can do this is by blocking the receptors of the cell so the intrinsic drug cannot bind with and activate the receptor. An extrinsic drug that blocks the receptor site of a cell, which prevents the naturally occurring body substance from binding to the receptor and decreases the cell's response, is called a receptor **antagonist**. An antagonist drug must be similar enough in shape to the intrinsic drug so it will bind with the receptor but not tightly enough or correctly enough to activate it. Antagonist action is like taking the key from one Honda Civic and trying to start the motor of a different Honda Civic with it. The key may fit into the ignition slot, but it will not turn on the motor. Instead, as long as the wrong key is in the ignition slot, the correct key cannot be placed into the slot, and the car's motor does not run. The antagonist competes with the intrinsic drug for the receptor sites, blocking the receptors and slowing or stopping the activity of the cell. Antagonists have effects that are opposite of agonists. Fig. 1.4 shows how antagonist drugs exert their effects on cells.

Receptors are the sites of direct action for many drugs. The final cell action when a drug binds to its receptor depends on both the nature of the drug (agonist or antagonist) and the nature of the receptor. Some drugs can act as agonists for certain cells and as antagonists for other cells. For example, epinephrine acts like an agonist when it binds to its receptors on heart muscle cells, making them contract more strongly and quickly. However, when epinephrine binds to muscle cells in the airways, it acts like an antagonist, causing these cells to relax rather than contract. Thus sometimes the same drug speeds up the activity of some cells and at the same time slows the activity of other cells. This is why you need to know the mechanism of action for each drug to understand both its intended actions and side effects. For example, when a person uses an epinephrine inhaler to widen the lung airways and breathe more easily, this is the intended action of the drug. The side effects are a more rapid heart rate and higher blood pressure because the drug is absorbed into the body and acts on a variety of cells and tissues.

Nonreceptor Actions

Not all drugs use receptors to exert their effects. Some drugs, such as antibacterial drugs, cancer chemotherapy drugs, and many drugs that reduce blood clotting, do not activate or inactivate cell receptors to exert their effects. The exact mechanism of action varies for each drug type that does not use receptors. For example, the targets of antibacterial drugs are bacteria. These drugs are either **cytotoxic** and directly kill these organisms or prevent them from reproducing.

PHYSIOLOGIC EFFECTS

The physiologic effect of a drug is the result of its mechanism of action on cells, tissues, organs, and the whole body. Usually, this effect can be felt by the patient or measured or observed by another person. For example, a drug that binds to airway receptors and dilates the airways has the physiologic effect of improving airflow in the airways. The improved airflow leads to better gas exchange. The patient notices easier breathing and you can observe improved oxygen saturation.

Physiologic effects are the expected and unexpected patient responses, including intended actions, side effects, and adverse effects. Two specific types of adverse effects are allergic responses and unique or personal responses (sometimes called *idiosyncratic* responses).

Intended Actions

The intended actions or therapeutic responses are the desired effect (main effect) of a drug on specific body cells or tissues and are the reason a drug is prescribed. All approved drugs have at least one expected intended action, and many have more than one.

Side Effects

Side effects are any minor effects of a drug on body cells or tissues that are not its intended action. All drugs have side effects, which generally are the most common mild changes that occur in at least 10% of patients receiving a drug. These effects are expected to occur in most patients taking a specific drug but vary in intensity from one person to another. Although side effects are expected, not all patients taking the same drug will experience them. Many are related to the mechanism of action of the drug and are temporary, resolving when the drug is discontinued. For example, people who take an oral penicillin for more than 5 days often develop diarrhea. This problem usually stops within 2 to 3 days after the drug is no longer taken. Although some side effects may be uncomfortable and may cause the patient to avoid a specific drug, they usually are not harmful. Examples of common side effects include:

- Constipation with the use of opioid analgesics
- Sexual disinterest or impotency with the use of certain antidepressants
- Diarrhea with the use of penicillin and many other antibacterial drugs
- Drowsiness with the use of certain antihistamines
- Increased bleeding and bruising with the use of aspirin
- Increased eyelash growth with the use of prostaglandins agonists for glaucoma therapy

Some drug side effects may even become a therapeutic effect. For example, topical prostaglandins agonists are now used to thicken eyelashes. The aspirin side effect of reduced blood clotting is now a common reason for why it is prescribed for people with coronary artery disease to reduce the risk for a heart attack.

Adverse Effect/Adverse Drug Reaction

A drug adverse effect or an adverse drug reaction (ADR) is a harmful side effect that is more severe than expected and has the potential to damage tissue or cause serious health problems. It may also be called a *toxic effect* or a *toxicity*. Often these effects occur with higher drug doses and are rare when the patient is taking normal doses of a specific drug. For example, many patients have the side effect of diarrhea when taking an antibacterial drug for 10 to 14 days. A few may have such severe diarrhea that they become dehydrated. At higher doses, a very few patients may develop the adverse effect of pseudomembranous colitis, which is profound bloody diarrhea and infection that can lead to complications such as perforation of the colon.

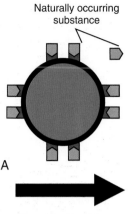

Naturally occurring substance

A

Rate of cell activity when each specific receptor is bound with the naturally occurring substance (intrinsic drug).

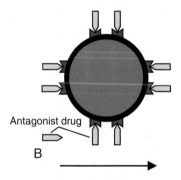

Antagonist drug

B

Rate of cell activity when each specific receptor is bound with an antagonist drug.

FIG. 1.4 Comparison of cell activity when receptor sites are bound with the naturally occurring substance (intrinsic drug) (A) and with an extrinsic drug that is an antagonist (B) (blocks the receptor site, preventing the naturally occurring substance from binding).

 Memory Jogger

Drug side effects are expected, are mild, may not occur in all patients, and often do not require either discontinuation of the drug or changing the dosage.

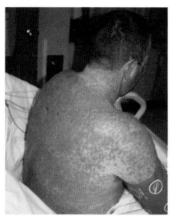

FIG. 1.5 Stevens-Johnson syndrome.

Memory Jogger

An ADR is rare and serious and has the potential to damage organs (cause toxicities). Usually when a patient has an ADR, the drug is stopped to prevent organ damage.

Memory Jogger

Anaphylaxis is a severe, life-threatening inflammatory response with these symptoms:
- Chest tightness
- Difficulty breathing
- Low blood pressure
- Hives
- Swelling of the face, mouth, and throat (angioedema)
- Weak, thready pulse
- A sense that something bad is happening

Drug Alert

Administration Alert

When a person has a true allergic response to a drug, **do not administer** that drug or any drug from the same drug family without additional precautions.

QSEN: Safety

Although adverse effects are not common, it is important to know what types of ADRs and their signs and symptoms are associated with a specific drug so any problems that do occur are identified and managed early. Examples of ADRs include:
- Angioedema with swelling of the mouth, face, lips, and tongue associated with angiotensin-converting enzyme inhibitors for hypertension therapy
- Muscle breakdown with the use of "statin-type" cholesterol-lowering drugs
- Lung fibrosis with the use of amiodarone
- Pseudomembranous colitis with the use of antibacterial drugs such as amoxicillin and vancomycin
- Stevens-Johnson syndrome, a rare and severe skin reaction that can occur with any drug (Fig. 1.5)

Usually when a patient has an adverse effect to a drug, he or she is taken off the drug. However, at times the patient requires the intended action, and the drug cannot be discontinued. In such cases, other precautions then are taken to limit tissue and organ damage.

Some adverse effects occur so commonly with a specific drug that the drug is removed from the market. Other drugs may continue to be prescribed but carry a black box warning. A **black box warning** is a notice from the FDA that a drug may produce serious or even life-threatening effects in some people, in addition to its beneficial effects. This warning is printed on the package insert sheet and is bordered in black. Prescribers must make certain that such drugs are prescribed only for patients who meet strict criteria and who understand the serious nature of the possible adverse effects. The drugs may be used in patients for whom the potential benefits outweigh the possible risks.

Allergic responses. An **allergic response** is a type of adverse effect in which the presence of the drug stimulates the release of histamine and other body chemicals that cause inflammatory reactions. It may be as mild as a skin rash or as severe and life threatening as anaphylaxis.

If not recognized and treated quickly, anaphylaxis can lead to vascular collapse, shock, and death. The patient who develops a skin rash, hives, or mild throat swelling within minutes, hours, or days of taking a drug may develop a more severe response and anaphylaxis the next time he or she takes the same drug. Usually when the person has a true allergic response to a drug, that drug and any from the same drug family should not be prescribed for him or her. This is known as a **contraindication**, which is a personal or health-related reason for not administering a specific drug to a patient or group of patients. Not all contraindications are for allergies. For example, a drug known to cause birth defects is considered an absolute contraindication for anyone who is pregnant. Another example is when two drugs interact very badly; one may be contraindicated for the time a patient is prescribed to take the other drug.

Another allergic reaction that can occur after days, weeks, months, and even years of therapy with a specific drug is *angioedema*. Although angioedema can occur in any part of the body, it is most serious when it occurs in the face and neck. The tongue, lips, and lower face swell to the point that the person has a hard time talking and may not be able to swallow (Fig. 1.6). The swelling can extend to the throat, which is life threatening because the airway can become too narrow to breathe. People may not associate the problem with a drug they are taking because they may have been taking the drug for a long time before angioedema occurs.

Unique/personal responses. *Unique* and *personal responses*, also known as *idiosyncratic responses*, are unexpected adverse effects that are unique to the patient and not related to a drug's mechanism of action. They are not true allergies but are related to the person's genetic differences. Some unique responses may occur within members of one family or are more common within a specific ethnicity. For example, patients who have a deficiency of the enzyme glucose-6-phosphate dehydrogenase, which is more common among men of African or Mediterranean descent, develop hemolytic anemia when they take drugs such as primaquine to prevent malaria, sulfonamide antibiotics, or thiazide diuretics. Other unique responses may occur only in one person, such as developing hiccups after every time a certain drug is taken.

Although the exact cause of personal responses is not always known, the effects can be severe and life threatening. For purposes of prevention, they are documented in the patient's chart in the same way as severe drug allergies.

HOW THE BODY AFFECTS AND CHANGES DRUGS (PHARMACOKINETICS)

Except for some topical drugs used to manage some skin problems, drugs must enter the body to produce their intended actions. Once a drug enters a person, **pharmacokinetics** occur, which is the process of how the body changes the drug through metabolism. So, after absorption, the body is affecting the drug at the same time the drug is affecting the body. Through metabolism, the body changes the structure of the drug so it can be processed, inactivated, and eliminated from the body. Metabolizing drugs by the body is why drugs must be taken repeatedly (for days and sometimes more than once each day) to continue to exert their intended actions. If drugs were never inactivated or eliminated, one dose would remain in the body for years and continue to exert both its intended actions and its side effects.

A drug must enter the body and reach a high enough constant level as a steady state in the blood or target tissue to produce the intended action. The lowest blood drug level needed to result in a measurable intended action is the **minimum effective concentration (MEC)** (Fig. 1.7). If the body eliminates the drug faster than it enters the body, the drug level at any given time will not be high enough to produce the intended action. If the body eliminates the drug more slowly than it enters the body, the drug level could become high enough to cause more side effects or adverse effects. A **steady-state** blood level is the point at which drug elimination is balanced with drug entry, resulting in a constant effective drug blood level (Fig. 1.8). Calculation of the MEC is based on the "average" response of the drug when it was given to a large number of test subjects. The same drug may have a different MEC in some patients because of differences in age, size, gender, race/ethnicity, metabolism, genetic differences, and health and the presence of other drugs. The body processes drugs through the stages of absorption, distribution, metabolism, and elimination.

A drug's **duration of action** is the length of time a single dose of a drug is present in the blood at or greater than the level needed to produce an effect or response. The duration of action is one way to assess the potency of a drug. Drug **potency** is the strength of the intended action produced at a given drug dose. Drugs that have higher potency need lower doses to produce an intended action. Drugs that are less potent require higher doses to produce the same intended action. The longer a drug dose stays active in the body at or above the MEC, the more potent it is. In general, less-potent drugs have fewer expected side effects but may need to be taken more often. A more potent drug may need to be taken only once or twice daily to achieve the intended action.

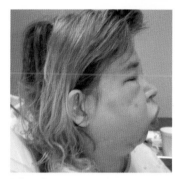

FIG. 1.6 Angioedema of the face, lips, and mouth.

 Drug Alert

Action/Intervention Alert

Ask the patient about any adverse reactions, including allergic and personal reactions, and record these in the patient's chart.

QSEN: Safety

 Memory Jogger

At the same time that a drug is having an effect on the body, the body is also having an effect on the drug.

 Memory Jogger

Drugs that have higher potency need lower doses to produce an intended action. Drugs that are less potent require higher doses to produce the same intended action.

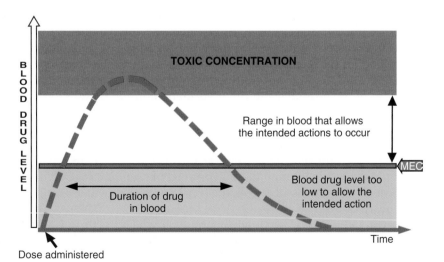

FIG. 1.7 Minimum effective concentration and blood level needed to allow the intended action to occur.

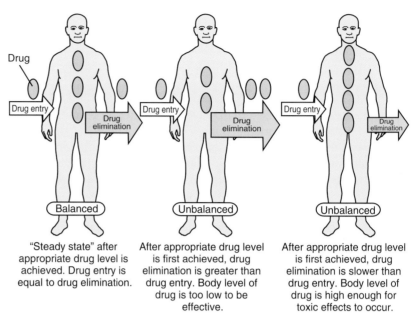

FIG. 1.8 Comparison of body levels of drug when drug entry and elimination are balanced and unbalanced.

ABSORPTION

For a drug to be able to change target cell activity, the drug must come into direct contact with these target cells. Thus extrinsic drugs must first enter the body and get into the bloodstream to find their target cells. **Absorption** is the movement of a drug from the outside of the body into the bloodstream. The percentage of a drug dose that actually reaches the blood is its **bioavailability**. If an entire drug dose reaches the bloodstream, its bioavailability is 100%. When only part of a drug dose gets into the blood, that drug is less than 100% bioavailable.

Drugs can enter the body in many ways:
- The **percutaneous route** means that the drug enters through the skin or mucous membranes.
- The **enteral route** is the movement of drugs into the body using the gastrointestinal (GI) tract.
- The **parenteral route** is the movement of drugs into the body by injection (intra-arterial, intravenous [IV], intramuscular, subcutaneous, intradermal, intracavitary, intraosseous, intrathecal).

Table 1.2 lists the different routes of drug entry and their advantages and disadvantages. Chapter 2 describes how to administer drugs by these routes, along with any specific precautions needed.

Drugs are designed and prepared differently by the manufacturer, depending on their intended routes. For example, drugs given by the parenteral route must be sterile, but those given by the enteral route only need to be clean, not sterile. Some drugs prepared for the enteral route may have special coatings (enteric coatings) on them. These coatings either prevent the drugs from harming the stomach lining or prevent some of the enzymes and other substances in the digestive tract from destroying the drug before it can be absorbed.

Percutaneous Route

The percutaneous route of drug entry is the movement of the drug from the outside of the body to the inside through the skin or mucous membranes. Only lipid-soluble drugs—those that easily dissolve in lipids (fats) rather than water—can be absorbed percutaneously.

Transdermal delivery is a percutaneous route in which the drug is applied to the skin, passes through the skin, and enters the bloodstream to affect an internal organ. Although drugs are placed on the skin, the skin is not the target for the drug. For

---

★ Critical Point for Safety

Do **not** give a drug that is prepared to be given by one route by any other route.

QSEN: Safety

Table 1.2	Advantages and Disadvantages of Drug Entry Routes	
ROUTE	**ADVANTAGES**	**DISADVANTAGES**
Percutaneous	Convenient	Absorption dependent on circulation
Transdermal	Bypasses gastrointestinal tract Large selection of body areas	Absorption less predictable Can lead to skin breakdown
Sublingual	Less invasive Rapid absorption	Effect is reduced when patient eats or drinks
Buccal	Less invasive/obtrusive	Effect is reduced when patient eats or drinks
Rectal[a]	Usually painless	Embarrassing
Enteral	Convenient High patient acceptance Least expensive Drugs need only to be clean, not sterile Large surface area for absorption	Can cause gastrointestinal disturbance First-pass loss Can bind to other substances in the tract and not get absorbed Absorption dependent on motility; has great individual variation
Parenteral	Speed 100% bioavailability Decreased first-pass loss	Speed Invasive administration Increased cost because drugs need to be sterile rather than just clean Discomfort

[a]Rectal drug delivery can be either percutaneous or enteral depending on how far into the rectum the drug is placed. Drugs placed within the lowest 1.5 inches are considered delivered by the percutaneous route. Those placed higher in the rectum are considered delivered by the enteral route.

example, nitroglycerin paste applied to the skin dissolves through the skin, then enters the bloodstream, and finally exerts its effect on blood vessels in the heart. Other drugs that are often given by this route using skin patches include certain types of pain medications and continuous hormone treatments.

Some drugs can be given through the mucous membranes of the mouth, nose, lungs, rectum, or vagina and have effects on deeper tissues. Mucous membranes have many blood vessels close to the surface, making movement of the drug through the membranes and into the bloodstream rapid and easy. Drugs given this way can be placed as tablets under the tongue or between the gum and the cheek, sprayed in the nose or under the tongue, inhaled through the nose or mouth, or placed as a liquid or a suppository in the rectum or vagina, as shown in Chapter 2. Examples of drugs that can be given this way include hormones, pain medications, drugs for nausea and vomiting, and anesthetic agents.

Enteral Route

The **enteral route** of drug delivery is the movement of drugs from the outside of the body to the inside using the gastrointestinal (GI) tract. It is the most commonly used route of drug administration, and drugs are swallowed as liquids, tablets, or capsules. Most drugs that can be taken by mouth can also be placed directly into the stomach or intestines through a tube or into the rectum (when prescribed to do so). Once the drug is in the GI tract, it must dissolve and enter the bloodstream before it can exert its effects on target cells. Usually not all of a drug taken enterally enters the blood, and thus these drugs have less bioavailability than those given by the parenteral route. Enteral drugs are often given in higher doses than the same drug given parenterally just for this reason.

The GI tract is long, and issues within it can affect oral drug absorption. Diarrhea can move drugs through the intestine so quickly that they are eliminated rather than absorbed and do not exert a therapeutic effect. Food in the stomach or intestines slows or delays absorption. For this reason, some drugs such as the tetracycline antibiotics are not to be taken with food or milk. On the other hand, taking some oral drugs when the stomach is empty can cause such rapid absorption that the effects can occur too quickly and harm the patient.

 Memory Jogger

Mucous membranes have many blood vessels close to the surface, making movement of the drug through the membranes and into the bloodstream rapid.

 Memory Jogger

Many drugs given by mouth usually require higher doses than the same drugs when given intravenously, because they are less bioavailable.

Rectal drug delivery with drugs placed within the lowest 1.5 inches is considered delivered by the percutaneous route. Those placed higher in the rectum are considered delivered by the enteral route. The reason for this difference is the way venous blood leaves these areas. Venous blood from the last half of the mouth, the esophagus, the stomach, the intestines, and the higher part of the rectum drains into the liver before it returns to the heart as part of systemic circulation. This means that the liver has a chance to metabolize drugs from the GI tract before they get to their target tissues. Blood from the lowest part of the rectum does not first enter the GI circulation, and drugs absorbed there do not get metabolized before they reach their target tissues.

Parenteral Route

The parenteral route involves giving drugs by injection, which bypasses the intestinal tract and other organs of digestion such as the liver, placing drugs more directly into the blood or target cells. Drugs can be injected into many structures:

- An artery, called an *intra-arterial injection* (administered by the prescriber)
- A vein, known as *IV injection*
- The skin, known as *intradermal injection*
- The fatty tissue below the skin, called a *subcutaneous injection*
- A muscle, or *intramuscular injection*
- A body cavity, known as *intracavitary injection* (administered by the prescriber)
- A joint, known as *intra-articular injection* (administered by the prescriber)
- A bone, or *intraosseous injection* (administered by the prescriber)
- The fluid of the brain or spinal cord, known as *intrathecal injection* (administered by the prescriber)
- Directly into specific tissues or organs (administered by the prescriber)

The parenteral route gets the drug into the bloodstream more quickly and more completely than other routes. For example, the dose of a drug given IV is entirely in the blood immediately after injection and then is 100% bioavailable. Not only do drugs work more quickly when given this way, but any problems the drugs may cause also occur more quickly. The parenteral route is more invasive and more dangerous to the patient than other routes. Give drugs parenterally only if they are made to be given by the parenteral route. In addition, because the IV route directly enters the bloodstream, care must be taken during administration to prevent infection and sepsis.

DISTRIBUTION

After drugs have been placed or absorbed into the blood, they must be distributed to their target tissues, where the intended action is supposed to occur. Most drugs do not exert their mechanisms of action while in the blood. The bloodstream is just the "roadway" used by the body to get the drug to its target cells. Drugs can be distributed or spread to different body areas. Drug **distribution** is the extent that a drug spreads into three specific compartments. The bloodstream or blood volume (sometimes called the plasma volume) is the first drug compartment. This area is made up of the spaces in all the arteries, veins, and capillaries. The second drug compartment includes both the blood volume and the watery spaces between all body cells, also known as the interstitial space. The third drug compartment is the largest, including the blood volume, the watery spaces between the cells, and the space inside the cells (intracellular space).

The size and chemical nature of the drug determine how widely a drug distributes within the body. Physically smaller drugs are able to fit through cell channels and tend to distribute widely into tissues and cells. Large drugs do not fit easily through cell pores or channels and often have a much more limited distribution within the body.

Some drugs bind to proteins in the blood. These drugs do not touch or enter other cells; they can exert their effects only on cells in the blood. An example of this type of drug is an antibiotic that stays in the blood and affects only the microorganisms that are also in the blood. Drugs that distribute only to the blood volume are eliminated more rapidly than those that are distributed more widely and may need to be taken three or four times a day to keep the drug level high enough to be effective.

Very small drugs and those that easily dissolve in fats (are lipid soluble) can cross cell membranes and enter cells. These drugs are distributed the most widely, staying in the body longer and affecting more tissues and organs.

Some places in the body are more difficult for drugs to enter (e.g., the brain, inside the eye, sinuses, and prostate gland). In addition, some body conditions can reduce drug distribution, such as when the patient is dehydrated or has low blood pressure *(hypotension).* If a person is taking more than one drug, the drugs can interact (meaning that the presence of one drug can change the distribution of another drug). This issue is a type of drug interaction and must be considered whenever the patient is taking more than one drug.

Another issue affecting drug distribution is the "trapping" of drugs in certain tissues. This is called *sequestration*. Lipid-soluble drugs often enter body fat cells and are sequestered there, with the drug being slowly released over time, like a "time-release" capsule. Completely eliminating these drugs may take a long time. Thus the effects of sequestered drugs may be present for weeks or longer after the person has stopped taking the drug, especially in people who have a higher percentage of body fat.

METABOLISM

Metabolism is a set of physiologic body actions by enzymes that change the chemical shape and content of a drug, most commonly to prepare it for inactivation and elimination. Metabolism is needed because any drug that enters the body is a "foreign" substance, and the body tries to eliminate it. Before most drugs can be eliminated, they must first be degraded to some degree through metabolism. Usually, the changing of a drug by the body inactivates the drug and makes it easier to eliminate. A few drugs are actually first activated by body metabolism by removing a part of the drug that is inactive before the drug can exert its effects. After such a drug has exerted its mechanism of action, it is then remetabolized or reprocessed for elimination.

Enzyme Activity for Metabolism

Drugs can be metabolized to different degrees by enzymes in different body tissues. The organs and cells most involved in drug metabolism are the liver, kidneys, lungs, and white blood cells (WBCs). All these tissues contain special enzymes that break down and change the chemicals in the drugs. Two common enzymes and enzyme systems for drug degradation and metabolism are lactate dehydrogenase and the very large cytochrome P-450 family of enzymes. Cytochrome p is abbreviated as CYP (pronounced "sip"). There are at least 300,000 different CYP enzymes, many of which have important roles in drug metabolism. Small genetic changes in these enzymes affect how well an individual person is able to metabolize a specific drug. Other personal issues that influence the activity of enzymes for drug metabolism include age, organ health, and exposure to other drugs and chemicals.

Pharmacogenetics/Pharmacogenomics

Enzymes are proteins the body makes using different DNA genes as the instructions for assembling long chains of amino acids in the correct order to make them. For example, insulin is a protein containing 51 amino acids in a specific order. If even one amino acid is out of place or missing, the insulin will not work as well or may not work at all. DNA contains the genes that code for the exact sequence of amino acids needed for active insulin. Although the DNA gene for insulin should be identical in all people, some may have a variation in the gene that slightly changes the insulin's amino acid sequence, which then alters how well that person's insulin works. The same is true for the DNA genes that code for metabolizing enzymes.

Gene function influences drug effectiveness and metabolism through pharmacogenetics and pharmacogenomics. These two similar terms are often used interchangeably, but one is more personal than the other. **Pharmacogenomics** refers to

Memory Jogger

Physically smaller drugs and those that are lipid soluble are more widely distributed and enter cells more easily than larger or water-soluble drugs.

Memory Jogger

Drug distribution and activity are reduced in a patient who is dehydrated or has a very low blood pressure.

Memory Jogger

Metabolism changes the chemical structure of drugs; it can activate drugs, inactivate them, and prepare them for elimination.

how the general expression of all genes and gene variations influence the effects of drug therapy. This term is broad and reflects all of what is known currently about the relationship between enzyme differences based on gene changes and possible drug responses. Pharmacogenetics is more specific to an individual person. Thus **pharmacogenetics** refers to how differences or variations in one person's specific gene or genes affect the physiologic action of a drug or drugs. The most well-studied gene variations are associated with the CYP family of enzymes.

Not only are there thousands of CYP enzymes, they are also quite large with many amino acids. Genetic-based variations in these amino acid sequences are common, and some can make the resulting enzyme less active than normal or more active than normal. Many of these changes are harmless and do not affect drug therapy. Some genetic differences allow patients to make more active forms of the enzymes used in drug metabolism. These patients may need higher-than-average doses of drugs for the drugs to work well and may also need to take the drugs more often to keep a steady-state level. Other patients have genetic differences that reduce the amount or activity of enzymes they make for drug metabolism. These patients need lower doses for the same effect compared with the "average" person. Thus, either way, a change in activity of any one of these enzymes can affect a person's response to drug therapy.

One common example of how gene variation for metabolizing enzymes affects drug function is the anticoagulant drug warfarin, which reduces blood clotting. This drug is metabolized for elimination primarily by two enzymes from the CYP system, CYP2C9 and CYP2C19. About 17% to 37% of White people have a small variation in CYP2CP that slows the metabolism of warfarin. This means that warfarin remains in the patient's system longer, greatly increasing the risk for bleeding and other side effects. For people who have this gene mutation, warfarin doses need to be much lower than those for the general population.

Whenever patients do not have the expected response to drug therapy, such a gene variation may be responsible. When the response to drug therapy is far less than expected or there is no response, a different drug therapy is needed. When the response to drug therapy is greater than expected or causes toxic reactions, the dose may need to be reduced or a different drug prescribed. Research into gene variation for metabolizing enzymes continues and new variation are discovered often. At this time, genetic testing for specific gene variations are not routine but may become so in the future. Nurses need to remain alert for differences in patient responses to drug therapy. When such differences are observed, be sure to inform the prescriber. Information regarding specific known examples and problems for variation in drug responses are discussed in the appropriate clinical chapter.

The liver and kidneys are the most important organs for drug metabolism (Fig. 1.9). If a patient has a problem with either the liver or the kidneys, drugs may be metabolized slowly and remain active longer. In this situation, high levels of a drug can quickly build up in the patient, often leading to toxic side effects.

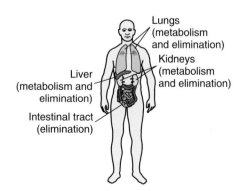

FIG. 1.9 Major sites of drug metabolism and elimination.

ELIMINATION

Elimination is the removal of drugs from the body accomplished by certain enzyme metabolizing systems and organs. The most active routes for drug elimination are the intestinal tract, the kidneys, and the lungs (see Fig. 1.9). Drugs leave the body in the feces, urine, exhaled air, sweat, tears, saliva, and breast milk.

Drugs metabolized by the liver are sent to either the intestinal tract or the blood and then to the kidney for elimination. Even drugs given parenterally can be eliminated through the intestinal tract. When a drug is given orally, some of the drug is metabolized quickly by the liver and rapidly eliminated from the body. The rapid inactivation and elimination of oral (enteral) drugs by liver metabolism is called **first-pass loss**. This is the reason an enteral drug is less bioavailable and the dosage is higher compared with the same drug given intravenously.

Drugs that are dissolved in the blood may leave the body in the urine. The drugs may change the color or smell of the urine. (This is why urine tests can determine whether a person is using certain illegal drugs.)

A few types of drugs are metabolized and eliminated through the lungs and leave the body in the exhaled air. Drugs that are small can be **vaporized**, which is changed into a gas or mist. In addition to vaporized drugs being able to enter the body through the lungs, they can also be eliminated by the lungs during exhalation. This is why a Breathalyzer test can measure blood alcohol levels.

Just as for metabolism, the liver and kidneys are the most important organs for drug elimination. The liver metabolizes the drug to make it ready for elimination, which often is performed by the kidney. If a patient has a problem with either the liver or the kidneys, drugs may take a longer time to be eliminated from the body and can build up to toxic levels quickly. In addition, some drugs cause liver or kidney damage. Drugs that can cause liver damage are called *liver toxic* or *hepatotoxic*. Drugs that can cause kidney damage are called *kidney toxic*, *renal toxic*, or *nephrotoxic*.

Half-Life

A drug's **half-life** is the time span needed for one half of a single drug dose to be eliminated from the body. When multiple doses are given over time, the half-life for the total dosage also can be calculated. For example, the antiinflammatory drug naproxen has a half-life of 12 hours. Suppose the first dose of the drug was 220 mg. Twelve hours after the drug was given, 110 mg of the drug remains in the body. Half of the remaining 110 mg is eliminated in the next 12 hours so that, 24 hours after the first dose, 55 mg of the drug remains in the patient's body. Thus, if you received only a single 220-mg dose of a drug that has a half-life of 12 hours, it would take almost 48 hours for you to completely eliminate the drug (Table 1.3). The drug is considered

Did You Know?

Drugs administered intravenously can be eliminated through the intestinal tract because the blood circulates nearly everywhere, including the GI system.

Table 1.3	Time Needed to Completely Eliminate a Single-Dose Drug with a Half-Life of 6 Hours	
TIME PASSED (H)	**AMOUNT OF DRUG REMAINING IN THE BODY (MG)**	
0 (time of drug administration)	500	
6	250	
12	125	
18	62.5	
24	31.25	
30	15.625	
36	7.813	
42	3.906	
48	1.953	
54	0.976	
60	0.488	

Memory Jogger

A drug with a half-life of 4 hours is not eliminated in 8 hours. Each portion remaining after a half-life time has passed is eliminated one half at a time.

 Memory Jogger

Loading doses are generally needed and used for drugs that have a long half-life to increase the drug's effectiveness and prevent toxicities or adverse reactions at the same time.

eliminated when less than 10% of the drug remains, which would be between 36 and 48 hours for this example. For most drugs, at least five half-lives after the last dose are needed to eliminate a drug.

The half-life of a drug is determined by how fast it is normally eliminated. Drugs that are eliminated rapidly have a short half-life; drugs eliminated slowly have a long half-life. The half-life is used to determine how much drug should be prescribed and how often it should be taken to get to and stay at a steady-state level to be maintained at or greater than the MEC. Although the MEC and half-life of a specific drug are generally known based on research, they may be different in some patients because of differences in age, size, gender, race/ethnicity, metabolism, genetic heritage, and health and the presence of other drugs.

Drugs with a short half-life are often prescribed to be taken more than once per day to get to and keep a steady-state level long enough to make the drug effective (produce its therapeutic effect). Drugs with a long half-life may be prescribed with a **loading dose**, which is a first dose that is larger than all subsequent doses of the same drug. It is used to get the blood level up to the MEC as fast as possible. However, if subsequent doses were as large as the loading dose for drugs with a long half-life, toxicities and adverse reactions would be more likely to occur. Once the MEC is achieved, all other doses can be smaller and still maintain the MEC because the drug has a long half-life and is eliminated slowly. One example of a drug that is usually prescribed with a higher loading dose than a maintenance dose is amikacin, an antibiotic with a long half-life that is prescribed for serious life-threatening infections.

Peaks and Troughs

Peaks and troughs describe the relationship between the actual dose of drug given and the blood drug level over time (Fig. 1.10). The **peak** is the maximum or highest blood drug level that can be measured (like the top of a mountain), and the **trough** is the lowest or minimal blood drug level that can be measured (like the bottom of a water trough for animals).

When patients have no severe health problems or unusual reactions to a drug and its metabolism, the peaks and troughs of a specific drug are already known (they have been worked out for the average person).

LIFE SPAN CONSIDERATIONS

SIZE

Children are smaller than most adults, and prescribed drugs, with a few exceptions, are usually given in smaller doses in proportion to the child's size, especially weight.

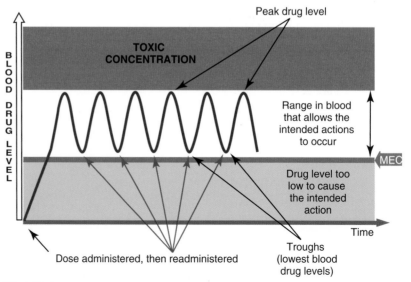

FIG. 1.10 Peaks and troughs of blood drug levels. *MEC,* Minimum effective concentration.

Some drugs are prescribed in milligrams (mg) per kilogram (kg). Some prescribed drug doses are based on body surface area (BSA) that are calculated in or milligrams per square meter (m^2) based on both height and weight. Either calculation must be made carefully and accurately because a math error of even one decimal place results in tremendous overdosing or underdosing. Follow these rules for pediatric drug administration:

- Always compare the drug dose prescribed for an infant or child with the recommended dose for the child's size.
- Question any drug prescription for a child in which the prescribed dose is greater or less than the recommended dose.
- Double check your drug dose calculation for an infant or child with another health care profession who is licensed to administer drugs or with a pharmacist.

Drugs that have a specific type of effect or response on adults may have the opposite effect on children (these effects are called *paradoxical*). For example, the drug methylphenidate stimulates the central nervous system of an adult and causes an overall increase in excitability and activity. This same drug reduces excitability and activity in children. Some drugs that cause drowsiness in adults may cause hyperactive behavior in some children.

Other drug side effects that occur in children but not in adults can be related to the growth and maturity of specific tissues. For example, when teeth are developing, the antibiotic tetracycline changes the density of the tooth enamel and can result in tooth darkening and staining. After teeth are mature, they are no longer at risk for this side effect. As a result, the drug tetracycline is rarely used for pregnant women (when the first teeth are forming) or in children under the age of 12 years (when the permanent teeth are forming). Another example of a drug affecting development is the quinolone type of antibiotics. These drugs damage bone growth in children and are not prescribed for them unless an infection is life threatening and the organism responds only to a quinolone.

 Memory Jogger

Children may have completely different responses to a drug than an adult would have to the same drug.

ORGAN HEALTH

The health of the organs most involved in drug distribution, metabolism, and elimination affects drug actions, especially the liver and kidneys. Along with physical immaturity and age-related changes in organ function, diseases can have an effect on organ function.

Liver Health

A healthy liver is important for good drug metabolism and elimination. Not only do preexisting liver problems change drug metabolism, some drugs can cause liver damage or worsen existing liver problem. The liver health status of any person should be known before drug therapy is started. Table 1.4 lists the normal values for tests of liver function. A serious response as a result of reduced liver function is the prevention of the pigment bilirubin incorporation into bile. Bilirubin levels build up in the blood and eventually deposit into all tissues, especially the skin, sclera of the

Table **1.4**	Laboratory Values for Liver Function in Adults	
TEST	**NORMAL VALUES**	**SIGNIFICANCE OF ABNORMAL VALUES**
Albumin	3.5–5.0 g/dL	*Decreased*: possible liver disease
Alanine aminotransferase	4–36 IU/L	*Increased*: possible liver disease
Aspartate aminotransferase	10–35 units/L	*Increased*: possible liver disease
Lactate dehydrogenase	100–190 IU/L	*Increased*: possible liver disease
Alkaline phosphatase	30–120 units/L	*Increased*: possible liver disease
Bilirubin total serum	0.3–1.0 mg/dL	*Increased*: possible liver disease
Ammonia	10–80 mcg/dL	*Increased*: possible liver disease

IU, International units.

From Pagana, K., & Pagana, T. (2018). *Mosby's manual of diagnostic and laboratory tests* (6th ed.). St. Louis: Elsevier.

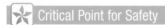
eyes, and mucous membranes. Bilirubin also enters the urine. Symptoms of excessive bilirubin include *jaundice* (yellowing of the skin, sclera, and mucous membranes), *pruritus* (itchiness), and dark or coffee-colored urine. Lack of bilirubin in the bile causes stools to lose color and appear white or clay colored. Patients with reduced liver function also experience fatigue, nausea, and increased bleeding.

Pediatric considerations. Drug metabolism in children varies depending on age and organ maturity. A premature infant or newborn may have a slower rate of metabolism than an adult because the enzyme systems of the liver may not yet be fully active. Toddlers, preschool children, school-age children, and adolescents usually have higher rates of metabolism than do adults. A child may receive a much lower dose of a drug than an adult, but the dose may need to be given more often because it is metabolized and eliminated more rapidly.

Considerations for older adults. Many older adults have reduced liver function as a result of liver damage or the aging process, making drug metabolism and elimination slower. Thus older adults often metabolize and eliminate drugs more slowly than younger adults, although this problem is greater in adults who have actual organ damage. Slow metabolism and elimination increase the half-life of a drug and make it easier to develop toxic drug levels in older adults.

In addition, often an older adult may be prescribed many different drugs to take every day. New drugs may be prescribed and old ones may be discontinued. An important consideration to ensure that any patient is receiving the correct drugs at the correct dosages in any setting is the issue of medication reconciliation. It is the responsibility of the prescriber and the health care professional administering the drugs, especially nurses, to ensure that all of a patient's active drugs are properly listed in the patient record. More information on medication reconciliation is discussed in Chapter 2.

Kidney Health

Some drugs are metabolized and eliminated by the kidney. Others are metabolized elsewhere and just eliminated by the kidney. Thus a healthy kidney is important for drug elimination and prevention of toxic drug levels. The kidney (renal) health status of any person should be known before drug therapy is started. Table 1.5 lists the normal values for tests of kidney function. When kidney function is reduced, drugs normally eliminated in the urine remain in the body longer and can build up to dangerous levels.

Pediatric considerations. An infant's kidneys do not concentrate fluids well. In addition, infants have a greater proportion of total body water than older children or adults. This means that drugs easily dissolved in water spread through proportionally

Table 1.5	Laboratory Tests Assessing Kidney Function in Adults
SUBSTANCE	**NORMAL VALUES**
Blood urea nitrogen	10–20 mg/dL
Creatinine	*Males:* 0.6–1.3 mg/dL *Females:* 0.5–1 mg/dL
Sodium	136–145 mEq/L
Potassium	3.5–5 mEq/L
Calcium	9.0–10.5 mg/dL
Chloride	98–106 mEq/L
Magnesium	1.3–2.1 mEq/L
Bicarbonate	21–28 mEq/L

From Pagana, K., & Pagana, T. (2018). *Mosby's manual of diagnostic and laboratory tests* (6th ed.). St. Louis: Mosby.

more water, and drugs are lost by the kidney route more rapidly. Thus an infant may need a higher dose for these drugs in terms of milligrams per kilogram than would a toddler or an older child. Water-soluble drugs are eliminated more rapidly in infants and young children than they are in adults.

Considerations for older adults. Kidney function slowly decreases with age, which can increase drug half-life. This means that one dose of a drug stays in the body longer and continues to have intended actions, as well as side effects, in an older adult than in a younger adult.

Cardiopulmonary Health

Together the heart, blood, and lungs promote the health of all organs by ensuring adequate oxygenation. The cardiovascular system ensures that drugs reach their target sites of action and sites for metabolism and elimination. The lungs and pulmonary system help to metabolize and eliminate some drugs. Red blood cells (RBCs) carry oxygen, and WBCs are sites of drug metabolism. Thus a healthy heart, adequate blood pressure, healthy lungs, and good oxygenation are needed for optimal drug therapy. Table 1.6 lists normal values for tests of cardiac, blood, and lung function.

 Memory Jogger

Older adults may need a lower drug dosage than younger adults because of reduced kidney or liver function, and they are at a higher risk for dosage-related side effects.

Table 1.6	Laboratory Tests Assessing Cardiovascular Function and Oxygenation in Adults
TEST	**RANGE**
Blood Cells	

Red blood cells
  Women
  Men
	4.2–5.4 million per cubic millimeter (mm^3) of blood
	4.7–6.1 million/mm^3 of blood

Platelets	150,000–400,000/mm^3 of blood
White blood cells, total	5000–10,000/mm^3 of blood
Oxygenation	

Hematocrit
  Women
  Men
  Newborn to 6 months
  Older than 6 months
	37%–47%
	42%–45%
	44%–64%
	30%–44%

Hemoglobin
  Women
  Men
  Newborn to 6 months
  Older than 6 months
	12–16 g/dL
	14–18 g/dL
	10–17 g/dL
	10–15.5 g/dL

Oxygen saturation (Spo_2)	95%–100%
Arterial oxygen (Pao_2)	80–100 mm Hg
Arterial carbon dioxide ($Paco_2$)	35–45 mm Hg
Cardiac Function	
Brain natriuretic peptide	Less than 100 pg/mL

Creatine kinase
  Women
  Men
  Newborns
  Children
	30–135 units/L
	55–170 units/L
	68–580 units/L
	Same as adults

Creatine kinase-MM	100%
Creatine kinase-MB	0%
Creatine kinase-BB	0%

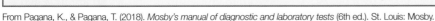 From Pagana, K., & Pagana, T. (2018). *Mosby's manual of diagnostic and laboratory tests* (6th ed.). St. Louis: Mosby.

Considerations for older adults. Many adults older than age 70 years have some degree of heart failure and poor blood flow to the liver and other body areas. This reduced blood flow both decreases drug effectiveness and limits how well drugs are distributed, metabolized, and eliminated.

The respiratory changes that occur with aging reduce lung volume and function to some degree in all older patients. These effects are made worse by a lifetime of exposure to inhaled irritants such as cigarette smoke, bacteria, air pollutants, and industrial fumes, reducing lung metabolism and elimination of some drugs. Lung problems may reduce the effectiveness of drugs taken by inhalation.

Older adults often have fewer RBCs and WBCs than younger adults. These changes reduce oxygenation of all organs and limit drug metabolism.

SPECIAL POPULATIONS

Pregnancy

Pregnancy is the time for development of a new human being. Nearly every organ forms in the 9 months before birth. Although during pregnancy the mother's bloodstream is separated from the unborn baby's bloodstream by the placenta, it is not a perfect barrier. Some drugs can cross the placenta and may affect the unborn baby. Regardless of the presumed safety of a drug, no prescribed or OTC drug should be taken during pregnancy unless it is clearly needed and its benefits outweigh any risks to the fetus.

Drugs that can cause birth defects are *teratogenic* or *teratogens*. Some drugs are more teratogenic than others, and even one dose can cause a severe birth defect. Other drugs are less teratogenic and require either many doses or very high doses to cause even a minor birth defect. Not all pregnant women who take a teratogenic drug during pregnancy have a child with birth defects, but the *risk* for birth defects is higher. Usually drugs are avoided during pregnancy; however, certain health problems may need to be managed with drug therapy.

Drugs have the same effects on the fetus as on the mother but can cause more problems. For example, when a pregnant woman takes the anticoagulant warfarin, the unborn baby's blood is also less able to clot, and the fetus can bleed to death. Drugs that lower blood pressure can lower the fetus's blood pressure so much that the brain does not receive enough oxygen, and brain damage results.

The FDA has revised guidelines for the "information for prescribers" section of the drug package inserts under the Physician Labeling Rule for "Use in Special Populations." This section has the subsections of "pregnancy" (including labor and deliver), "lactation" (breastfeeding), and "females and males of reproductive potential." Package inserts must contain all appropriate information regarding when and how a drug may affect these special populations. This information is presented as a risk summary when a drug is known to be absorbed systemically, and risk is classified in the following manner:

- Not predicted to increase risk
- Low likelihood of increasing risk
- Moderate likelihood of increasing risk
- High likelihood of increasing risk
- Insufficient data to assess the likelihood of increasing risk

This classification is used for risk to the fetus, risk to the pregnant woman (for problems when taking the drug, as well as problems that could occur from not taking the drug), risk for affecting the production of milk, risk for affecting the health of the nursing infant, and risk for affecting the fertility of females and males. It is the responsibility of the prescriber to know this information and to ensure that patients for whom the drugs are prescribed understand the risks versus the benefits of the prescribed therapy.

Lactation

Some drugs taken by a breastfeeding woman cross into the milk and are ingested by the infant. The effects of the drugs on the baby are the same as on the mother. For example, lipid-lowering drugs taken by a breastfeeding woman will lower her

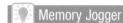
Memory Jogger

No prescribed or OTC drug is considered to be completely safe to take during pregnancy.

Critical Point for Safety

Before administering any newly prescribed drug, ask any female patient between the ages of 10–60 years if she is pregnant, likely to become pregnant, or breastfeeding. If she is pregnant or breastfeeding, ensure that the prescriber is aware of these conditions.

QSEN: Safety

| Box 1.1 | Recommended Methods of Reducing Infant Exposure to Drugs During Breastfeeding |

- For drugs that should not be given to infants:
  - Switch the infant to formula feeding temporarily or to breast milk obtained when you were not taking the drug.
  - Maintain your milk supply by pumping your breasts on a regular schedule, and discard the pumped milk.
  - When you are no longer taking the drug and it has been eliminated, resume direct breastfeeding.
  - When long-term therapy is needed, breastfeeding may have to be discontinued.
- For drugs that do not have to be avoided but should have levels reduced:
  - Nurse your baby right before taking the next dose of the drug.
  - Drink plenty of liquids to dilute the amount of drug in the breast milk.
  - Take the drug immediately after breastfeeding and just before the baby's longest sleep period.

infant's blood lipid levels. Although the mother may need to lower her blood lipid levels, the infant does not. Low lipid levels in an infant may cause poor brain development and permanent cognitive deficits.

When a breastfeeding woman has an infection, usually the infant does not; however, the antibiotic the mother takes can enter the breast milk and affect the infant. Some antibiotics such as penicillin may not cause a problem. Other antibiotics such as the quinolones, even taken for a short time, can disrupt bone development.

Before a drug is selected and prescribed for a breastfeeding woman, the effects on the infant must be considered. The mother's prescriber, the infant's health care provider, and the mother must discuss the issues together.

Breastfeeding is not recommended for mothers with chronic disorders that require daily drug therapy (e.g., seizures, hypertension, and high blood lipid levels). For short-term health problems that require less than 2 weeks of drug therapy (e.g., infection), the breastfeeding woman can make adjustments to reduce the infant's exposure to the drug (Box 1.1).

Females and Males with Reproductive Potential

People with reproductive potential include teenagers and adults who are capable of becoming pregnant (females) or are capable of causing a pregnancy (males). Some drugs reduce fertility temporarily, and others can reduce it permanently. A few drugs can increase fertility. Any person who is prescribed to take a drug that can affect fertility should have full knowledge about such effects.

DRUG INTERACTIONS

Drugs can interact with other drugs, food, vitamins, and herbal compounds. These interactions can change the way a drug works or the timing of its action. Some interactions actually increase the activity of the drug, whereas others decrease it. Some drugs and herbal compounds are not compatible with each other and can lead to adverse effects. Always ask patients who are being prescribed a new drug what other drugs (prescribed or OTC), vitamins, and herbal supplements they are taking currently. Because the number of possible problem interactions is huge, always check with the pharmacy or a drug reference for potential drug interactions.

A few common examples of interactions between drugs and between drugs and other agents include:

- Cimetidine enhances the action of quinidine, increasing the risk for adverse effects.
- Ciprofloxacin increases the blood concentration of warfarin, increasing the risk for bleeding.
- Ibuprofen and naproxen reduce the effectiveness of some antihypertensives such as captopril and lisinopril, increasing the risk for heart failure and strokes.
- Grapefruit juice greatly decreases the activity of the metabolizing enzyme CYP3A, which results in slower breakdown of many drugs, including felodipine, midazolam, and many statin-types of cholesterol lowering drugs. This change increases the risks for overdose and adverse effects. For some other drugs, grapefruit juice can decrease rather than increase their activity.

 Critical Point for Safety

If a woman is breastfeeding, urge her to discuss any drugs that she may be taking with her pediatrician.

QSEN: Safety

 Critical Point for Safety

Warn patients taking prescribed drugs to check with the prescriber or a pharmacist before starting any OTC drugs, vitamins, or herbal supplements.

QSEN: Safety

- St. John's wort, an herbal preparation, reduces the effectiveness of many drugs, including digoxin, warfarin, and oral contraceptives (birth control pills). Reducing the effectiveness of digoxin may worsen heart failure; reducing the effectiveness of warfarin increases the risk for clot formation, strokes, and pulmonary embolism; reducing the effectiveness of oral contraceptives may lead to unplanned pregnancies.

Get Ready for the NCLEX® Examination!

Key Points

- The prescriber's role in drug therapy is to select and order specific drugs. Prescribers may include physicians, dentists, podiatrists, advanced practice nurses, and physician's assistants.
- The health care professionals most responsible for teaching patients about their drugs include the prescriber, the pharmacist, and the nurse.
- Nurses who administer drugs to patients have responsibility for understanding the purposes, actions, side effects, problems, delivery methods, usual dosages, and necessary follow-up care for different drugs.
- When possible, always check the order and dosage calculation of a high-alert drug with a licensed health care professional or pharmacist.
- OTC drugs can be harmful when directions for dosage and schedule are **not** followed.
- When taking a history, always ask what specific herbal products the patient uses daily, including the brand names and the amounts.
- Anaphylaxis is a severe, life-threatening inflammatory response with symptoms of chest tightness; difficulty breathing; low blood pressure; hives; swelling of the face, mouth, and throat (angioedema); weak, thready pulse; a sense that something bad is happening.
- When a person has a true allergic response to a drug, **do not administer** that drug or any drug from the same drug family without additional precautions.
- Ask the patient about any adverse reactions, including allergic and personal reactions, and record these in the patient's chart.
- At the same time that a drug is changing body activity, the body is processing the drug for elimination.
- Drugs must reach a high enough level in the blood to exert their effects.
- Do **not** give a drug that is prepared to be given by one route by any other route.
- Know the manufacturer's recommendations for timing of any oral drug administered with regard to meals, specific foods, and liquids. If there are any restrictions or requirements, ensure that patients and families understand the reasons for these directions.
- Any problem with the GI tract can interfere with how fast a drug is absorbed.
- Never give by injection any drug made to be given by the enteral route.

- The most rapid drug entry route commonly used by nurses is the IV route. This rapid entry makes the IV route more dangerous because any adverse reaction would also happen more quickly. Always monitor patients closely during the first 15 to 30 minutes following the initial administration of a newly prescribed IV drug.
- The most important organs for drug metabolism and elimination are the liver and kidneys.
- Loading doses are generally needed and used for drugs that have a long half-life to increase the drug's effectiveness and prevent toxicities or adverse reactions at the same time.
- Although the expected actions and patient responses are known for all approved drugs, some patients may react differently than expected. Whenever a patient receives the first dose of a drug, be alert to the possibility of unique responses.
- Before administering any newly prescribed drug, ask any female patient between the ages of 10 to 60 years if she is pregnant, likely to become pregnant, or breastfeeding. If she is pregnant or breastfeeding, ensure that the prescriber is aware of these conditions.
- Unless a serious health problem exists in the pregnant woman, all types of drugs should be avoided (except for prenatal vitamins and iron supplements).
- When a female patient is prescribed to take a drug that is known to cause birth defects, be sure that she understands the risks, that her pregnancy test is negative, and that she is using one or more reliable methods of birth control (or completely abstains from sex) during treatment.
- Urge breastfeeding women to consult with their infant's health care provider before taking any prescribed or OTC drug.
- Always ask patients who are being prescribed a new drug what other drugs (prescribed or OTC), vitamins, and herbal supplements they are taking currently.
- Check with the pharmacy or a reliable drug reference for potential drug interactions.
- Warn patients taking prescribed drugs to check with the prescriber before starting any OTC drugs, vitamins, or herbal supplements.

Additional Learning Resources

🌐   Be sure to visit your Evolve website (http://evolve.elsevier.com/Workman/pharmacology/) for additional online resources.

[SG]   Go to your Study Guide for additional learning activities to help you master this chapter content.

Review Questions

See *Answers to In-Text Review Questions* in the back of the book for answers to these questions.

1. How are drugs different from medications?

   A. Medications are totally safe, but drugs more frequently have one or more side effects.
   B. Drugs are available over-the-counter whereas all medications require a prescription.
   C. The terms have the same meaning and drugs are not different from medications.
   D. Medications have a lower risk potential for addiction than do drugs.

2. Why is morphine categorized in the United States as a "schedule II" drug rather than a "schedule I" drug?

   A. It has a high potential for addiction and dependence.
   B. It has a currently accepted use for standard treatment.
   C. It is a synthetic product rather than a naturally occurring substance.
   D. It is usually combined with nonopioid drugs for use in pain management.

3. A patient tells the nurse that a mistake has been made because she was given Furocot instead of her usual Lasix. What is the nurse's **best** response?

   A. "Don't worry. Lasix is just a different brand of the same drug."
   B. "I will report this to your prescriber right away so corrective action can be taken."
   C. "Drink a lot of water, and report any shortness of breath or unusual sensation you have right away."
   D. "I am so sorry. The nurse who gave you the wrong drug is new and inexperienced. It is not likely one dose will harm you."

4. Which patient condition will the nurse expect to be considered a contraindication for a specific drug?

   A. Loose stools occurred previously when a patient took an oral antibiotic for 2 weeks.
   B. The patient who is prescribed to take penicillin for an infection is 7 months pregnant.
   C. The patient prescribed to take the antihistamine diphenhydramine reports that he gets a very dry mouth when taking the drug.
   D. The patient prescribed to take an antibiotic with a similar makeup to penicillin has a documented adverse drug reaction to penicillin.

5. A patient newly prescribed to take an anticoagulant drug along with other cardiac drugs reports that she also takes St. John's Wort daily. What is the nurse's **best** action?

   A. Documenting the information as the only action
   B. Asking the patient about any new or unusual bruising/ bleeding
   C. Consulting with the pharmacist about any potential interactions
   D. Instructing the patient to avoid taking the anticoagulant at the same time of day as the St. John's Wort

6. A patient is prescribed to take a cardiac drug that is an adrenaline antagonist. How does the nurse expect the effects of the patient's natural adrenaline to change with this therapy?

   A. Natural effects of adrenaline are decreased.
   B. Natural effects of adrenaline are increased.
   C. Natural effects of adrenaline are unchanged.
   D. Natural effects of adrenaline are completely eliminated.

7. A patient prescribed to take an antibiotic reports all of the following changes after 3 days on the drug. For which change does the nurse instruct the patient to seek medical attention or call 911 immediately? **Select all that apply.**

   A. Shortness of breath
   B. Increased number of daily stools
   C. Loss of interest in sexual activity
   D. Change in the taste of some foods
   E. Chest pain that extends to the jaw
   F. Sunburn after moderate sun exposure

8. The patient has a genetic variation in an enzyme that increases its rate for metabolizing and eliminating drugs and other compounds. What changes in drug therapy does the nurse expect will be needed as a result of these factors?

   A. More frequent monitoring because of the increased risk for adverse drug reactions
   B. Use of a large loading dose followed by smaller daily maintenance doses
   C. Increased drug dosages with more frequent scheduled doses
   D. Issuance of a black box warning

9. Which patient response to a newly prescribed drug will the nurse consider *paradoxical*?

   A. Increased insomnia after taking a sedative
   B. Increased gum bleeding with aspirin therapy
   C. Reduced taste sensation with an antihypertensive drug
   D. Blurred vision for a few minutes after instilling eyedrops

10. A patient who has rheumatoid arthritis and is breastfeeding a 2-month-old infant is prescribed to receive an IV drug monthly that is poorly absorbed from the GI tract. Which is the best advice for the nurse to give the patient to minimize the infant's exposure to the drug?

   A. "Switch your baby to formula during the week that you receive the IV drug."
   B. "Stop breastfeeding your baby now completely. You have already given her a healthy start."
   C. "Drink lots of fluids to dilute the drug in the breast milk and reduce your baby's exposure to it."
   D. "Because the drug is poorly absorbed from the GI tract, no changes in breastfeeding are needed."

Safely Preparing and Giving Drugs

http://evolve.elsevier.com/Workman/pharmacology/

Learning Objectives

The content presented in this chapter should help you to:

1. List the eight "rights" of giving drugs.
2. Describe how four types of drug orders differ.
3. Explain methods of preventing drug errors.
4. List important principles related to preparing and giving drugs.
5. Describe responsibilities related to giving enteral drugs.
6. Describe responsibilities related to giving parenteral drugs.
7. Describe responsibilities related to giving drugs through the skin and mucous membranes.
8. Describe responsibilities related to giving drugs through the ears and eyes.
9. Identify priority nursing responsibilities for before and after a drug has been given.

Key Terms

buccal route (BŬK-ŭl ROWT) (p. 41) Application of a drug within the cheek or the cavity of the mouth.

drug error (DRŬG ĀR-ŭr) (p. 29) Any preventable event that may cause inappropriate drug use or patient harm while the drug is in the control of the health care professional or the patient. A drug error may cause a patient to receive the wrong drug, the right drug in the wrong dose, the wrong route, or at the wrong time.

intradermal route (ĭn-tră-DŬR-mŭl ROWT) (p. 35) Injection of drugs within or between the layers of the skin.

intramuscular (IM) route (ĭn-tră-MŬS-kyŭ-lŭr ROWT) (p. 38) Injection of drugs into a muscle.

medication reconciliation (mĕ-dĭ-KĀ-shŭn rĕ-kŭn-sĭl-ē-ā-shŭn) (p. 30) The process of identifying the most accurate list of all medications that the patient is taking, including name, dosage, frequency, and route, by comparing the medical record to an external list of medications obtained from a patient, hospital, or other provider.

onset of action (ŎN-sĕt ŭv ĂK-shŭn) (p. 32) The length of time it takes for a drug to start to work.

oral route (ŌR-ŭl) (p. 32) Administration of drugs by way of the mouth.

per os (PO) (PŬR ŎS) (p. 32) Giving drugs by way of the mouth.

PRN order (p. 29) An order written to administer a drug to a patient as needed.

rectal route (RĔK-tŭl ROWT) (p. 34) Movement of a drug from outside of the body to the inside of the body through the rectum.

single-dose order (SĬN-gŭl DŌS ŌR-dŭr) (p. 29) An order written to administer a drug one time only.

standing order (STĂN-dĭng) (p. 29) An order written when a patient is to receive a drug on a regular basis. Also called a routine order.

STAT order (STĂT) (p. 29) An order written to administer a drug once and immediately.

subcutaneous route (sŭb-kū-TĂN-ē-ŭs ROWT) (p. 36) Injection of drugs into the tissues between the skin and muscle.

sublingual (SL) route (sŭb-LĬN-gwŭl ROWT) (p. 41) Administration of drugs by placing them underneath the tongue.

suppository (sŭ-PŎZ-ĭ-tōr-ē) (p. 34) A small medication plug designed to melt at body temperature within a body cavity other than the mouth, usually the rectum or vagina.

topical route (TŎP-ĭ-kŭl ROWT) (p. 40) Application of drugs directly to the skin.

transdermal route (trănz-DŬR-mŭl ROWT) (p. 40) A type of percutaneous drug delivery in which the drug is applied to the skin, passes through the skin, and enters the bloodstream.

unit-dose drugs (YŪ-nĭt DŌS) (p. 30) Drugs that are dispensed to fill each patient's drug orders for a 24-hour time period.

OVERVIEW

Nurses are responsible for providing competent and safe patient care. A major role is to give drugs safely. Because all drugs have side effects and the possibility of adverse effects, nurses have responsibility for the drug therapy process and must be knowledgeable about any drug administered to a patient. Essential knowledge about drugs includes the purpose, action, side effects, abnormal reactions (e.g., side effects, adverse effects), delivery methods, and necessary follow-up care.

Nurses, along with prescribers and pharmacists, are responsible for teaching patients about any drugs that are prescribed.

Although administering drugs to patients is one of the nurse's most important responsibilities, safely administering ("giving") drugs includes much more. Every nurse must be familiar with the professional practice act for the state in which he or she works.

To give drugs safely, you must understand the basic principles of drug administration. Check the expiration date to be sure that the drug is not outdated. Look carefully at intravenous (IV) drugs for any sediment or discoloration that may indicate that the drug is unstable and should not be used. Be sure to wash your hands and follow the eight "rights" of drug administration.

After giving a drug, you must check the patient for the expected results and for any side effects or adverse effects. You also have a duty to teach patients and their families about drugs, including the desired action, side effects, and when to call the prescriber.

THE EIGHT RIGHTS OF SAFE DRUG ADMINISTRATION

When preparing and giving drugs to patients, safety requires that you always follow the eight "rights" for drug administration:
1. Right patient
2. Right drug
3. Right dose
4. Right route
5. Right time
6. Right documentation
7. Right diagnosis
8. Right response

The Right Patient

The Joint Commission recommends checking two unique patient identifiers (e.g., name and birth date) before any medication is given to ensure that the right patient is receiving the drug that has been prescribed. An alert and oriented patient can be asked directly. If a patient is confused, hard of hearing, unconscious, or otherwise unable to reply, wash your hands first and then check the name, birth date, and identification number on his or her wristband. Some long-term care facilities such as nursing homes use pictures of patients to ensure that the correct patient receives the correct drugs. If a patient does not have an identification wristband, have one made and place it on his or her wrist. As an added safety measure, be sure to check the medication administration record (MAR) and the label on the patient's medication box with the wristband.

The Right Drug

Whenever a drug is prescribed there is a particular intended action. Be sure that the drug being given for that action is correct. Carefully compare the drug you are about to administer with the drug order. Be sure to give the drug in the form ordered by the prescriber (e.g., pill, capsule, liquid). Thousands of drugs are available today, and many of their names are so similar that they can be confusing. Be aware of these easily confused drug names. For more information about them, see "Confusing Drug Name Lists" later in this chapter.

The Right Dose, Route, and Time

The US government requires specific information to be included whenever a drug is prescribed. The drug order should be in written form and include the date, patient's name, name and address of the prescriber, generic or brand name of the drug, strength and number of times per day the drug should be taken, specific instructions for use, number of doses and refills, and the prescriber's signature. Verbal orders should be accepted only in emergency situations. As soon as the emergency has been resolved, verbal orders must be written and signed.

 Memory Jogger

Safe drug administration requires that the person administering the drug be knowledgeable about these drug features:
- Purpose(s)
- Actions
- Side effects
- Abnormal reactions
- Delivery methods
- Necessary follow-up care

 Memory Jogger

Be sure to review the professional practice act (e.g., nurse practice act) for your state on the state board website.

 Critical Point for Safety

Remember to use the eight "rights" every time you prepare and administer drugs.

QSEN: Safety

 Critical Point for Safety

Be sure to always check two unique identifiers (e.g., name and birth date) to ensure that you are giving the right drug to the right patient.

QSEN: Safety

Memory Jogger

Minimum information required by the US government for a written prescription:
- Date
- Patient's name
- Name and address of the prescriber
- Generic or brand name of the drug
- Strength of the drug
- Number of times per day that the drug is to be taken
- Any specific instructions for use
- Number of doses to be dispensed
- Number of refills allowed
- Prescriber's signature

Critical Point for Safety

Never document a drug dose until after it is given!

QSEN: Safety

Contact the prescriber whenever a drug order seems unclear or if a drug dosage is higher or lower than expected. For safety, when you contact the prescriber by telephone or follow a verbal order, be sure to write the order, read it back, and ask for confirmation that what you wrote is correct before administering any drug. Be sure to document that you read back the order to the prescriber.

The Right Documentation

After giving a drug, immediately record that it has been administered. This is essential for all drugs, but it is especially important for drugs given on an as-needed (PRN) basis. Many pain-relieving drugs are prescribed to be given as needed. These drugs often require 20 to 30 minutes to take effect. If you fail to document giving one of these drugs, a patient may request and receive a second dose from another nurse. When a patient is receiving a narcotic (opioid) pain drug, a second dose can cause complications such as a decreased respiratory rate. Documenting that a drug has been given may prevent the mistake of repeating the dose as well as possible complications.

The Right Diagnosis

Before giving a drug, check the patient's medical diagnosis, which should match the purpose of the drug. If the diagnosis does not match the drug's purpose, question the prescription.

Also check any related laboratory tests before giving a drug. For example, if a patient's diagnosis is digoxin toxicity, be sure to check the serum digoxin level before giving this drug. If the drug you are giving may cause adverse effects on a major body organ, be sure to check laboratory values related to that organ. For example, before giving an aminoglycoside drug such as gentamicin, you must check kidney function test results such as creatinine and blood urea nitrogen.

Check the patient's vital signs before giving drugs that affect blood pressure, heart rate, or respiratory rate. If the patient's vital signs are outside of the normal limits, hold the drug and notify the prescriber. Often prescribers include ranges for when to give or hold one of these drugs when writing the prescription. For example, a beta (β)-blocker given to slow down the heart rate may be held for a heart rate less than 50 bpm. Be sure to check the patient's vital signs again after giving these drugs.

The Right Response

After giving any drug, check the patient to make sure that the drug has the desired effect. For example, check the blood pressure for improvement after giving an antihypertensive drug within 30 minutes to an hour. Be sure to document what you monitored and any other appropriate interventions.

The Right to Refuse

An additional right cited by some sources when giving drugs is the patient's right to refuse any drug. When this occurs, be sure that the patient understands why the drug has been prescribed and the consequences of refusing to take it. If a patient refuses to take a drug, document the refusal, including the fact that the patient understands what may happen if the drug is not taken. When a drug is essential to the patient's plan of care, it is also important to notify the prescriber.

TYPES AND INTERPRETATION OF DRUG ORDERS

Reading and Interpreting Drug Labels

Reading and interpreting drug labels for prescription or over-the-counter drugs are important to ensure that medications are used correctly. Learning this skill and teaching patients how to care for and use medications are essential.

Drug labels provide important information (Fig. 2.1) including:
- Trade (brand) name
- Generic name

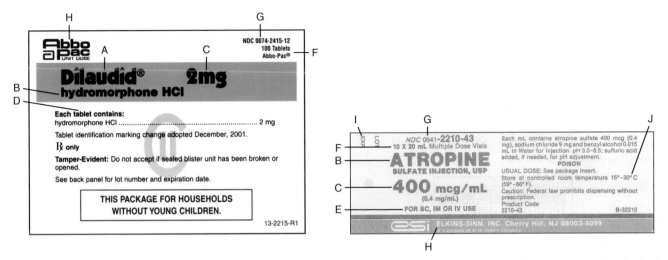

FIG. 2.1 Drug labels. *A*, Trade name; *B*, generic name; *C*, drug strength; *D*, drug form; *E*, route of administration; *F*, total amount of medication in container; *G*, national drug code; *H*, manufacturer's name; *I*, expiration date; *J*, storage temperature. (From Fulcher, E. M., Fulcher, R. M., & Soto, C. D. [2012]. *Pharmacology: Principles and applications* [3rd ed.]. St. Louis: Saunders.)

- Drug strength (e.g., milligrams, micrograms, milliequivalents)
- Drug form (e.g., tablet, capsule, powder, solution, cream, suppository)
- Route of administration (e.g., subcutaneous, intramuscular [IM], intravenous [IV])
- Total amount of medication in the container (e.g., number of tablets)
- Directions for reconstitution (if needed before administration)
- National drug code (number assigned to identify the manufacturer, product, and size of container)
- Manufacturer's name
- Expiration date
- Controlled drug symbol (warning that drug may be habit forming) if needed

Drug labels may also include abbreviations that indicate modifications of drug forms such as SR (slow release), CR (controlled release), LA or XL (long acting), DS (double strength), TR (time released), and XR or ER (extended release).

Types of Drug Orders

A drug order from a qualified prescriber is necessary before you administer any drug to a patient. Drug orders may be written by different types of health care providers, including physicians, dentists, some advanced practice nurses, and physician assistants. Common types of drug orders include standing (routine) orders, PRN orders, single-dose orders, and immediate (STAT) orders.

When a patient is to receive a drug on a regular basis, a **standing (routine) order** is written. These drugs are prescribed for a specific number of days or until discontinued by the prescriber. Certain drugs such as narcotics (opioids) can be prescribed as standing orders only for a certain number of days. If the patient is to continue taking the drug after that number of days, the prescription must be renewed.

When a patient is to receive a drug once only, a **single-dose order** is written by the prescriber. A **PRN drug order** is given to the patient as needed. Prescribers usually designate a time interval between doses of these drugs. **STAT orders** are given one time immediately.

DRUG ERRORS

A **drug error** is a preventable event that leads to inappropriate drug use or patient harm. An error can occur while the drug is in the control of health care professionals (e.g., in the hospital, pharmacy, or prescriber's office) or the patient. There are eight categories of drug errors.

 Memory Jogger

There are four common types of drug orders: standing (routine), single-dose, as needed (PRN), and immediate (STAT).

 Memory Jogger

Eight categories of drug errors include:
- Omission
- Wrong patient
- Wrong dose
- Wrong route
- Wrong rate
- Wrong dosage form
- Wrong time
- Error in preparation of dose

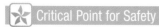

Drug errors are one of the five most common medical errors and are a leading cause of death and injury. Medication errors cause at least one death every day and injure as many as 1.3 million people annually in the United States. Errors can occur when the prescriber writes the drug order, when the pharmacist dispenses the drug, when the nurse administers the drug, or when a patient takes a drug at home. *Because nurses give most drugs to patients in care facilities, they are the final defense for detecting and preventing drug errors.*

PREVENTING DRUG ERRORS

Medication Reconciliation

The five-step process of **medication reconciliation** has been developed to prevent drug errors. Medication reconciliation is the process of identifying the most accurate list of all medications that a patient is taking, including name, dosage, frequency, and route, by comparing the medical record to an external list of medications obtained from a patient, hospital, or other health care provider. When a patient visits a primary care provider, is admitted to the hospital, or is transferred from unit to unit in the hospital, it is common to receive new prescriptions or to have changes made in currently prescribed drugs. The process of medication reconciliation is used during these transitions of patient care to avoid drug errors such as omissions, duplications, dosing errors, and drug interactions.

The medication reconciliation process consists of five steps:
1. Develop a list of current medications
2. Develop a list of medications being prescribed
3. Compare the medications on the two lists
4. Make clinical decisions based on the comparison
5. Communicate the new list to appropriate caregivers and the patient

Always follow the eight "rights" when administering drugs. Many drug errors occur because one or more of the "rights" are not followed. If a drug prescription does not make sense, contact the prescriber to ensure that the order is correct. Always check drug dosage calculations with another nurse. Listen to the patient's questions about a drug or a drug dose. Administer drugs only after the patient's questions have been researched and answered appropriately. While giving drugs, concentrate and focus on the task at hand. Often drug errors result from distractions or interruptions.

Bar-Code Systems

Computerized charting is used by most health care facilities and care providers. Computers are located in physician's offices, patient rooms, and nursing stations for ease in documentation of patient care. Facility computer systems are integrated to include the various departments (e.g., pharmacy, radiology, dietary) and patient care units. Most hospitals now use bar-code systems, with bar codes added to each patient's identification wristband on admission. **Unit-dose drugs** (drugs dispensed to fill a patient's drug orders for a 24-hour period) and IV fluids are all bar coded. A bar-code scanner is used to ensure that each patient receives the right drug doses at the right time. Take the scanner to each patient's bedside to scan the identification band and the drugs that are given (Fig. 2.2). Scanning automatically documents the drugs that have been given into the facility's computer system. Standing order, one-time, PRN, and STAT drugs are scanned. The bar-code system instantly tells the nurse when the scanned drug is incorrect. Research shows that bar-code systems dramatically decrease the number of drug errors.

Confusing Drug Name Lists

Confused drug names can be found in lists of drug names that have involved in drug errors and are published by organizations such as the Institute for Safe Medication Practices (ISMP). A partial list is provided in Box 2.1. As you read through this text, be sure to check the "Do Not Confuse" boxes for additional hints on how to avoid confusing drug names.

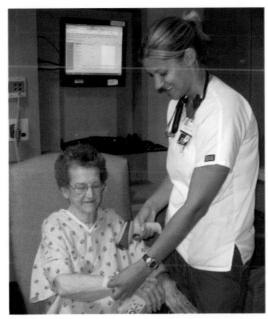

FIG. 2.2 Checking a patient's wristband with a bar-code scanner. (From Perry, A., Potter, P., Osterdorf, W., & Laplante, N. [Eds.]. [2022]. *Clinical nursing skills & techniques* [10th ed.]. St. Louis: Elsevier.)

Box **2.1**	Examples of Easily Confused Drug Names

FOSAMAX (alendronate) for osteoporosis
FLOMAX (tamsulosin) for enlarged prostate
LAMICTAL (lamotrigine) for epilepsy
LAMISIL (terbinafine) for fingernail fungus
OXYCONTIN (oxycodone) for pain
Ditropan (**OXYBUTYNIN**) for urinary incontinence

SINGULAIR (montelukast) for asthma
SINEQUAN (doxepin) for depression and anxiety
XANAX (alprazolam) for anxiety
ZANTAC (ranitidine) for heartburn and ulcers

Reporting Drug Errors

Immediately report any drug errors! After a drug error, carefully watch the patient for any signs of an adverse reaction. Drug errors may result in life-threatening complications such as coma or death. Most patient care facilities have a form and standard procedures that are used to report drug errors. The patient's prescriber must also be notified.

PRINCIPLES OF ADMINISTERING DRUGS

Essential knowledge before giving any drug includes its uses, actions, common adverse reactions, and any special precautions. You will probably become familiar with the drugs given most often in your institution or on your specialized unit. However, many drugs are not given on a daily basis, and new drugs are constantly being developed. Before giving a drug that you are not familiar with, seek out information from dependable sources such as pharmacists, drug inserts, and manufacturers' websites. In addition, *be sure to know the patient's drug history, allergies, previous adverse reactions, pertinent laboratory values, and any important changes in his or her condition before administering a drug.*

Often prescribers put limitations on when a drug should be given. For example, the prescriber may order that the drug be given only if the patient's blood pressure is greater than or less than a particular value. Similar limitations may be based on heart rate, respiratory rate, or pain level. Be aware of the prescribed limitations, and check them before giving the drug. If the patient's condition or vital signs are outside of the set limits, you must hold the drug, document the reason for your action, and in some cases notify the prescriber.

 Critical Point for Safety

Always report drug errors *immediately* so appropriate actions can be taken to counteract possible adverse reactions to the drug.

QSEN: Safety

 Critical Point for Safety

Know the patient's drug history, allergies, previous adverse reactions, pertinent laboratory values, and any important changes in his or her condition before administering any drug.

QSEN: Safety

Always listen to your patient when giving drugs. Patient comments give clues to adverse reactions such as nausea, dizziness, unsteady walking, and ringing in the ears. These comments indicate that the patient may be having an adverse reaction, and you need to hold the drug while you notify the prescriber. In addition, a patient may tell you that they never have taken two of these tablets before, which is a "red flag" that there may be a dosage error.

GETTING READY TO GIVE DRUGS

Important guidelines to follow before preparing to give any drug include:
- Always follow the eight "rights."
- Always check the written order.
- Check the patient's identification wristband, and ask the patient's name and birthdate.
- Limit interruptions and distractions (Focus on what you are doing!).
- Wash your hands, and wear clean gloves when needed (e.g., parenteral, rectal routes).
- Keep drugs in their containers or wrappers until at the patient's bedside.
- Avoid touching pills or capsules.
- Never give drugs prepared by someone else.
- Follow sterile technique when handling syringes and needles.
- Remain alert to drug names that sound or look alike. Giving the wrong drug can have serious adverse effects.

When pills and capsules are prepared for slow absorption, follow special precautions. These drugs are often labeled enteric coated, time release, or slow release. If chewed, crushed, or opened, these drugs may be absorbed too rapidly. This can irritate the gastrointestinal (GI) system or cause symptoms of overdose. If a patient cannot take pills or capsules, a liquid form of the drug may be a better option. A prescriber's order is needed to change the drug form.

Giving drugs to children can be challenging and difficult. Tips that may help you give drugs to children are listed in Box 2.2.

GIVING ENTERAL DRUGS

When a drug is delivered from the outside of the body to the inside of the body using the GI tract, it is given by the **enteral route**. Enteral drugs enter the body in one of three ways: through the mouth (oral), by feeding tube (e.g., nasogastric [NG] tube or percutaneous endoscopic gastrostomy [PEG]), or through the rectum.

Oral Drugs Given by Mouth

The oral route, when a drug is given by mouth, is the most common enteral route. Prescriptions for oral drugs are sometimes written as the abbreviation "PO," which means *per os* or "by mouth." Most drugs are available in one or more oral forms (e.g., tablets, capsules, and liquids). Oral drugs are easy to give as long as a patient can swallow. A major advantage of PO drugs is that if a patient receives too much, the drug can be removed by pumping the stomach or causing the patient to vomit. Oral drugs do not work well for patients suffering from nausea and vomiting. Onset of action for these drugs is slow because they must be absorbed through the GI tract.

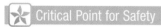

⭐ *Priority actions to take* before *giving oral drugs.* Assess the patient to be sure that he or she can swallow. Position the patient upright, and have a full glass of water ready. Tell him or her what drugs you will be giving, and answer any questions asked. Tell the patient if there are any special instructions related to the drugs (e.g., getting up slowly from bed after new antihypertensive drugs are given). Ask him or her to place the tablets or capsules in the back of the mouth, take a few sips of water, and swallow the drugs. Unless the patient is on a fluid restriction, have him or her drink the entire glass of water because oral drugs dissolve better and cause less GI discomfort when they are given with enough water. Stay at the bedside until the drugs are swallowed. Do **not** leave drugs at the patient's bedside to be taken later.

| Box **2.2** | **Tips for Administering Drugs to Children** |

DOS

- Keep drugs in their original containers and never in dishes, cups, bottles, or other household containers.
- When dosage calculations are needed, have another nurse, prescriber, or pharmacist also perform the calculation to ensure accuracy.
- Check with a drug guide for information on dosage by milligrams per kilogram, and ensure that the calculated dosage is within the guidelines.
- Question any order in which the prescribed dosage does not match the recommended dosage for body weight or size.
- Use appropriate measuring devices (see Fig. 2.3) to ensure accurate doses of liquid drugs.
- Work with the pharmacist to ensure that a liquid oral drug or a crushed oral tablet is mixed with a small amount of pleasant, delicious-tasting liquid.
- Keep all drugs out of reach of children.
- Before crushing a tablet, check with the pharmacist or drug resource book to determine whether it should be crushed.
- Apply transdermal patch drugs to a child's back between the shoulder blades.
- Use two identifiers, including the child's name band, to identify him or her before administering any drug (this can include asking a parent the child's full name and date of birth).
- Position children in a sitting or semisitting position when administering an oral drug (to avoid aspiration or choking).
- Help a child rinse his or her mouth after taking an oral liquid drug.
- Watch an infant or child closely (at least every 15 min) for the first 2 h after giving the first dose of a newly prescribed drug for expected and unexpected or unusual responses to the drug.
- Offer creative choices for the child who is old enough to understand, such as:
  - Which drug to take first if more than one drug will be administered at the same time
  - Which type of drink the child would like as a follow-up after a drug is administered
  - Which leg or arm (when appropriate) the child would prefer be used for an injection
  - Which toy to hold during an injection
- When an infant or child is prescribed to take a drug at home, demonstrate to the parents exactly how to measure and give the drug. Have the parents demonstrate these acts back to you.
- Obtain the assistance of another adult when administering a parenteral drug, drops or ointment to the eye, or drops to the ear of an infant or child.
- Select the smallest gauge and shortest needle that will safely deliver the injection.
- If possible, change needles after pulling the drug from the vial into the syringe before injecting it into the child (prevents any irritating drug residue from contacting the child's tissues).
- Follow agency policy for site selection of injectable drugs for a child.
- Use diversion during an injection.
- Try to avoid having the child see the needle or the actual injection.

DON'TS

- Don't refer to drugs as "candy."
- Don't place liquid drugs in a large bottle of formula (unless the child drinks the entire amount, he or she will not receive the correct dose).
- Don't place crushed drugs into the child's *favorite* food or snack (he or she may never eat that food again).
- Don't threaten a child with an injection in place of an oral drug.
- Don't lie to a child.

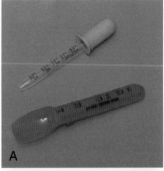

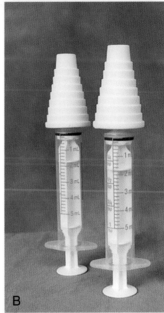

FIG. 2.3 Calibrated devices for delivery of liquid oral drugs. (A) Calibrated dropper and calibrated spoon. (B) Calibrated oral syringes. (A, From Hockenberry, M. J., & Wilson, D. [2006]. *Wong's nursing care of infants and children* [8th ed.]. St. Louis: Mosby. B, Courtesy Paul Vincent Kuntz, Texas Children's Hospital, Houston.)

An exception may be made for antacids or nitroglycerin tablets *if* there is an order permitting this. You are responsible for documenting when drugs have been taken and must witness that this has occurred.

When an oral drug is in suspension form, be sure to shake it well. When giving oral liquid drugs, be sure to use a calibrated device to measure the correct dose (Fig. 2.3) because household devices such as spoons or cups vary widely in size and their use

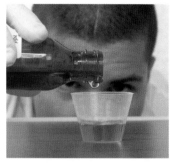

FIG. 2.4 Checking the drug dose in a medicine cup. (From Perry, A. G., & Potter, P. [2009]. *Clinical nursing skills and techniques* [7th ed.]. St. Louis: Mosby.)

 Critical Point for Safety

Do *not* give a drug by nasogastric tube if CO_2 is present when the tube is tested with an end-tidal CO_2 detector.

QSEN: Safety

 Critical Point for Safety

Always check for correct placement of a feeding tube before giving drugs by this route to ensure that the drugs do not go into the lungs.

QSEN: Safety

 Memory Jogger

Vasovagal reactions are a common cause of fainting from a decrease in heart rate and blood pressure. This reaction can be stimulated during rectal manipulation, such as when a suppository is inserted.

can result in giving inaccurate doses. Always hold a calibrated medicine cup at eye level to measure the dose (Fig. 2.4).

⭐ *Priority actions to take* after *giving oral drugs.* Be sure to document that the drug was given. If a drug was refused or not given, document the reason (e.g., abnormal blood pressure or heart rate, patient refusal). Be sure to check the patient later for side effects, adverse effects, and the desired effect. For example, check the patient taking antihypertensive drugs for decreased blood pressure or change in heart rate. Document your findings.

Oral Drugs Given by Feeding Tube

Oral drugs may be given by feeding tubes. When a patient is unable to swallow, oral drugs may be given by a temporary or long-term feeding tube (e.g., NG tube, PEG tube). An NG tube delivers drugs by a tube inserted through the nostrils to the stomach. A PEG tube is a feeding tube that is surgically implanted through the abdomen into the stomach.

⭐ *Priority actions to take* before *giving drugs by NG or PEG tube.* As with all drugs, check the drug orders, which may be written as PO or by feeding tube. Check a valid drug reference or check with the pharmacist before crushing tablets or opening capsules. Wash your hands, and place the patient upright. Check to make sure that the tube is located in the stomach by withdrawing *(aspirating)* stomach contents with a syringe, or you can attach an end-tidal carbon dioxide (CO_2) detector to the feeding tube. The presence of carbon dioxide indicates that the tube is in the trachea rather than the stomach, and the drugs must not be given.

If the patient is receiving a tube feeding, check the amount of tube feeding remaining in the stomach *(residual)*. Some drugs are not well absorbed when food is in the stomach (e.g., phenytoin [Dilantin]), and the tube feeding must be stopped for a period before and after drug administration. Liquid drugs are first diluted and then flushed through the tube. Crushed tablets and the contents of opened capsules are first dissolved in water before being given through the tube. To give the drugs, attach a large syringe to the tube, pour the liquid or dissolved drug into the syringe, and let it run in by gravity.

⭐ *Priority actions to take* after *giving drugs by NG or PEG tube.* After giving drugs by feeding tube, flush the tube well to make sure it is clear. Use at least 50 mL of water to prevent the tube from becoming clogged. If the patient's NG tube is connected to suction, the tube is clamped for at least 30 minutes after administering drugs before reattaching it to suction. This allows time for the drugs to be absorbed from the GI system. As with any drug, document what has been given and watch the patient for side effects, adverse effects, and the desired effects. Document your findings.

Rectal Drugs

When a patient is unable to swallow or has severe nausea and vomiting, drugs may need to be given by the **rectal route** (movement of a drug from outside the body to inside the body through the rectum). These drugs may come as suppositories or in the form of an enema. A **suppository** is a small drug plug designed to melt at body temperature when placed within the rectum or vagina. With drugs given by this route, absorption is not as dependable or predictable as when drugs are given orally. The patient with diarrhea cannot hold a suppository long enough for absorption to take place. The rate of absorption is also affected by the amount of stool present.

⭐ *Priority actions to take* before *giving rectal drugs.* Assess if the patient has any health problems (e.g., diarrhea) that may make using this route undesirable. Other reasons for not giving a rectal drug include recent rectal surgery or trauma and a history of *vasovagal reactions* (slowed heart rate and dilation of blood vessels, which can lead to fainting, sometimes called *syncope*).

Bring the drug, some lubricant, and a pair of disposable gloves to the bedside. Assist the patient to turn to the side with one leg bent over the other (modified left lateral recumbent position) (Fig. 2.5). The modified left lateral recumbent position is best for giving rectal suppositories.

Protect the patient's privacy by closing doors or drapes and keeping as much of the patient covered as possible. Explain what you will be doing, and be sure to include any special instructions such as how long the drug must be held inside the rectum. Put on your gloves. Take the wrapper off the suppository, and coat the pointed end with a small amount of water-soluble lubricant. Also apply a small amount of lubricant to the finger that you will be using to insert the drug. Hold the suppository next to the anal sphincter, and explain that you are ready to insert the drug. Ask the patient to take a deep breath, and bear down a little. With the pointed end first, push the suppository into the rectum about 1 inch (Fig. 2.6).

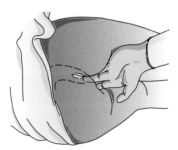

FIG. 2.5 Modified left lateral recumbent position. For this position, the patient lies on one side with the knee and thigh drawn upward toward the chest.

⊛ ***Priority actions to take** after **giving rectal drugs.*** Remind the patient to remain on his or her side for about 20 minutes. Clean the patient's anal area, and cover the patient. Remove gloves, and wash your hands. Immediately document that the drug was given. Check the patient for any expected or unexpected responses, and chart these. For example, if the patient was given a suppository to relieve constipation, be sure to note whether the patient later had a bowel movement.

GIVING PARENTERAL DRUGS

Giving drugs by injection through the skin is called the **parenteral route.** Drugs may be injected intradermally, subcutaneously, intramuscularly, or intravenously. The four primary reasons for giving drugs parenterally include:

- Patient is unable to take oral drugs.
- Patient needs a drug to act rapidly.
- Patient needs a constant blood level of a drug.
- Patient needs drugs such as insulin or heparin, which are not made in an oral form.

Standard precautions from the Centers for Disease Control and Prevention (CDC) recommend wearing gloves whenever you are exposed to blood or other body fluids, mucous membranes, or any area of broken skin.

Safe use of needles and syringes is essential when giving parenteral drugs. Do **not** recap needles, and always dispose of needles and syringes in labeled containers. "Sharps" containers are located in every patient room. Many hospitals use needleless systems, retractable needles, or needles with plastic guards that slip over the needle to protect against needlesticks.

The Needlestick Safety and Prevention Act was signed into law in November 2000. In 2001, the Occupational Safety and Health Administration (OSHA) developed guidelines to help prevent needlesticks. OSHA advises that *prevention* of needlesticks is best and recommends that health care employers select safer needle devices. Needlestick injuries are tracked using a Sharps Injury Log. The purpose of this log is to identify problem areas. In addition, OSHA recommends that employers have a written Exposure Care Plan that is updated on an annual basis.

▶ Intradermal Drugs

When a drug is given by injection between the layers of skin, it is called the **intradermal route** or an intradermal injection. The most common site for intradermal injections is the inner part of the forearm. The primary uses of intradermal injections are for:

- Allergy testing
- Local anesthetics
- Tuberculosis (TB) testing

A TB test is done with purified protein derivative by injecting a small amount of the drug into the space between the epidermis and the dermis layers of the skin (Fig. 2.7). This results in a bump *(bleb)* that looks like an insect bite. The volume of drug injected is very small (0.01 to 0.1 mL), and the needle used is short and small ($^3/_8$ inch, 25 gauge).

FIG. 2.6 To administer a rectal suppository, push the suppository into the rectum about 1 inch.

✦ Critical Point for Safety

Always wear gloves when giving parenteral drugs to avoid exposure to blood and other body fluids.

QSEN: Safety

✦ Critical Point for Safety

To avoid needlesticks, do **not** recap needles.

QSEN: Safety

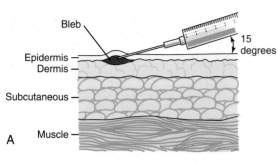

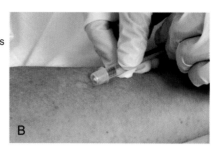

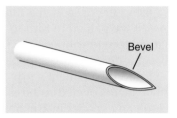

FIG. 2.8 Close-up of a needle with the bevel up.

FIG. 2.7 (A and B) Intradermal injection. (B, From Harkreader, H., Thobaben, M., & Hogan, M. A. [2007]. *Fundamentals of nursing: Caring and clinical judgment* [3rd ed.]. Philadelphia: Saunders.)

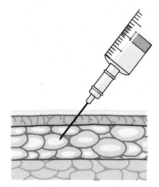

FIG. 2.9 Subcutaneous injection.

> ### Critical Point for Safety
> Use a small needle and a 5- to 15-degree angle for intradermal drugs. Do **not** aspirate before injecting the drug or massage afterward.
>
> QSEN: Safety

> ### Critical Point for Safety
> Be sure *not* to aspirate when giving subcutaneous heparin. Aspirating causes a vacuum and can lead to tissue damage and bruising when the heparin is injected.
>
> QSEN: Safety

⭐ *Priority actions to take* before *giving intradermal drugs.* Put on gloves. Cleanse the injection site in a circular motion, beginning from the center and moving outward. Insert the needle at a 5- to 15-degree angle with the bevel facing up (Fig. 2.8). Do not pull back (aspirate) on the plunger of the syringe. Inject the drug so a little bump forms, and remove the needle. *Do not massage the area.* If the little bump does not form, the drug has probably been injected too deeply into the subcutaneous tissue, and test results will not be accurate. When this happens, discard the used equipment and chose a different site with a new sterile needle and syringe for the intradermal injection

⭐ *Priority actions to take* after *giving intradermal drugs.* Do not massage the area after injecting the drug. Massaging can disperse the drug too widely and prevent an accurate tissue response. Document the drug administration immediately after the injection. Check the patient for allergic or sensitivity reactions to the injection. These reactions may take several hours to days. Making a circle around the injection site with a pen may help to accurately check the site. Document any reactions and notify the prescriber. TB tests must be checked and read 2 to 3 days (48 to 72 hours) after the injection.

Subcutaneous Drugs

A subcutaneous drug is given by the subcutaneous route and is injected into tissues between the skin and muscle (Fig. 2.9). Although several drugs are given by this route, two drugs commonly given subcutaneously are insulin and heparin. Subcutaneous drugs are absorbed more slowly than intramuscular drugs. Usually, these injections are from 0.5 to 1 mL. If a larger volume of drug is ordered, give the injection in two different sites with different syringes and needles. Small, short needles are used (³/₈ inch, 25 to 27 gauge). Sites for subcutaneous injections include the upper arms, the abdomen, and the upper back. Some sources also recommend use of the anterolateral thigh. Rotate the sites for the injections to avoid damage to the patient's tissues.

⭐ *Priority actions to take* before *giving subcutaneous drugs.* Check the MAR order. Put on clean gloves. Select and cleanse the site. Insert the needle at a 45-degree angle for most patients. If the patient is obese, you may need to use a 90-degree angle. If the patient is thin, you may need an angle that is less than 45 degrees. Before giving any subcutaneous injection, do *not* aspirate (pull back on the plunger of the syringe). Inject the drug, and remove the needle.

⭐ *Priority actions to take* after *giving subcutaneous drugs.* Apply pressure to prevent bleeding, but do not massage the site. If a patient has a bleeding disorder or is receiving anticoagulation therapy, you may need to apply pressure longer until the bleeding has stopped. Document giving the drug immediately, including the site used for injection. Check the patient for side effects, adverse effects, and expected effects. Document your findings. If the patient will be self-injecting to give a subcutaneous drug, use the steps in Box 2.3 to teach him or her how to perform self-injection.

Box **2.3**	Steps for Teaching a Patient to Self-Inject a Subcutaneous Drug

- Explain about the parts of the injection syringe:
  - There are three parts to a syringe: the needle, barrel, and plunger. The needle goes into your skin. The barrel holds the medicine and has markings on it like a ruler. The markings are for milliliters (mL). The plunger is used to get medicine into and out of the syringe.

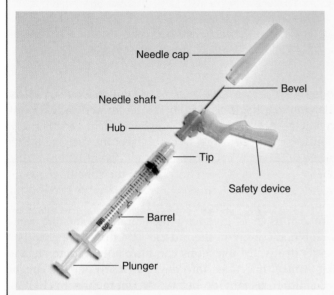

(From Lilley, L. L., Collins, S. R., & Snyder, J. S. [2023]. *Pharmacology and the nursing process* [10th ed.]. St. Louis: Elsevier.)

- Wash your hands before preparing to give your injection.
- Inspect the medication container, and check the expiration date. Do **not** use if expired.
- Clean the bottle stopper with an alcohol sponge (leave out this step if you are using a prefilled pen or cartridge).
- Remove the cover from the needle, and pull back the plunger to draw in the same amount of air into the syringe as the amount of medication you will be withdrawing from the bottle.
- Push the needle through the rubber stopper, and inject the air into the medication bottle with the bottle in the upright position.
- With the needle still in the bottle stopper, turn the bottle upside down and withdraw the same amount of medication from the bottle as the air you put into the bottle.
- Make sure that the tip of the plunger is on the line of the syringe for your medication dose.
- If air bubbles are present, tap the syringe while holding it upside down, letting the bubbles come to the top of the syringe where the needle is attached. Push out any air bubbles, and recheck to ensure that the tip of the plunger is on the same line as your medication dose.
- Remove the needle from the bottle stopper, and recap the needle until you are ready to inject the insulin.
- Select and inspect the site for your subcutaneous injection:
  - **Abdomen:** Uncover your abdomen. You may give an injection within the following area: below the waist to just above the hip bone and from the side to about

2 inches from the umbilicus (belly button). Avoid the belly button.
  - **Thigh:** Uncover the entire leg. Find the area halfway between the knee and hip and slightly to the side. Gently grasp the area to make sure you can pinch 1–2 inches of skin.
- **Keep track of where the injections are given:** Make a list of the sites you can use. Write down the date, time, and the site each time you give an injection.
- **Change sites for the injections:** It is important to use a different site each time you give an injection. This prevents scars and skin changes. The sites where injections are given should be at least 1 inch away from each other. Ask your health care provider if you need to inject the medicine in a certain site.
- Tell the patient what equipment is needed to give a subcutaneous injection:
  - One alcohol wipe
  - One sterile 2 × 2 gauze pad
  - A new needle and syringe that are the correct size
  - Disposable gloves, if you have them
- Instruct the patient on steps to give a subcutaneous injection:
  - **Open the alcohol wipe:** Wipe the area where you plan to give the injection. Let the area dry. Do not touch this area until you give the injection.
  - **Prepare the needle:** Hold the syringe with your writing hand, and pull the cover off with your other hand. Place the syringe between your thumb and first finger. Let the barrel of the syringe rest on your second finger.
  - **Grasp the skin:** With your other hand, grasp the skin.
  - Pinch up a fold of skin in the area you cleaned.
  - **Insert the needle into the skin at a 90-degree angle:** Hold the syringe barrel tightly and use your wrist to inject the needle into the skin. Once the needle is all the way in, push the plunger down to inject the medicine.

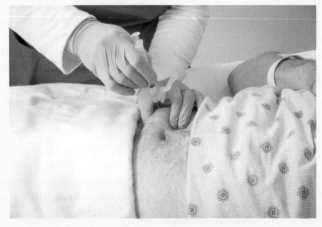

(From Lilley, L. L., Collins, S. R., & Snyder, J. S. [2023]. *Pharmacology and the nursing process* [10th ed.]. St. Louis: Elsevier.)

- **Do not** aspirate for some injections such as insulin and heparin, because it can cause tissue damage. **Do** aspirate with other injection such as direct-acting monoclonal antibodies to ensure the solution will not be injected into a blood vessel.

Continued

Box 2.3   Steps for Teaching a Patient to Self-Inject a Subcutaneous Drug—cont'd

- **Pull out the needle:** Remove the needle at the same angle you put it in. Gently wipe the area with the gauze pad.
- Tell the patient how to dispose of the needle and syringe:
  - It is important to dispose of the needles and syringes correctly. Do not throw needles into the trash. You may receive a hard plastic container made especially for used syringes and needles. You can also use a soda bottle or other plastic bottle with a screw lid. Make sure that both the syringe and needle fit into the container easily and cannot break through the sides. Ask your health care provider or a pharmacist what your state or local requirements are for getting rid of used syringes and needles.
- Discuss risks of subcutaneous injections:
  - You may get an infection, have the needle break in your skin, or hit a nerve. You may have scarring, lumps, or dimpling of the skin from a subcutaneous injection.

- Explain when to contact the health care provider after giving a subcutaneous injection:
  - A fever, sneezing, or coughing develops after the injection is given.
  - There is a lump, swelling, or bruising where the injection was given that does not go away.
  - You have questions about how to give an injection.
- Explain when to seek immediate care:
  - A rash or itching develops after the injection is given.
  - Shortness of breath develops after the injection is given.
  - The mouth, lips, or face swells after the injection is given.

⭐ **Critical Point for Safety**

IM injections of more than 3 mL are rare. To ensure that the drug dose is correct, carefully calculate and check it with another nurse.

QSEN: Safety

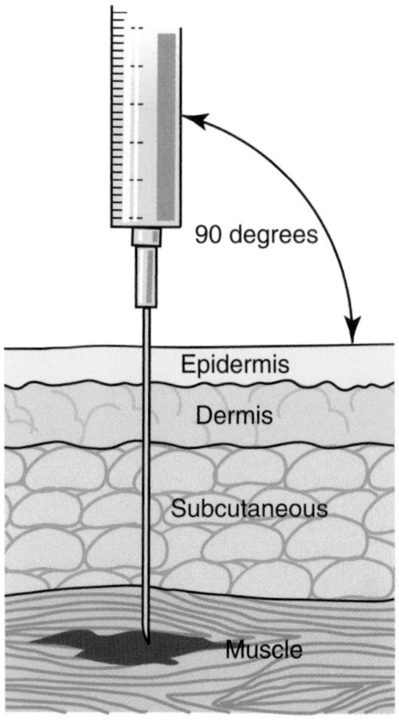

FIG. 2.10 Intramuscular injection.

(labels: 90 degrees, Epidermis, Dermis, Subcutaneous, Muscle)

Intramuscular Drugs

A drug injected deeper into a muscle is given by the **intramuscular (IM) route** (Fig. 2.10). Because of the rich blood supply in the muscles, IM drugs are absorbed much faster than subcutaneous drugs. IM injections can also be much larger than subcutaneous injections (1 to 3 mL). Injections into an adult's arm should not be more than 2 mL. Infants and children usually do not receive more than 1 mL. If an injection order is for more than 3 mL, divide the dose and give two injections. Injections of more than 3 mL are not as well absorbed.

Needles for these injections are longer (1 to 1.5 inches) and larger (20 to 22 gauge). Sites for IM injections include the upper arm deltoid muscle, the thigh vastus lateralis muscles, and the ventrogluteal muscle in the hip (Figs. 2.11 through 2.13). The dorsogluteal site is *not* favored because of the presence of nerves and major blood vessels. This site is avoided in obese patients because research has shown that injections do not reach the muscle. Be sure to rotate injection sites when multiple IM injections are prescribed. Table 2.1 describes the advantages and disadvantages of IM injection sites.

⭐ *Priority actions to take* **before** *giving intramuscular drugs.* Help the patient into a comfortable position that is appropriate for the site you plan to use. Select the injection site by identifying the correct anatomic landmarks. Wash your hands, and be sure to wear clean gloves. Cleanse the injection site. Using a 90-degree angle, insert the needle firmly into the muscle. *Aspiration is not recommended for IM injection of vaccines or immunizations.* For drugs such as penicillin, aspiration may be indicated. When indicated, aspirate the syringe (pull back on the plunger) to make sure that the needle is not in a vein. If the needle is in a vein, blood will appear in the syringe. Remove the needle, and discard the drug if this happens. Get a new dose of the drug and a sterile needle and syringe, and give the injection in another site. Once you have determined that the needle is not in a blood vessel, inject the drug at a rate of 1 mL per 10 seconds and remove the needle.

The Z-track method of IM injection is used for drugs that are irritating to subcutaneous tissue or that may permanently stain the tissues (Fig. 2.14). After drawing the drug into the syringe, draw in 0.1 to 0.2 mL of air. The air follows the drug into the muscle and stops it from oozing through the path of the needle. Wash your hands, and put on clean gloves. After you select and cleanse the site, pull the tissue laterally and hold it. Insert the needle into the muscle; inject the drug and release the tissue as you remove the needle. Releasing the tissue allows the skin to slide over the injection and seal the drug in the muscle.

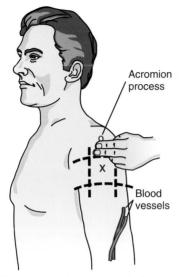

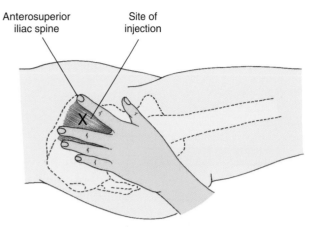

FIG. 2.12 Ventrogluteal intramuscular injection site landmarks. (From Potter, P. A., & Perry, A. G. [2013]. *Fundamentals of nursing: Concepts, process, and practice* [8th ed.]. St. Louis: Mosby.)

FIG. 2.11 Deltoid (arm) intramuscular injection site landmarks.

Table **2.1**	Intramuscular Injection Site Advantages and Disadvantages	
Injection Site	**Advantages**	**Disadvantages**
Deltoid (upper arm)	Easily accessible Useful for vaccinations in adolescents and adults	Poorly developed in young children Only small amounts (0.5–1 mL) can be injected
Vastus lateralis (thigh)	Preferred site for infant injections Relatively free of large blood vessels and nerves Easily accessible	Intake or medication is slower than the arm but faster than buttocks
Ventrogluteal (hips)	Used for children age 7 or older and adults Less likely to be inadvertently injected subcutaneously	Patient anxiety due to unfamiliarity with site and visibility of site during injection

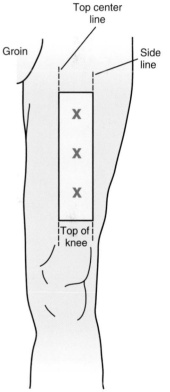

FIG. 2.13 Vastus lateralis (thigh) intramuscular injection site landmarks.

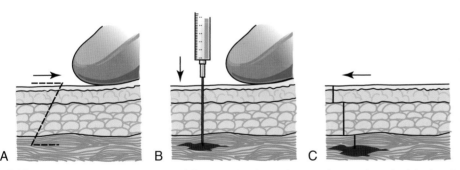

FIG. 2.14 Z-track intramuscular injection. (A) Displace the tissue downward, away from the injection site. (B) Inject while holding the tissue away. (C) Allow the displaced tissue to move back into place.

⭐ *Priority actions to take* after *giving intramuscular drugs.* Apply pressure after removing the needle, to prevent bleeding. When documenting the drug administration, be sure to include the injection site. Check the patient for adverse effects, side effects, and expected effects of the drug. Document your findings.

Intravenous Drugs

When a drug needs to enter the bloodstream rapidly or a large dose of a drug must be given, the intravenous **(IV) route** is used to inject the drug directly into a vein (Fig. 2.15).

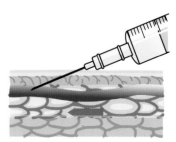

FIG. 2.15 Intravenous injection.

The rates of absorption and action are very rapid with this route. Emergency drugs may be given by a needle and syringe directly into a vein; however, most IV drugs are given slowly through a needle or an IV catheter that has been inserted into a vein. The needle or catheter is attached to IV tubing with an injection port. IV drugs may be pushed slowly over 1 or more minutes, pushed rapidly over a few seconds, or given slowly by IV piggyback. They may be given through an IV line or a saline lock.

⭐ *Priority actions to take* **before** *giving intravenous drugs.* Wash your hands, and put on clean gloves. Check the IV site to make sure that it is patent. Assess and document the condition of the IV site. When a drug is to be given IV push, draw up the dose into an appropriate syringe, gently tap the syringe to remove any air by pushing the plunger, and replace the syringe cap. To give the drug through a saline lock, scrub the needleless connector, flush with saline to be sure the line is patent, attach the medication syringe, unclamp the line and inject the drug as directed, remove the syringe, and flush the line with saline to be sure all of the medication is injected. If the drug has been added to IV fluid, be sure to remove all air from the tubing. (This is called *priming* the IV tubing.) If the drug is to be administered in a continuous IV infusion or an IV piggyback, it should be placed on an infusion pump to control the rate (see Chapter 5).

In most cases, registered nurses will give IV push and IV piggyback drugs. Be sure to check the scope of practice laws of your state. In some states, licensed practical nurses or licensed vocational nurses may administer IV drugs with additional training.

⭐ *Priority actions to take* **after** *giving intravenous drugs.* Document that the drug has been given, including the site and flow rate. Continue to check the IV site for signs of these conditions:
- Infection
- Escape of fluid from the vein into tissue (*extravasation*)
- Collection of fluid in the tissues (*infiltration*)

If fluid escapes or collects in the tissues, the IV catheter must be discontinued and replaced in a different vein. As with administration of any drug, check the patient for side effects, adverse effects, or expected effects of the drug. Document these effects. To learn more about IV fluids, see Chapter 5.

GIVING PERCUTANEOUS DRUGS

Drugs given by the **percutaneous route** are applied to and absorbed through the skin and mucous membranes. Absorption of these drugs is affected by several factors:
- Size of area covered by the drug
- Concentration or strength of the drug
- Time the drug remains in contact with the skin or mucous membranes
- Condition of the skin (e.g., breakdown, thickness, hydration, nutrition, and skin tone)

Topical and Transdermal Drugs

Drugs given by the **topical route** are applied directly to the skin for local effects. These drugs include creams, lotions, and ointments. They soften or lubricate the skin. Some are used to treat superficial infections of the skin. Topical drugs are applied in a thin, even layer over the affected area of skin.

A drug given by the **transdermal route** is applied to the skin, but it is absorbed and enters the bloodstream. The transdermal route allows the patient to maintain a steady blood level of the drug. For this reason, toxicity and adverse effects can usually be avoided. Examples of transdermal drugs are:
- Nitroglycerin to treat cardiac problems
- Scopolamine to treat dizziness and nausea
- Birth control
- Nicotine patches for smoking cessation
- Long-term pain drugs

These medications are applied as patches or ointments. Drug patches have a semi-permeable membrane and an adhesive that attaches to the skin (Fig. 2.16). Common sites of application include the chest, flank, back, and upper arms.

⭐ *Priority actions to take* **before** *giving topical or transdermal drugs.* Wash your hands, and put on clean gloves. Clean the area of skin where the drug will be applied. Apply topical drugs in a smooth, thin layer, and cover the area. When administering transdermal drugs, remove old patches or doses of the drug. Be sure to remove all traces of the drug from the previous dosage site, and rotate sites to avoid skin irritation or breakdown.

Do not shave skin before applying topical or transdermal drugs. Shaving may cause skin irritation and change the absorption of the drug. If body hair must be removed, use scissors.

⭐ *Priority actions to take* **after** *giving topical or transdermal drugs.* Document that the drug has been given, including the application site. Be sure to write the date, time, and your initials on the new patch. Check the patient for adverse effects or expected effects, and document these. For example, headache and dizziness related to decreased blood pressure are common side effects of nitroglycerin ointment.

GIVING DRUGS THROUGH THE MUCOUS MEMBRANES

Drugs may be absorbed through the mucous membranes. The following are examples of drug forms used for the different mucous membranes found in the body:
- Buccal or sublingual drugs are used in the mouth.
- Drops and ointments are applied to the eyes, nose, or ears.
- Inhalation drugs are drawn into the lungs.
- Suppositories and creams are used in the vagina.

Drugs are usually well absorbed through these areas; however, the blood supply to mucous membranes varies. When administering drugs through the mucous membranes, be sure to use sterile procedure before placing eye drops or ointments and clean procedure before giving drugs into the ears, nose, mouth, or vagina.

⭐ *Priority actions to take* **before** *giving drugs through the mucous membranes.* Always check the order and the patient's identity. Wash your hands, and put on clean gloves. Follow the eight "rights."

Buccal and sublingual drugs. Drugs given by the buccal route (e.g., lozenges) are placed between the cheek and molar teeth of the upper jaw (Fig. 2.17). When a drug such as nitroglycerin is given by the sublingual route, it is placed under the tongue (Fig. 2.18). The blood supply is very good in the mouth; therefore these drugs dissolve and are absorbed quickly. Instruct the patient to not eat or drink until the drug is completely dissolved. Teach the patient not to swallow or chew while the drug is in the mouth, because these drugs are not effective when absorbed through the GI tract.

Ear drops. Ear drops are drugs given to treat local infection or inflammation. Keep ear drops at room temperature because if they are too cold or hot, the drops can cause a patient to feel dizzy or disoriented. Help the patient to lie on one side with the affected ear up. For children younger than 3 years, pull the ear lobe (pinna) down and back. For older children and adults, pull the ear lobe up and out (Fig. 2.19). This straightens the ear canal. Do not let the ear dropper touch the ear. Have the patient stay in the same position for at least 5 minutes so the drug can coat the inner ear canal. Sometimes a cotton ball is ordered to be placed in the ear canal. Repeat this procedure for the other ear when both ears are affected.

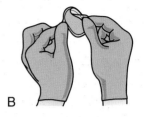

A

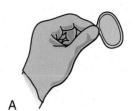

B

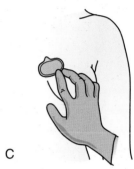

C

FIG. 2.16 Applying a transdermal patch. (A) Nitroglycerin patch. (B) Remove plastic backing carefully, taking care not to touch the medication. (C) Place the medication side of the patch on the patient's skin and press the adhesive to stay in place.

⭐ Critical Point for Safety

When giving a transdermal drug, always remove old patches and all traces of the drug to prevent excessive dosages!

QSEN: Safety

⭐ Critical Point for Safety

Teach the patient to avoid swallowing any buccal or sublingual drugs.

QSEN: Safety

⭐ Critical Point for Safety

Before giving ear drops to children younger than 3 years, pull the ear lobe down and back to straighten the ear canal. Before giving ear drops to older children and adults, pull the ear lobe up and out to straighten the ear canal.

QSEN: Safety

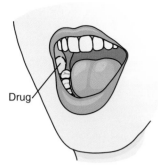

FIG. 2.17 Giving buccal drugs.

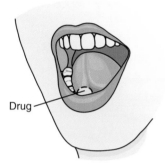

FIG. 2.18 Giving sublingual drugs.

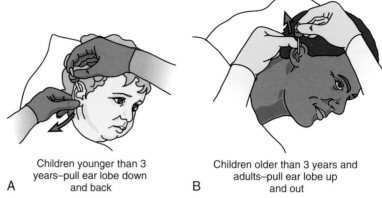

Children younger than 3 years–pull ear lobe down and back

A

Children older than 3 years and adults–pull ear lobe up and out

B

FIG. 2.19 Giving ear drops. (A) Children younger than 3 years: pull ear lobe down and back. (B) Children older than 3 years and adults: pull ear lobe up and out.

Eye drops and ointments. Administration of eye drops and ointments is discussed in detail in Chapter 27.

Nose drops. Nose drops or sprays are most often used to treat nasal congestion or infection. To give nose drops, draw the drops into a dropper. Ask the patient to gently blow his or her nose and then lie down with the head hanging over the edge of the bed. Hold the dropper over a nostril, and give the prescribed number of nose drops. Do not let the dropper touch the nose. Repeat for the second nostril if needed.

To give a nasal spray, position the patient sitting up with one nostril blocked by a finger. Place the tip of the spray in the other nostril. Ask the patient to take a deep breath. During the deep breath, squeeze a puff of spray into the nostril. Wipe the spray bottle tip if it is to be used with both nostrils. Nasal sprays are absorbed quickly from the nasal mucosa. Do not use the same spray container for any other patient.

Inhalers. Drugs may be inhaled through the respiratory tract. Different types of devices are used for delivery of inhaled drugs. Specific techniques for administering inhaled drugs are presented in Chapter 18.

Vaginal drugs. Vaginal drugs are given to treat irritation or infection. Types of vaginal drugs include creams, jellies, tablets, foams, or suppositories. These drugs should be kept at room temperature. Ask the patient to empty her bladder then lie down. Be sure to put on clean gloves after washing your hands. Suppositories are lubricated and given in the same way as rectal suppositories. Creams, jellies, tablets, and foams are given with a special applicator that is placed in the vagina as far as possible. The plunger of the applicator is pushed to give the drug. Be sure to have the patient lie down for 10 to 15 minutes after receiving these drugs.

⭐ *Priority actions to take after giving drugs through the mucous membranes.* Always document that the drugs have been given, including the route. Check the patient for any expected or unexpected actions of the drug that you have given. Document these effects.

Get Ready for the NCLEX® Examination!

Key Points

- Always follow the procedures of the eight "rights" when giving drugs (right patient, right drug, right dose, right route, right time, right documentation, right diagnosis, and right response).
- The patient has the right to refuse to take a drug.
- Be sure to always check two unique identifiers (e.g., name and birth date) to ensure that you are giving the right drug to the right patient.
- Never document a drug dose until after it is given!
- The four types of drug orders are standing (routine), single dose, PRN, and STAT.
- Most drug errors occur while giving drugs. Following the procedure of the eight "rights" helps to prevent drug errors.
- Nurses give most drugs to patients and are the final defense for detecting and preventing drug errors.
- Medication reconciliation and bar-code systems for giving drugs have led to decreases in drug errors.
- Always report a drug error immediately so actions can be taken to counteract any possible adverse drug reactions.
- Always listen to patients for clues to adverse effects when giving drugs.
- Know the patient's drug history, allergies, previous adverse reactions, pertinent laboratory values, and any important changes in his or her condition before administering any drug.
- Always check the written order and pertinent laboratory values and vital signs before giving a drug.
- Always check the patient for expected effects, side effects, and adverse effects after giving a drug.
- Never crush tablets or open capsules without first checking with a valid drug reference or pharmacist.
- Never leave drugs at the bedside for the patient to take at a later time or ask someone else to administer drugs that you have prepared.
- Check the patient's ability to swallow before giving oral drugs.
- Do *not* give a drug by NG tube if CO_2 is present when the tube is tested with an end-tidal CO_2 detector.

- Always check for correct placement of a feeding tube before giving drugs by this route to ensure that the drugs do not go into the lungs.
- Always wear gloves and use Standard Precautions to protect yourself from the risk of exposure to body fluids when giving drugs.
- To avoid needlesticks, do not recap needles.
- Use a small needle and a 5- to 15-degree angle for intradermal drugs. Do **not** aspirate before injecting the drug or massage afterward.
- Be sure *not* to aspirate when giving subcutaneous heparin. Aspirating causes a vacuum and can lead to tissue damage and bruising when the heparin is injected.
- IM injections of more than 3 mL are rare. To ensure that the drug dose is correct, carefully calculate and check it with another nurse.
- With the Z-tract IM injection, draw up 0.1 to 0.2 mL of air after drawing up the drug. Injection of air keeps the drug in the muscle, and the drug does not ooze through the path of the needle.
- Always check the IV site before administering IV drugs. If an IV line is not patent, the drug will go into the tissue instead of the vein and may cause tissue damage.
- When giving a transdermal drug, always remove old patches and all traces of the drug to prevent excessive dosages!
- Teach patients to avoid swallowing any buccal or sublingual drugs.
- Before giving ear drops to children younger than 3 years, pull the ear lobe down and back to straighten the ear canal. Before giving ear drops to older children and adults, pull the ear lobe up and out to straighten the ear canal.

Additional Learning Resources

🌐 Be sure to visit your Evolve website (http://evolve.elsevier.com/Workman/pharmacology/) for additional online resources.

SG Go to your Study Guide for additional learning activities to help you master this chapter content.

Review Questions

See *Answers to In-Text Review Questions* in the back of the book for answers to these questions.

1. **When is it acceptable for the nurse to take a verbal order from the prescriber before giving a drug to a patient?**

   A. During the night shift when the prescriber is not at the hospital

   B. In an emergency situation such as a cardiac arrest

   C. When a patient is experiencing severe pain

   D. At any time it is necessary

2. **The nurse is giving morning medications to a patient who refuses to take an oral dose of docusate (Colace). What is the nurse's best response?**

   A. "Your prescriber ordered that you must take this drug twice a day."

   B. "Docusate will soften your bowel movements so that you do not strain."

   C. "This drug will help prevent constipation while you are on bed rest."

   D. "Can you tell me why you do not want to take the docusate?"

3. **What is the most important role of the nurse in preventing drug errors?**

    A. Always checking the patient's diagnosis before giving a drug

    B. Always following the "eight rights" of drug administration

    C. Being the only defense for detecting and preventing drug errors

    D. Being most likely to detect a drug error that has occurred

4. **A patient is prescribed an omeprazole (Prilosec) 20 mg capsule once a day orally. The patient is having difficulty with swallowing and has a feeding tube in place. What is the nurse's best action?**

    A. Open the capsule, mix the contents with water, and then give the drug through the feeding tube.

    B. Raise the head of the bed 90 degrees, and mix the capsule in applesauce for easier swallowing.

    C. Contact the prescriber and pharmacist about using another drug or another form of the drug.

    D. Hold the tube feeding for at least 30 minutes before and after giving the drug.

5. **A patient with severe postoperative pain is prescribed morphine 2 mg intravenously. The patient asks the nurse if the drug could be taken by mouth instead. What is the nurse's best response?**

    A. "Giving the drug intravenously will give you faster pain relief."

    B. "I will call your prescriber and ask if the order can be changed."

    C. "Your surgeon wants you to receive the drug intravenously."

    D. "We can substitute the intravenous drug with an oral drug."

6. **Which administration technique does the nurse use to give a 2-year-old child ear drops?**

    A. Pull the earlobe down and back.

    B. Pull the earlobe up and out.

    C. Keep the earlobe straight.

    D. Hang the patient's head over the side of the bed.

7. **What instruction must the nurse be sure to provide for a patient after a vaginal drug is administered?**

    A. "This drug should be refrigerated."

    B. "You may take this drug at home while sitting on the toilet."

    C. "Be sure to empty your bladder after receiving this drug."

    D. "Remain lying down for 10 to 15 minutes after taking this drug."

8. **The health care provider prescribes all of the following drugs for a patient who had surgery 2 days ago. Which drug order will the nurse administer first?**

    A. Cyanocobalamin 100 mcg intramuscularly once

    B. Diphenhydramine 25 mg orally every 8 hours

    C. Prochlorperazine 10 mg orally STAT

    D. Flurazepam 30 mg orally at night PRN

9. **The nurse preparing to administer an intravenous (IV) push drug notices that the skin around the patient's IV site is swollen and red. The patient states that the area hurts, and no blood return is obtained when the nurse aspirates the IV setup. What is the nurse's best action?**

    A. Start IV administration of the drug as ordered.

    B. Discontinue IV administration then notify the prescriber.

    C. Dilute the drug in saline before injecting it into the current IV site.

    D. Reassure the patient that this is an expected reaction.

10. **A patient is to receive an acetaminophen suppository for an elevated temperature of 102.8°F. What actions must the nurse take? Select all that apply.**

    A. Ask if the patient is having any diarrhea.

    B. Lubricate the blunt end of the suppository.

    C. Put on a pair of sterile gloves.

    D. Place the patient in the modified left lateral recumbent position.

    E. Ask the patient to take a deep breath and bear down.

    F. Push the suppository into the rectum about 1 inch.

11. **When compared with the subcutaneous route, what are the advantages of giving drugs intramuscularly (IM)? Select all that apply.**

    A. IM injections require a smaller, shorter needle.

    B. IM drugs are absorbed faster than subcutaneous drugs.

    C. IM injections can be much larger than subcutaneous injections.

    D. IM injections do not require the rotation of injection sites.

    E. IM injections are less painful than subcutaneous injections.

    F. IM injections are given deeper than subcutaneous injections.

12. **Which question is most important for the nurse to ask a patient before administering a new drug to prevent harm?**

    A. "Are you allergic to any drugs?"

    B. "Do you know what this drug is for?"

    C. "When was the last time you ate or drank?"

    D. "What other drugs have you taken in the last 24 hours?"

Mathematics Review and Introduction to Dosage Calculations

3

http://evolve.elsevier.com/Workman/pharmacology/

Learning Objectives

The content presented in this chapter should help you to:

1. Identify the numerator and denominator of a fraction.
2. Identify a proper and an improper fraction.
3. Change a whole number into a fraction.
4. Change a mixed number into a fraction.
5. Reduce a fraction to its lowest terms.
6. Calculate the lowest common denominator of a series of fractions.
7. Add two or more fractions and subtract two or more fractions.
8. Multiply two fractions and divide two fractions.
9. Identify the divisor and the dividend of a decimal problem.
10. Multiply two decimals and divide two decimals.
11. Change a fraction into a decimal and a decimal into a fraction.
12. Calculate a given percentage of a number.
13. Compare the dose on hand (what you have) with the dose that has been prescribed (what you want).
14. Calculate the number of tablets or amount of liquid drug needed to make the prescribed dose.
15. Convert a set of fractions into a proportion.
16. Solve for "*X*" (the unknown) in a math problem.

Key Terms

decimal (DĔS-ĭ-mŭl) (p. 52) The part of a whole number based on a system of units of 10 (for example, 0.5 is 5 tenths of 1).

decimal point (DĔS-ĭ-mŭl PŌYNT) (p. 52) The dividing point between whole numbers and parts of numbers in a system based on units of 10.

denominator (dē-NŎM-ĭn-ā-tŭr) (p. 48) The bottom number in a fraction, the dividing number (for example, in $\frac{3}{4}$ the denominator is 4); same as divisor.

dividend (DĬ-vĭ-dĕnd) (p. 54) The number to be divided in a division problem (for example, in $\frac{3}{4}$ the dividend is 3); same as numerator.

divisor (dĭ-VĪ-zŭr) (p. 54) The number the dividend is divided by (or that is divided into the dividend) (for example, in $\frac{3}{4}$ the divisor is 4); same as denominator.

fraction (FRĂK-shŭn) (p. 48) A part of a whole number obtained by dividing one number by a larger number.

improper fraction (ĭm-PRŎ-pŭr FRĂK-shŭn) (p. 49) A fraction that has a top number (numerator) that is larger than the bottom number (denominator). The final answer to an improper fraction is always greater than the number 1.

mixed-number fractions (MĬKST NŬM-bŭr FRĂK-shŭnz) (p. 49) Whole numbers with a fraction attached.

numerator (NŪ-mŭr-ā-tŭr) (p. 48) The top number in a fraction that is divided by the bottom number (denominator) (for example, in $\frac{3}{4}$ the numerator is 3; same as dividend).

percent (pŭr-SĔNT (p. 55) The expression of how a number is related to 100; literally "for each hundred."

proper fraction (PRŎ-pŭr FRĂK-shŭn) (p. 48) A fraction in which the top number is smaller than the bottom number. The final answer to a proper fraction is always less than the number 1.

proportion (prō-PŌR-shŭn) (p. 58) An equal mathematic relationship between two sets of numbers.

quotient (KWŌ-shĕnt) (p. 54) The answer to a division problem.

reduced fractions (rē-DŪST FRĂK-shŭnz) (p. 49) Fractions that have been changed to their lowest common denominator (that is, both the numerator and the denominator of a fraction have been divided by the same number evenly).

scored tablet (SKŌRD TĂB-lĕt) (p. 57) A tablet that has a line etched into it, marking the exact midpoint. Cutting (or breaking) a tablet along this line gives you two halves with known dosages.

WHY NURSES NEED MATHEMATICS

Clinical nursing requires the use of math in many ways. The most important is the use of math to give drugs to others safely and accurately, including the *right dose*. This is one of the eight rules for drug administration known as the *eight rights* (see Chapter 2). Understanding math helps to ensure that a drug is given at the right dose.

 Memory Jogger

Use math correctly to calculate or check drug dosages, which is an important "right" of correct drug administration.

Although some drugs come from the pharmacy prepared in exactly the right dose to give to a patient, not every drug is prepared this way. For those that are not, you will need to calculate *how much to give* from what you *have on hand* (available). Dosage calculations are performed in the same way whether the drug is a tablet, oral liquid, injectable liquid, or suppository.

This chapter and Chapters 4 and 5 contain all the basic skills and equivalencies needed to solve any drug dosage problem. Traditional math terms are used only when they help you to understand the dosage calculation concept. If you already have a good working knowledge of the principles of basic math, check yourself by working the problems in the following "MATH CHECK" section.

MATH CHECK

If you work these problems correctly, you probably do not need to review the chapter. If you have a weakness in any specific area, review the content and principles for that area. The answers to these math check problems are located at the end of the chapter.

MATH CHECK PROBLEMS

MC-1: Change these mixed-number fractions into improper fractions.

a. $3\dfrac{5}{8}$

b. $7\dfrac{1}{3}$

MC-2: Reduce each of these fractions to their lowest common denominators.

a. $\dfrac{25}{75}$

b. $\dfrac{115}{130}$

MC-3: How many zeros can you chop and drop?

a. $\dfrac{180}{2200}$

b. $\dfrac{50,000}{100,000}$

MC-4: Which fraction represents the largest part of the whole for a and b? What is the lowest common denominator for each set of three fractions?

a. $\dfrac{1}{3}, \dfrac{10}{15},$ or $\dfrac{12}{24}$

b. $\dfrac{2}{4}, \dfrac{6}{8},$ or $\dfrac{3}{24}$

Which fraction represents the smallest part of the whole for c and d? What is the lowest common denominator for each set of three fractions?

c. $\dfrac{6}{8}, \dfrac{6}{12},$ or $\dfrac{2}{3}$

d. $\dfrac{8}{9}, \dfrac{1}{3},$ or $\dfrac{3}{27}$

MC-5: Add these fractions. If a sum is an improper fraction, convert it to either a whole number or to a mixed-number fraction.

a. $\dfrac{1}{3}+\dfrac{2}{3}+\dfrac{3}{3}$

b. $\dfrac{9}{9}+\dfrac{5}{9}+\dfrac{7}{9}+\dfrac{4}{9}$

MC-6: Add these fractions. If the sum is an improper fraction, convert it to either a whole number or a mixed-number fraction. Reduce the answers to their lowest common denominators.

a. $\dfrac{2}{3}+\dfrac{6}{12}+\dfrac{6}{8}$

b. $\dfrac{1}{9}+\dfrac{3}{4}+\dfrac{2}{3}$

MC-7: Subtract these fractions. If a fraction is a mixed-number fraction, first convert it to an improper fraction. Reduce answers to their lowest common denominators.

a. $\dfrac{5}{6}-\dfrac{2}{6}$

b. $2\dfrac{5}{6}-1\dfrac{3}{6}$

MC-8: Subtract these fractions. If a fraction is a mixed-number fraction, first convert it to an improper fraction. Reduce answers to their lowest common denominators.

a. $\dfrac{7}{8} - \dfrac{2}{3}$

b. $6\dfrac{1}{3} - 2\dfrac{1}{2}$

MC-9: Multiply these fractions.

a. $1\dfrac{22}{24} \times \dfrac{1}{2}$

b. $4\dfrac{5}{8} \times \dfrac{2}{3}$

MC-10: Divide these fractions.

a. $\dfrac{7}{8} \div \dfrac{2}{3}$

b. $6\dfrac{3}{4} \div 2\dfrac{1}{3}$

MC-11: Decimals as parts of a whole:

a. 0.50 = How many parts of a whole?

b. 2.48 = How many whole numbers and how many parts of a whole?

MC-12: Multiply these decimals.

a. 16.5×0.5

b. 1.2×1.2

MC-13: Divide these decimals.

a. $52.8 \div 12$

b. $1.4 \div 1.4$

MC-14: Change the following fractions to decimals and decimals to fractions.

a. 0.065

b. $\dfrac{300}{650}$

MC-15: Work to three places and then round to two places.

a. $\dfrac{128.5}{80}$

b. $\dfrac{26.8}{13.4}$

MC-16: Convert the following percents into fractions.

a. $\frac{2}{3}\%$

b. 7%

MC-17: Find the percentages of the whole number.

a. 0.6% of 50

b. 20% of 120

MC-18: How many tablets should you give?

a. *Want* carvedilol 25 mg; *Have* carvedilol 6.25 mg

b. *Want* estrogen 0.0625 mg; *Have* estrogen 0.125 mg

MC-19: How many milliliters should you give?

a. *Want* diphenhydramine (Benadryl) 50 mg; *Have* diphenhydramine 25 mg/5 mL

b. *Want* chloral hydrate syrup 100 mg; *Have* chloral hydrate syrup 500 mg/5 mL

MC-20: How many milliliters should you give by injection?

a. *Want* penicillin 50,000 units; *Have* penicillin 1,000,000 units/ 50 mL

b. *Want* prochlorperazine (Compazine) 10 mg; *Have* prochlorperazine 5 mg/mL

MC-21: Express the following problems as a fractional proportion.

a. If one box of eggs has 18 eggs, then two boxes have 36 eggs.

b. If one chewable tablet of diphenhydramine contains 12.5 mg, then four chewable tablets have 50 mg.

MC-22: How many milliliters should you give?

a. *Want* carbamazepine (Tegretol) 75 mg oral suspension; *Have* carbamazepine 100 mg/5 mL

b. *Want* acetaminophen (Tylenol) 100 mg; *Have* acetaminophen 160 mg/5 mL

GETTING STARTED

Some nurses prefer to use a calculator to work all math problems. However, for a calculator to provide the correct answer, you must be sure to set the problem up correctly. This involves entering the numbers into the calculator in the right order, known as the order of operation. If you understand the math principle, you will be more likely to enter the numbers correctly. Calculator keys differ from one brand to another. Be sure to practice with your calculator before you use it at work to calculate drug dosages. *Practice makes perfect!*

Remember that math problems are punched into a calculator just like they are written or just like you would say them aloud. For example, 24 × 12 is punched in as 2, 4, ×, 1, 2 = *answer*. If you punch in any of the numbers backwards (e.g., 4, 2, ×, 1, 2 or 2, 4, ×, 2, 1), the answer will be wrong.

Always use common sense when calculating drug dosages. Always ask yourself, *DOES IT MAKE SENSE?* Some people refer to this thinking as the "DIMS test." If the answer doesn't look right (e.g., give 15 tablets), it probably isn't right! Think about it again and rework the problem.

Some types of drugs are *high-alert drugs* and are very dangerous if the dosage is miscalculated. As described in Chapter 1, these include the "PINCH" drugs of *p*otassium, *i*nsulin, *n*arcotics, *c*hemotherapy and cardiac drugs, and *h*eparin or other anticlotting drugs. After you calculate one of these drug doses, always have another health care professional independently double check your calculation.

WHOLE NUMBERS VERSUS A PART OF A NUMBER

If you are comfortable with the difference between whole numbers and a part of a number, just skip to the next section. Let's review whole numbers versus fractions. A fraction is a part of a whole number obtained by dividing one number by a larger number. The simplest way to do this is to think about money. A $1 bill represents the whole number one (1). A $1.25 amount is both a whole dollar (1) and a part of another dollar. The 25 cents is a fraction of the second $1. If you wrote it out, it would be 25 out of 100 cents, or $\frac{25}{100}$. The same amount written as a decimal would be $0.25. Both express the exact same amount of money. So, the dollar is a *whole number,* and the 25 cents is a *part* or *fraction* of another whole number. Fig. 3.1 shows the relationship of a fraction (part of a whole number) to a whole number.

FRACTIONS

A **fraction** is a part of a whole number obtained by dividing one number by a larger number. Any fraction (e.g., $\frac{25}{100}$) is actually a division problem. The fraction is the same as $100\overline{)25}$ or 25 ÷ 100. So any number *over* another number is a fraction. The top number in a fraction, in this example 25, is called the **numerator**. Remember the numerator as being "numero uno," No. 1, the best! The number on the bottom in a fraction is the **denominator**. In the example $\frac{25}{100}$, the denominator is 100.

Any number can be expressed as a fraction, even a whole number. To make a whole number a fraction, simply make the denominator of the fraction 1. Thus, the whole number 2 has the same value when written as the fraction $\frac{2}{1}$. When any whole number is written as a fraction, the whole number is always on top (numerator), and the denominator (1) is always on the bottom. Remembering this concept will help you solve drug dosage problems using fractions.

Different Types of Fractions

There are several types of fractions, including proper fractions, improper fractions, mixed-number fractions, and reduced fractions. The differences are simple, and you can do it!

Proper fractions. A **proper fraction** is one in which the top number is smaller than the bottom number. So $\frac{25}{100}$ is a proper fraction. A proper fraction is the most common

---

 Drug Alert

Administration Alert

Use the DIMS ("does it make sense") test when calculating a drug dose. If your answer requires more than four tablets or more than one syringe, it is probably wrong.

QSEN: Safety

 Memory Jogger

High-alert or PINCH drugs include potassium, insulin, narcotics (also known as opioids), chemotherapy and cardiac drugs, and heparin or other anticlotting drugs.

 Memory Jogger

Remember the word NUDE. The top number in a fraction is the numerator (NU), and the bottom number is the denominator (DE): NU/DE

Memory Jogger

Whenever a whole number is written as a fraction, the whole number is on top, and the denominator is always 1.

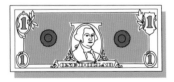

A one-dollar bill representing the whole number one

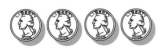

Four quarters, each representing 1/4 or 25% (0.25) of the whole one-dollar bill

FIG. 3.1 Comparison of part of a number to a whole number.

type of fraction. The value of a proper fraction is always less than the number 1. For example, the answer to $\frac{25}{100}$ (which is really $100\overline{)25}$ or $25 \div 100$) is **0.25,** a number less than 1.

Improper fractions. Improper fractions didn't do anything wrong. They are just different from proper fractions, which represent only part of a whole number. A fraction can also have a top number (numerator) that is *bigger* than the bottom number (denominator) (for example, $\frac{125}{100}$). This number is still a fraction, but it represents *more* than the number 1. So, an **improper fraction** is a fraction that has a top number (numerator) that is larger than the bottom number (denominator), meaning that the value is greater than 1. For example, $\frac{125}{100}$ is really $100\overline{)125}$ or $125 \div 100$, and the answer is **1.25.**

Mixed-number fractions. **Mixed-number fractions** are whole numbers with a fraction attached. For example, $1\frac{2}{4}$ is a mixed-number fraction; 1 is a whole number, and $\frac{2}{4}$ is a fraction. A mixed-number fraction can be changed into an improper fraction by multiplying the denominator (4) times ($\times$) the whole number (1) and adding the numerator (2). $4 \times 1 = 4 + 2 = 6$. Now make 6 the new numerator (top number) with the same denominator (4) and you get $\frac{6}{4}$, an improper fraction. Being able to convert mixed-number fractions into improper fractions is useful when you have to multiply proper and improper fractions together.

Reducing Fractions
Reducing fractions is a way to make fractions "simpler" and easier to use. **Reduced fractions** have been changed to their lowest common denominator. This means that both the top number (numerator) and the bottom number (denominator) of a fraction have been divided evenly by the same number. For example, the part of a dollar ($\frac{25}{100}$, or 25 cents out of 100 cents in a dollar) is also equal to $\frac{1}{4}$ of a dollar. To change $\frac{25}{100}$ into $\frac{1}{4}$, *divide both* the numerator and the denominator by the largest number possible that will go evenly into both numbers. In this example both 25 and 100 can be divided evenly by 25. You have just *reduced* this fraction to its lowest common denominator! When you are working with a drug dosage problem, wouldn't it be easier to work with $\frac{1}{4}$ rather than with $\frac{25}{100}$? The final dosage answer is the same either way.

   If you find it hard to think of a large number that can be divided evenly into both the numerator and the denominator, start with several small numbers. For example, in $\frac{25}{100}$ each number can be divided evenly by 5. This answer, $\frac{5}{20}$, can then be divided by 5 again to get to $\frac{1}{4}$. Does this make sense? Do whatever is easier for you. The final answer is the same.

Reducing Special Fractions
How do you manage fractions with larger numbers, such as $\frac{240}{120}$? You could reduce it the way it is (dividing 240 by 120), and the answer is 2. There is a way to make it a little easier. Because *both* the top number (numerator) and the bottom number (denominator) end in *zero,* you can "chop off" both zeros and be left with $\frac{24}{12}$. By chopping off the zeros, you are actually dividing both the numerator (240) and the denominator (120) by 10, resulting in a new numerator of 24 and a new denominator of 12. The answer is still 2 because you divided both the numerator and the denominator by 10. *However, be careful because this shortcut only applies to zeros.* You can use it with any number of zeros as long as there are an *equal* number of them on both the top and bottom of a fraction. For example, $\frac{3500}{4600}$ can be chopped off to $\frac{35}{46}$. The answer to reducing both fractions is the same! When reducing a fraction by 10, chop off one zero from both the numerator and the denominator. For example, this reduces $\frac{30}{50}$ to $\frac{3}{5}$. When reducing a fraction by 100, chop off two zeros from both the numerator and the denominator. For example, this reduces $\frac{300}{500}$ to $\frac{3}{5}$. When reducing a fraction by 1000, chop off three zeros from both the numerator and the denominator (for example, $\frac{3000}{5000}$ is reduced to $\frac{3}{5}$).

 Memory Jogger

The value of a proper fraction is always less than 1; for example, $\frac{1}{5}$.

 Memory Jogger

The value of an improper fraction is always <u>greater</u> than 1; for example, $100\overline{)125}$, or 1.25.

 Try This!

TT-1 Change these mixed-number fractions into improper fractions.

a. $1\frac{3}{4}$ c. $4\frac{1}{5}$

b. $2\frac{5}{8}$

Answers are at the end of this chapter.

 Try This!

TT-2 Reduce each of these fractions to their lowest common denominators.

a. $\frac{10}{24}$ c. $\frac{36}{84}$

b. $\frac{50}{100}$

Answers are at the end of this chapter.

 Memory Jogger

When dividing a fraction with both the top and bottom numbers ending in zero, you can chop off the same number of zeros from both numbers.

 Try This!

TT-3 How many zeros can you chop and drop?

a. $\frac{230}{3500}$ c. $\frac{20}{500}$

b. $\frac{1400}{10}$

Answers are at the end of this chapter.

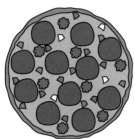

Whole pizza
(1/1)

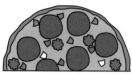

1/2 pizza
slice

1/4 pizza
slice

1/8 pizza
slice

FIG. 3.2 Fraction sizes.

 Memory Jogger

When the numerator of a fraction is 1, the bigger the denominator, the smaller the fraction.

Try This!

TT-4 Which fraction represents the *largest* part of the whole for a and b? What is the lowest common denominator for each set of three fractions?

a. $\dfrac{1}{2}$, $\dfrac{3}{4}$, or $\dfrac{7}{8}$

b. $\dfrac{1}{5}$, $\dfrac{5}{15}$, or $\dfrac{6}{45}$

Which fraction represents the *smallest* part of the whole for c and d? What is the lowest common denominator for each set of three fractions?

c. $\dfrac{1}{3}$, $\dfrac{1}{5}$, or $\dfrac{1}{6}$

d. $\dfrac{1}{2}$, $\dfrac{3}{8}$, or $\dfrac{3}{4}$

Answers are at the end of this chapter.

Comparing Fractions

There may be times when you must compare several drugs and determine which dose is the strongest (or weakest). What if the dose comes in $\frac{1}{4}$, $\frac{1}{2}$, and $\frac{1}{8}$ strengths? How are you going to decide which is the strongest dose?

If the numerators (top numbers) are all 1, you can just think of slices of a pizza. Would you get a bigger slice if you had $\frac{1}{8}$ or $\frac{1}{4}$ of the pizza? Fig. 3.2 shows the comparison of sizes by fractions. Don't be fooled into thinking that the biggest denominator gives the biggest slice. It is actually the other way around! As you can see in Fig. 3.2, if the numerators are all the same (in this case they are all equal to 1), the *smallest* denominator gives the biggest slice (or the strongest dose).

But what if the denominators AND the numerators are different? Consider the fractions $\frac{2}{3}$ and $\frac{3}{4}$. How can these fractions be compared? Because they are different, you cannot compare them until you first rewrite the fractions to find the lowest common denominator. As you recall from the section on reducing fractions, this means that, to be able to compare the two strengths, you first have to convert both of them to the same denominator. Once you convert them to the same denominator, you can figure out exactly how they are related by comparing their numerators.

The best way to make them have a common denominator is to determine the *lowest* bottom number that both can be divided into evenly. For 3 and 4, that number is 12. To determine the lowest common denominator, start writing all the multiples of both denominators. Multiples of 3 are 3, 6, 9, 12, 15, 18, and so on because $1 \times 3 = 3$, $2 \times 3 = 6$, $3 \times 3 = 9$, $4 \times 3 = \mathbf{12}$, $5 \times 3 = 15$, and $6 \times 3 = 18$. Multiples of 4 are 4, 8, 12, 16, 20, 24, and so on because $1 \times 4 = 4$, $2 \times 4 = 8$, $3 \times 4 = \mathbf{12}$, $4 \times 4 = 16$, $5 \times 4 = 20$, and $6 \times 4 = 24$. When you compare the multiples of 3 with the multiples of 4, the first number that appears on both lists is **12**. For denominators of 3 and 4, then, the lowest common denominator is 12. This means that you will now use 12 as the *new* denominator for both fractions. Now, take each original denominator (3 and 4) and divide it into 12. Take each answer and multiply it by its numerator. That number becomes the *new* numerator for each fraction. For example, for the first fraction $\frac{2}{3}$, when you divide the new denominator 12 by the old denominator (3), you get 4. Now multiply the old numerator (2) by 4, and you get 8. So, when the common denominator is 12, $\frac{2}{3}$ is equal to $\frac{8}{12}$. Those of you who love math may have noticed that the cross products are equal (2×12 is equal to 3×8)! This will tell you that your answer is correct.

Next try the fraction $\frac{3}{4}$. Did you get $\frac{9}{12}$? Now that both the original fractions have the same denominator ($\frac{8}{12}$ and $\frac{9}{12}$), you can easily see which one is the strongest or biggest ($\frac{9}{12}$)! Do you see that $\frac{9}{12}$ (or $\frac{3}{4}$) has more parts of the whole ($\frac{12}{12}$) than $\frac{8}{12}$ (or $\frac{2}{3}$), and so it is the strongest dose?

Adding Fractions

Adding fractions that have the same denominator is as simple as adding whole numbers. The math symbol for addition is a plus sign (+). When adding fractions that have the same denominator, you only add the numerators (top numbers). For example, when adding $\dfrac{2}{4} + \dfrac{1}{4}$, just add the numerators ($2 + 1 = 3$) and place that answer (the sum) on top of the original denominator. (The denominator does not change.) The result is $\dfrac{2}{4} + \dfrac{1}{4} = \dfrac{3}{4}$. You can add any amount of fractions with the same denominators in this way. For example, the answer to the addition problem $\dfrac{2}{6} + \dfrac{2}{6} + \dfrac{4}{6} + \dfrac{5}{6}$ is $\dfrac{13}{6}$. When the sum of fractions is an improper fraction, convert it to a mixed fraction. In this case the answer ($\frac{13}{6}$) can be converted to the mixed-number fraction of $2\frac{1}{6}$.

Adding fractions that have different denominators requires that they all first be converted to the same lowest common denominator, just as is necessary when comparing fractions. Then the numerators can be added in the same way as for fractions that started out with the same denominators. How would you add $\frac{1}{2}+\frac{4}{5}+\frac{3}{4}$? First, calculate the multiples of each denominator. For the denominator of 2 the multiples are 2, 4, 6, 8, 10, 12, 14, 16, 18, **20**, 22, 24, and so on. For the denominator of 5 the multiples are 5, 10, 15, **20**, 25, 30, 35, and so on. The numbers 10 and 20 are common to both 2 and 5. However, the multiples of 4 are 4, 8, 12, 16, **20**, 24, 28, and so on. The number 10 is not a multiple of 4, but **20** is a multiple of all three denominators. So, **20** is now our common denominator. To make the fraction $\frac{1}{2}$ have a common denominator of 20, multiply both its numerator (1) and its denominator (2) by 10 to get $\frac{10}{20}$. To make the fraction $\frac{4}{5}$ have a common denominator of 20, multiply both its numerator (4) and its denominator (5) by 4 to get $\frac{16}{20}$. To make the fraction $\frac{3}{4}$ have a common denominator of 20, multiply both its numerator (3) and its denominator (4) by 5 to get $\frac{15}{20}$. Next add $\frac{10}{20}+\frac{16}{20}+\frac{15}{20}$, which equals $\frac{41}{20}$. Then change this improper fraction to the mixed-number fraction of $2\frac{1}{20}$.

Subtracting Fractions

The need to subtract fractions is rare for drug calculations or drug preparation, so this review of subtracting fractions is brief. Not only is subtracting fractions rare in drug calculation, negative numbers are not used. This means that you would not need to subtract the larger numerator from the smaller numerator.

The math symbol for subtraction is a minus sign ($-$). When subtracting two fractions that have the same denominator (bottom number), subtract the smaller numerator (top number) from the larger one. For example, when subtracting $\frac{2}{4}-\frac{1}{4}$, simply subtract 1 from 2 (2 − 1) and place that answer on the original denominator. The result is $\frac{2}{4}-\frac{1}{4}=\frac{1}{4}$.

Subtracting fractions that have different denominators first requires their conversion to the same lowest common denominator, just as you did when adding fractions with different denominators. After they have been converted to the lowest common denominator, the numerators can be subtracted in the same way as for fractions that began with the same denominators. For example, to subtract $\frac{4}{7}-\frac{2}{5}$, first find the lowest common denominator (as described under "Comparing Fractions" on p. 50), which is 35. Then multiply the numerators by the amount needed to make their denominators become 35. (That would be 5 for the first fraction and 7 for the second fraction.) Multiply the numerator (4) in $\frac{4}{7}$ by 5 and place that number on the new denominator to get $\frac{20}{35}$. Then multiply the numerator (2) in $\frac{2}{5}$ by 7 and place that number on the new denominator to get $\frac{14}{35}$. Subtract $\frac{14}{35}$ from $\frac{20}{35}$ ($\frac{20}{35}-\frac{14}{35}=\frac{6}{35}$).

Multiplying Fractions

Multiplying fractions is straightforward. The math symbol for multiplication is "×." Look at all the fractions in an equation that you need to multiply. For example, multiply $\frac{3}{9}\times1\frac{5}{6}$. First make sure that all the fractions are reduced to their lowest possible terms (but you do not have to find the lowest *common* denominator). So, reduce $\frac{3}{9}$ to $\frac{1}{3}$. Then see if there are any mixed-number fractions and change them to improper fractions. For this example, change the mixed-number fraction $1\frac{5}{6}$ into an improper

TT-9 Multiply these fractions.

a. $1\dfrac{3}{4} \times 5\dfrac{6}{7}$ c. $\dfrac{3}{4} \times 9\dfrac{11}{16}$

b. $2\dfrac{2}{4} \times 6\dfrac{7}{8}$

Answers are at the end of this chapter.

TT-10 Divide these fractions.

a. $3 \div \dfrac{1}{2}$ c. $5\dfrac{1}{4} \div \dfrac{6}{8}$

b. $\dfrac{3}{4} \div \dfrac{1}{2}$

Answers are at the end of this chapter.

Memory Jogger

Decimal places are always written in (and represent) multiples of 10.

Critical Point for Safety

The places to the right or left of the decimal point determine the value of a number. So always put a zero before the decimal point of any proper fraction written as a decimal. If you don't, 0.25 g of a drug written as .25 could be misread as 25 g of a drug: a BIG overdose. For example, an adult morphine dose of 5 mg is normal, but a pediatric morphine dose might be .5 mg and should be written as 0.5 mg. If this dose is read as 5 mg, it is 10 times the normal dose, which could be lethal.

QSEN: Safety

fraction ($6 \times 1 + 5 = \dfrac{11}{6}$). Now you have $\dfrac{1}{3} \times \dfrac{11}{6}$. To get the answer, simply multiply all the numerators (top numbers) straight across the top ($1 \times 11 = 11$). Doing this makes a *new* numerator. Now do the same thing with the denominators ($3 \times 6 = 18$). Doing this makes a *new* denominator. The new total is now $\frac{11}{18}$. That's it!

Dividing Fractions

Fractions that need to be divided are usually written out with the math symbol for division ($\div$), (for example, $\dfrac{5}{8}$ divided by $\dfrac{2}{3}$, or $\dfrac{5}{8} \div \dfrac{2}{3}$). To divide these fractions, flip (invert) the second fraction so the problem now reads $\dfrac{5}{8} \times \dfrac{3}{2}$. Multiply across the numerators and denominators as you did when multiplying two fractions. The answer is $\frac{15}{16}$. If possible, reduce the fraction answer to its lowest terms. In this case, $\frac{15}{16}$ cannot be reduced further.

If your division involves a whole number to be divided by a fraction (for example, $2 \div \dfrac{3}{4}$), change the whole number 2 into a fraction by putting it over 1. The whole number 2 is the fraction $\dfrac{2}{1}$. (Remember that all whole numbers can be expressed as fractions by putting the whole number over 1.) Therefore, the problem is now $\dfrac{2}{1} \div \dfrac{3}{4}$. After you invert (flip) the second fraction, the problem is $\dfrac{2}{1} \times \dfrac{4}{3} = \dfrac{8}{3}$. Reduce this fraction to $2\frac{2}{3}$. That's it!

Dividing a fraction by a whole number works the same way. For the problem $\dfrac{1}{3} \div 4$, first convert it to $\dfrac{1}{3} \div \dfrac{4}{1}$ and flip (invert) the second fraction, converting the problem to $\dfrac{1}{3} \times \dfrac{1}{4}$. The answer is $\dfrac{1}{12}$!

DECIMALS

A **decimal**, like a fraction, describes parts of a whole. Decimals and fractions are related because decimals can be written as fractions and fractions can be written as decimals. To understand how to change from one to the other, you must first understand that the place value of decimals is based on multiples of 10. We will talk about the relationship between fractions and decimals a little later.

The key to understanding decimals is to understand the way they are written. A **decimal point** is the dividing point between whole numbers and parts of numbers in a system based on units of 10 (Table 3.1). It is located between the whole number and the part of the whole number.

Any number to the *left* of a decimal point is a *whole* number. So, the whole number 125 is written from left to right as 1 one hundred, 2 tens, and 5 ones (or right to left as 5 ones, 2 tens, and 1 one hundred). By now you do this instinctively because you started doing it in first grade!

Any number to the *right* of the decimal point is a *part* of the whole number. So, the decimal 0.25 is 25 parts of 100 because the place value of the 5 is hundredths, and 0.025 is 25 parts of a thousand because the third place after the decimal point (in this case the 5) has a place value of thousandths. The place to the right or left of the decimal determines the value of a number.

When working with drug dosages, *always* put a *zero before* the decimal point of any number less than 1 to indicate that there are no whole parts (for example, write .5 mg as 0.5 mg). When you are tired, reading a fax order, or reading an order written on no-carbon-required (NCR) paper, the numbers may not be clear; a decimal point could easily be missed, leading to a serious drug dosage error.

Never put any extra zeros, known as *trailing zeros*, at the end of a decimal when writing a drug dose. Trailing zeros are useless and can be confusing. For example,

Table **3.1** Decimal Table and Conversions		
WORD DESCRIPTION	**NUMBER**	**FRACTION**
Hundred thousands	100,000	$\dfrac{100,000}{1}$
Ten thousands	10,000	$\dfrac{10,000}{1}$
Thousands	1,000	$\dfrac{1,000}{1}$
Hundreds	100	$\dfrac{100}{1}$
Tens	10	$\dfrac{10}{1}$
Ones/units	1	$\dfrac{1}{1}$
Decimal point	.	
Tenths	0.1	$\dfrac{1}{10}$
Hundredths	0.01	$\dfrac{1}{100}$
Thousandths	0.001	$\dfrac{1}{1,000}$
Ten thousandths	0.0001	$\dfrac{1}{10,000}$
Hundred thousandths	0.00001	$\dfrac{1}{100,000}$
Millionths	0.000001	$\dfrac{1}{1,000,000}$

although 0.25 is equal to 0.250, 0.250 could be easily misread as 250 instead of 25 parts when measuring drugs. *Always* chop off those trailing zeros to the right of the decimal point (but only the *end* zeros).

Adding and Subtracting Decimals

Adding and subtracting decimals is exactly the same as adding and subtracting whole numbers. The key to ensuring that you obtain the correct answer when adding or subtracting decimals is to keep the decimal points in all the numbers that you are adding in the same position. For example, when adding 7.25, 9.3, and 11.71, position the decimal points as shown in the following problem.

$$
\begin{array}{r}
7.25 \\
+9.3 \\
+11.71 \\
\hline
28.26
\end{array}
$$

Follow the same procedure when subtracting decimals (e.g., 42.22 from 98.61).

$$
\begin{array}{r}
98.61 \\
-42.22 \\
\hline
56.39
\end{array}
$$

 Try This!

TT-11 Decimals as parts of a whole:
a. 0.3 = How many parts of a whole?
b. 0.75 = How many parts of a whole?
c. 5.1 = How many whole numbers, and how many parts of a whole?

Answers are at the end of this chapter.

Multiplying Decimals

Multiplying decimals is almost as easy as multiplying whole numbers. The only difference is that your answer has to contain the right number of decimal places for it to make sense. The key is to count the total number of decimal places (the number of digits after the decimal point) in the whole problem and then make sure that the same amount of decimal places are in the answer. So, you do not need to keep track of the decimals until you have an answer!

To multiply 2.4 × 4, treat the numbers as 24 × 4 and multiply, which equals 96. Now add the number of decimal places in both numbers. There is only one decimal place for this problem (it is in 2.4). Starting from the far right of 96, count one space to the left and place the decimal point; 9.6 is the correct answer. Try multiplying a decimal by another decimal. For example, when multiplying 2.4 × 3.6, treat it as 24 × 36; 964 is the correct answer. Add the number of decimal places in both numbers that were multiplied. There is one decimal place in 2.4 and one decimal place in 3.6, for a total of two decimal places. Starting from the far right of 964, count two spaces to the left and place the decimal point; 9.64 is the correct answer. Now multiply 4.3 × .21 by treating it as 43 × 21, with 903 being the answer. There are three decimal places in the number being multiplied (one in 4.3 and two in .21). So, starting from the far right of 903, count spaces to the left, and place the decimal point for 0.903 as the correct answer. Remember, just as when you multiply whole numbers, it is important to line up your numbers properly when you are doing the problem without a calculator.

Dividing Decimals

Let's start by dividing a decimal by a whole number: $\frac{36.48}{2}$, or, to put it another way, $2\overline{)36.48}$ or 36.48 ÷ 2. The number being divided (or divided into) is 36.48 and is known as the **dividend**. The number doing the dividing (in this case 2) is the **divisor**. The answer to a division problem is the **quotient.**

The problem works like any other division problem except that *you must be sure that the decimal point in the answer is placed exactly above the one in the dividend.* So first put the decimal point for the answer *exactly above* the one in the dividend (36.48):

$2\overline{)36.48}$ Then complete the division: $2\overline{)36.48}^{\,18.24}$ Does this make sense?

To check division, multiply the divisor (2) and the quotient (18.24). Your answer should equal the dividend (36.48). If you don't get the dividend, your division was wrong, and you must redo it.

Dividing a decimal by a decimal is a little harder, but the principle is the same. Keep in mind that you always have to *divide by a whole number*. If your divisor is a decimal, you have to move the decimal point all the way to the right to make it a whole number. Whatever you do to the divisor, you also must do to the dividend. So, move the decimal point in the dividend the *same number* of decimal spaces. For example, in the problem $\frac{32.4}{1.6}$ or $1.6\overline{)32.4}$, moving the decimal point in the divisor all the way to the right involves moving it one place: changing 1.6 to the whole number 16. Now move the decimal point in the dividend (32.4) one place to the right (an equal number of places) so 32.4 becomes 324, giving you $16\overline{)324}$. Divide as usual, and you should get $16\overline{)324.00}^{\,20.25}$. Check your answer in the same way as mentioned previously: multiply the divisor (16) and the answer (quotient, 20.25). The result should equal the dividend (324).

Dividing a whole number by a decimal also requires moving the decimal points to make things even. In a whole number, the decimal point is located at the *end* of the number. For example, the whole number 4 actually equals 4. Using $\frac{4}{2.5}$, which is the same as $2.5\overline{)4}$ or 4 ÷ 2.5, move the decimal point one place to the right in the divisor. *Add* a decimal place after 4 and move it one place to the right, making it 40. The resulting problem is $25\overline{)40.0}$. Now work the problem the way you would any division problem. Did you get $25\overline{)40.0}^{\,1.6}$? To divide a whole number by a decimal, add as many

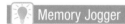

Try This!

TT-12 Multiply these decimals.
a. 100 × 0.25
b. 51.2 × 2.1
c. 15.5 × 10

Answers are at the end of this chapter.

Memory Jogger

Divisor × Quotient (answer)
= Dividend
(if you divided correctly).

extra zeros to the whole number after the decimal as you need until the division ends or repeats. For drug calculations, you will not need to work a decimal problem through more than the thousandth (third) place.

Changing Fractions into Decimals

Decimals and fractions are related because they are both parts of a whole. For example, decimals change the fraction $\frac{25}{100}$ into 0.25 (see Table 3.1). Because both decimals and fractions are a part of the whole, you can change fractions into decimals and decimals into fractions. You do this every time you turn $\frac{25}{100}$ into 0.25. To do this, just divide the numerator (in this case 25) by the denominator (in this case 100). This step is written as $100\overline{)25}$ or $25 \div 100$. To divide, place a decimal point after the 25 and add zeros until the division ends. The answer is .25, but when writing drug dosages, remember to write it as 0.25 to avoid any confusion.

Changing Decimals into Fractions

To change a decimal to a fraction, drop the decimal point and make this number the numerator (top number) of the fraction. The denominator (bottom number) of the fraction is the place value of the last digit (number) of the decimal. Determine the place value of the last number (digit) after the decimal point. For example, the decimal 0.25 is 25 parts of 100 because the place value of the 5 is hundredths. Then reduce the fraction to its lowest terms. For example, to change 0.25 to a fraction, drop the decimal point and make 25 the numerator. The denominator becomes 100 because the place value of the 5 in 0.25 is hundredths and 0.25 is 25 out of 100 (see Table 3.1). Therefore, the fraction is written as $\frac{25}{100}$ and is reduced to $\frac{1}{4}$. Another example is the conversion of the decimal 5.017 into a fraction. It becomes $5\frac{17}{1000}$ because the place value of the 7 in .017 is thousandths.

ROUNDING PARTS OF NUMBERS

When giving drugs, it may be necessary to decide how many milliliters to give if your calculated dose is uneven. For example, if you get an answer such as 2.17 mL, you must decide whether to give 2 mL or more than 2 mL because the .17 is part of the next whole number. How do you decide which number to give? Usually liquid dosages are rounded to the tenth place rather than to a whole number.

The key concept in rounding decimals is to remember the number **5**! Any answer that ends in a number *below* .05 is *rounded down* to the next lower tenth. Any answer that ends in the number .05 or higher is *rounded up* to the next higher tenth. So, if your answer is 2.82 mL, you give 2.8 mL *(rounded down)*. If your answer is 2.17 mL, you give 2.2 mL *(rounded up)*. In clinical practice with drugs that come in tablet form, there is an exception. Some tablets can be cut in half.

PERCENTS

You are probably familiar with percents from using them to decide how much money to tip a waiter in your favorite restaurant (10%, 15%, or 20%). **Percent** expresses a number as part of a hundred. The word *percent* literally means "for each hundred." In health care, percents are used to calculate drug doses and the strength of solutions (for example, the percent [%] of salt in a salt-and-water solution).

Percents express the same idea as a fraction or decimal. They can be written as a whole number (20%), a mixed-number fraction ($12\frac{1}{2}$%), a decimal (0.9%), or a proper fraction ($\frac{1}{2}$%).

Converting a Percent to a Decimal

Let's say we have a 9% salt solution. To change 9% to a decimal, drop the percent sign and multiply the number in the percent by 0.01. The 9% can then be written as 0.09, or 9 parts salt per 100 parts of water. A 0.9% salt solution (commonly called "normal saline" in the health care setting) when multiplied by 0.01 results in 0.009 or 0.9 parts of salt per 100 parts of water (also 9 parts of salt per 1000 parts of water).

 Memory Jogger

Add as many extra zeros (decimal places) to the right of the dividend (whole number) as you need to make the answer accurate.

 Try This!

TT-13 Divide these decimals.
a. 630 ÷ 0.3
b. 0.125 ÷ 0.5
c. 2.5 ÷ 0.75

Answers are at the end of this chapter.

 Memory Jogger

To turn a fraction into a decimal, always divide the numerator (top number) by the bottom number (denominator).

 Try This!

TT-14 Change the following fractions to decimals and the decimals to fractions.

a. $\frac{3}{4}$ d. 1.25

b. 0.55   e. $\frac{7}{8}$

c. 0.075

Answers are at the end of this chapter.

 Critical Point for Safety

The exception to the rounding principle is when you get an answer of exactly half (0.5 or $\frac{1}{2}$) of a tablet. If the tablet can be cut, give $\frac{1}{2}$ tablet (see guidelines under Dosage and Calculation problems).

QSEN: Safety

 Try This!

TT-15 Work to three places and then round to two places.

a. $\frac{58.4}{33}$ c. $\frac{27.5}{3.4}$

b. $\frac{6}{3.4}$

Answers are at the end of this chapter.

Try This!

TT-16 Convert the following percents into fractions.

a. $\frac{1}{2}$%   c. $5\frac{3}{4}$%

b. 3%

Answers are at the end of this chapter.

 Try This!

TT-17 Find the percentages of the whole numbers.
a. 25% of 300
b. 10% of $5.00
c. 0.2% of 10

Answers are at the end of this chapter.

 Drug Alert

Administration Alert

Whenever you read a drug order, check and double check carefully for decimal points and zeros.

QSEN: Safety

 Memory Jogger

You can use the calculation formulas only when the drug dose that you have on hand is in the same measurement unit as the drug dose you want to give.

You can change the 9% to a decimal just by moving the decimal point that is behind the 9 two places to the *left*. Thus 9% = 0.09 (see Table 3.1).

To change a decimal to a percent, reverse the process by moving the decimal point two places to the *right* (e.g., 0.09 = 9%).

Be careful to move the decimal point in the correct direction. Moving it in the wrong direction can result in a serious error. Work it out or *call the pharmacist if you are not sure*.

Converting a Percent to a Fraction

The process of converting a percent to a fraction is the same whether you have a whole number, a mixed number, or a fraction of a percent.

To convert a whole number percent to a fraction, drop the percent sign and divide the percent whole number by 100. For example, to convert 20% to a fraction, drop the percent sign and divide 20 by 100 ($\frac{20}{100}$). Reduce this number to its lowest common denominator, $\frac{1}{5}$. So 20% of a pizza is the same as $\frac{1}{5}$ of a pizza (remember that 5% of a pizza is the same as $\frac{1}{20}$ of a pizza).

To convert a mixed number to a fraction, first drop the percent sign and change the mixed number to an improper fraction. Then divide that fraction by 100. So, to convert $12\frac{1}{2}$% to a fraction, convert it to an improper fraction ($\frac{25}{2}$) and divide that fraction by 100: $\frac{25}{2} \div \frac{100}{1} = \frac{25}{2} \times \frac{1}{100} = \frac{25}{200}$, which can then be reduced to $\frac{1}{8}$. So, 12.5% or $12\frac{1}{2}$% of a pizza is $\frac{1}{8}$ of a pizza!

You can use the same process to make a fraction of a percent. For example, to express $\frac{1}{4}$% as a fraction, divide it by 100 (which means multiplying it by $\frac{1}{100}$). $\frac{1}{4} \times \frac{1}{100} = \frac{1}{400}$, a mere crumb of a pizza!

Finding the Percentage of a Number

Let's begin with what you already know: 50% of a number is $\frac{1}{2}$ of that number, right? In other words, 50% of 84 is 42. How did you get that answer? You either multiplied 84 by 0.50 or you divided 84 by 2.

What is 30% of 150? This "word" problem is the same as the one you just did in your head. You already know that 30% is equal to 0.3. So, to find 30% of 150, just multiply 150 × 0.3. The answer is 45! Remember to count the total number of decimal places and put the decimal in the correct place in your answer.

SOLVING DOSAGE AND CALCULATION PROBLEMS

As stated earlier, most drugs come from the pharmacy in the correct dose, ready to give to the patients. However, remember that you are the *last check* in the system and are responsible for making sure that the patient not only gets the right drug but also gets the right dose. Always read each drug order carefully, watching for decimal points and zeros.

Sometimes a drug dose that you have on hand does not equal what you *want* to administer to the patient. You will need to calculate the correct drug dose from what you *have* on hand. The first thing you must do is write down all the information that you have and then *label* each number (that is, categorize each number as either *have* or *want*). For example, if you *have* Catapres (clonidine) 0.1 mg and you *want* to give 0.2 mg, first label all the information. Then you may proceed to plug the numbers into the following formulas and do the math. *Finally, do the DIMS (does it make sense?) test to see if the answer makes sense!* You can use these formulas only when the drug dose that you have on hand is in the same measurement unit (for example, milligrams and milligrams) as the drug dose that you want to give.

ORAL DRUGS

Formula 1

This formula works for drug calculations involving dry pills (tablets, capsules, caplets). If the drug order is for 440 mg of naproxen and you have tablets that each contain 220 mg of naproxen, how many tablets should you give? Here is the easy way to know: divide the number you *want* by the number you *have*.

$$\frac{Want}{Have} = \text{Number of tablets to give!}$$

$$\text{So, } \frac{440\,mg}{220\,mg} = (\text{chop off the end zeros}) \frac{44}{22} = 2 \text{ tablets!}$$

What happens if the dose of diazepam (Valium) you *want* is 15 mg and you *have* Valium 10-mg tablets? Use the formula:

$$\frac{15\,mg}{10\,mg} = 1\frac{1}{2} \text{ tablets}$$

You can cut a tablet in half and give a half tablet only if the tablet is scored. A **scored tablet** is one that has a line etched into it marking the exact center (Fig. 3.3). Cutting (or breaking) a tablet along this line gives you two halves of equal known dosages. If you cut or break a tablet that is not scored, the dose will not be correct, and you will have uneven halves. If tablets are not scored, call the pharmacy to see if the drug comes either in a smaller strength or as a liquid.

Other types of drugs that should not be cut or broken include capsules, long-acting or sustained-release capsules or tablets, and enteric-coated tablets. Cutting a capsule allows the powder or tiny beads inside to spill. Long-acting or sustained-release drugs are made so that small amounts of drug are released continuously throughout the day. Cutting this type of drug allows all of the drug to enter the patient's system rapidly and may cause an overdose. Enteric-coated drugs are meant to dissolve and be absorbed in the intestine rather than in the stomach. Cutting or crushing these drugs not only may cause stomach irritation, but the acid in the stomach may inactivate the drugs so they won't work. Always look up any new drug or one you are not familiar with to see if there is any reason that it should not be cut.

Formula 2

This formula works for drug calculations involving oral liquids. These drugs may be called a *suspension* or an *elixir* (an old word for an alcohol-based liquid).

$$\frac{Want}{Have} \times Liquid = \text{Amount of liquid to give}$$

If an order reads, "Give Benadryl (diphenhydramine) 50 mg," and the diphenhydramine liquid comes in 25 mg/5 mL, 5 mL is the amount of liquid in one dose that you have on hand. In this example:

$$\frac{50\,mg}{25\,mg} \times 5\,mL = 2 \times 5\,mL = \text{Give 10 mL}$$

Be sure to label both the numerator and the denominator of the formula to double check that the two dosage measurements you are working with are the same.

DRUGS GIVEN BY INJECTION

There are three major types of injectable drugs: *intramuscular (IM)*, which is injected into a muscle; *subcutaneous*, which is injected into the fat below the skin; and *intradermal (ID)*, which is injected just under the top part of the skin. All three types are *parenteral* forms of drug delivery that do not go through the gastrointestinal tract (see Chapters 1 and 2 for more information about parenteral drug delivery). These drugs may come in either single-dose containers (syringes, vials, or ampules) or multiple-dose bottles (vials).

All injectable drugs are liquids, so they follow the same formula as formula 2 for liquid drugs. For example, the unit-dose syringe that you *have* contains meperidine (Demerol) 100 mg/mL, and you are ordered *(want)* to give 50 mg IM.

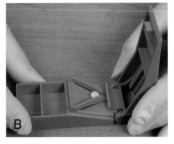

FIG. 3.3 (A) A scored tablet. (B) A cutter for scored tablets.

Critical Point for Safety

Do not attempt to cut drugs that come in these forms:
- Tablet that is not scored
- Capsule
- Gelcap
- Enteric-coated (EC) tablet
- Long-acting (LA), sustained-release (SR), or extended-release (ER) tablet

QSEN: Safety

Try This!

TT-18 How many tablets should you give?
a. *Want* digoxin (Lanoxin) 0.25 mg; *Have* digoxin 0.125 mg
b. *Want* alendronate sodium (Fosamax) 5 mg; *Have* alendronate 10 mg
c. *Want* alprazolam (Xanax) 1.5 mg; *Have* alprazolam 0.5 mg

Answers are at the end of this chapter.

Try This!

TT-19 How many milliliters should you give?
a. *Want* dextromethorphan (Robitussin) 7 mg; *Have* dextromethorphan 3.5 mg/5 mL
b. *Want* acetaminophen (Tylenol) 240 mg; *Have* acetaminophen 80 mg/2.5 mL
c. *Want* ibuprofen (Advil) 100 mg; *Have* ibuprofen 50 mg/1.25 mL

Answers are at the end of this chapter.

Memory Jogger

When dividing a fraction with both the top number (numerator) and the bottom number (denominator) ending in zero, the same number of zeros can be chopped off of both numbers.

Try This!

TT-20 How many milliliters should you give by injection?
a. *Want* hydromorphone (Dilaudid) 1 mg; *Have* a unit-dose syringe with 4 mg/mL
b. *Want* heparin 5000 units; *Have* a unit-dose syringe with 10,000 units/mL
c. *Want* trimethobenzamide 200 mg; *Have* a 20-mL vial with 100 mg/mL

Answers are at the end of this chapter.

Try This!

TT-21 Express the following problems as a fractional proportion.
a. If 3 boats have 6 sails, then 9 boats have 18 sails.
b. If 1 case of IV fluids holds 12 bags, then 3 cases hold 36 bags.
c. If 5 mL have 325 mg of acetaminophen, then 2 mL have 130 mg.

Answers are at the end of this chapter.

Memory Jogger

Remember to label your problem correctly or you might not know what the answer you get actually means!

How should you set up the problem? You would set it up the same way as for other liquid drugs.

$$\frac{Want}{Have} \times Liquid = Amount\ to\ pull\ up\ into\ a\ syringe$$

$$\frac{50\ mg}{100\ mg} \times 1\ mL = \frac{1}{2} = 0.5\ mL\ IM$$

USING PROPORTIONS TO SOLVE FOR *X*

A fraction uses a division line (called a *bar*) or slash to describe a mathematic relationship between two numbers (e.g., $\frac{1}{2}$ or ½). A **proportion** describes an *equal* mathematic relationship between two *sets* of numbers (for example, $\frac{1}{2} = \frac{2}{4}$). If you look closely, you will see that, when you multiply *diagonally* across the equal sign, 1×4 equals 2×2! Another way of thinking of the proportion is that 1 is related to 2 in the same way as 2 is related to 4.

You can use proportions to solve for *X*, the unknown, as an alternate approach to drug calculations, especially if you don't want to memorize a formula. When you write a proportion as a set of fractions, be careful to label each piece of the equation. For example:

$$\frac{1\ case}{12\ bottles} = \frac{3\ cases}{36\ bottles}$$

Notice that in the fractions, *both* numerators identify the number of "cases," and *both* denominators identify the number of bottles. All fractional proportions must be set up this way for you to obtain the correct answer.

What if a piece of the proportion is missing? This is what happens when the prescriber orders a drug strength that is different from the one you have on hand. To figure out how many of the drug tablets you have on hand will be equal to the strength that is ordered, set up a proportion to solve for the missing piece.

For example, an order reads, "Give 500 mg of primidone orally," and you have on hand primidone 250 mg per one caplet. How many caplets will you have to give the patient to equal 500 mg? Set the problem up as:

$$\frac{250\ mg}{1\ caplet} = \frac{500\ mg}{X\ caplets}$$

The *X* is what you need to give. By figuring out the "*X*" correctly, both sides of the proportion will be equal. You can cross out ("cancel") the word "mg" in the proportion equation because they are both known numbers. That leaves you with the word "caplets" as the missing part of the proportion. Therefore, your answer must be the number of *caplets* needed.

Maybe you can do this in your head, but you need to understand how you get the 2 caplets. First, cross multiply to set up the equation $250\ X = 500$. An easy way to work the problem is to remember that any time you bring the number in front of the *X* (250 in this case) across the equals sign (or bring the 250 to the other side of the equals sign), it means *divide*.

$$So,\ X = \frac{500}{250} = 2\ caplets$$

Solving liquid drug problems by proportion involves two steps, but they are relatively easy. First label what you *have* and what you *want*, as usual. Then, set up the proportion. For example, you *want* to give diphenhydramine (Benadryl) 100 mg, and you *have* diphenhydramine 50 mg per mL. How would the proportion be set up?

Step 1:

$$\frac{50\,mg}{1\,mL} = \frac{100\,mg}{X\,mL} \text{ (cancel the mg)}$$

$$50\,X = 100 \text{ or } \frac{100}{50} \text{ (chop the zeros)}; 5\,X = 10 \text{ or } \frac{10}{5}; 10 \div 5 = 2$$

Step 2: Take the answer from step 1 and multiply that times the liquid dose that you have:

$$(\text{Liquid} = 1\,mL) : 2 \times 1\,mL = 2\,mL$$

Try This!

TT-22 How many milliliters should you give?
a. *Want* dextromethorphan (Robitussin) 7 mg; *Have* dextromethorphan 3.5 mg/5 mL
b. *Want* ibuprofen (Advil) 100 mg; *Have* ibuprofen 50 mg/1.25 mL
c. *Want* digoxin (Lanoxin) 0.03 mg; *Have* digoxin 0.05 mg/1 mL

Answers are at the end of this chapter.

Get Ready for the NCLEX® Examination!

Key Points

- The top number of a fraction is the numerator and the bottom number is the denominator.
- If the numerator of a fraction is 1, then the larger the denominator, the smaller a part of the whole it is.
- A whole number is turned into a fraction by making the whole number the numerator and making "1" the denominator.
- Reducing fractions to their lowest terms (1 is the only number that can be evenly divided into the numerator and the denominator) helps simplify working with fractions.
- Adding fractions that have the same denominator involves only adding the numerators; the denominator remains the same.
- Adding fractions that have different denominators requires calculating the lowest common denominator, changing the numerators to proportionately match their new denominators, and adding the numerators.
- Subtracting fractions that have the same denominator involves only subtracting the smaller numerator from the larger numerator; the denominator remains the same.
- Subtracting fractions that have different denominators requires calculating the lowest common denominator, changing the numerators to proportionately match their new denominators, and subtracting the smaller numerator from the larger numerator.
- Multiplying fractions involves multiplying the numerators with one another and then multiplying the denominators with one another.
- When dividing fractions, the second fraction is inverted and multiplied by the first fraction.
- When dividing a fraction with both the top number and the bottom number ending in one or more zeros, the same number of zeros can be "chopped off" *both* numbers.
- Decimal places are always written in multiples of 10.

- The places to the right or left of the decimal determine the value of a number.
- Place a zero before the decimal point of any proper fraction written as a decimal.
- Never put a meaningless zero ("trailing zero") at the end of a decimal.
- To change a fraction into a decimal, always divide the bottom number into the top number.
- To check division of a decimal, multiply the divisor by your answer. If the division was performed correctly, you will get the dividend.
- Moving the decimal point in error to the right will make a drug dose too high and may cause serious or even lethal side effects.
- Moving a decimal point in error to the left will make a drug dose too small to be effective.
- If your drug calculation for tablets results in a decimal number less than 0.5, round down to the next lowest whole number. If the calculation results in a decimal number greater than 0.5, round up to the next highest whole number.
- Do not attempt to cut a tablet that is not scored, a capsule, a gelcap, a drug that is enteric coated, or one that is long acting.
- When reading a drug order, check and double check carefully for decimal points and zeros.
- Remember to label proportion problems so that you know the correct units for your final answer.

Additional Learning Resources

🌐 Be sure to visit your Evolve website (http://evolve.elsevier.com/Workman/pharmacology/) for additional online resources.

SG Go to your Study Guide for additional learning activities to help you master this chapter content.

Review Questions

See *Answers to In-Text Review Questions* in the back of the book for answers to these questions.

1. In the formula $X = \dfrac{100}{25}$, which element of the formula represents the denominator?

   A. X
   B. $=$
   C. The top number
   D. The bottom number

2. Why is $\frac{165}{33}$ an "improper" fraction?

   A. The answer is an odd number.
   B. Neither number can be divided evenly by 2.
   C. The numerator is greater than the denominator.
   D. The denominator is greater than the numerator.

3. Which fraction represents the whole number 16?

   A. $\dfrac{16}{1}$

   B. $\dfrac{16}{16}$

   C. $\dfrac{1}{16}$

   D. $\dfrac{16}{2}$

4. What fraction accurately represents $4\frac{1}{2}$?

   A. $\dfrac{9}{2}$

   B. $\dfrac{5}{16}$

   C. $\dfrac{16}{5}$

   D. $\dfrac{8}{1}$

5. Which fraction is reduced to its lowest terms?

   A. $\dfrac{5}{25}$

   B. $\dfrac{17}{29}$

   C. $\dfrac{2}{8}$

   D. $\dfrac{12}{16}$

6. What is the lowest common denominator for this series of fractions: $\frac{3}{4}, \frac{1}{4}, \frac{3}{5}$?

   A. 12
   B. 15
   C. 20
   D. 30

7. What is the sum of the fractions $\frac{3}{4}, \frac{1}{4}$, and $\frac{3}{5}$?

   A. $\dfrac{32}{20}$ or $1\dfrac{3}{5}$

   B. $\dfrac{35}{20}$ or $1\dfrac{3}{4}$

   C. $\dfrac{64}{40}$ or $1\dfrac{3}{5}$

   D. $\dfrac{70}{40}$ or $1\dfrac{3}{4}$

8. What is the quotient of $\dfrac{1}{3} \div \dfrac{1}{2}$?

   A. $\dfrac{1}{6}$

   B. $\dfrac{1}{3}$

   C. $\dfrac{2}{3}$

   D. $\dfrac{6}{1}$

9. In the equation $75.5 \div 125.5 = 0.6016$, which element is the divisor?

   A. 0.6016
   B. 75.5
   C. 125.5
   D. $\div$

10. What is the quotient of $26.4 \div 16.22$ rounded to the tenth place?

    A. 0.163
    B. 1.628
    C. 16.280
    D. 162.800

11. Which number expresses the fraction $\frac{5}{8}$ as a decimal?

    A. 0.625
    B. 40.05
    C. 1.6
    D. 0.2

12. How much is 18% of 52?

    A. 2.889
    B. 9.36
    C. 288.89
    D. 936

13. The drug and dose prescribed are prednisone 20 mg. The dose of the drug on hand is prednisone 3-mg tablets. What is the relationship between the dose prescribed and the dose on hand?

    A. There is no relationship.
    B. Dose on hand is greater than dose prescribed.
    C. Dose prescribed is greater than dose on hand.
    D. Dose on hand is proportional to dose prescribed.

14. A patient is ordered 1000 mg of penicillin orally. Available are 250-mg tablets. How many tablets should you give to the patient?

   A. $\frac{1}{4}$ of a tablet

   B. $\frac{1}{2}$ of a tablet

   C. 2 tablets
   D. 4 tablets

15. Which response expresses the relationship "50 mL of morphine contains 500 mg of morphine" as a proportion?

   A. 1 mL of morphine contains 5 mg of morphine.
   B. 5 mL of morphine contains 100 mg of morphine.
   C. 10 mL of morphine contains 50 mg of morphine.
   D. 15 mL of morphine contains 150 mg of morphine.

16. You are ordered to give a patient with an allergic reaction 60 mg of diphenhydramine (Benadryl) by IM injection. The vial contains 10 mL of diphenhydramine solution with a concentration of 25 mg/mL. Exactly how many milliliters of diphenhydramine should you give to this patient? _____ mL

Answers to *Math Check* Problems

MC-1 Change these mixed-number fractions into improper fractions.

a. $3\frac{5}{8} = \frac{29}{8}$

b. $7\frac{1}{3} = \frac{22}{3}$

MC-2 Reduce each of these fractions to their lowest common denominators.

a. $\frac{25}{75} = \frac{1}{3}$

b. $\frac{115}{130} = \frac{23}{26}$

MC-3 How many zeros can you chop and drop?

a. $\frac{180}{2200}$ Chop off one zero from the top and bottom to make

   $\{\frac{18}{220}\}$ (reduced to $\{\frac{9}{110}\}$).

b. $\frac{50,000}{100,000}$ Chop off four zeros from the top and bottom to

   make $\frac{5}{10}$ (reduced to $\frac{1}{2}$).

MC-4 Which fraction represents the largest part of the whole for a and b? What is the lowest common denominator for each set of three fractions?

a. $\frac{1}{3}, \frac{10}{15}$, or $\frac{12}{24}$? $\frac{10}{15}$ is the largest part of the whole ($\frac{2}{3}$). The lowest common denominator is 3.

b. $\frac{2}{4}, \frac{6}{8}$, or $\frac{3}{24}$? $\frac{6}{8}$ is the largest part of the whole. The lowest common denominator for these fractions is 4.

   Which fraction represents the smallest part of the whole for c and d? What is the lowest common denominator for each set of three fractions?

c. $\frac{6}{8}, \frac{6}{12}$, or $\frac{2}{3}$? $\frac{6}{12}$ is the smallest part of the whole. The lowest common denominator is 24.

d. $\frac{8}{9}, \frac{1}{3}$, or $\frac{3}{27}$? $\frac{3}{27}$ is the smallest part of the whole. The lowest common denominator for these fractions is 3.

MC-5 Add these fractions. If a sum is an improper fraction, convert it to either a whole number or to a mixed-number fraction.

a. $\frac{1}{3} + \frac{2}{3} + \frac{3}{3} = \frac{6}{3} = 2$

b. $\frac{9}{9} + \frac{5}{9} + \frac{7}{9} + \frac{4}{9} = \frac{25}{9} = 2\frac{7}{9}$

MC-6 Add these fractions. If the sum is an improper fraction, convert it to either a whole number or a mixed-number fraction. Reduce the answers to their lowest common denominators.

a. $\frac{2}{3} + \frac{6}{12} + \frac{6}{8} = \frac{46}{24}$; reduced to $1\frac{22}{24}$; further reduced to $1\frac{11}{12}$

b. $\frac{1}{9} + \frac{3}{4} + \frac{2}{3} = \frac{4}{36} + \frac{27}{36} + \frac{24}{36} = \frac{55}{36}$; reduce to $1\frac{19}{36}$

MC-7 Subtract these fractions. If a fraction is a mixed-number fraction, first convert it to an improper fraction. Reduce answers to their lowest common denominators.

a. $\frac{5}{6} - \frac{2}{6} = \frac{3}{6}$; reduce to $\frac{1}{2}$

b. $2\frac{5}{6} - 1\frac{3}{6} = \frac{17}{6} - \frac{9}{6} = \frac{8}{6} = 1\frac{2}{6} = 1\frac{1}{3}$

MC-8 Subtract these fractions. If a fraction is a mixed-number fraction, first convert it to an improper fraction. Reduce answers to their lowest common denominators.

a. $\frac{7}{8} - \frac{2}{3} = \frac{21}{24} - \frac{16}{24} = \frac{5}{24}$

b. $6\frac{1}{3} - 2\frac{1}{2} = \frac{19}{3} - \frac{5}{2} = \frac{38}{6} - \frac{15}{6} = \frac{23}{6} = 3\frac{5}{6}$

MC-9 Multiply these fractions.

a. $1\frac{22}{24} \times \frac{1}{2} = \frac{46}{24} \times \frac{1}{2} = \frac{46}{48}$; reduce to $\frac{23}{24}$

b. $4\frac{5}{8} \times \frac{2}{3} = \frac{37}{8} \times \frac{2}{3} = \frac{74}{24} = 3\frac{2}{24}$; reduce to $3\frac{1}{12}$

MC-10 Divide these fractions.

a. $\dfrac{7}{8} \div \dfrac{2}{3} = \dfrac{7}{8} \times \dfrac{3}{2} = \dfrac{21}{16}$ or $1\dfrac{5}{16}$

b. $6\dfrac{3}{4} \div 2\dfrac{1}{3} = \dfrac{27}{4} \div \dfrac{7}{3} = \dfrac{27}{4} \times \dfrac{3}{7} = \dfrac{81}{28}$ or $2\dfrac{25}{28}$

MC-11 Decimals as parts of a whole:

a. $0.50 = 50$ parts of 100

b. $2.48 = 2$ whole numbers and 48 parts of 100

MC-12 Multiply these decimals.

a. $16.5 \times 0.5 = 165 \times 5 = 825$, two decimal places, final answer is 8.25

b. $1.2 \times 1.2 = 12 \times 12 = 144$, two decimal places, final answer is 1.44

MC-13 Divide these decimals.

a. $52.8 \div 12 = 120\overline{)528}$, then divide $120\overline{)528}^{\,4.4}$

b. $1.4 \div 1.4 = 14\overline{)14}$, then divide $14\overline{)14}^{\,1}$

MC-14 Change the following fractions to decimals and the decimals to fractions.

a. $0.065 = \dfrac{65}{1000}$; reduced to $\dfrac{13}{200}$

b. $\dfrac{300}{650} = 650\overline{)300}$ $\left(\text{or } 65\overline{)30}\right) = 0.4615$

MC-15 Work to three places and then round to two places.

a. $\dfrac{128.5}{80} = 80\overline{)128.5} = 80\overline{)128.500} = 1.505 = 1.51$

b. $\dfrac{26.8}{13.4} = 13.4\overline{)26.8} = 134\overline{)268} = 2$

MC-16 Convert the following percents into fractions.

a. $\dfrac{2}{3}\% = \dfrac{2}{3} \div \dfrac{100}{1} = \dfrac{2}{3} \times \dfrac{1}{100} = \dfrac{2}{300}$ reduced to $\dfrac{1}{150}$

b. $7\% = 7 \div 100 = \dfrac{7}{100}$ (cannot be reduced further)

MC-17 Find the percentages of the whole number.

a. 0.6% of $50 = 0.006 \times 50 = 0.3$

b. 20% of $120 = 0.2 \times 120 = 24$

MC-18 How many tablets should you give?

a. *Want* carvedilol 25 mg; *Have* carvedilol 6.25 mg: $\dfrac{25\text{ mg}}{6.25\text{ mg}}$

= 4 tablets

b. *Want* estrogen 0.0625 mg; *Have* estrogen 0.125 mg tablet:

$\dfrac{0.0625\text{ mg}}{0.125\text{ mg}} = \dfrac{1}{2}$ tablet

MC-19 How many milliliters should you give?

a. *Want* diphenhydramine (Benadryl) 50 mg; *Have* diphenhydramine 25 mg/5 mL: $\dfrac{50\text{ mg}}{25\text{ mg}} \times 5\text{ mL} = 2 \times 5\text{ mL}$

= give 10 mL

b. *Want* chloral hydrate syrup 100 mg; *Have* chloral hydrate syrup 500 mg/5 mL: $\dfrac{100\text{ mg}}{500\text{ mg}} \times 5\text{ mL} = \dfrac{1}{5} \times 5\text{ mL} =$ give 1 mL

MC-20 How many milliliters should you give by injection?

a. *Want* penicillin 50,000 units; *Have* penicillin 1,000,000 units/50 mL:

$\dfrac{50,000\text{ units}}{1,000,000\text{ units}} \times 50\text{ mL} = \dfrac{1\text{ unit}}{20\text{ units}} \times 50\text{ mL} =$ inject 2.5 mL

b. *Want* prochlorperazine (Compazine) 10 mg; *Have* prochlorperazine 5 mg/mL: $\dfrac{10\text{ mg}}{5\text{ mg}} \times 1\text{ mL} = 2 \times 1\text{ mL}$

= inject 2 mL

MC-21 Express the following problems as a fractional proportion.

a. If one box of eggs has 18 eggs, then two boxes have 36 eggs. $\dfrac{1}{18} = \dfrac{2}{36}$

b. If one chewable tablet of diphenhydramine contains 12.5 mg, then four chewable tablets have 50 mg.

$\dfrac{1\text{ tablet}}{12.5\text{ mg}} = \dfrac{4\text{ tablets}}{50\text{ mg}}$

MC-22 How many milliliters should you give?

a. *Want* carbamazepine (Tegretol) 75 mg oral suspension; *Have* carbamazepine 100 mg/5 mL

$\dfrac{100\text{ mg}}{5\text{ mL}} = \dfrac{75}{X\text{ mL}}$; (cancel mg), $100\,X = 375$ mL; $X = \dfrac{375}{100}$;

$X = 3.75$ mL, give 3.75 mL

b. *Want* acetaminophen (Tylenol) 100 mg; *Have* acetaminophen 160 mg/5 mL:

$\dfrac{160\text{ mg}}{5\text{ mL}} = \dfrac{100\text{ mg}}{X\text{ mL}}$; (cancel mg), $160\,X = 500$ mL; $X = \dfrac{500}{160}$;

$X = 3.125$; (round down), give 3 mL

Answers to *Try This!* Problems

TT-1 Change these mixed-number fractions into improper fractions.

a. $1\dfrac{3}{4} = \dfrac{7}{4}$

b. $2\dfrac{5}{8} = \dfrac{21}{8}$

c. $4\dfrac{1}{5} = \dfrac{21}{5}$

TT-2 Reduce each of these fractions to their lowest common denominators.

a. $\dfrac{10}{24} = \dfrac{5}{12}$

b. $\dfrac{50}{100} = \dfrac{1}{2}$

c. $\dfrac{36}{84} = \dfrac{3}{7}$

TT-3 How many zeros can you chop and drop?

a. $\dfrac{230}{3500}$ Chop off one zero from the top and bottom to make $\dfrac{23}{350}$.

b. $\dfrac{1400}{10}$ Chop off one zero from the top and bottom to make $\dfrac{140}{1}$.

c. $\dfrac{20}{500}$ Chop off one zero from the top and bottom to make $\dfrac{2}{50}$.

TT-4 Which fraction represents the largest part of the whole?

a. $\dfrac{1}{2}$, $\dfrac{3}{4}$, or $\dfrac{7}{8}$? $\dfrac{7}{8}$ is the largest part of the whole. The lowest common denominator for these fractions is 8.

b. $\dfrac{1}{5}$, $\dfrac{5}{15}$, or $\dfrac{6}{45}$? $\dfrac{5}{15}$ is the largest part of the whole. The lowest common denominator for these fractions is 15. (Hint: $\dfrac{6}{45}$ is not in lowest terms.)

Which fraction represents the smallest part of the whole?

c. $\dfrac{1}{3}$, $\dfrac{1}{5}$, or $\dfrac{1}{6}$? $\dfrac{1}{6}$ is the smallest part of the whole. The lowest common denominator for these fractions is 30.

d. $\dfrac{1}{2}$, $\dfrac{3}{8}$, or $\dfrac{3}{4}$? $\dfrac{3}{8}$ is the smallest part of the whole. The lowest common denominator for these fractions is 8.

TT-5 Add these fractions. If a sum is an improper fraction, convert it to a mixed-number fraction.

a. $\dfrac{1}{7} + \dfrac{5}{7} = \dfrac{6}{7}$

b. $\dfrac{1}{5} + \dfrac{2}{5} + \dfrac{1}{5} = \dfrac{4}{5}$

c. $\dfrac{6}{8} + \dfrac{1}{8} + \dfrac{3}{8} + \dfrac{5}{8} = \dfrac{15}{8} = 1\dfrac{7}{8}$

TT-6 Add these fractions. If the sum is an improper fraction, convert it to either a whole number or a mixed-number fraction.

a. $\dfrac{4}{7} + \dfrac{2}{5} = \dfrac{20}{35} + \dfrac{14}{35} = \dfrac{34}{35}$ (cannot be reduced further)

b. $\dfrac{3}{4} + \dfrac{1}{3} + \dfrac{5}{6} = \dfrac{9}{12} + \dfrac{4}{12} + \dfrac{10}{12} = \dfrac{23}{12}$; convert to $1\dfrac{11}{12}$

c. $\dfrac{1}{2} + \dfrac{1}{6} + \dfrac{1}{5} = \dfrac{15}{30} + \dfrac{5}{30} + \dfrac{6}{30} = \dfrac{26}{30}$; reduce to $\dfrac{13}{15}$

TT-7 Subtract these fractions. If a fraction is a mixed-number fraction, first convert it to an improper fraction. Reduce answers to their lowest common denominators.

a. $\dfrac{4}{5} - \dfrac{1}{5} = \dfrac{3}{5}$

b. $1\dfrac{1}{3} - \dfrac{2}{3} = \dfrac{4}{3} - \dfrac{2}{3} = \dfrac{2}{3}$

c. $\dfrac{3}{4} - \dfrac{1}{4} = \dfrac{2}{4}$; reduce to $\dfrac{1}{2}$

TT-8 Subtract these fractions. If a fraction is a mixed-number fraction, first convert it to an improper fraction. Reduce answers to their lowest common denominators.

a. $\dfrac{3}{4} - \dfrac{2}{3} = \dfrac{9}{12} - \dfrac{8}{12} = \dfrac{1}{12}$ (cannot be reduced further)

b. $2\dfrac{2}{3} - 1\dfrac{1}{2} = \dfrac{8}{3} - \dfrac{3}{2} = \dfrac{16}{6} - \dfrac{9}{6} = 1\dfrac{1}{6}$

c. $\dfrac{4}{5} - \dfrac{1}{3} = \dfrac{12}{15} - \dfrac{5}{15} = \dfrac{7}{15}$ (cannot be reduced further)

TT-9 Multiply these fractions.

a. $1\dfrac{3}{4} \times 5\dfrac{6}{7} = \dfrac{7}{4} \times \dfrac{41}{7} = \dfrac{287}{28}$; reduce to $10\dfrac{1}{4}$

b. $2\dfrac{2}{4} \times 6\dfrac{7}{8} = \dfrac{10}{4} \times \dfrac{55}{8} = \dfrac{550}{32}$, or $\dfrac{275}{16}$; reduce to $17\dfrac{3}{16}$

c. $\dfrac{3}{4} \times 9\dfrac{11}{16} = \dfrac{3}{4} \times \dfrac{155}{16} = \dfrac{465}{64}$; reduce to $7\dfrac{17}{64}$

TT-10 Divide these fractions.

a. $3 \div \dfrac{1}{2} = \dfrac{3}{1} \div \dfrac{1}{2} = \dfrac{3}{1} \times \dfrac{2}{1} = \dfrac{6}{1}$ or 6

b. $\dfrac{3}{4} \div \dfrac{1}{2} = \dfrac{3}{4} \times \dfrac{2}{1} = \dfrac{6}{4} = 1\dfrac{2}{4}$ or $1\dfrac{1}{2}$

c. $5\frac{1}{4} \div \frac{6}{8} = \frac{21}{4} \div \frac{6}{8} = \frac{21}{4} \times \frac{8}{6} = \frac{168}{24}$ or 7

TT-11 Decimals as parts of a whole.

a. 0.3 = 3 parts of 10

b. 0.75 = 75 parts of 100

c. 5.1 = 5 whole numbers and 1 part of 10

TT-12 Multiply these decimals.

a. $100 \times 0.25 = 100 \times 25 = 2500$, two decimal places, final answer is 25

b. $51.2 \times 2.1 = 512 \times 21 = 10752$, two decimal places, final answer is 107.52

c. $15.5 \times 10 = 155 \times 10 = 1550$, one decimal place, final answer is 155

TT-13 Divide these decimals.

a. $630 \div 0.3 = 3\overline{)6300}$, then divide $3\overline{)6300}^{2100}$

b. $0.125 \div 0.5 = 5\overline{)1.25}$, then divide $5\overline{)1.25}^{0.25}$

c. $2.5 \div 0.75 = 75\overline{)250}$, then divide $75\overline{)250}^{3.33}$

TT-14 Change the following fractions to decimals and the decimals to fractions.

a. $\frac{3}{4} = 4\overline{)3} = 0.75$

b. $0.55 = \frac{55}{100}$; reduced to $\frac{11}{20}$

c. $0.075 = \frac{75}{1000}$; reduced to $\frac{3}{40}$

d. $1.25 = 1\frac{25}{100}$ or $1\frac{1}{4}$

e. $\frac{7}{8} = 8\overline{)7} = 0.875$

TT-15 Work to three places and then round to two places.

a. $\frac{58.4}{33} = 33\overline{)58.4} = 330\overline{)584.000} = 1.769 = 1.77$

b. $\frac{6}{3.4} = 3.4\overline{)6} = 34\overline{)60.000} = 1.764 = 1.76$

c. $\frac{27.5}{3.4} = 3.4\overline{)27.5} = 34\overline{)275.000} = 8.088 = 8.09$

TT-16 Convert the following percents into fractions.

a. $\frac{1}{2}\% = \frac{1}{2} \div \frac{100}{1} = \frac{1}{2} \times \frac{1}{100} = \frac{1}{200}$

b. $3\% = 3 \div 100 = \frac{3}{100}$ (cannot be reduced further)

c. $5\frac{3}{4}\% = \frac{23}{4} \div \frac{100}{1} = \frac{23}{4} \times \frac{1}{100} = \frac{23}{400}$ (cannot be reduced further)

TT-17 Find the percentages of the whole numbers.

a. 25% of 300 = 0.25 × 300 = 75

b. 10% of $5.00 = 0.1 × $5.00 = $.50

c. 0.2% of 10 = 0.002 × 10 = 0.02

TT-18 How many tablets should you give?

a. *Want* digoxin (Lanoxin) 0.25 mg; *Have* digoxin 0.125-mg tablet: $\frac{0.25 \text{ mg}}{0.125 \text{ mg}}$ = two tablets

b. *Want* alendronate sodium (Fosamax) 5 mg; *Have* alendronate 10-mg tablet: $\frac{5 \text{ mg}}{10 \text{ mg}} = \frac{1}{2}$ tablet

c. *Want* alprazolam (Xanax) 1.5 mg; *have* alprazolam 0.5-mg tablet: $\frac{1.5 \text{ mg}}{0.5 \text{ mg}}$ = three tablets

TT-19 How many milliliters should you give?

a. *Want* dextromethorphan (Robitussin) 7 mg; *Have* dextromethorphan 3.5 mg/5 mL: $\frac{7 \text{ mg}}{3.5 \text{ mg}} \times 5 \text{ mL} = 2 \times 5 \text{ mL}$ = give 10 mL

b. *Want* acetaminophen (Tylenol) 240 mg; *Have* acetaminophen 80 mg/2.5 mL: $\frac{240 \text{ mg}}{80 \text{ mg}} \times 2.5 \text{ mL} = 3 \times 2.5 \text{ mL}$ = give 7.5 mL

c. *Want* ibuprofen (Advil) 100 mg; *Have* ibuprofen 50 mg/1.25 mL: $\frac{100 \text{ mg}}{50 \text{ mg}} \times 1.25 \text{ mL} = 2 \times 1.25 \text{ mL}$ = give 2.5 mL

TT-20 How many milliliters should you give by injection?

a. *Want* hydromorphone (Dilaudid) 1 mg; *Have* a unit-dose syringe with 4 mg per mL: $\frac{1 \text{ mg}}{4 \text{ mg}} \times 1 \text{ mL} = 0.25 \times 1 \text{ mL}$ = inject 0.25 mL

b. *Want* heparin 5000 units; *Have* a unit-dose syringe with 10,000 units/mL: $\frac{5000 \text{ units}}{10,000 \text{ units}} \times 1 \text{ mL} = 0.5 \times 1 \text{ mL}$ = inject 0.5 mL

c. *Want* trimethobenzamide 200 mg; *Have* 20 mL vial with 100 mg/mL: $\frac{200 \text{ mg}}{100 \text{ mg}} \times 1 \text{ mL} = 2 \times 1 \text{ mL}$ = inject 2 mL

TT-21 Express the following problems as a fractional proportion.

a. If three boats have 6 sails, then nine boats have 18 sails.

$\frac{3}{6} = \frac{9}{18}$

b. If one case of IV fluids holds 12 bags, then three cases hold 36 bags. $\frac{1}{12} = \frac{3}{36}$

c. If 5 mL have 325 mg of acetaminophen, then 2 mL have 130 mg. $\dfrac{5\ \text{mL}}{325\ \text{mg}} = \dfrac{1\ \text{mL}}{65\ \text{mg}} = \dfrac{2\ \text{mL}}{130\ \text{mg}}$

TT-22 How many milliliters should you give?

a. *Want* dextromethorphan (Robitussin) 7 mg; *Have* dextromethorphan 3.5 mg/5 mL:

$\dfrac{3.5\ \text{mg}}{5\ \text{mL}} = \dfrac{7\ \text{mg}}{X\ \text{mL}}$; (cancel mg), 3.5 X = 35; $X = \dfrac{7}{3.5} = 2$;

2 × 5 mL = give 10 mL

b. *Want* ibuprofen (Advil) 100 mg; *Have* ibuprofen 50 mg/1.25 mL:

$\dfrac{50\ \text{mg}}{1.25\ \text{mL}} = \dfrac{100\ \text{mg}}{X\ \text{mL}}$; (cancel mg), 50 X = 125; $X = \dfrac{100}{50} = 2$;

2 × 1.25 mL = give 2.5 mL

c. *Want* digoxin (Lanoxin) 0.03 mg; *Have* digoxin 0.05 mg/1 mL:

$\dfrac{0.05\ \text{mg}}{1\ \text{mL}} = \dfrac{0.03\ \text{mg}}{X\ \text{mL}}$; (cancel mg), 0.05 X = 0.03; X = 0.6;

0.6 × 1 mL = give 0.6 mL

4

Medical Systems of Weights and Measures

Learning Objectives

The content presented in this chapter should help you to:

1. Define common units of measure for liquids and solids.
2. Convert from the household system of measurement to the metric system of measurement.
3. Identify the three basic units of measure in the metric system.
4. Identify the unit of measure using a prefix and a root word.
5. Convert milliliters to liters; convert liters to milliliters.
6. Convert ounces and pounds to grams and kilograms.
7. Solve dosage problems using the metric system.
8. Solve drug calculation problems using units.

Key Terms

centigrade or Celsius (SĔN-tĭ-grād, SĔL-sē-ŭs) (p. 68) Metric or hospital scale of temperature measurement based on 100. Zero (0) degrees is the freezing point of water, and 100° is the boiling point of water. Normal human body temperature ranges between 36.1° and 37.8°.

dimensional analysis (dĭ-MĒN-shŭn-ăl ă-NĂL-ă-sĭs) (p. 73) A method of comparing and equating different physical quantities by using simple algebraic rules along with known conversion factors (called equivalency ratios).

equivalent (ē-KWĬV-ĕ-lĕnt) (p. 66) To be equal in amount or to have equal value.

Fahrenheit (FĂR-ĕn-hīt) (p. 68) System of temperature measurement used in the United States in which the freezing point of water is 32° above zero and the boiling point of water is 212°. Normal human body temperature ranges between 97° and 100°.

gram (g) (GRĂM) (p. 70) The basic metric unit for measurement of weight.

liter (L) (LĒ-tŭr) (p. 70) The basic metric unit for measurement of liquids.

meter (m) (MĒ-tŭr) (p. 70) The basic metric unit for measurement of length or distance.

OVERVIEW

Systems of weights and measures standardize the ways of comparing two or more objects for size and strength. The first measuring system discussed in this chapter is for temperature. All systems that follow are used in prescribing drugs. For solving the conversion problems in this chapter, you will need to apply the math principles presented in Chapter 3, including using proportions.

Most drugs are measured by weight (e.g., an extra-strength acetaminophen [Tylenol] tablet contains 500 mg of drug) or liquid volume (5 mL or 1 tsp of diphenhydramine [Benadryl]). This chapter identifies which units are used for *dry weights* and which are used for *liquids* for each measuring system. After each system is presented, there will be practice problems to work so you can see exactly how each system is used.

To convert from one system to another, values that are equal to each other, known as **equivalents**, are used. You need to understand and either memorize the equivalents in each system or carry a conversion card with you so you can convert from one system to another quickly and easily.

MATH CHECK

You may already be familiar with weights and measures, as well as converting from one system to another. Use the following math check problems to determine your understanding of specific concepts for weights and measures and your skill level in converting from one system to another. The answers to these problems are listed at the end of the chapter. If you are accurate in your math for these problems, you may not need to review some of the content in this chapter. If you have a weakness in any specific area, review the content and principles for that area.

MATH CHECK PROBLEMS

MC-1 Convert the Fahrenheit temperature to Centigrade and the Centigrade temperature to Fahrenheit.

a. 101.4°F = _____ °C

b. 40°C = _____ °F

MC-2 Calculate the response in teaspoons or drops. (Note: "How to" math steps for conversion of *Want* versus *Have* problems are in Chapter 3.)

a. *Want* Benadryl 5 mg; *Have* Benadryl 12.5 mg/5 mL _____ drops (gtts)

b. *Want* acetaminophen 200 mg; *Have* acetaminophen 40 mg/mL _____ teaspoons

MC-3 Convert the following weights in pounds to kilograms and the weights in kilograms to pounds.

a. 25 lb

b. 260 lb

c. 45 kg

d. 90 kg

MC-4 Convert these household measures into metric equivalents, rounding to the nearest tenth when necessary.

a. 3 tablespoons

b. 8.8 lb

c. 20 inches

d. 4 ounces

e. 4 teaspoons

MC-5 Convert these metric measures into household equivalents.

a. 75 kg

b. 180 mL

c. 75 g

d. 500 mL

MC-6 Calculate how much drug you should administer.

a. *Want* potassium 20 mEq in extended-release tablet; *Have* potassium 5 mEq in extended-release tablet

b. *Want* potassium gluconate 30 mEq oral solution; *Have* potassium gluconate 20 mEq/15 mL oral solution.

MC-7 Calculate how many milliliters you should give.

a. *Want* heparin 1250 units subcutaneously; *Have* heparin 1000 units/mL

b. *Want* heparin 1250 units intravenously; *Have* heparin 500 units/mL

MC-8 Calculate how many milligrams in how many teaspoons you will give to a child who weighs 26.8 lb.

Want acyclovir 20 mg/kg; *Have* acyclovir 200 mg/5 mL oral suspension

MC-9 Using dimensional analysis and showing your work, calculate the dosages for these problems.

a. Dilantin (phenytoin) 100 mg is prescribed to give a child orally. The drug available is Dilantin 125 mg/5 mL. How many milliliters of this solution should be administered to equal the ordered dose?

b. A patient who weighs 154 lb is prescribed to receive 50,000 units of penicillin intravenously per kg of weight. The penicillin solution you have on hand is 1,000,000 units/25 mL. How many milliliters should you give by intravenous (IV) injection?

MEASURING SYSTEMS FOR TEMPERATURE: FAHRENHEIT AND CELSIUS

When measuring temperature, the symbol ° is used in place of the word "degree." Some hospitals use the metric system for measuring temperature (Celsius [C]), and other settings use the Fahrenheit (F) system. Nurses must be familiar with both

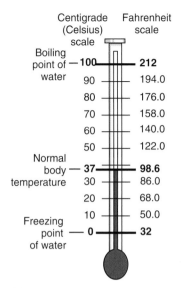

FIG. 4.1 Comparing Centigrade to Fahrenheit values with a mercury thermometer.

systems of measurement. In the **Fahrenheit** system, the freezing point of water is 32° above zero, and the boiling point of water is 212°. The normal human body temperature ranges between 97° and 100°. The **centigrade** or **Celsius** system is based on the number 100. Zero (0) degrees is set as the freezing point of water, and 100° is used for the boiling point of water. Normal human body temperature ranges between 36.1° and 37.8°.

Digital thermometers are often used to check body temperature and can be set for either system. For learning purposes, picture the old mercury thermometers such as the one shown in Fig. 4.1. As you can see in the figure, there is a big difference in ranges between centigrade (Celsius) and Fahrenheit temperatures. To change from one system to another, use the following two equations or a conversion chart. Conversion is often necessary because patients usually report their temperatures from home using a thermometer with a Fahrenheit scale.

EQUATION 1: FAHRENHEIT TO CENTIGRADE

$$(\text{Fahrenheit temperature} - 32) \times \frac{5}{9} = \text{Degrees Centigrade}$$

First, subtract 32° from 102° (102° − 32°) for an answer of 70 and plug that number into the formula:

$$70 \times \frac{5}{9}$$

Multiply 70 by 5, which equals 350. Divide 350 by 9, which equals 38.88°.

If the answer has more than one decimal place, round to the nearest tenth of a degree (e.g., 38.9°, not 38.88°).

EQUATION 2: CENTIGRADE TO FAHRENHEIT

$$(\text{Centigrade temperature}) \times \frac{9}{5} + 32 = \text{Degrees Fahrenheit}$$

Place the centigrade temperature of 41°C into the formula:

$$41 \times \frac{9}{5} + 32$$

Multiply 41 by 9, which equals 369. Divide 369 by 5, which equals 73.8. Add 32, which makes the answer 105.8.

If the answer has more than one decimal place, round to the nearest tenth of a degree (e.g., 100.6°, not 100.59°).

HOUSEHOLD SYSTEM FOR LIQUID AND DRY MEASUREMENTS

Household measurements are used in measuring ingredients for cooking. This same system is the often used by patients when they are taking *liquid* drugs at home.

The household system uses drops (gtts), teaspoons (tsp), tablespoons (Tbs), ounces (oz), and cups (c) to measure liquids. Note that a liquid ounce is *not* equal to a dry ounce such as flour. In cooking, liquid ounces are measured in a one-piece measuring cup (often made of glass), and dry ounces are measured in nested cups (Fig. 4.2). In health care, liquid drugs have their own special measuring tools. Table 4.1 lists household abbreviations and equivalents.

The only *dry* measures used in the household system for health care purposes are ounces and pounds. In the United States, patients report their weight in pounds (lb). Weight in pounds often must be converted to kilograms (kg) in the hospital or other health care setting.

Larger liquid household measures include the pint, quart, and gallon. These larger measures are discussed later in the chapter under the metric system.

Table 4.1	Abbreviations and Equivalents for the Household System of Measure	
ABBREVIATION	**MEANING**	**EQUIVALENT**
Dry Measure (Smallest to Largest)		
Oz	Ounce	16 oz = 1 lb
Lb	Pound	1 lb = 16 oz
Liquid Measure (Smallest to Largest)		
gtts	Drops	60 gtts = 1 tsp
tsp	Teaspoon	3 tsp = 1 Tbs
Tbs	Tablespoon	2 Tbs = 1 oz
fl oz	Fluid ounce	8 oz = 1 c 16 oz = 1 pt 32 oz = 1 qt 64 oz = ½ gal 128 oz = 1 gal
c	Cup	2 c = 1 p 4 c = 1 qt 8 c = ½ gal 16 c = 1 gal
pt	Pint	2 pt = 1 qt 4 pt = ½ gal 8 pt = 1 gal
qt	Quart	4 qt = 1 gal
gal	Gallon	1 gal = 4 qt
Length (Smallest to Largest)		
in	Inch	12 in = 1 ft
ft	Foot	3 ft = 1 yd 5280 ft = 1 mile
yd	Yard	1 yd = 3 ft 1760 yd = 1 mile

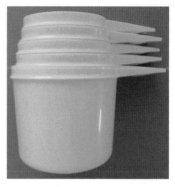

FIG. 4.2 Nested cups used to measure dry ingredients in the household system.

Teaching Alert

Teach patients who are taking liquid drugs to buy and use only measuring tools that are designed and calibrated for liquid drugs rather than using tableware spoons to measure liquid drugs.

QSEN: Safety

Administration Alert

When using a dropper to administer liquid drugs, place it into the side of the patient's mouth rather than in the middle, where it can move down the throat too quickly and cause choking.

QSEN: Safety

Administration Alert

Always double check the amount of drug in any measuring device against the amount ordered to prevent giving an overdose.

QSEN: Safety

 Try This!

TT-2 Calculate the response in teaspoons or drops. (Note: "How to" math steps for conversion of *Want* versus *Have* problems are in Chapter 3.)
a. *Want* ampicillin 750 mg; *Have* ampicillin 250 mg/tsp
b. *Want* guaifenesin 50 mg; *Have* guaifenesin 100 mg/60 gtts
c. *Want* milk of magnesia 1 Tbs; *Have* milk of magnesia 1 tsp

Answers are at the end of this chapter.

Patients often use the teaspoons and tablespoons from tableware to measure liquid drugs. However, these spoons are *not* accurate, and patients should be instructed *not* to use them to measure drugs. It is best to use measuring tools that are designed and *calibrated* (marked in accurate units) for liquid drugs. These include the dropper, oral syringe, medication spoon, and small medicine cup (see Fig. 2.3 in Chapter 2). All of these can be purchased in any pharmacy or drugstore and even in many grocery stores.

Droppers are marked in both teaspoons and milliliters (mL; metric). Check the drug order carefully to determine which measurement is correct.

The most common device for measuring oral drugs in the hospital is the *oral syringe* (similar to a dropper). Oral syringes are marked in both teaspoons and milliliters. The rubber stopper is small enough to be aspirated (inhaled) into the lungs, so be sure to remove the stopper before you attempt to use the syringe.

Medication spoons have calibrated hollow handles and are useful for giving small doses between 1 and 2 tsp (5 to 10 mL). Mark the desired dose with your finger and hold the spoon at eye level to ensure that the dose you pour is accurate.

Medicine cups are useful to measure and give liquid doses from 1 tsp to 1 oz. The cup is marked around its sides in teaspoons, tablespoons, and ounces. Note that the ounce is marked "FL OZ" to indicate that this cup is for liquids only. The other marks indicate the liquid unit of the metric system: the milliliter (mL).

To use the cup accurately, fill while holding it at eye level. Either place the cup on a table and bend to look straight at the mark or hold it up to your eyes as you fill it (see Fig. 2.4 in Chapter 2). Looking down at the mark or from an angle will result in an inaccurate dose.

Box **4.1**	Metric Equivalents				

DRY		**LIQUID**		**LENGTH**	
1 kg	= 1000 g	1 L	= 1000 mL	1 m (meter)	= 100 cm
1 g	= 1000 mg	1 mL	= $\dfrac{1}{1000}$ L		= 1000 mm
	= $\dfrac{1}{1000}$ kg			1 cm	= 10 mm
					= $\dfrac{1}{100}$ meter
1 mg	= $\dfrac{1}{1000}$ g			1 mm	= $\dfrac{1}{10}$ cm
					= $\dfrac{1}{1000}$ meter

METRIC SYSTEM

The metric system is the most used system worldwide for drug prescriptions because it is accurate even in small doses. This system is based on the number 10 and uses the decimal system (multiples of 10) (see Chapter 3 for a review of decimals). In giving drugs, only a few metric measurements are used. For a more complete discussion of the metric system, consult a mathematics text. This system is not difficult, and you *can* learn it!

METRIC BASICS

The three basic units of the metric system are the **meter** (length), the **liter** (liquid), and the **gram** (weight). Each of these three words forms the *root* (that part or parts of a multiple-part word that indicates the basic meaning) of every metric measuring unit. Always look for these root words in each metric measurement. They indicate whether you are measuring a length, liquid volume, or weight. For example:

- Your height can be measured in either inches or centi*meters*.
- Your weight can be measured in pounds or kilo*grams*.
- Penicillin is prescribed in 250-milli*gram* tablets.
- A household quart is slightly less than a *liter*.

Box 4.1 lists basic metric equivalents.

Just as in decimals, there are measurements for *less than* and *more than* the basic unit. These descriptive words are called *prefixes* because they come before the root of a word. Which prefix is attached to the root explains how much larger or smaller each unit is in relation to the basic unit. For example, weight can be written in *kilo*grams, in which a kilogram is 1000 times heavier or *larger* than a gram. Drugs are often prescribed using the *milli*gram, which is 1000 times *smaller* than a gram. See Table 4.2 for a list of the prefixes most commonly used in health care, listed from large to small.

METRIC ABBREVIATIONS

The basic metric unit abbreviations are meter (m), liter (L), and gram (g). Note that the "L" for liter is capitalized to avoid confusion with other abbreviations. Table 4.2 lists the abbreviations most often used.

The metric units for liquids are used for liquid oral drugs and intravenous (IV) fluids. The metric units for weight are used for drug doses and to weigh objects, including the human body. Two prefixes for weights are very small, the microgram (mcg) and the nanogram (ng). Both micrograms and nanograms are the exceptions to the "three decimal place" rule discussed in Chapter 3.

SWITCHING BETWEEN HOUSEHOLD AND METRIC SYSTEMS

As a nurse you are often the medical interpreter for your patients and must be able to quickly switch or convert between metric and household measurements. Only practice will make you comfortable with the conversion (switching) process. Begin with the smaller equivalents, and move to the larger ones. Box 4.2 shows

Drug Alert

Administration Alert

The milligram is 1000 times stronger than the microgram. Confusion could lead to a BIG overdose. If any drug dose order is written using an abbreviation, always clarify with the prescriber which unit is meant before giving the drug.

QSEN: Safety

Memory Jogger

Remember from the drug dosage calculations that **L** stood for liquid dose. This will help you to remember that liters (L) are a way of measuring liquids.

Table **4.2**	Metric Prefixes and Abbreviations	
PREFIX	**ABBREVIATION**	**MEANING**
Weight (Gram) (g)		
kilo	kg	1000 g
milli	mg	0.001 or $\dfrac{1}{1000}$ of a gram
micro	mcg	0.000001 or $\dfrac{1}{1,000,000}$ of a gram
		$\dfrac{1}{1000}$ of a milligram
nano	ng	0.000000001 or $\dfrac{1}{1,000,000,000}$ of a gram
Liquids (Liter)		
deci	dL	100 mL
		0.1 or $\dfrac{1}{10}$ of a liter
milli	mL	0.001 or $\dfrac{1}{1000}$ of a liter
Length (Meter)		
kilo	km	1000 meters
centi	cm	0.01 or $\dfrac{1}{100}$ of a meter
milli	mm	0.001 or $\dfrac{1}{1000}$ of a meter

 Memory Jogger

Because 1 kg is equal to 2.2 lb, a person's weight in kilograms is *always* less than half his or her weight in pounds.

Box **4.2**	Household-to-Metric Equivalents

DRY WEIGHT

1 oz	= 30 g (30,000 mg)
16 oz	= 1 lb
	= 454 g
2.2 lb	= 1 kg

LENGTH

1 in	= 2.54 cm
1 ft	= 30.48 cm

LIQUID

15 gtts	= 1 mL
1 tsp	= 5 mL
1 Tbs	= 15 mL
2 Tbs	= 30 mL
1 fl oz	= 30 mL
8 fl oz	= 1 c
	= 240 mL
1 pt	= 500 mL (slightly less)
	= 0.5 L (slightly less)
1 qt	= 1000 mL (slightly less)
	= 1 L

household-to-metric equivalents. Remember that metric measurements are precise, and household measurements are only approximate, at best. When using household measuring instruments for drugs, the dose is not exact. One of the most common switching situations is changing a patient's weight between pounds and kilograms. One kilogram is equal to 2.2 lb. So, a person's weight in kilograms is *always* less than half of his or her weight in pounds. To obtain the kilogram weight, first weigh the patient on a standard pound scale and then *divide* this number by 2.2. For example, a patient who weighs 232 lb weighs 105.45 kg (round to 105.5 kg). A patient who weighs 120 lb weighs 54.5 kg. To change weight in kilograms to pounds, *multiply* the

 Try This!

TT-3 Convert the following weights in pounds to kilograms and the weights in kilograms to pounds.
a. 98 lb
b. 54 lb
c. 315 lb
d. 2.9 lb
e. 145 lb
f. 68 kg
g. 12 kg
h. 128 kg
i. 52 kg
j. 80 kg

Answers are at the end of this chapter.

Administration Alert

Switching from one measuring system to another is only approximately right. Always apply the DIMS test ("does it make sense?") when converting between systems. If an answer does not make sense to you (e.g., give 50 tsp), redo the math and ask for help.

QSEN: Safety

TT-4 Convert these household measures into metric equivalents, rounding to the nearest tenth when necessary.
a. 250 lb
b. 10 oz (liquid)
c. 17 in
d. 5 Tbs
e. 2 tsp

Answers are at the end of this chapter.

TT-5 Convert these metric measures into household equivalents.
a. 45 g
b. 120 mL
c. 1500 mL
d. 110 kg
e. 780 g

Answers are at the end of this chapter.

TT-6 Calculate how much drug you should administer.
a. *Want* potassium 24 mEq in extended-release tablet; *Have* potassium 8 mEq in extended-release tablet
b. *Want* potassium 10 mEq effervescent tablet; *Have* potassium 20 mEq scored effervescent tablet
c. *Want* potassium 10 mEq in an oral solution; *Have* potassium 20 mEq dissolved in 8 oz of water

Answers are at the end of this chapter.

Administration Alert

To prevent insulin dose errors, check the specific markings on the syringe rather than relying on the color of the cap, needle hub, or box label.

QSEN: Safety

kilogram number by 2.2. For example, the patient who weighs 90 kg weighs 198 lb. The infant who weighs 1.6 kg weighs 3.5 lb.

MILLIEQUIVALENT MEASURES

Milliequivalents (mEq) are used to measure electrolytes. *Electrolytes* are minerals and chemicals in the body that have a positive or negative charge. The electrolytes most often calculated in milliequivalents are potassium chloride (KCl), potassium phosphate (KPO_4), potassium gluconate, sodium, and some types of calcium (Ca^{++}). The electrolyte most often prescribed is KCl, which can be given orally or mixed with IV fluid. Whichever way it is given, it is irritating to the body.

Potassium can be given as a tablet, an extended-release tablet, or an effervescent (fizzy) tablet, in a liquid, as a powder, or dissolved in IV fluids. The different types are *NOT interchangeable*. Do not substitute a different potassium type for the one prescribed.

Although drugs measured and prescribed in milliequivalents sound different from those measured and prescribed in milligrams, the dosage calculations are performed exactly the same way. Once again, you are determining the amount of tablets or milliliters to administer based on what you *want* versus what you *have* on hand. (If necessary, review drug dosage calculations in Chapter 3.) For example, the order reads "potassium chloride (Slow-K) 40 mEq orally," and you have Slow-K tablets that contain 20 mEq/tablet. Divide the number you *want* by the number you *have*.

$$\frac{\text{Want}}{\text{Have}} = \text{Number of tablets to give! Want 40 mEq; Have 20 mEq.}$$

$$\text{So,} \frac{40\,\text{mEq}}{20\,\text{mEq/1 tablet}} = (\text{chop off the end zeroes}) \frac{4}{2} = 2\,\text{tablets!}$$

UNIT MEASURES

Drugs measured in units come in either plain or international units. The most common drugs measured in units are insulin and heparin (a drug to reduce blood clotting). Others include injectable penicillin and some vitamins.

INSULIN

Insulin is a drug used by some patients with diabetes to replace the insulin their bodies no longer make. (Chapter 21 has more information about diabetes and insulin.) The drug insulin is very concentrated and requires special syringes. The most common insulin syringe holds 50 units in one small 0.5-mL syringe. Each unit on the syringe is marked up to 50. However, there are many different types of insulin syringes. Some are measured up to 100 units, and others are measured up to 500 units. These syringes *cannot* be interchanged with one another or with noninsulin syringes. Carefully check the concentration of insulin in the bottle with the type of syringe chosen to make sure that you have the correct syringe. Do not go by the color of the syringe to determine whether the syringe is a 50-unit insulin syringe. *There is no common color for insulin syringe types.* Check the specific markings on the syringe rather than going by the color of the cap, needle hub, or box label. If the incorrect dose of insulin is given, severe hypoglycemia and death can result. Chapter 21 discusses safe insulin administration in detail.

HEPARIN

Heparin is a fast-acting anticoagulant (drug to slow or prevent blood clotting) that leaves the body quickly. A discussion of heparin and heparin-like drugs can be found in Chapter 17.

Heparin is only given by subcutaneous injection or into an IV site. It comes in single- and multiple-dose vials. In addition, weaker solutions of heparin are available already loaded in single-use syringes. Strengths of heparin vary from 10 units/mL to 40,000 units/mL.

Although drugs measured and prescribed in units sound different from those measured and prescribed in milligrams, the dosage calculations are performed exactly the same way. Once again, you are determining the milliliters to administer based on what you *want* versus what you *have* on hand. (If necessary, review drug dosage calculations in Chapter 3.) For example, the order reads "heparin 2000 units subcutaneously," and you have heparin 5000 units/mL. Divide the number you *want* by the number you *have*.

$$\frac{\text{Want}}{\text{Have}} = \text{Number of milliliters!}$$

$$\text{Want } 2000 \text{ units, Have } 5000 \text{ units}$$

$$\frac{2000}{5000/\text{mL}} (\text{chop the zeroes}) = \frac{2}{5} = 0.4 \text{ mL}$$

TWO-STEP DRUG DOSAGE CALCULATIONS

When you have two measurements that are in different systems, dosage calculation becomes a two-step problem similar to the proportion calculations presented in Chapter 3. First find how the two measurements are related to one another.

The equivalent tables shown earlier will help convert one measurement into another. For example, dextromethorphan comes in solutions of 3.5 mg per 5 mL (or written as a ratio of $\frac{3.5 \text{ mg}}{5 \text{ mL}}$). You want to give 7 mg, but you need the final dose expressed in teaspoons. How do you determine how many teaspoons to give?

The Household-to-Metric Equivalents table (see Box 4.2) tells us that 1 tsp = 5 mL.

Step 1: Convert the system you *have* into the system you *want* using proportion calculations.

$$1 \text{ tsp} = 5 \text{ mL, then } 3.5 \text{ mg} = 5 \text{ mL} = 1 \text{ tsp}$$

Step 2: Plug the numbers into the formula for liquids.

$$\frac{\text{Want}}{\text{Have}} \times \text{Liquid} = \frac{7 \text{ mg}}{3.5 \text{ mg}} \times 1 \text{ tsp} = 2 \text{ tsp}$$

DIMENSIONAL ANALYSIS

Instead of using ratio and proportion to solve dosage problems, some people use dimensional analysis. **Dimensional analysis** is a method of comparing and equating different physical aspects and quantities by using simple algebraic rules along with known conversion factors (called *equivalency ratios*). Although this type of mathematical calculation is more commonly used in engineering computations when several different dimensions are being compared, it can be applied to dosage calculations; however, it does require additional steps. Only physical quantities measuring the same phenomenon can be solved this way; physical quantities such as length, speed, weight, and, importantly, dosage size conversions can be determined using this math problem-solving technique. Dimensional analysis is often used to convert from one set of measurement units to another set of units via conversion factors in such a way that unwanted units are canceled out and a person comfortable with the calculation can always account for these units.

A simple example of this method is how many pounds are in 20 kilograms of a given substance? One kilogram is equivalent to 2.2 lb (in medical measurement), so the conversion factor from kilograms to pounds is 2.2 pounds per kilogram (2.2 lb/kg). So,

 Drug Alert

Administration Alert

Always write out the word *unit* or the words *international units.*

QSEN: Safety

 Try This!

TT-7 Calculate how many milliliters you should give.
a. *Want* heparin 5000 units subcutaneously; *Have* heparin 10,000 units/mL
b. *Want* heparin 1000 units; *Have* heparin 5000 units/mL
c. *Want* heparin 300 units/kg body weight; *Have* heparin 20,000 units/mL. The patient weighs 250 lb.

Answers are at the end of this chapter.

 Try This!

TT-8 Calculate how many milligrams in how many teaspoons you should give to an infant who weighs 13 lb.
Want amoxicillin 50 mg/kg; *Have* amoxicillin 50 mg/mL (Remember to round up or down.)

Answers are at the end of this chapter.

multiplying the 20 kilograms by the conversion factor, 20 kg × 2.2 lb/kg, or expressed as the following equation:

$$\frac{20\,kg}{1}\times\frac{2.2\,lb}{1\,kg}\,(\text{now cancel out the kg because this unit is in both the}$$

$$\text{numerator and the denominator}),\frac{20}{1}\times\frac{2.2\,lb}{1}=\frac{44\,lb}{1}=44\,lb$$

As you can see, the kilogram unit is canceled out through simple algebra.

What about going the other way? How many kilograms are in 315 pounds? Flip the conversion factor over, so 1 kg/2.2 lb, multiply the weight in pounds by the new conversion factor, 315 lb × 1 kg/2.2 lb, which results in 143.2 kg. The equation would look like this:

$$\frac{315\,lb}{1}\times\frac{1\,kg}{2.2\,lb}\,(\text{cancel the pound units})=\frac{315}{1}\times\frac{1\,kg}{2.2}=\frac{315\,kg}{2.2}=143.2\,kg$$

Once again, the weight unit (this time pounds unit) was factored out.

These two simple examples highlight how this method could be used for longer problems and how it allows the practitioner to keep an eye on the units involved.

Here is a dosage example:

A patient who weighs 220 lb is prescribed a dose of medication at 12.5 mg/kg of body weight. The concentration of the medication on hand is 125 mg/mL, and the patient wants to take the medication orally, by teaspoon. How many teaspoons of medication will the patient need to take per dose?

Use the following dimensional analysis steps for the conversions and accounting:

Step 1: 1 kg = 2.2 lb, so the weight conversion ratio is 1 kg/2.2 lb; the patient weighs 100 kg, 220 lb × 1 kg/2.2 lb or

$$\frac{220\,lb}{1}\times\frac{1\,kg}{2.2\,lb}=\text{the patient weighs 100\,kg}$$

Step 2: The weight (amount) of medication needed based on body mass is 12.5 mg/kg × 100 kg = 1250 mg or

$$\frac{12.5\,mg/kg}{1}\times\frac{100\,kg}{1}=\frac{1250\,mg}{1}=1250\,mg$$

Step 3: 1 tsp = 5 mL, so the volumetric conversion ratio is 5 mL/tsp
The concentration in teaspoons is now 125 mg/mL × 5 mL/tsp = 625 mg/tsp or

$$\frac{125\,mg}{1\,mL}\times\frac{5\,mL}{1\,tsp}\,(\text{cancel out the mL})=\frac{625\,mg}{1\,tsp}=625\,mg/tsp$$

Step 4: The final dose in teaspoons is 1250 mg divided by 625 mg/tsp = 2 tsp or

$$\frac{1250\,mg}{625\,mg/tsp}\,(\text{cancel out the mg})=\frac{1250}{625/tsp}=2\,\text{teaspoons}$$

Steps 1 and 3 were conversions in which dimensional analysis was explicitly used. Steps 2 and 4 were simple calculations, but using dimensional analysis to solve for them allows for a higher degree of accountability and understanding of the units involved.

 Try This!

TT-9 Using dimensional analysis and showing your work, calculate the dosages for these problems.
a. Heparin 25 units is ordered to be administered subcutaneously. The solution available is heparin 40 units/mL. How many milliliters of this solution should be administered to equal the correct ordered dose?
b. A patient (an infant) who weighs 22 lb is prescribed to receive 50,000 units of penicillin intravenously per kilogram of weight. The penicillin solution you have on hand is 1,000,000 units/50 mL. How many milliliters should you give by IV injection?

Answers are at the end of this chapter.

Get Ready for the NCLEX® Examination!

Key Points

- A liquid ounce is not equal to a dry ounce.
- Always double check the amount of drug in a measuring device with the amount ordered to prevent giving an overdose.
- The household measurement system is not as precise as the metric system.
- Do not substitute one type of potassium for another.
- When calculating doses for drugs that are manufactured in milliequivalents or units, determine the amount of tablets or milliliters to administer based on what you *want* versus what you *have* on hand, in the same way as for drugs manufactured in milligrams.

- To prevent insulin dose errors, check the specific markings on the syringe rather than going by the color of the cap, needle hub, or box label.
- Always write out the word *unit* or the words *international units* rather than using abbreviations.

Additional Learning Resources

⊕ Be sure to visit your Evolve website (http://evolve.elsevier.com/Workman/pharmacology/) for additional online resources.

[SG] Go to your Study Guide for additional learning activities to help you master this chapter content.

Review Questions

See *Answers to In-Text Review Questions* in the back of the book for answers to these questions.

1. If there are 60 gtts in a teaspoon, how many gtts are there in two tablespoons?
   - A. 360
   - B. 240
   - C. 180
   - D. 120

2. You prepare to mix dry amoxicillin into a solution by adding 150 mL of water to the bottle containing the dry amoxicillin. How many ounces of water will you add to the bottle?
   - A. 30
   - B. 20
   - C. 10
   - D. 5

3. A patient is to take 45 mg of a drug that comes as 5 mg/tsp. How many tablespoons is this? _____ Tbs

4. Which weight is the *smallest*?
   - A. 1 kg
   - B. 10 mg
   - C. 100 mcg
   - D. 1000 g

5. Convert 0.25 L into milliliters. _____ mL

6. The patient weighs 175 lb. Convert this weight to kilograms. _____ kg

7. The drug and dose prescribed is morphine 15 mg by intramuscular injection. The dose available is 10 mg/mL. How many milliliters will you draw up into the syringe? _____ mL

8. The patient is to receive 12,000 units of heparin intravenously. The vial contains heparin 20,000 units/mL. How many milliliters will you draw up into the syringe? _____ mL

Answers to *Math Check* Problems

MC-1 Convert the Fahrenheit temperature to Centigrade and the Centigrade to Fahrenheit.
- a. 101.4°F = 38.6°C
- b. 40°C = 104°F

MC-2 Calculate the response in teaspoons or drops. (Note: "How to" math steps for conversion of *want* versus *have* problems are in Chapter 3.)
- a. *Want* Benadryl 5 mg; *Have* Benadryl 12.5 mg/5 mL
  30 drops (gtts) or 2 mL
- b. *Want* acetaminophen 200 mg; *Have* acetaminophen 40 mg/mL
  5 mL or 1 teaspoon

MC-3 Convert the following weights in pounds to kilograms and the weights in kilograms to pounds.
- a. 25 lb = 11.36 kg
- b. 260 lb = 117.9 kg
- c. 45 kg = 99 lb
- d. 90 kg = 198.4 lb

MC-4 Convert these household measures into metric equivalents, rounding to the nearest tenth when necessary.
- a. 3 tablespoons = 45 mL
- b. 8.8 lb = 4 kg
- c. 20 inches = 50.8 cm
- d. 4 ounces (liquid) = 120 mL
- e. 4 teaspoons = 20 mL

MC-5 Convert these metric measures into household equivalents.
- a. 75 kg = 165.3 lb
- b. 180 mL = 6 ounces
- c. 75 g = 2.5 ounces (dry weight)
- d. 500 mL = 1 pint liquid

MC-6 Calculate how much drug you should administer.
- a. *Want* potassium 20 mEq in extended-release tablet; *Have* potassium 5 mEq in extended-release tablet. Administer four tablets.

b. *Want* potassium gluconate 30 mEq oral solution; *Have* potassium gluconate 20 mEq/15 mL oral solution. Administer 22.5 mL.

MC-7 Calculate how many milliliters you should give.
   a. *Want* heparin 1250 units subcutaneously; *Have* heparin 1000 units/mL. Give 1.25 mL.
   b. *Want* heparin 1250 units intravenously; *Have* heparin 500 units/mL. Give 2.5 mL.

MC-8 Calculate how many milligrams in how many teaspoons you will give to a child who weighs 26.8 lb.
   Want acyclovir 20 mg/kg. *Have* acyclovir 200 mg/5 mL oral suspension.
   A 26.8-lb child weighs 12.16 kg. Total dose wanted = 12.16 (kg) × 20 (mg) = 243.2 mg.
   If 5 mL contain 200 mg, then 1 mL contains 40 mg. 243.2 mg divided by 40 mg/mL = 6 mL of drug to be administered.

MC-9 Using dimensional analysis and showing your work, calculate the dosages for these problems.
   a. Dilantin (phenytoin) 100 mg is prescribed to give a child orally. The drug available is Dilantin 125 mg/5 mL. How many milliliters of this solution should be administered to equal the ordered dose?

$$\frac{100\ mg}{1} \div \frac{125\ mg}{5\ mL} = \frac{100\ mg}{1} \times \frac{5\ ml}{125\ mg}\ (\text{cancel the mg})$$

$$= \frac{500\ ml}{125} = 4\ mL$$

   b. A patient who weighs 154 lb is prescribed to receive 50,000 units of penicillin intravenously per kilogram of weight. The penicillin solution you have on hand is 1,000,000 units/25 mL. How many milliliters should you give by IV injection?

Step 1 Convert the patient's weight in pounds to kilograms.

$$\frac{154\ lb}{1} \times \frac{1\ kg}{2.2\ lb}\ (\text{cancel the pounds}) = \frac{154\ kg}{2.2} = 70\ kg$$

Step 2 Calculate the amount of penicillin needed based on the patient's weight in kilograms.

$$\frac{50,000\ units}{1\ kg} \times \frac{70\ kg}{1}\ (\text{cancel out the kilograms})$$

$$= \frac{3,500,000\ units}{1} = 3,500,000\ units$$

Step 3 Convert penicillin to units per milliliter.

   25 mL = 1,000,000 units. So 1,000,000 divided by 25 = 40,000 units per mL.

$$\frac{1,000,000\ units}{25\ mL} = 40,000\ units\ per\ mL$$

Step 4 Using the conversion factor of 40,000 units per milliliter, the desired dose of 50,000 units/kg, and the patient's weight in kilograms, calculate the volume of drug to administer in milliliters. Multiply the patient's weight by 50,000 units, and divide the total by 40,000 = 87.5 mL.

$$\frac{50,000\ units}{1} \times \frac{70\ kg}{1} = 3,500,000\ units\ \frac{3,500,000\ units}{40,000\ units/mL}$$

   (cancel out the units) = 87.5 mL

Answers to *Try This!* Problems

TT-1 Convert the Fahrenheit temperature to Centigrade and the Centigrade to Fahrenheit.
   a. 99°F = 37.2°C
   b. 102.6°F = 39.2°C
   c. 35°C = 95°F
   d. 39.2°C = 102.6°F

TT-2 Calculate the response in teaspoons or drops.
   a. *Want* ampicillin 750 mg; *Have* ampicillin 250 mg/tsp
       3 tsp = 750 mg
   b. *Want* guaifenesin 50 mg; *Have* guaifenesin 100 mg per 60 gtts
       50 mg in 30 gtts or in 0.5 tsp
   c. *Want* milk of magnesia 1 Tbs; *Have* milk of magnesia 1 tsp
       3 tsp of milk of magnesia = 1 Tbs

TT-3 Convert the following weights in pounds to kilograms and the weights in kilograms to pounds.
   a. 98 lb = 44.5 kg
   b. 54 lb = 24.5 kg
   c. 315 lb = 143.2 kg
   d. 2.9 lb = 1.3 kg

   e. 145 lb = 65.8 kg
   f. 68 kg = 149.6 lb
   g. 12 kg = 26.4 lb
   h. 128 kg = 281.6 lb
   i. 52 kg = 114.4 lb
   j. 80 kg = 176 lb

TT-4 Convert these household measures in metric equivalents, rounding to the nearest tenth when necessary.
   a. 250 lb = 113.6 kg
   b. 10 oz (liquid) = 300 mL
   c. 17 in = 43.2 cm
   d. 5 Tbs = 75 mL
   e. 2 tsp = 10 mL

TT-5 Convert these metric measures into household equivalents.
   a. 45 g = 1.5 oz (dry weight)
   b. 120 mL = 4 oz
   c. 1500 mL = 1 qt and 1 pt, or 6 c
   d. 110 kg = 242 lb
   e. 780 g = 1.6 lb

TT-6 Calculate how much drug you should administer.

  a. *Want* potassium 24 mEq in extended-release tablet; *Have* potassium 8 mEq in an extended-release tablet

  Give three extended-release tablets.

  b. *Want* potassium 10 mEq effervescent tablet; *Have* potassium 20 mEq scored effervescent tablet

  Give one half ($\frac{1}{2}$) of the effervescent tablet.

  c. *Want* potassium 10 mEq in an oral solution; *Have* potassium 20 mEq dissolved in 8 oz of water as an oral solution

  Give 4 oz of the oral solution.

TT-7 Calculate how many milliliters you should give.

  a. *Want* heparin 5000 units subcutaneous; *Have* heparin 10,000 units/mL

  $$\frac{5000}{10,000/mL} = \frac{50}{100} = 0.5 \text{ mL}$$

  b. *Want* heparin 1000 units; *Have* heparin 5000 units/mL

  $$\frac{1000}{5000/mL} = \frac{1}{5} = 0.2 \text{ mL}$$

  c. *Want* heparin 300 units/kg body weight; *Have* heparin 20,000 units/mL. The patient weighs 250 lb.

  250 lb = 250 divided by 2.2 = 113.6 kg, round to 114 kg

  114 kg × 300 units = need 34,200 units

  34,200 divided by 20,000 = 1.71 mL, round to 1.7 mL

TT-8 Calculate how many milligrams in how many teaspoons you should give to an infant who weighs 13 lb.

  Want amoxicillin 50 mg/kg; *Have* amoxicillin 50 mg/mL (Remember to round up or down.)

  13 lb = 5.89 kg, round to 5.9 kg

  50 mg × 5.9 kg = 295 mg; want 295 mg

  5 mL = 1 tsp; 50 mg/mL = 250 mg/5 mL (1 tsp)

  $\frac{295}{250}$ × 1 tsp = 1.14 tsp; not easy to measure, better to use

  a medicine dropper (in mL)

  $$\frac{\text{Want}}{\text{Have}} \times 1\,mL = \frac{295 \text{ mg}}{50 \text{ mg}} \times 1\,mL = 5.9 \text{ mL}$$

TT-9 Using dimensional analysis and showing your work, calculate the dosages for these problems.

  a. Heparin 25 units is ordered to be administered subcutaneously. The solution available is heparin 40 units/mL. How many milliliters of this solution should be administered to equal the correct ordered dose?

  $$\frac{25 \text{ units}}{1} \div \frac{40 \text{ units}}{1\,mL} = \frac{25 \text{ units}}{1} \times \frac{1\,mL}{40 \text{ units}}$$

  (cancel out the units) $= \frac{25 \text{ mL}}{40} = 0.625 \text{ mL}$

  Round down to 0.6 mL.

  b. A patient (infant) who weighs 22 lb is prescribed to receive 50,000 units of penicillin intravenously per kg of weight. The penicillin solution you have on hand is 1,000,000 units/50 mL. How many milliliters should you give by intravenous injection?

  Step 1: Convert the patient's weight in pounds to kilograms.

  $$\frac{22 \text{ lb}}{1} \times \frac{1 \text{ kg}}{2.2 \text{ lb}} \text{ (cancel out the lb)} = \frac{22}{1} \times \frac{1 \text{ kg}}{2.2} = \frac{22 \text{ kg}}{2.2} = 10 \text{ kg}$$

  Step 2: Calculate the amount of penicillin needed based on the infant's body mass.

  $$\frac{50,000 \text{ units}}{1 \text{ kg}} \times \frac{10 \text{ kg}}{1} \text{ (cancel out the kg)} = \frac{50,000 \text{ units}}{1} \times \frac{10}{1}$$
  $$= 500,000 \text{ units}$$

  Step 3: Convert penicillin to units per milliliter.

  50 mL = 1,000,000 units. So 1,000,000 divided by 50 = 20,000 units per mL.

  $$\frac{1,000,000 \text{ units}}{50 \text{ mL}} = 20,000 \text{ units per mL}$$

  Step 4: Using the conversion factor of 20,000 units per milliliter, the desired dose of 50,000 units/kg, and the infant's weight in kilograms, calculate the volume of drug to administer in milliliters. Multiply the patient's weight by 50,000 units and divide the total by 20,000 = 25 mL.

  $$\frac{50,000 \text{ units}}{1} \times \frac{10}{1} = 500,000 \text{ units} \quad \frac{500,000 \text{ units}}{20,000 \text{ units/mL}}$$

  (cancel out the units) = 25 mL

Dosage Calculation of Intravenous Solutions and Drugs

http://evolve.elsevier.com/Workman/pharmacology/

Learning Objectives

The content presented in this chapter should help you to:

1. Explain how the size of an intravenous (IV) fluid drop determines the flow rate for IV fluid infusion.
2. Describe the parts of an order for IV fluids that are considered a valid prescription and are necessary to determine the correct infusion rate.
3. Explain three potential patient problems associated with IV therapy.
4. Correctly calculate IV drug infusion problems when provided with the volume, hours to be infused, and drip factor.
5. Use the "15-second" rule to determine an IV flow rate.

Key Terms

administration set (ăd-mĭn-ĭ-STRĂ-shŭn SĔT) (p. 79) The tubing and drip chamber used to administer an IV infusion.

drip chamber (DRĬP CHĂM-bŭr) (p. 79) The clear cylinder of plastic attached to the IV tubing. It is filled no more than half-way so you can see the fluid dripping.

drip rate (DRĬP RĀT) (p. 80) The number of drops per minute needed to make an IV solution infuse in the prescribed amount of time.

drop factor (DRŎP FĂK-tŭr) (p. 79) The number of drops (gtts) needed to make 1 mL of IV fluid. The larger the drop, the fewer drops needed to make 1 mL.

duration (dŭr-Ā-shŭn) (p. 78) How long in minutes or hours an IV infusion is prescribed to run.

extravasation (ĕks-tră-vă-SĀ-shŭn) (p. 81) Condition in which an IV needle or catheter pulls out from the vein and causes

tissue damage by leaking irritating IV fluids into the surrounding tissue.

flow rate (FLŌ RĀT) (p. 79) How fast an IV infusion is prescribed to run—the number of milliliters (mL) delivered in 1 hour.

infiltration (ĭn-fĭl-TRĀ-shŭn) (p. 81) Condition in which an IV needle or catheter pulls out from the vein and begins to leak IV fluids into the surrounding tissue, resulting in tissue swelling.

infuse (infusion) (ĭn-FYŪZ) (p. 78) To run IV fluids into the body.

volume (VŎL-yūm) (p. 78) Amount of fluids prescribed to be in-fused (e.g., 1000 mL).

VI (p. 80) IV pump abbreviation for "volume infused."

VTBI (p. 80) IV pump abbreviation for "volume to be infused."

 Memory Jogger

IV infusions are most often used for drugs or fluids that:
- Must get into the patient's system quickly.
- Need to be given at a steady rate.
- Are patient-controlled (e.g., IV drugs for pain).

OVERVIEW

Providing drug and fluids by the intravenous (IV) route, or IV therapy, is *parenteral* drug delivery method. The IV fluids, along with any drugs, go directly into a vein and thus *immediately* into the bloodstream. This process is called an **infusion**, which means to run (**infuse**) IV fluids into the body. IV fluids may be given alone to hydrate the patient, or they may be used to place drugs directly into the patient's system. The **volume** is the amount of fluids prescribed, and the **duration** is how long in minutes or hours an IV infusion is prescribed to run.

Fluids given by IV are also used for drugs that would not be absorbed if taken by mouth and for when the patient is unable to take drugs or fluids orally. However, because IV drugs act immediately, there is always the potential for an immediate and severe problem if there is an adverse drug reaction. As discussed in Chapter 1, an *adverse drug reaction* is a severe, unusual, or life-threatening patient response to a drug that requires intervention.

How fast an IV infusion is prescribed to run depends on the reason for having it. For example, if a patient is dehydrated, the prescriber might want to run the fluids faster than if the IV is present just in case a problem occurs. So not only must you know how fast an IV infusion is prescribed to run, you must know *why* it was prescribed.

▶ IV MECHANICS

The IV **flow rate** is how fast the IV infusion is prescribed to run (i.e., the number of milliliters delivered in 1 hour). The rate of an IV depends on the diameter of the tubing. Compare the tubing to a straw. A fat straw will suck up a larger amount of soda in 10 seconds compared with a thinner straw in the same 10 seconds. When you use your finger to make the soda drip out of the straw, the fatter the straw, the larger the drop. Ten fat drops have more fluid in them than 10 thin drops. The same principle applies to IV fluids. Tubing with a larger diameter will let bigger drops into the vein and a larger amount of fluid into the body. The number of drops needed to make a milliliter of fluid is called the **drop factor.**

The diameter of the tubing varies by the tubing manufacturer. Tubing sizes are divided into macrodrip and microdrip and have different types of drip chambers. A **drip chamber** is the clear cylinder of plastic attached to the IV tubing. It is filled not quite halfway so you can see the fluid dripping (Fig. 5.1). The complete set of tubing and drip chamber used to infuse IV fluids is the **administration set.** A *microdrip* tubing set delivers very small drops. It is most often used for children, older patients, and patients who cannot tolerate a fast infusion rate or a high volume of fluids. On the other hand, *macrodrip* sets deliver larger drops and are used when faster infusion rates or larger quantities of fluids or drugs are needed. Fig. 5.1 shows the difference in drop size between a macrodrip chamber and a microdrip chamber.

Each manufacturer puts its drop factor (sometimes called *drip factor*) on every IV fluid administration set. Depending on the brand, macrodrip tubing delivers 10 drops/mL, 15 drops/mL, or 20 drops/mL. Microdrip tubing is more standard and is always 60 drops/mL, regardless of which manufacturer makes it. *You must use the drop factor in every IV calculation.* Fig. 5.2 shows different IV tubing administration sets. Administration sets for blood transfusions are larger to prevent damage to blood cells and also have some differences in the drip chamber. This chapter does not discuss infusing blood or blood products; however, flow rate calculations for any blood product are the same as for any other type of IV fluid.

IV drug therapy is an invasive procedure that requires a prescriber's order (prescription). Always double check the prescription (order) before starting the procedure. Remember that the prescription must contain the specific drug concentration or IV solution to be infused, the dosage or volume, the duration, and the rate of infusion to be considered valid.

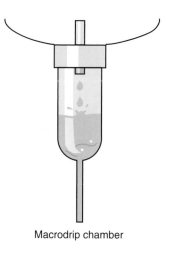

Macrodrip chamber

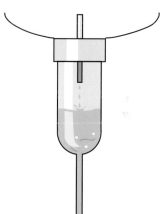

Microdrip chamber

FIG. 5.1 Drop size differences between a macrodrip chamber and a microdrip chamber on IV tubing.

💡 Memory Jogger

The larger the diameter of the IV tubing, the larger the drops.

💡 Memory Jogger

For a prescription to start IV therapy to be valid, it must contain the specific drug or IV solution to be infused, the dosage or volume, the duration, and the rate of infusion.

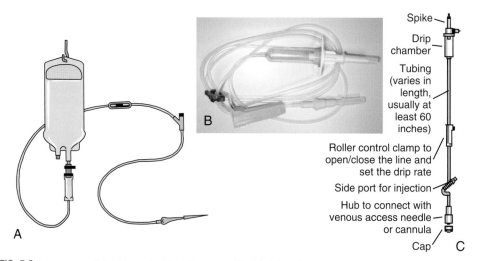

Spike

Drip chamber

Tubing (varies in length, usually at least 60 inches)

Roller control clamp to open/close the line and set the drip rate

Side port for injection

Hub to connect with venous access needle or cannula

Cap

FIG. 5.2 Intravenous (IV) tubing administration sets. **(A)** Administration set connected to an IV solution bag. **(B)** Photo of an actual IV tubing administration set. **(C)** Detail of IV tubing administration set.

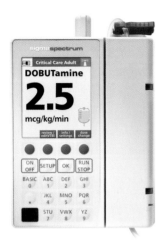

FIG. 5.3 Example of an IV infusion pump. (Copyright Baxter Healthcare Corp., Deerfield, IL)

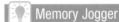
Memory Jogger

The four basic parts of IV fluid regulation are what type of fluid, how much (volume), for how long (duration), and how fast the fluids should be infused (rate).

Memory Jogger

Adding the VI and the VTBI should equal the total amount of fluid that was in the bag when it was first hung.

REGULATING IV FLUIDS

IV therapy involves calculating the **drip rate**, the number of drops per minute needed to make the IV infuse in the prescribed amount of time. Calculations for drip rates are precise and must be made carefully. Although IV infusion rates can be controlled by adjusting the roller clamp, the vast majority of IV fluids nowadays are regulated by either a pump or a controller. A *controller* is a simple device that uses gravity to control the flow of an IV infusion. An *IV infusion pump* is a computer-based machine that pushes fluid into the vein by low pressure. The buttons used to program an IV pump are much like the ones you use to work the remote control to your television. Fig. 5.3 shows an example of an IV infusion pump. All pumps have at least the following buttons:

- **ON/OFF** switch
- **Start/Enter**
- **STOP**
- **Delete or Clear**
- **Direction arrows:** ↑↓ → ←
- **Silence (MUTE)**
- **IV lock** (prevents patients and visitors from tampering with the IV pump)
- **Primary** (controller for the main IV bag—the bag hanging at the lowest point)
- **IVPB** (piggyback or secondary bag controller—the bag hanging at the highest point)

Because each brand of control device differs, always read and follow the manufacturer's directions. Even if you are not directly responsible for starting or maintaining the IV infusion, you may be responsible for checking that it is running smoothly and on time.

To understand the basics of IV fluid regulation, you need to understand these four important concepts:

- *What:* What type of fluid should be infused
- *Volume:* How much of the fluid should be infused
- *Duration:* For how long the fluid should be infused
- *Rate:* How fast the fluid should be infused

For example, a prescription reads "1000 mL of normal saline (NS) to be infused over 8 hours." The order already gives you the "What," "Volume," and "Duration." Using this information, you can calculate the flow rate. As you prepare the IV infusion, check the clock to determine the start and stop time.

Once you know what type of fluids to give, how much, and for how long, you can use this information to program the pump. Just remember that the accuracy of the pump depends on the information that you punch into it. Remember "GIGO!": "Garbage in, garbage out!" *If you make an error programming the pump, at least one factor will be incorrect, and a drug administration error will result.*

Be sure to understand all the abbreviations that are used and that may show up on the IV monitor screen. For example, a pump may use the abbreviations "VI" and "VTBI." The **VI** stands for "volume infused" and tells you how much has been infused up to that minute. **VTBI** means the "volume to be infused," or the amount that is left in the bag at any point. As the VI increases, the VTBI decreases. At any given time, if you add what has been infused (VI) to what is left in the bag (VTBI), you should have the total amount of fluid that was prescribed.

How will you know how much is really in the IV bag at any time during the infusion? Fig. 5.4 shows a standard IV bag for NS (0.9% saline in water, known as "normal saline"). In this illustration, the red markings on the clear plastic bag are repeated in the box next to the bag so that you can read them more easily. Note that there are numbers with horizontal lines going down the right side of the bag (and the label). These numbers indicate how much fluid has been infused from the bag. For example, if the fluid line of solution in the bag is even with the line next to the number 4, 400 mL have been infused, and 600 mL (1000 mL−400 mL) remain in the bag to be infused.

Mark the top line of the bag with the *start time* (the actual time when the IV infusion is started), and put a thick line with a pen or marker on the bag in 1-hour segments down the volume line, just like a ruler. Each hour marked should be right next

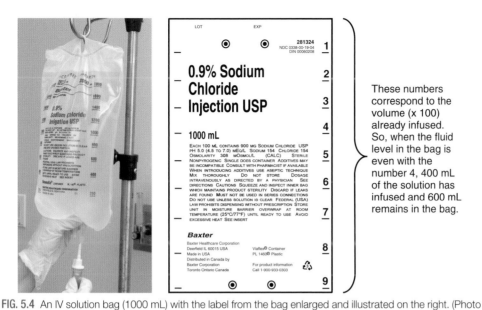
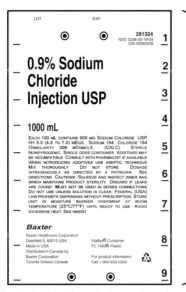
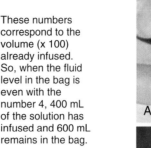

LOT   EXP

281324
NDC 0338-00-19-04
DIN 00060208   1

**0.9% Sodium
Chloride
Injection USP**   2

3

4

1000 mL

EACH 100 mL CONTAINS 900 mg SODIUM CHLORIDE USP   5
pH 5.0 (4.5 to 7.0) mEq/L SODIUM 154 CHLORIDE 154
OSMOLARITY 308 mOsmol/L (CALC) STERILE
NONPYROGENIC SINGLE DOSE CONTAINER ADDITIVES MAY
BE INCOMPATIBLE CONSULT WITH PHARMACIST IF AVAILABLE
WHEN INTRODUCING ADDITIVES USE ASEPTIC TECHNIQUE
MIX THOROUGHLY DO NOT STORE DOSAGE
INTRAVENOUSLY AS DIRECTED BY A PHYSICIAN SEE   6
DIRECTIONS CAUTIONS SQUEEZE AND INSPECT INNER BAG
WHICH MAINTAINS PRODUCT STERILITY DISCARD IF LEAKS
ARE FOUND MUST NOT BE USED IN SERIES CONNECTIONS
DO NOT USE UNLESS SOLUTION IS CLEAR FEDERAL (USA)
LAW PROHIBITS DISPENSING WITHOUT PRESCRIPTION STORE
UNIT IN MOISTURE BARRIER OVERWRAP AT ROOM   7
TEMPERATURE (25°C/77°F) UNTIL READY TO USE AVOID
EXCESSIVE HEAT SEE INSERT

Baxter

Baxter Healthcare Corporation
Deerfield IL 60015 USA   Viaflex® Container   8
Made in USA   PL 146®® Plastic
Distributed in Canada by
Baxter Corporation   For product information
Toronto Ontario Canada   Call 1-900-933-0303   9

These numbers
correspond to the
volume (x 100)
already infused.
So, when the fluid
level in the bag is
even with the
number 4, 400 mL
of the solution has
infused and 600 mL
remains in the bag.

FIG. 5.4 An IV solution bag (1000 mL) with the label from the bag enlarged and illustrated on the right. (Photo from Perry, A., & Potter, P. [2009]. *Clinical nursing skills & techniques* [7th ed.]. St. Louis: Mosby.)

to the volume to be infused (VTBI) for that hour. End with the *stop time*, the time when the IV bag is supposed to be empty (fluid is totally infused).

Always calculate both the start and stop times, and mark the IV bag, even when it is on a controller or pump. Many things can happen to disturb the flow rate. For example, the tubing may kink, or the IV needle may get out of place and lead to infiltration. **Infiltration** is a condition that occurs when an IV needle or catheter pulls from the vein and begins to leak (infiltrate) the fluids into the surrounding tissue. Not only does this condition prevent the patient from receiving the right dose of fluid or drug, it also causes swelling in the surrounding tissues. When the fluid or drug that infiltrates is irritating and leads to tissue damage or loss, the condition is termed **extravasation**. Fig. 5.5 shows the appearance of the tissue around an IV infusion that has infiltrated and the appearance of tissue where extravasation has occurred.

Unless specifically prescribed to do so, never speed up an IV infusion to make up for lost time when the infusion is behind schedule. Playing "catch up" can cause fluids to enter the patient too quickly. This can lead to fluid overload and other complications.

An IV infusion on a pump or controller can develop flow problems just as an IV infusion without a pump can. A *controller* stops dripping if it an obstruction is present. On the other hand, a *pump* actually uses pressure to push the drops in to get past the blockage. *This means that pumps can continue to push in drops even if the needle is no longer in the vein.* Thus, if an infiltration has occurred, a controller stops, but a pump continues to push IV fluid into the surrounding tissue. All pumps have a set limit to the pressure that can be used. This limit is displayed on the IV screen (e.g., "Limit 600 mm Hg" [millimeters of mercury]). If the IV pump has to exert more pressure than the 600 mm Hg of pressure that was set to force the fluid into the vein, it will BEEP—loudly!

IV CALCULATIONS

To correctly calculate the flow rate, every IV prescription must include (1) the total volume to be infused (VTBI) and (2) the length of time the IV should run (in hours). You then use the particular drop factor of the tubing that you are using to calculate how many *drops per minute* are needed to make the IV fluid infuse in the ordered time. All IV rates that are controlled using the control roller or the control slide on the tubing are calculated by drops per minute. Some pump rates are calculated by drops per minute, and others are programmed by the pump computer in terms of milliliters per hour to be infused.

Now that you know the theory, let's work with the formula.

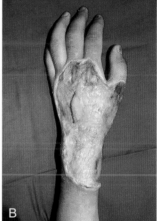

A

B

FIG. 5.5 Appearances of tissues after IV fluid infiltration **(A)** and after extravasation **(B)**. (A, From Hockenberry, M. J., & Wilson, D. [2006]. *Wong's nursing care of infants and children* [8th ed.]. St. Louis: Mosby; B, From Weinzweig, J., & Weinzweig, N. [2005]. *The mutilated hand.* St. Louis: Mosby.)

 Drug Alert

Administration Alert

Always calculate both the start and stop times and then mark the IV bag, even when the IV bag is on a controller or pump.

QSEN: Safety

 Critical Point for Safety

Unless specifically prescribed to do so, **never** speed up an IV to make up for lost time when the infusion is behind schedule.

QSEN: Safety

 Memory Jogger

If an infiltration has occurred, a controller stops, but a pump can continue to push IV fluid into the surrounding tissue and is capable of causing more tissue damage.

Try This!

TT-1 Calculate the milliliters to be infused in 1 h given each of the following prescriptions.
a. 500 mL in 6 hours
b. 125 mL in 2 hours
c. 1000 mL in 6 hours
d. 1000 mL in 24 hours

Answers are at the end of this chapter.

Try This!

TT-2 Use the macrodrip tubing shortcut to calculate the drip rate for each of these prescriptions.
a. 1000 mL D$_5$W in 4 hours, drop factor 10
b. 500 mL lactated Ringer's in 5 hours, drop factor 15
c. 1000 mL NS in 24 hours, drop factor 20

Answers are at the end of this chapter.

Try This!

TT-3 Calculate the drops per minute needed to get the right volume per hour for each of these prescriptions.
a. 500 mL D$_5$W in 24 hours with microdrip tubing
b. 1000 mL lactated Ringer's solution in 12 hours, drop factor = 15
c. 250 mL D$_5$W in 2 hours, drop factor = 10

Answers are at the end of this chapter.

Memory Jogger

Remember that the 15-sec drip rate check works only for *manually* controlled IV bags, not those on a pump.

Try This!

TT-4 Calculate the 15-sec drip rate for each of these problems.
a. 20 gtts/min
b. 84 gtts/min
c. 28 gtts/min

Answers are at the end of this chapter.

Macrodrip Formula

The basic formula for determining how fast to run an IV infusion is $\dfrac{\text{Drop factor}}{\text{Minutes}}$.

Now let's break it down to make it easier.

Step 1: An IV infusion of 1000 mL is prescribed to run for 8 hours.

First find out how many milliliters should run in 1 hour *(flow rate)*. It is much easier to work with 1 hour than with 8 hours!

$$\text{Divide 1000 by 8:} \quad \frac{1000}{8} = 125 \text{ mL/1 hr. Does it make sense (DIMS)?}$$

Step 2: Now calculate how many drops per minute are needed to make the IV fluid infuse at 125 mL/h (or 125 mL/60 min). This depends on the drop factor (drops/mL) of the IV tubing and drip chamber.

$$\frac{\text{Volume (milliliters)}}{\text{Time (minutes)}} \times \text{Drop factor (drops/milliliters)} = \text{Drops per minute}$$

You check the label information on the administration set, and find that the drop factor is 15.

$$\frac{125}{60} \times 15 = 2.08 \times 15 = 31.2 \text{ drops/min, round down to 31 drops/min.}$$

The Macrodrip Tubing Shortcut

Now that you know the macrodrip formula, here is a shorter way to calculate the drops per minute with macrodrip tubing. Because all of the diameters of tubing and drip chamber (10, 15, or 20) can be evenly divided into 60, you can use this relationship to calculate drip rates. Let's use these to calculate the original prescription of 1000 mL to infuse over 8 hours, which equals 125 mL/hr.

- Sets with 10 gtts/mL, divide milliliters per hour by 6 (because 6 × 10 = 60 minutes); 125 ÷ 6 = 12.5 drops/min, round to 13 drops/min
- Sets with 15 gtts/mL, divide milliliters per hour by 4 (because 4 × 15 = 60 minutes); 125 ÷ 4 = 31.2 drops/min, round to 31 drops/min
- Sets with 20 gtts/mL divide milliliters per hour by 3 (because 3 × 20 = 60 minutes); 125 ÷ 3 = 41.6 drops/min, round to 42 drops/min

Get the idea?

Microdrip Formula

The microdrip formula is much easier. When using microdrip tubing, the drop factor of 60 drops/mL is the same as the number of minutes in 1 hour (60). Using the same formula as for macrodrip, you can see that the two 60s cancel each other out.

$$\frac{125}{60} \times \frac{60}{1} \text{ (drop factor)} = \frac{125}{1} = 125 \text{ microdrops/min.}$$

This is why the flow rate for microdrip tubing always equals the drop rate. Just calculate the milliliters needed per hour, and you have the drops per minute!

The 15-Second Rule

To see if the drip rate (e.g., 42 gtts/min) is accurate, technically you should stand at the bedside and count the drops in the drip chamber for a full minute. When you are busy, a minute can seem like a long time! Because a minute has 60 seconds, you can divide the drop rate by 4, round off the answer, and then count that number of drops for 15 seconds. Your answer will be close to what it would have been if you had counted for the whole 60 seconds. For example, if the drop rate is the 31 gtts/min using the macrodrip tubing shortcut, divide 31 by 4: $\dfrac{31}{4} = 7.75$, and round that up to 8.

If you count 8 gtts when you count for 15 seconds, the IV infusion rate is correct! Be sure to check the IV rate every time that you are in the room. It takes only 15 seconds! Remember that this method works only for *manually* controlled IV bags, not those on a pump.

Get Ready for the NCLEX® Examination!

Key Points

- Always double check the order before starting an IV infusion.
- For a prescription to start IV therapy to be valid, it must contain the specific drug or IV solution to be infused, the dosage or volume, the duration, and the rate of infusion.
- The four basic parts of IV regulation are what type of fluid, how much (volume), for how long (duration), and how fast the fluids should be infused (rate).
- The rate of an IV infusion depends on the diameter of the tubing. The larger the diameter of IV tubing, the larger the drops.
- Because each brand of IV pump or control device differs, always read and follow the manufacturer's directions.
- Always calculate both the start and stop times and then time-tape the IV bag, even when it is on a controller or pump.
- Unless prescribed to do so, never speed up an IV to make up for lost time when the infusion is behind schedule.
- Adding the VI and the VTBI should equal the total amount of fluid that was in the bag when it was first hung.
- Remember that the 15-second drip rate check works only for *manually* controlled IV bags, not those on a pump.

Additional Learning Resources

Be sure to visit your Evolve website (http://evolve.elsevier.com/Workman/pharmacology/) for additional online resources.

SG   Go to your Study Guide for additional learning activities to help you master this chapter content.

Review Questions

See *Answers to In-Text Review Questions* in the back of the book for answers to these questions.

1. How does the administration set "drop factor" affect IV infusions?
   - A. Fluid with a larger drop factor infuses more slowly than fluid with a smaller drop factor.
   - B. Smaller drop factors occur with smaller needles (or cannulas) and larger drop factors occur with larger needles.
   - C. The larger the drop factor, the fewer the number of drops needed to administer 1 mL of infusion fluid.
   - D. The smaller the drop factor, the fewer the number of drops needed to administer 1 mL of infusion fluid.

2. A nurse is caring for four patients who each have IV infusions of 1000 mL of normal saline (NS) running at a drip rate of 31 gtts/min, and each patient's administration set is different. If the drip rates remain the same, which infusion will the nurse expect to take the *longest* amount of time to complete?
   - A. Microdrip tubing with 60 gtts/mL
   - B. Macrodrip tubing with 20 gtts/mL
   - C. Macrodrip tubing with 15 gtts/mL
   - D. Macrodrip tubing with 10 gtts/mL

3. Which parts of a patient's prescription for IV therapy does the nurse recognize as necessary for the prescription to be valid? *Select all that apply.*
   - A. Administration drip rate
   - B. Drop factor
   - C. Drug to be infused
   - D. Duration of infusion
   - E. gtts/min
   - F. Rate of infusion
   - G. Volume/dosage to be infused

4. Which potentially harmful adverse reaction or patient response is the nurse most likely to *prevent* by examining the IV infusion site at least hourly when an irritating fluid is being infused?
   - A. Anaphylaxis
   - B. Extravasation
   - C. Infiltration
   - D. Fluid overload

5. A patient is to receive 1000 mL intravenously of dextrose 5% in lactated Ringer solution in 6 hours. Four hours after the start of the infusion, the nurse finds the VBTI reading on the pump at 250 mL. How many milliliters have already infused?
   - A. 750
   - B. 500
   - C. 250
   - D. 150

6. A patient is prescribed to receive 125 mL of intravenous fluid per hour and the drop factor is 10 gtt/mL. The nurse counts 15-second drip rate to be 8 gtt/min. What is the nurse's best action?
   - A. Nothing, the IV flow rate is correct.
   - B. Turn the rate up to 11 gtt/15 seconds.
   - C. Turn the rate up to 15 gtt/15 seconds.
   - D. Turn the rate down to 5 gtt/15 seconds.

7. Calculate the flow rate for 1000 mL of dextrose 5% in NS to be infused over 8 hours. The tubing that is available has a drop factor of 10 gtts/mL. _____ gtts/min

8. An infant is prescribed to receive 150 mL of fluid intravenously over 5 hours using a microdrip administration set. Calculate the drop rate per minute needed to accurately deliver the prescribed volume of fluid per hour. Drop rate_____gtt/min

Answers To *Try This!* Problems

TT-1 Calculate the milliliters to be infused in 1 hour given the following orders.

a. 500 mL in 6 hours: $\dfrac{500}{6}$ = 83 mL in 1 hour

b. 125 mL in 2 hours: $\dfrac{125}{2}$ = 62.5 mL, round to 63 mL in 1 hour

c. 1000 mL in 6 hours: $\dfrac{1000}{6}$ = 166.66 mL, round to 167 mL in 1 hour

d. 1000 mL in 24 hours: $\dfrac{1000}{24}$ = 41.66 mL, round to 42 mL in 1 hour

TT-2 Calculate the drip rate using the macrodrip tubing shortcut.

a. 1000 mL D$_5$W in 4 hours, drop factor 10: $\dfrac{1000}{4}$ = 250 mL/h ÷ 4 = 41 gtts/min

b. 500 mL lactated Ringer solution in 5 hours, drop factor 15: $\dfrac{500}{5}$ = 100 mL/hr ÷ 4 = 25 gtts/min

c. 1000 mL NS in 24 hours, drop factor 20: $\dfrac{1000}{24}$ = 42 mL/hr ÷ 3 = 14 gtts/min

TT-3 Calculate the drops per minute needed to get the right volume per hour.

a. $\dfrac{500}{24}$ mL D$_5$W in 24 hours with microdrip tubing
= 20.8 mL/h, round up to 21 mL/hr and 21 gtts/min

b. 1000 mL lactated Ringer solution in 12 hours, drop factor 15: $\dfrac{1000}{12}$ = 83.33 mL/hr, round down to 83 mL/hr

$\dfrac{\text{Volume (milliliters)}}{\text{Time (minutes)}} \times$ drop factor (drops per milliliter)

= drops per minute: $\dfrac{83}{60} \times 15$ = 1.38 × 15
= 20.7 gtts/min, round up to 21 gtts/min

c. 250 mL D$_5$W in 2 hours, drop factor = 10 $\dfrac{250}{2}$ = 125 mL/hr

$\dfrac{\text{Volume (milliliters)}}{\text{Time (minutes)}} \times$ drop factor (drops per milliliter)

= drops per minute: $\dfrac{125}{60}$ = 2.08 × 10 = 20.8 gtts/min, round up to 21 gtts/min

TT-4 Calculate the 15-second drip rate for each of these problems.

a. 20 gtts/min = 5 gtts/15 seconds

b. 84 gtts/min = 21 gtts/15 seconds

c. 28 gtts/min = 7 gtts/15 seconds

Antiinfectives: Antibacterial Drugs

6

http://evolve.elsevier.com/Workman/pharmacology/

Learning Objectives

The content presented in this chapter should help you to:

1. Explain the names, actions, usual adult dosages, possible side effects, and adverse effects of the different types of antibacterial drugs.
2. Describe priority actions to take before and after giving any of the different types of antibacterial drugs.
3. Prioritize essential information to teach patients taking any of the different types of antibacterial drugs.
4. Explain appropriate life span considerations for the different types of antibacterial drugs.

Key Terms

antibiotic resistance (ăn-tī-bī-Ŏ-tĭk rē-ZĬS-tĕns) (p. 86) The ability of a bacterium to resist the effects of antibacterials.

bactericidal (băk-tēr-ĭ-SĪD-ŭl) (p. 87) A drug that reduces the number of bacteria by killing them directly.

bacteriostatic (băk-tēr-ē-ō-STĂT-ĭk) (p. 87) A drug that reduces the number of bacteria by preventing them from dividing and growing rather than directly killing them.

cell wall synthesis inhibitors (SĔL WŎL SĬN-thě-sĭs ĭn-HĬB-ĭ-tŭrz) (p. 91) A class of antibacterial drugs that kills susceptible bacteria by preventing them from forming strong, protective cell walls.

drug generation (DRŬG jěn-ŭr-Ā-shŭn) (p. 91) Stage of drug development in which later generations are changed slightly to improve their effectiveness or means of administration.

fluoroquinolones (flŏr-ō-KWĬN-ă-lōnz) (p. 101) A group of drugs from the DNA synthesis inhibitor class that enter bacterial cells and prevent bacteria reproduction by suppressing the action of two enzymes important in making bacterial DNA.

metabolism inhibitors (mă-TĂS-bo-lizm ĭn-HĬB-ĭ-tŭrz) (p. 99) A class of antibacterial drugs that interfere with bacterial reproduction by preventing the bacteria from making folic acid.

protein synthesis inhibitors (PRŌ-tēn SĬN-thě-sĭs ĭn-HĬB-ĭ-tŭrz) (p. 94) A large class of antibacterial drugs that includes amino-glycosides, macrolides, and tetracyclines, which prevent bacteria from making proteins important to their life cycles and infective processes.

spectrum of efficacy (SPĔK-trŭm of ĔF-ĭ-kě-sē) (p. 87) A measure of how many different types of bacteria a drug can kill or prevent from growing.

susceptible organisms (sŭ-SĔP-tĭ-bŭl ŌR-găn-ĭ-zĭmz) (p. 86) Bacteria or other organisms that either can be killed by or have their reproduction reduced by an antibacterial drug.

virulence (VĬR-ŭl-ĕns) (p. 86) The measure of how well bacteria can invade and spread despite a normal immune response.

A major scientific accomplishment of the 20th century was the development of drugs that are antiinfectives known as *antibiotics* and *antibacterials*. These drugs originally targeted infections caused by invading bacteria that have the potential to lead to death or permanent health problems. Newer drugs now target additional microorganisms, including viruses, fungi, and protozoa. Bacterial infections are the most common cause of disease, sepsis, and death worldwide.

REVIEW OF RELATED PHYSIOLOGY AND PATHOPHYSIOLOGY OF BACTERIAL INFECTION

As living creatures, we interact constantly with various types of microorganisms, especially bacteria. Some of these bacteria are harmless *(nonpathogenic),* and others are or can become *pathogenic,* which means these bacteria can cause infection, systemic disease, and tissue damage. Some nonpathogenic bacteria coexist with us, causing no systemic disease or tissue damage, and are helpful *normal flora,* also

Memory Jogger

Pathogenic bacteria are those that can cause tissue damage or disease. Nonpathogenic bacteria do not cause disease or damage unless they overgrow or are present in a susceptible body area. Opportunistic bacteria cause disease or tissue damage only when the immune system is impaired.

known as a person's *microbiome*. These are bacteria that we always have on skin, mucous membranes, in the lungs, and in the digestive tract. They are helpful in digestion of food, and some provide protection by "crowding out" pathogenic organisms and preventing them from entering the body or overgrowing in a body area. The composition of normal flora changes as we age and is also influenced by where we live, what we eat, what drugs we take, what illnesses we experience, and even what pets we have. These bacteria are kept in check by our immune system and, as long as they remain in their normal body locations, do not cause harm or illness. *Opportunistic* bacteria cause disease and tissue damage only in someone whose immune system is not working well. So there are differences in bacteria that make some types more dangerous to humans than others.

BACTERIAL FEATURES

Bacteria are single-cell organisms that have their own genetic material (DNA and genes), cytoplasm, some organelles, and membranes (Animation 6.1). Unlike human cells, bacterial cells may also have several layers of membranes, cell walls, and capsules or coats (Fig. 6.1). Bacterial types vary in their ability to invade a person and avoid that person's immune and inflammatory responses. The **virulence** of bacteria is a measure of how well they can invade and spread despite a normal immune response. Bacteria are also classified according to whether they change color when a dye called Gram stain is applied. Those that change color are called gram positive, and those that do not are called gram negative. In general, gram-negative bacteria are more virulent and harder to kill or control because they are surrounded by a protective capsule.

ANTIBACTERIAL DRUG RESISTANCE

When antibacterials are overused, prescribed for conditions not responsive to these drugs, or taken improperly, drug-resistant strains of bacteria may develop. **Antibiotic resistance** is the ability of a bacterium to resist the effects of antibacterial drugs. Bacteria that can either be killed by antibacterials or have their reproduction suppressed are called **susceptible organisms.** Those that are neither killed nor suppressed by antibacterial drugs are called *resistant* organisms. Some bacteria are resistant to one type of antibacterial drug but susceptible to other types. The concern now is that many bacteria species and strains that were once susceptible to many types of antibacterial drugs are becoming resistant to most types. When a bacterium becomes

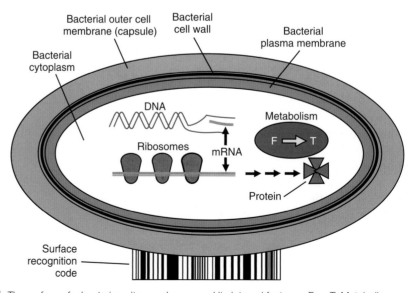

FIG. 6.1 The surface of a bacterium, its membrane, and its internal features. $F \rightarrow T$, Metabolic conversion of folic acid to thymine.

Table **6.1**	Drug Resistance Threat Categories and Current Organisms	
Urgent Threats	**Serious Threats**	**Concerning Threats**
Carbapenem-resistant *Acinetobacter* (B)	Drug-resistant *Campylobacter* (B)	Erythromycin-resistant Group A *Streptococcus* (GAS) (B)
Candida auris (F)	Drug-resistant *Candida* Species (F)	Clindamycin-resistant Group B *Streptococcus* (GBS) (B)
Clostridioides difficile (C. diff) (B)	Extended-spectrum β-lactamase-producing Entero-bacterales (ESBL-producing Enterobacterales) (B)	
Carbapenem-resistant *Enterobacterales* (CRE) (B)	Vancomycin-resistant *Enterococcus* (VRE) (B)	
Drug-resistant *Neisseria gonorrhoeae* (B)	Multidrug-resistant *Pseudomonas aeruginosa* (B)	
	Drug-resistant nontyphoidal *Salmonella* (B)	
	Drug-resistant *Salmonella* serotype Typhi (B)	
	Drug-resistant *Shigella* (B)	
	Methicillin-resistant *Staphylococcus aureus* (MRSA) (B)	
	Drug-resistant *Streptococcus pneumoniae* (B)	
	Drug-resistant *Mycobacterium tuberculosis* (also known as multidrug-resistant TB [MDR TB] or ex-tensively drug-resistant TB [XDR TB]) (B)	

resistant to three or more different types of antibacterial drugs, it is called a *superbug* or a *multidrug-resistant (MDR) organism*. The fear is that common bacteria that are not particularly hard to treat will become superbugs and cause *superinfections* that are difficult or impossible to control or cure. According to the Centers for Disease Control and Prevention, more than 2.8 million antibiotic-resistant infections occur in the United States each year, accounting for more than 35,000 deaths. This report lists 18 bacteria and fungi that are now resistant and separates these into serious, urgent, and concerning categories. Examples of resistant organisms and their class of threat are listed in Table 6.1. The infections caused by resistant organisms cost more to treat, increase the lengths of hospital stays, and lead to higher death rates.

OVERVIEW OF ANTIBACTERIAL THERAPY

Regardless of immune protections and normal barriers, sometimes bacteria are able to enter your body in sufficient numbers to multiply, damage tissues, and cause disease. Some bacterial infections are minor and can be suppressed and cured by the immune system. Others are more severe and could cause serious harm and even death. (Usually more virulent bacteria cause more serious infections.) Antibacterial drugs are used to prevent bacteria from spreading infection throughout your body and causing severe damage.

BACTERICIDAL AND BACTERIOSTATIC DRUGS

Some antibacterial drugs are **bactericidal,** which means that they kill bacteria directly. Other antibacterial drugs are **bacteriostatic,** which means that they prevent bacteria from reproducing until the body's own white blood cells (WBCs) and antibodies get rid of them (eradicate the infection). So, if a person's immune system is not working well, he or she would benefit from a bactericidal drug and not a bacteriostatic drug. Some drugs are bactericidal at high dosages but are only bacteriostatic at lower dosages.

SPECTRUM OF EFFICACY

One way to describe antibacterial drugs is by their **spectrum of efficacy,** which is a measure of how many different types of bacteria the drug can kill or prevent from growing. Each drug is judged by how many types of bacteria are susceptible to it. A *narrow-spectrum antibacterial drug* is effective against only a few types of bacteria. An

 Memory Jogger

Bactericidal drugs directly kill bacteria, whereas bacteriostatic drugs stop them from reproducing while the immune system kills the bacteria.

extended-spectrum antibacterial drug is effective against more types of bacteria. A *broad-spectrum antibacterial drug* is effective against a wide range of bacteria, both gram positive and negative.

Identifying the type of bacteria causing an infection is important for selecting the appropriate drug to treat the infection. The most common method to identify bacteria is culture and sensitivity (C&S). Culturing bacteria means to transfer it from an infected site and place it in a sterile nutritious broth to grow for 24 to 48 hours. By allowing the bacteria to multiply, more bacteria can be examined microscopically and tested with other procedures for identification. Culturing may be done alone or along with sensitivity testing, which is done by placing discs containing a specific antibacterial drug into the culture with the bacteria. When a drug is effective against the bacteria, the bacteria do not grow in the area where the disc was placed.

A perfect antibacterial drug would kill bacteria and not harm the patient. As discussed in Chapter 1, there are no perfect drugs. Because bacteria have some of the same cell structures as human cells (e.g., DNA, proteins, and cellular metabolism), some of the drug effects on bacteria also have the same effects on your cells. The goal of antibacterial drug therapy is to use a dose that kills the bacteria or suppresses its growth as much as possible without serious harm to the patient. However, sometimes, when an infection is life threatening, it may be necessary to use higher doses or combinations of drugs that together have more serious side effects.

TYPES OF ANTIBACTERIAL DRUGS

Antibacterial drugs are classified according to the action they use to either kill bacteria or slow bacterial reproduction. The four major classes of antibacterial drugs are cell wall synthesis inhibitors, protein synthesis inhibitors, metabolism inhibitors, and DNA synthesis inhibitors. Within each class there are several types of drugs. Table 6.2 lists the actions of the different types of antibacterial drugs. Fig. 6.2 shows the specific areas of a bacterium that are targeted by different types of antibacterial drugs. The decision to use one type of drug over another is based on whether the actual bacterium causing

Memory Jogger

The goal of antibacterial therapy is to eradicate the infection without harming the patient.

Table 6.2 Antibacterial Categories and Mechanisms of Action

Drug Category and Class	Mechanisms of Action
Cell Wall Synthesis Inhibitors	Binding to cell wall proteins and prevent them from being incorporated into bacterial cell wall units.
Penicillins	
Cephalosporins	Inhibiting bacterial enzymes needed to cross-link the cell wall components, making the walls loose.
Monobactams	
Carbapenems	Inappropriately activating autolysin maintenance enzymes in the bacterial cell walls, which eat holes in the walls, making them leaky.
Glycopeptide inhibitors	
Protein Synthesis Inhibitors	Interfere with protein synthesis by binding to the large (50S) subunit of bacterial ribosomes, preventing them from "reading" the mRNA for placement of the correct amino acid in the new protein.
Aminoglycosides	
Macrolides	Interfere with protein synthesis by binding to the small (30S) subunit of ribosomes, preventing them from "reading" the mRNA for placement of the correct amino acid into the new protein.
Tetracyclines	
Lincosamides	
Oxazolidinones	Interfere with protein synthesis by binding to the enzyme aminoacyl transfer RNA (tRNA) needed to bring the amino acids into contact with the mRNA and link them together.
Streptogramins	
Metabolism Inhibitors	Suppress the activity of the enzymes (dihydropteroate synthase and dihydrofolate reductase) needed to convert other substances (PABA and pteridine) into folic acid in bacteria. As a result, the bacteria do not have enough folic acid to be able to make DNA and reproduce.
Sulfonamides	
Trimethoprim	
Combinations	*Generally bacteriostatic*
DNA Synthesis Inhibitors	Enter bacterial cells and suppress the action of two enzymes (gyrase and topoisomerase) that are most important in allowing the bacteria to make DNA.
Fluoroquinolones	Bactericidal

mRNA, Messenger RNA; *PABA,* para-aminobenzoic acid; *tRNA,* transfer RNA.

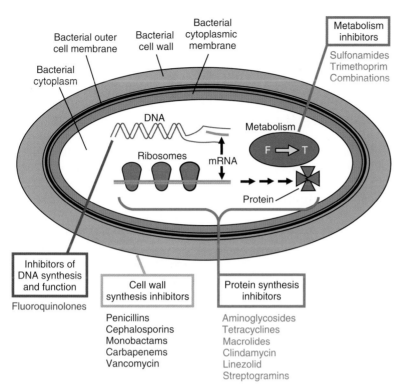

FIG. 6.2 Bacterial targets of different types of antibacterial drugs. $F \rightarrow T$, Metabolic conversion of folic acid to thymine.

the infection is known, how serious the infection is, which drugs are known to kill it or slow its growth, how well the patient's immune system is working, his or her overall health, and whether he or she has any known drug allergies.

GENERAL ISSUES IN ANTIBACTERIAL THERAPY

Each drug type used for antibacterial therapy has both distinctive and common actions and effects. A discussion of general side effects, adverse effects, and responsibilities for antibacterial drugs follows. Additional intended responses, specific side effects, adverse effects, and responsibilities are listed with each individual drug class.

Intended Responses for All Antibacterial Drugs
- Eradication of the infectious bacteria
- Normal body temperature
- WBC count between 5000 and 10,000 cells/mm³
- Absence of drainage and redness or other symptoms of infection.

Common Side Effects for Any Antibacterial Drug
- Intestinal disturbances, especially diarrhea
- Oral and vaginal yeast infection

Possible Adverse Effects of Any Antibacterial Drug
Severe allergic reactions and anaphylaxis are possible, especially when the drug is given intravenously (IV). The major symptom of an allergic reaction to an oral drug is a skin rash that may appear days after starting the drug. A more severe allergic reaction to an IV drug is difficulty breathing and shock, which is called *anaphylaxis*. If not recognized and treated quickly, anaphylaxis can lead to vascular collapse, shock, and death.

Before giving any antibacterial drug, ask patients if they have any drug allergies. Notify the prescriber if the patient has an allergy to the drug. If a patient does have an allergy to a drug and is to receive it anyway, check with the prescriber about first giving diphenhydramine and epinephrine to reduce any serious reaction. Place the emergency cart close to the door of the patient's room.

 Memory Jogger

The four classes of antibacterial drugs are:
- Cell wall synthesis inhibitors
- Protein synthesis inhibitors
- Metabolism inhibitors
- DNA synthesis inhibitors

 Memory Jogger

When helpful normal flora are killed by antibiotic therapy, the microbiome is changed and the patient may develop diarrhea and the overgrowth of yeast in the mouth and vagina. Antibacterial-induced diarrhea is **not** an allergic reaction and is usually not a reason to stop therapy unless it is severe.

 Memory Jogger

Signs and symptoms of an anaphylactic reaction to a drug are:
- Tightness in the chest and trouble breathing
- Low blood pressure, weak pulse
- Hives around the IV site
- Swelling of the face, mouth, and throat
- Hoarse voice

Pseudomembranous colitis is a complication of antibacterial therapy that causes severe inflammation in areas of the colon (large intestine). Other names for this problem include antibiotic-associated colitis and necrotizing colitis. The cause is overgrowth of the intestinal organism *Clostridioides difficile* (*C. diff*). This organism is not killed by most antibacterial drugs, and it can take over the patient's intestinal tract when normal flora are killed off. This organism releases a powerful toxin that damages the intestines. The lining of the colon becomes raw and bleeds. Other symptoms include watery diarrhea, abdominal cramps, low-grade fever, and bloody stools. If patients lose so much water and electrolytes in the watery diarrhea that they become dehydrated, the drug is stopped. Any antibacterial drug can cause the problem if it is taken long enough, but more powerful drugs often allow it to happen sooner.

Priority Actions to Take *Before* Giving Any Antibacterial Drug

Antibacterial drugs often suppress the growth of WBCs in the bone marrow. Check the patient's WBC count (see Table 1.6 in Chapter 1) before drug therapy begins and use the value as a baseline in detecting side effects and drug effectiveness.

Also check the patient's vital signs (including temperature) and mental status before starting any antibacterial drug. These too can help detect side effects and drug effectiveness.

Many IV antibacterial drugs can interact with other drugs and irritate the tissues. Make sure that the IV infusion is running well and has a good blood return. Either flush the line before giving the drug, or use fresh tubing to give it. Check the recommended infusion rate for the specific drug. Most should be given slowly over at least 30 to 60 minutes.

Priority Actions to Take *After* Giving Any Antibacterial Drug

The dosages listed in the drug tables are the recommended dosages for the most common infections. Specific infections may require higher or lower dosages than those listed. Always double check a prescribed dosage that is higher or lower than the average recommended dosage.

Ask the patient about the number of daily bowel movements and their character. Although all antibacterial drugs change the normal flora of the intestines and can cause diarrhea, this symptom is also a sign of the more serious pseudomembranous colitis. The diarrhea of colitis is more watery and intense.

When giving the first IV dose of an antibacterial drug, check the patient every 15 minutes for any signs or symptoms of an allergic reaction. If the patient is having an anaphylactic reaction, your first priority is to prevent any more drug from entering. Stop the drug from infusing, but keep the IV access open. Change the IV tubing after stopping the drug, and do not let any drug remaining in the tubing run into the patient.

Monitor the patient for the effectiveness of the antibacterial drug in treating the infection. Signs and symptoms of a resolving infection include reduced or absent fever; no chills; wound drainage that is no longer thick, foul smelling, brown, green, or yellow; wound edges that are not red and raw looking; and a WBC count that is in the normal range.

Assess the patient's mouth daily for a white, cottage cheese–like coating on the gums, roof of the mouth, or insides of the cheeks. This substance is an overgrowth of yeast called *thrush*.

Assess the IV site at least every 2 hours for symptoms of phlebitis, which include a change in blood return, any redness or pain, or the feeling of hard or cordlike veins above the site. If any of these occur, follow the policy of your agency concerning removal of the IV access.

Teaching Priorities for Patients Taking Any Antibacterial Drug

- Take the drug for as long as it was prescribed, not just until you feel better. Stopping too early can cause the infection to come back and increase the risk for bacteria to become drug resistant.

- Take the drug evenly throughout a 24-hour day to keep your blood level of the drug high enough to be effective. For example, if you are to take the drug twice daily, take it every 12 hours. For three times a day, take it every 8 hours. For four times a day, take it every 6 hours.
- If you develop a rash or hives, stop taking the drug and call your prescriber immediately.
- If you have trouble breathing or have the feeling of a "lump in your throat," call 911 immediately because these are signs of a serious allergic reaction.

SPECIFIC CLASSES OF ANTIBACTERIAL DRUGS

Penicillins, Cephalosporins, and Other Cell Wall Synthesis Inhibitors

Penicillin was the first antibacterial drug developed for general use and was a natural by-product of mold. Some penicillins are still made as a product of mold, and others are made synthetically from chemicals. In addition to penicillin, this drug class includes the cephalosporins, carbapenems, monobactams, and glycopeptide inhibitors (vancomycin).

How cell wall synthesis inhibitors work. Some bacteria have a cell wall, and others do not (see Figs. 6.1 and 6.2). **Cell wall synthesis inhibitors** are able to kill susceptible bacteria by preventing them from forming strong, protective cell walls. Although the penicillins are just one type of drug in this class, many people refer to any cell wall synthesis inhibitor as a "penicillin-like drug."

These drugs usually act in at least one of three ways. Think of a cell wall as made up of individual bricks composed of glycopeptides. The bricks are first held together with certain penicillin-binding proteins (PBPs) that maintain the bricks in the proper alignment. Other PBPs act as mortar between the bricks and cross-link them to both hold the wall together tightly and keep them connected to other bacterial structures. One way these drugs interfere with cell walls is that they bind to the bricks, keeping them from being placed in the wall. The second way these drugs work is by preventing the mortar from being made, which results in the bricks just lying loosely on top of each other so the wall is easy to break. The third way these drugs work is by excessively activating enzymes *(autolysins)* that normally remove damaged wall components so that they can be replaced with newer, stronger components. When autolysin activity is greater than wall-building activity, the cell wall is leaky and does not protect the bacteria.

Cell wall synthesis inhibitors are most effective against bacteria that divide rapidly and are usually found on the skin and mucous membranes, respiratory tract, ear, bone, and blood. Common infections for which these drugs are prescribed include strep throat, tonsillitis, otitis media, simple urinary tract infections, wound infections, upper and lower respiratory infections, prostatitis, and gonorrhea. The more powerful drugs in this class, such as the carbapenems and glycopeptide inhibitors, are used for severe infections such as sepsis, endocarditis, abscesses, and infections that involve multiple types of bacteria.

Some cell wall synthesis inhibitors, especially the cephalosporins, have more than one drug generation. **Drug generation** is the stage of development of a drug in which later generations are changed slightly to improve their effectiveness or means of administration. For example, the cephalosporins have five drug generations. Box 6.1 lists the cephalosporins in each generation. Even though a later-generation drug may have effectiveness against more types of bacterial, earlier-generation drugs are still used to treat specific bacterial infections that remain susceptible to them.

The activity of some cell wall synthesis inhibitors can be enhanced when other agents are added to the drug. For example, penicillin can be destroyed by a bacterial enzyme called β-lactamase, which makes bacteria that have this enzyme resistant to penicillin. Combining penicillin with clavulanic acid (clavulanate) inhibits this bacterial enzyme and reduces penicillin resistance even though clavulanic acid alone has little if any effect on the bacteria. Another example is combining cilastatin with imipenem to extend the time imipenem remains in the body, for better antibacterial action.

There are many types of cell wall synthesis inhibitors, and within each type there are dozens of different brands and strengths. They all work in similar ways and

 Memory Jogger

Penicillin and other cell wall synthesis inhibitors are effective only against bacteria that have a cell wall, because that is the target of the actions of these drugs.

Critical Point for Safety

Although Kimyrsa and Orbactiv are both oritavancin, they have very different storage and dilution requirements and are **not** interchangeable.

QSEN: Safety

Memory Jogger

Of all the cell wall synthesis inhibitors, only the penicillins and cephalosporins have forms that can be given orally.

BOX 6.1 Cephalosporins by Drug Generation

FIRST GENERATION (EXTENDED SPECTRUM)
cefazolin (Ancef, Kefzol)
cephalexin (Biocef, Keflex)
cephradine (Velosef)

SECOND GENERATION (BROAD SPECTRUM)
cefaclor (Ceclor)
cefditoren (Spectracef)
cefoxitin (Cefoxitin, Mefoxin)
cefuroxime (Ceftin, Kefurox, Zinacef)
loracarbef (Lorabid)

THIRD GENERATION (BROAD SPECTRUM)
cefdinir (Omnicef)

cefixime (Suprax)
cefotaxime (Claforan)
cefotetan (Cefotan)
cefpodoxime (Vantin)
ceftazidime (Ceptaz, Fortaz, Tazicef, Tazidime)
ceftibuten (Cedax)
ceftizoxime (Cefizox)
ceftriaxone (Rocephin)

FOURTH GENERATION (BROAD SPECTRUM)
cefepime (Maxipime)

FIFTH GENERATION (BROAD SPECTRUM)
ceftaroline (Teflaro)

---

have similar effects. The more commonly prescribed drugs and their dosages are listed in the following table. Dosages may vary with infection severity and patient health. Consult a reliable drug reference for more information about other drugs in this class.

Usual Adult Dosages for Common Cell Wall Synthesis Inhibitors

Drug Category	Drug Name	Usual Maintenance Dose
Penicillins	amoxicillin (Amoxil, Dispermox, Moxatag, Moxilin)	500–1000 mg orally every 12 hr or 250 mg orally every 8 hr (immediate release) 775 mg orally once daily (extended release)
	amoxicillin/clavulanic acid (Amoclan, Augmentin)	500-875 mg amoxicillin with 125 mg clavulanic acid orally every 12 hr
	penicillin G benzathine; penicillin G procaine (Bicillin CR)	300,000–600,000 units IM
	penicillin V potassium (BeePen-VK, Veetids)	250–500 mg orally every 6 hr
	ticarcillin/clavulanic acid (Timentin)	3 g ticarcillin/0.1 g clavulanic acid IV every 4–6 hr
Cephalosporins	cefazolin (Ancef, Kefzol)	1 g IV or IM every 6–8 hr
	cefdinir (Omnicef)	300 mg orally every 12 hr or 600 mg orally every 24 hr for 5–7 days.
	ceftaroline (Teflaro)	600 mg IV every 12 hr for 5–14 days
	ceftriaxone (Rocephin)	1–2 g IM or IV every 12–24 hr
	cephalexin (Biocef, Daxbia, Keflex, Keftab, Panixine)	500 mg orally every 12 hr for 10 days
Monobactams	aztreonam (Azactam, Cayston)	1–2 g IV or IM every 8–12 hr
Carbapenems	doripenem (Doribax)	500 mg IV every 8 hr for 5–14 days
	ertapenem (Invanz)	1 g IV or IM daily for 10–14 days
	imipenem/cilastatin (Primaxin)	500 mg IV every 6 hr or 1 g IV every 8 hr
	meropenem (Merrem)	1–2 g IV every 8 hr
Glycopeptides	vancomycin (First-Vancomycin, FIRVANQ, Vancocin)	20–35 mg/kg/dose (max: 3000 mg/dose) IV loading dose; then 15–20 mg/kg/dose IV every 8–12 hr
	oritavancin (Kimyrsa, Orbactiv)	1200 mg IV once over a 1–3 hr infusion period
	telavancin (Vibativ)	10 mg/kg IV infusion over 60 min once every 24 hr for 7–21 days

Common side effects of cell wall synthesis inhibitors. Most cell wall synthesis inhibitors have fewer side effects than other types of antibacterial drugs. One reason for this is that human cells have no cell walls, so they are not targeted by these drugs. However, these drugs, especially penicillin, are more likely to cause allergic reactions.

The more powerful drugs in this class, especially the carbapenems and glycopeptides (e.g., vancomycin), have more side effects. These include nausea and vomiting, fever, chills, "red man syndrome" (with rash and redness of the face, neck, upper chest, upper back, and arms), pain at the injection site, reduced hearing, and greatly reduced kidney function.

Possible adverse effects of cell wall synthesis inhibitors. The carbapenems may cause central nervous system changes, including confusion and seizures. The cephalosporins, carbapenems, and glycopeptide antibiotics can greatly reduce kidney function. If a patient is being treated with two or more drugs from this class or with an aminoglycoside (discussed later), the risk for kidney damage and kidney failure increases.

⭐ ***Priority actions to take** before giving cell wall synthesis inhibitors.* In addition to the general responsibilities related to antibacterial therapy (p. 90), when giving a cell wall synthesis inhibitor for the first time, ask whether the patient has any known drug allergies, especially to the drug prescribed. If a patient is allergic to penicillin, the risk for a cephalosporin allergy is increased.

Oral cephalosporins are poorly absorbed with iron supplements and antacids. If a patient is receiving either of these drugs, the cephalosporin should be given 1 hour before or 4 hours after the dose of iron or antacid.

If a patient will receive IV penicillin, check that the injectable form can be given intravenously. One type of injectable penicillin, procaine penicillin, contains a local anesthetic and is **not** an IV drug. This drug is milky white rather than clear.

If a patient is to receive a carbapenem, ask whether he or she has ever had seizures. If so, notify the prescriber because this drug lowers the seizure threshold.

Glycopeptide antibiotics such as vancomycin have many adverse effects if given too fast. These include low blood pressure; a histamine release that causes dilation of blood vessels and a red appearance to the face, neck, chest, back, and arms (red man syndrome); and cardiac dysrhythmias. To reduce the risk for these problems, these drugs are given over at least 60 minutes and never as a bolus or a "push" dose.

⭐ ***Priority actions to take** after giving cell wall synthesis inhibitors.* In addition to general responsibilities related to antibacterial therapy (p. 90), check the patient hourly for the first 4 hours after the first oral dose and every 15 to 30 minutes for the first 2 hours after receiving the first IV dose. Remember that drugs from this class are more likely to cause an allergic reaction than are other types of antibacterials.

⭐ ***Teaching priorities for patients taking cell wall synthesis inhibitors.*** In addition to the general care needs and precautions related to antibacterial therapy (p. 91), include these teaching points and precautions:

- Take cephalosporin drugs at least 1 hour before or 4 hours after iron or an antacid.
- If you take the liquid oral form of penicillin or a cephalosporin, keep the drug tightly closed and refrigerated to prevent loss of drug strength.
- Shake liquid drugs well just before measuring them.

Life span considerations for cell wall synthesis inhibitors

Considerations for pregnancy and lactation. Penicillins and most of the cephalosporins have a low likelihood of increasing the risk for birth defects or fetal harm and can be used to treat infections during pregnancy. The more powerful drugs (carbapenems, monobactams, and glycopeptide antibiotics) have a low to moderate likelihood of

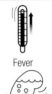
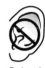

increasing the risk for birth defects or fetal harm and are also used, when needed, during pregnancy. All of these drugs pass into breast milk and will affect a nursing infant, possibly causing the infant to develop a drug allergy. These drugs are usually prescribed for only 5 to 14 days, and the breastfeeding mother should be urged to reduce infant exposure to the drug.

Considerations for older adults. The carbapenems and glycopeptide antibiotics can be both *ototoxic* (causing hearing problems) and *nephrotoxic* (causing kidney problems) at higher doses or when taken for many days in a row. Older adults may already have reduced hearing and kidney function that will be made worse with these drugs. Be alert for a decrease in hearing or for "ringing" in the ears *(tinnitus)*. Monitor intake and output daily, especially if the patient is also taking another drug known to affect kidney function.

Aminoglycosides, Macrolides, Tetracyclines, and Other Protein Synthesis Inhibitors

Protein synthesis inhibitors are a class of antibacterial drugs with several main subtypes that work on different parts of the process of protein synthesis (see Table 6.2). By slowing protein synthesis, these drugs prevent bacteria from making proteins important to their life cycles and infective processes. If any of the pieces and processes (e.g., gene expression, DNA replication, ribosome activity, and linking amino acids into a protein chain) needed for protein synthesis are not working, the bacterium cannot make the protein it needs to survive or reproduce.

How protein synthesis inhibitors work. *Aminoglycosides* actually go through the cell membrane and enter the bacterium. This process uses a transport system that requires oxygen. After entering, the drug binds to the ribosomes and prevents amino acids from forming proteins (see Fig. 6.2). Without these important proteins, bacteria, especially those that use oxygen, usually die.

Macrolides also enter the bacterium through the cell membrane and bind to ribosomes (see Fig. 6.2). The results are the same; no bacterial protein is made, and the bacteria either die or are unable to reproduce. At higher dosages with susceptible organisms, the macrolides are bactericidal. However, at usual and lower dosages, the macrolides are bacteriostatic. Macrolides have no effect on bacteria that do not require oxygen.

Tetracyclines use a special transporter or channel on the surface of the bacterium to pass through the cell's membrane and enter the bacterium. Once inside, tetracyclines act in two ways to inhibit protein synthesis (see Fig. 6.2). Their actions are usually only bacteriostatic rather than bactericidal except at high concentrations. If a bacterium does not have either of these entry mechanisms, it is not affected by tetracycline.

Lincosamides also use two actions to slow protein synthesis. They are usually bacteriostatic but can be bactericidal in high doses. *Oxazolidinones* prevent translation of messenger RNA (mRNA) into protein. They are bacteriostatic against staphylococci and enterococci and are bactericidal against most strains of streptococci. The *streptogramin* antibiotic in current use is made up of two streptogramins (dalfopristin and quinupristin) that work together to inhibit protein synthesis at both the beginning and the end of the process. This drug has many side effects, and its use is limited to severe systemic infections that are life threatening and resistant to vancomycin.

Each group of protein synthesis inhibitors is described separately in the following tables. Within each group, the listings include only the most commonly prescribed drugs and those most often used in acute care settings. Consult a reliable drug reference for more information about any other drugs in this category.

The *aminoglycosides* are powerful antibacterial drugs given IV or IM that have some uncomfortable side effects and serious adverse effects. They are most commonly used for burns, central nervous system infections, joint and bone infections, intra-abdominal infections, peritonitis, and sepsis. Streptomycin is also used in the treatment of tuberculosis.

Usual Adult Dosages for Common Aminoglycosides

Drug Name	Usual Maintenance Dose
amikacin (Amikin, Arikayce)	15–20 mg/kg/dose IV or IM at varying dosing intervals for 10–14 days
gentamicin (Garamycin)	5-7 mg/kg/day IV or IM once daily
streptomycin	1–2 g IM per day in divided doses every 6–12 hr 15 mg/kg/day IM once daily (tuberculosis)

Macrolides have extended- to broad-spectrum effects. Depending on the bacteria type, they are usually bacteriostatic but can be bactericidal at higher doses. These drugs are prescribed for common infections of the skin, mucous membranes, and other soft tissues, chlamydial infections, and respiratory infections. Macrolides are used for legionnaires disease, diphtheria, and mycobacterial infections. Azithromycin is part of the protocol for COVID-19 management.

Usual Adult Dosages for Common Macrolides

Drug Name	Usual Maintenance Dose
azithromycin (Azasite, Zithromax, Zmax)	500 mg orally on day 1; then 250 mg orally once daily for at least 5 days 500 mg IV once daily for 1–2 days, followed by oral therapy
clarithromycin (Biaxin)	250–500 mg orally every 12 hr for 5–7 days
erythromycin (E-mycin)	250 mg orally every 6 h or 500 mg orally every 12 hr

Tetracyclines are broad-spectrum drugs that are bacteriostatic against most of the organisms that are sensitive to penicillins. Because they are bacteriostatic, tetracyclines should be given only to patients with healthy immune systems. They are often prescribed for patients who are allergic to penicillins or cephalosporins. Infections most responsive to tetracyclines are acne, urinary tract infections, skin and mucous membrane infections, respiratory tract infections, sexually transmitted infections, Rocky Mountain spotted fever, syphilis, Lyme disease, and typhoid fever. In addition, they are used to prevent anthrax after exposure to the bacteria.

Usual Adult Dosages for Common Tetracyclines

Drug Name	Usual Maintenance Dose
doxycycline (Adoxa, Doryx, Monodox, Vibramycin, more)	200 mg IV on day 1, then 100–200 mg IV daily or 100 mg orally every 12 hr first day, then 100 mg once daily
minocycline (Arestin, Dynacin, Minocin, Solodyn, more)	200 mg IV initially, then 100 mg IV every 12 hr or 200 mg orally initially, then 100 mg orally every 12 hr
omadacycline (Nuzyra)	100–200 mg IV twice on first day as loading dose, then 100 mg IV daily for 7–14 days or 300 mg orally twice first day as loading dose, then 300 mg orally once daily
sarecycline (Seysara)	150 mg orally once daily for acne
tetracycline (Emtet-500, Panmycin, Sumycin)	500 mg orally every 6 hr for 14 days
tigecycline (Tygacil)	100 mg IV infusion loading dose (over 30–60 min), then 50 mg IV infusion (over 30–60 min) every 12 hr

The three remaining types of protein synthesis inhibitors are very powerful drugs with more severe side effects. These drugs are reserved for treating severe

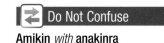

Do Not Confuse

Amikin *with* **anakinra**

An order for Amikin can be confused with anakinra. Amikin is an antibacterial drug, whereas anakinra is a biologic agent for rheumatoid arthritis.

QSEN: Safety

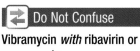

Do Not Confuse

Vibramycin *with* **ribavirin or vancomycin**

An order for Vibramycin can be confused with ribavirin or vancomycin. Vibramycin is a tetracycline antibacterial drug, whereas ribavirin is a strong antiviral agent known to cause birth defects. Vancomycin is a powerful cell wall synthesis inhibitor antibacterial.

QSEN: Safety

or life-threatening infections that do not respond well to other types of antibacterial drugs. The oxazolidinone and streptogramin classes are usually reserved for treating infections from vancomycin-resistant enterococcus (VRE) or methicillin-resistant *Staphylococcus aureus* (MRSA) and for infected diabetic foot ulcers. The third class, the lincosamides, in addition to topical therapy for acne, is used orally and parenterally for severe infections such as peritonitis, cellulitis, abscesses, malaria, and pneumonia caused by *Pneumocystis jirovecii*. The usual doses for all three drug types may be greatly increased when the infection is life threatening.

Usual Adult Dosages for Less Common Protein Synthesis Inhibitor Antibiotics

Drug Class	Drug Name	Usual Maintenance Dose
Oxazolidinones	linezolid (Zyvox)	600 mg IV or orally every 12 hr
	tedizolid (Sivextro)	200 mg IV or orally once daily for 6 days
Streptogramins	dalfopristin/ quinupristin (Synercid)	7.5 mg/kg IV (over 60 min) every 8–12 hr for at least 7 days
Lincosamides	clindamycin (Cleocin)	150–450 mg orally every 6 hr; 300–600 mg IM or IV every 6 or 12 hr
	lincomycin (Lincocin)	600 mg IM every 12–24 hr or 600–1000 mg IV every 8–12 hr

Common side effects of protein synthesis inhibitors. *Aminoglycosides* often cause nausea, vomiting, rash, lethargy, fever, and increased salivation. They also can increase the number of eosinophils (a type of WBC) in the blood. When given intravenously, these drugs are irritating to the vein.

Macrolides have side effects that occur more in the GI tract. They include nausea, vomiting, abdominal pain, diarrhea, loss of appetite, and changes in taste sensation. These drugs greatly increase sun sensitivity *(photosensitivity)*, making serious sunburns possible.

Tetracycline side effects include nausea, vomiting, diarrhea, a sore tongue *(glossitis)*, and rash. These drugs greatly increase sensitivity to the sun, making serious sunburns possible. Rarely do they cause esophageal irritation and ulcer formation. Although all antibacterial drugs can result in yeast overgrowth in the mouth and vagina, tetracycline is more likely to have this effect early in the course of treatment.

The less common protein synthesis inhibitors have many side effects. Lincosamides can cause rash, pain and redness at the injection site (when the drug is given IM), and thrombophlebitis in the vein where the drug infuses.

Oxazolidinones constrict blood vessels and can increase blood pressure in patients who have high blood pressure. Other side effects include nausea, diarrhea, and headaches.

Streptogramin side effects include muscle and joint pain, pain and inflammation at the IV site, rash, nausea, and vomiting.

Possible adverse effects of protein synthesis inhibitors. *Aminoglycosides* are highly toxic to the ears and kidneys, causing hearing loss and reduced kidney function when taken in high doses or for long periods. This is because the tissues of the inner ear and the kidney nephrons begin embryonic development at the same time. Because these tissues are similar in structure, both are at risk for damage by the same drugs.

Macrolides interfere with the metabolism of many drugs. For some, such as digoxin, macrolides keep the drug in the blood longer so digoxin side effects occur faster. Macrolides also increase the effects of warfarin (Coumadin), increasing the risk for bleeding. Combining many other drugs with a macrolide increases the risk for life-threatening cardiac dysrhythmias, especially long QT.

Parenteral forms of macrolides are irritating to veins and tissues. Symptoms of liver irritation or other problems have also been reported.

Common Side Effects

Aminoglycosides

Nausea/ Vomiting   Rash   Lethargy

Fever   Increased salivation

Common Side Effects

Macrolides

Abdominal pain, Nausea/ Vomiting   Taste changes   Photosensitivity

Common Side Effects

Tetracyclines

Nausea/ Vomiting   Sore tongue

Rash   Photosensitivity

Memory Jogger

Drugs that have adverse effects on the kidneys *(nephrotoxic)* almost always have adverse hearing and balance effects *(ototoxic)* on the ears.

Tetracyclines can increase pressure inside the brain (intracranial pressure). Symptoms occurring with this adverse reaction include dizziness, blurred vision, confusion, and ringing in the ears *(tinnitus).*

At high doses, tetracyclines can decrease kidney function and increase liver enzyme levels. These problems resolve when the drug is discontinued, but drugs from this class should be used with caution for any patient with reduced liver or kidney function.

Lincosamides can reduce liver function and decrease WBC counts. When they are given too rapidly by IV infusion, shock and cardiac arrest may occur.

Oxazolidinones reduce blood cell counts, especially red blood cells and platelets, and cause damage to the optic nerve. Usually, these problems occur only in patients who have been taking the drug for longer than 28 days.

Streptogramin increases the blood levels of many drugs, which can then lead to adverse effects of these drugs even when the patient is taking them at normal doses.

⭐ *Priority actions to take* **before** *giving protein synthesis inhibitors.* In addition to the general responsibilities related to starting antibacterial therapy (p. 90), these specific responsibilities are important before giving protein synthesis inhibitors.

Aminoglycosides. Check the patient's current laboratory work, especially blood urea nitrogen (BUN) and serum creatinine levels, because aminoglycosides are toxic to the kidneys. If laboratory values are higher than normal before starting the drug, the risk for kidney damage is greater. Use these data as a baseline to determine whether the patient develops kidney problems while taking aminoglycosides.

Assess the patient's hearing by whispering a phrase with your back turned toward the patient. Document how loudly you need to repeat the phrase until the patient hears it and can repeat it back correctly to you. Use these data as a baseline to determine whether the patient's hearing changes after taking the drug.

Make sure that the aminoglycoside is well diluted before giving it IV. Give the drugs slowly over 30 to 60 minutes to reduce the risk for vein irritation and adverse cardiac effects.

Macrolides. Check to see whether the patient is also taking digoxin, warfarin, pimozide, astemizole, terfenadine, or ergotamine. If so, notify the prescriber immediately because macrolides change the metabolism of these drugs, which can cause adverse effects.

When giving these drugs IV, infuse them slowly. For example, it is recommended that erythromycin be infused by slow continuous drip over 8 to 12 hours.

Tetracyclines. Food, antacids, and dairy products prevent oral tetracycline from being absorbed. Give drugs from this class 1 hour before or 2 hours after a meal. Do not give with milk. Give the patient a full glass of water to drink with tetracycline capsules or tablets, and urge him or her to drink more fluids throughout the day to prevent irritation to the esophagus.

Check the dosages for doxycycline and minocycline carefully because they are lower than for other tetracyclines and other types of antibacterial drugs.

Other protein synthesis inhibitors. Check the patient's current laboratory work, especially BUN and serum creatinine levels, because all of these drug classes are kidney toxic. If these values are higher than normal before starting the drug, the risk for kidney damage is greater.

All three drug classes are known to cause vein irritation and phlebitis. Give them slowly over 30 to 60 minutes, as prescribed, to reduce the risk for vein irritation and cardiac side effects.

When mixing and diluting streptogramins, use only dextrose 5% in water because a precipitate will form when mixed in anything else. The IV line used to give these drugs must either be fresh or flushed with only dextrose 5% in water and never with sodium chloride or heparin.

⭐ *Priority actions to take* **after** *giving protein synthesis inhibitors.* In addition to the general responsibilities related to antibacterial therapy (p. 90), see the specific responsibilities listed later by drug group for what to do after giving protein synthesis inhibitors.

Drug Alert

Administration Alert

Only use solutions of erythromycin that were mixed less than 8 h earlier.

QSEN: Safety

Drug Alert

Administration Alert

Check the dosages for doxycycline and minocycline carefully because they are lower than for other tetracyclines and other types of antibacterial drugs.

QSEN: Safety

Drug Alert

Administration Alert

Mix the parenteral form of streptogramins only with dextrose 5% in water.

QSEN: Safety

Aminoglycosides. Assess the patient's hearing daily as described above, and compare the findings with the patient's hearing before a drug from this class was started.

To determine whether the drug is effective and because aminoglycosides can also cause a fever as a side effect, check the patient's temperature every 4 to 8 hours.

Examine the patient's intake and output record daily to determine whether urine output is within 500 mL of the total fluid intake because these drugs can be kidney toxic. If blood work was done for kidney function, especially BUN and creatinine levels, compare the values before and after the drug was started. If the levels rise above the normal range, notify the prescriber.

Macrolides. For a patient taking a macrolide for the first time or for a patient with known cardiac rhythm problems, assess his or her heart rate and rhythm at least every shift during macrolide therapy. If a new change in rhythm develops, check the patient again in 15 minutes. If the change in rhythm persists or recurs, notify the prescriber.

Tetracyclines. The drugs increase the effects of warfarin (Coumadin). Assess the patient who is also taking warfarin daily for any signs or symptoms of increased bleeding such as bleeding from the gums, presence of bruising or petechiae, oozing of blood around IV insertions or other puncture sites, or the presence of blood in urine or stool.

Other protein synthesis inhibitors. Check the blood pressure of a patient taking an oxazolidinone at least every shift. These drugs can raise blood pressure, especially in patients who already have high blood pressure or are taking other drugs that also raise blood pressure.

⭐ *Teaching priorities for patients taking protein synthesis inhibitors.* In addition to the general care needs and precautions related to antibacterial therapy (p. 91), include the following specific teaching points for protein synthesis inhibitors:

For patients taking *macrolides*:
- Take the drug with food or within 1 hour of having eaten to reduce some of the intestinal side effects.
- Do not chew or crush tablets or capsules.
- Check with your prescriber before taking any other drug.
- Avoid direct sunlight, use sunscreen, and wear protective clothing (including a hat) whenever you are in the sun, to prevent a severe sunburn. Avoid tanning beds and salons.
- If you also take warfarin (Coumadin), keep all appointments to check blood clotting because these drugs increase the effects of warfarin and can increase your risk for bleeding.

For patients taking *tetracyclines*:
- Drink a full glass of water with the tetracycline capsules or tablets, and drink more fluids throughout the day to prevent irritation to the esophagus.
- Take the drugs 1 hour before or 2 hours after meals and do not take the drug with milk because food and milk interfere with absorption of oral tetracyclines.
- Avoid direct sunlight, use sunscreen, and wear protective clothing (including a hat) whenever you are in the sun, to prevent a severe sunburn. Avoid tanning beds and salons.

For patients taking oral forms of *oxazolidinones* or *lincosamides*:
- Drink a full glass of water with oral clindamycin and drink more fluids throughout the day to prevent irritation to the esophagus.
- If you take linezolid, avoid tyramine-containing food such as aged cheese, smoked meats, pickled food, beer, red wine, soy, and sauerkraut because these contain tyramine, which can increase your blood pressure to dangerous levels.

Life span considerations for protein synthesis inhibitors

Pediatric considerations. *Aminoglycosides* can cause severe respiratory depression in infants and children. In addition, because infants and children have immature kidney function, the risk for kidney damage is greater.

The use of *tetracyclines* during tooth development in infancy and early childhood can cause a permanent yellow-gray discoloration of the teeth and make the tooth enamel thinner. Therefore these drugs should not be used in children younger than 8 years of age except for anthrax exposure or a serious infection that is not likely to respond to other antibacterial drugs.

Considerations for pregnancy and lactation. IV and IM *aminoglycosides* have a moderate to high likelihood of increasing the risk for birth defects or fetal harm (except for gentamicin, which has a moderate likelihood) and should not be given to pregnant women unless the infection is life threatening and the organisms are susceptible only to these drugs. Because these drugs are known to cause hearing loss and reduced kidney function, a woman should not breastfeed while taking them.

Most *macrolides* have a low likelihood of increasing the risk for birth defects or fetal harm and can be taken during pregnancy if needed. These drugs pass into breast milk and affect the infant, often causing colic and diarrhea.

Tetracyclines have a moderate to high likelihood of increasing the risks for birth defects or fetal harm. Their use during tooth development in the last half of pregnancy and infancy can cause a permanent yellow-gray discoloration of the teeth and make the tooth enamel thinner. Therefore these drugs should not be used during pregnancy or when breastfeeding except for anthrax exposure or a serious infection that is not likely to respond to other antibacterial drugs.

Considerations for older adults. *Aminoglycosides* are both ototoxic and nephrotoxic at higher doses or when taken for many days in a row. Doses are usually lowered for the older adult. *Macrolides* may be ototoxic in older adults who are also taking a high ceiling or "loop" diuretic such as furosemide (Lasix). Be alert for patient reports of reduced hearing or tinnitus. Monitor the intake and output of older adults daily, especially if they are also taking other drugs known to affect kidney function.

Metabolism Inhibitors: Sulfonamides and Trimethoprim

Metabolism inhibitors are a class of antibacterial drugs that interfere with bacterial reproduction by interrupting critical metabolism. They include sulfonamides and trimethoprim and are bacteriostatic rather than bactericidal. Sulfonamides are based on sulfur and are known as "sulfa drugs." Trimethoprim is a synthetic drug compound that does not contain sulfur and is not a "sulfa drug." In addition to bacterial infections, metabolism inhibitors can be used to treat some nonbacterial infections, such as shigellosis, toxoplasmosis, and pneumocystis pneumonia. They are more commonly used to treat urinary tract infections, middle ear infections, pneumonia, and infectious diarrhea. They are also helpful in treating eye, skin, and vaginal infections and infections of the perineum.

How sulfonamides and trimethoprim work. Bacteria need a type of folic acid (tetrahydrofolate) to be able to make DNA and reproduce. Two specific enzymes are needed to convert para-aminobenzoic acid (PABA) into this type of folic acid in bacteria. The sulfonamides inhibit one enzyme (dihydrofolate synthetase) from working to convert PABA into folic acid, and trimethoprim prevents a different enzyme (dihydrofolate reductase) from converting PABA into folic acid. As a result, bacteria do not have enough folic acid to make DNA and reproduce. This does not kill the bacteria; it just limits their ability to reproduce (see Fig. 6.2). Some metabolism inhibitors combine a sulfonamide with trimethoprim for enhanced antibacterial effect.

The following table focuses on the oral and parenteral forms of these drugs. Dosages vary depending on the type and severity of the infection. Consult a reliable drug reference for more information about a specific drug in this drug group.

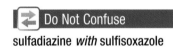

Do Not Confuse

sulfadiazine *with* **sulfisoxazole**

An order for sulfadiazine can be confused with sulfisoxazole. Although both drugs belong to the sulfonamide class of antibiotics, their dosages are different and they are **NOT** interchangeable.

QSEN: Safety

Usual Adult Dosages for Common Metabolism Inhibitor Drugs

Drug Class	Drug Name	Usual Maintenance Dose
Sulfonamides	sulfadiazine	2–4 g orally as a loading dose, then 500 mg to 1 g orally every 6–8 hr
	sulfamethoxazole (SMX)	2 g orally as a loading dose, then 1 g orally every 8–12 hr

Drug Class	Drug Name	Usual Maintenance Dose
	sulfisoxazole (Gantrisin)	2–4 g orally as a loading dose, then 1–2 g orally every 6 hr
Trimethoprim (TMP)	trimethoprim (Primsol, Proloprim, Trimplex)	100 mg orally every 12 hr or 200 mg orally once daily for 10–14 days
Combination Drugs: SMX-TMP, cotrimoxazole	(Bacter-Aid DS, Bactrim, Bactrim DS, Septra, Septra DS, Sulfatrim)	160 mg trimethoprim/800 mg sulfamethoxazole orally every 12 hr for 3–14 days

Common Side Effects

Metabolism Inhibitors

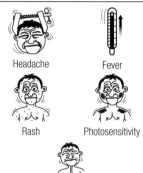

Headache   Fever

Rash   Photosensitivity

Nausea/ Vomiting

🌐 Cultural Awareness

Closely watch male patients who are of African-American or Mediterranean descent for anemia and jaundice when they are receiving a metabolism inhibitor.

Common side effects of metabolism inhibitors. Common side effects of sulfonamides are headache, fever, rash, and increased sun sensitivity. Serious sunburns are possible while taking drugs from this class. The most common side effects of trimethoprim are headache, nausea, vomiting, and a variety of skin rashes and eruptions.

Possible adverse effects of metabolism inhibitors. One of the most serious adverse effects of metabolism inhibitors is suppression of bone marrow cell division. This results in fewer red blood cells (anemia) and fewer WBCs. Some patients are affected in this way only slightly; for others the suppression can be so great that they are at risk for infection.

A simple skin rash can occur with metabolism inhibitors, but more serious skin problems are also possible. These include peeling and sloughing, blister formation, and a combination of many types of skin eruptions known as *Stevens-Johnson syndrome*. This problem is serious and can lead to life-threatening losses of fluids and electrolytes (see Chapter 1).

Metabolism inhibitors should be avoided in any person who has a genetic disorder called glucose-6-phosphate dehydrogenase (G6PD) deficiency. In a patient with this health problem the drug causes red blood cells to break. G6PD deficiency is most common among males of African-American or Mediterranean descent.

Trimethoprim can increase blood levels of potassium (hyperkalemia), especially when taken with other drugs that also increase potassium levels, such as angiotensin-receptor blockers (ARBs) and angiotensin-converting enzyme (ACE) inhibitors.

The sulfonamides are a type of chemical that can easily turn into crystals. Crystals that form and clump in the kidneys can cause kidney failure or kidney stones.

⭐ **Priority actions to take** before *giving metabolism inhibitors.* In addition to the general responsibilities related to antibacterial therapy (p. 90), ask patients about any known drug allergies, especially to sulfa drugs. Notify the prescriber about this issue.

Both the sulfonamides and trimethoprim interact with dozens of other drugs, including common drugs used for management of hypertension and cardiac problems. Be sure to obtain a complete list of all other drugs the patient takes on a regular basis.

If a patient is a male of African-American or Mediterranean descent, ask him if he or any member of his family has a genetic blood disorder. If he says yes, ask the prescriber whether a test for G6PD deficiency should be performed before starting the drug.

Check the patient's current laboratory work, especially liver function tests, because these drugs are irritating to the liver (see Table 1.4 in Chapter 1). If laboratory values are higher than normal before starting the drug, the risk for liver inflammation is greater. Also assess the patient's sclera and skin for yellowing (jaundice) because this problem occurs with liver inflammation. Use these data as a baseline to detect developing liver problems in patients taking metabolism inhibitors.

Check the patient's recent laboratory work for counts of WBCs, red blood cells, and platelets (see Table 1.6 in Chapter 1). Assess the patient's skin for bruises or petechiae.

Check whether the patient is also taking a thiazide diuretic, especially if he or she is older than age 65. If a thiazide diuretic is also ordered, notify the prescriber because combining these drugs greatly increases the risk for anemia and bleeding.

Give the patient a full glass of water to drink with an oral sulfonamide or trimethoprim. Urge him or her to drink more fluids to prevent crystals from forming in the kidneys.

 Priority actions to take after **giving metabolism inhibitors.** In addition to the general responsibilities related to antibacterial therapy (p. 90), offer the patient a full glass of water every 4 hours (day and night) to help prevent crystals from forming in the kidney tubules.

Check the complete blood count every time it is performed to determine whether WBC, red blood cell, and platelet levels have changed (see Table 1.6 in Chapter 1).

Assess the patient's skin every shift for rash, blisters, or other skin eruptions that may indicate a drug reaction. Ask whether he or she has noticed any itching or skin changes.

Assess the patient daily for yellowing *(jaundice)* of the skin or sclera, which is a symptom of liver problems and red blood cell breakdown *(lysis)*. The best places to check are the whites of the eyes closest to the iris, the roof of the mouth, and the skin of the chest. Avoid examining the soles of the feet or palms of the hands, especially in patients with darker skin, because these areas often appear yellow even when the patient is not jaundiced.

 Teaching priorities for patients taking metabolism inhibitors. In addition to the general care needs and precautions related to antibacterial therapy (p. 91), include these teaching points and precautions:

- Avoid direct sunlight, use sunscreen, and wear protective clothing (including a hat) whenever you are in the sun, to prevent a severe sunburn. Also avoid tanning beds and salons.
- Drink a full glass of water when you take the drug and drink more fluids throughout the day to prevent crystals from forming in the urine and clogging the kidneys.
- Notify your prescriber if yellowing of the skin or eyes, a sore throat, fever, rash, blisters, or multiple bruises develop. All these problems are signs of serious adverse effects.

Life span considerations for metabolism inhibitors

Pediatric considerations. Infants younger than 2 months of age are likely to become severely jaundiced when taking metabolism inhibitors, because of a less mature liver allowing free bilirubin levels to rise and cause possible brain damage. These drugs are not recommended for infants younger than 2 months of age except for life-threatening toxoplasmosis infections.

Considerations for pregnancy and lactation. Metabolism inhibitors have a low to moderate risk of increasing the risk for birth defects or fetal harm. Because these drugs can cause severe jaundice in infants, they should be avoided during the last 2 months of pregnancy to reduce the chance that the baby will be born while the mother is taking the drug. For the same reason, the breastfeeding mother should use alternate methods of infant feeding during the time that she is taking metabolism inhibitors.

Considerations for older adults. Metabolism inhibitors have more intense side effects, especially anemia and an increased risk for bleeding, in people older than age 65. When these drugs are taken by a person who also takes a thiazide diuretic, the risk for bleeding increases greatly.

DNA Synthesis Inhibitors: Fluoroquinolones

The primary drugs in the DNA synthesis inhibitors class are the fluoroquinolones. These drugs have many uses when taken systemically and in eye-drop and ear-drop forms. Their most common uses are for skin infections, urinary tract infections, respiratory tract infections, infectious diarrhea, and gonorrhea. Fluoroquinolones also are used to prevent and treat anthrax.

How fluoroquinolones work. Fluoroquinolones enter bacterial cells and prevent bacteria reproduction by suppressing the action of two enzymes important in making bacterial DNA. They are bactericidal to most bacteria that are sensitive to these drugs.

 Drug Alert

Administration Alert

Give patients a full glass of water to drink with an oral sulfonamide or trimethoprim to prevent crystals from forming in the kidneys, increasing the risk for kidney damage.

QSEN: Safety

Cultural Awareness

In patients with darker skin, assess for jaundice on the whites of the eyes closest to the iris and on the roof of the mouth. Do not examine the soles of the feet or palms of the hands for jaundice because these areas often normally appear slightly yellow.

Drug Alert

Teaching Alert

Teach patients taking sulfonamides or trimethoprim to protect themselves from sun exposure because these drugs greatly increase sun sensitivity, even among people with dark skin.

QSEN: Safety

 Critical Point for Safety

Sulfonamides and trimethoprim should not be used during the last 2 months of pregnancy or during breastfeeding because they can cause severe jaundice in the infant.

QSEN: Safety

The following table lists the usual adult dosages for the most commonly use fluoroquinolones. These drugs interact with many other drugs. Consult a reliable drug reference for information about the potential for such interactions.

Usual Adult Dosages for Common Fluoroquinolones

Drug Name	Usual Maintenance Dose
ciprofloxacin (Cetraxal, Ciloxan, Cipro, Cipro XR, ProQuin XR)	500–750 mg orally every 12 hr or 1000 mg orally once daily 200–400 mg IV every 12 hr
delafoxacin (Baxdela)	450 mg orally every 12 hr for 5–10 days 300 mg IV every 12 hr for 5–10 days
gemifloxacin (Factive)	320 mg orally once daily for at least 5 days
levofloxacin (Iquix, Levaquin, Quixin)	250–750 mg orally or IV daily for 5–14 days
moxifloxacin (Avelox, Avelox IV, Moxeza, Vigamox)	400 mg orally or IV daily for 5 days
ofloxacin (Floxin)	200–400 mg orally every 12 hr for 3–5 days

Common Side Effects

Fluoroquinolones

Rash

Nausea/Vomiting, Abdominal pain

Headache

Muscle and joint pain

Common side effects of fluoroquinolones. The most common fluoroquinolone side effects include rash, nausea and vomiting, abdominal pain, headache, and muscle and joint pain. Some also increase sun sensitivity, making serious sunburns possible.

These drugs can concentrate in urine, making the urine irritating to tissues. As a result, the patient may have pain or burning of the urethra and nearby tissues during urination. A patient who is incontinent may have skin irritation in the entire perineal area.

Possible adverse effects of fluoroquinolones. The fluoroquinolones are very effective against many bacterial infections. However, they have more potential adverse effects than most oral antibacterials. Thus prescribers must use caution when selecting these drugs for patients, and nurses must monitor them closely. In addition, patient and family education is critical to prevent problems or identify them early.

Many older patients (older than age 75) become temporarily confused about 2 hours after taking or receiving a fluoroquinolone. This acute confusion usually lasts only 2 to 3 hours but can have serious consequences if the patient is alone and unable to use good judgement. The drug carries a black box warning for mental status changes and impaired memory.

Fluoroquinolones can cause serious heart dysrhythmias, including prolonged QT interval. This serious problem is more common when patients are also taking other drugs for dysrhythmias (e.g., amiodarone, quinidine, procainamide, or sotalol) or when they also have a low blood potassium level (hypokalemia).

Development of peripheral neuropathy is possible while taking these drugs and may be irreversible. Signs and symptoms of this problem include tingling, burning, numbness, and pain in the hands or feet. This problem may become permanent.

For a patient with diabetes, these drugs raise or lower blood glucose levels, leading to either hyperglycemia or hypoglycemia. Hypoglycemia is more common.

A less common adverse effect of fluoroquinolones is the rupture of a tendon, most often in the shoulder, hand, wrist, or heel (Achilles tendon). This complication is more likely to occur in an older patient, particularly one who is also taking a corticosteroid.

⭐ ***Priority actions to take*** *before* ***giving fluoroquinolones.*** In addition to the general responsibilities related to antibacterial therapy (p. 90), the oral forms of some fluoroquinolones are poorly absorbed with iron supplements, multivitamins, and antacids. Give fluoroquinolones at least 2 hours before or 4 hours after the dose of a multivitamin, iron, or antacid.

Determine whether the patient also takes amiodarone, quinidine, procainamide, or sotalol. If so, notify the prescriber immediately because taking any of these drugs with a fluoroquinolone can lead to serious dysrhythmias.

Give patients a full glass of water to drink with oral fluoroquinolone capsules or tablets, and urge them to drink more fluids throughout the day. This action prevents forming a concentrated amount of drug in the urine that can irritate the urethra and perineum. Even the parenteral forms of the drug can concentrate in the urine. Make sure that patients receiving the drug by IV infusion also have a good fluid intake.

 Priority actions to take after giving fluoroquinolones. In addition to the general responsibilities related to antibacterial therapy (p. 90), assess the heart rate and rhythm every 4 hours during therapy of a patient who either has known cardiac dysrhythmias or is taking a fluoroquinolone for the first time. If a new change in rhythm develops, check the patient again in 15 minutes. If the change persists or recurs, notify the prescriber.

For a patient who also has diabetes, check the blood glucose level even more often than usual.

Monitor patients closely after giving the drug orally or parenterally for mental status changes, including acute confusion, especially among older patients. Ask family members to assist in this monitoring to prevent falls and interrupt other behaviors that may have harmful consequences.

 Teaching priorities for patients taking fluoroquinolones. In addition to the general care needs and precautions related to antibacterial therapy (p. 91), include the following teaching points and precautions:
- If you also take warfarin (Coumadin) keep all appointments to check blood clotting because this drug increases warfarin levels and the risk for bleeding.
- Take the drug at least 2 hours before or 4 hours after taking a multivitamin, iron supplement, or antacid because these agents interfere with this drug's absorption.
- Drink a full glass of water with the capsule or tablet and drink more fluids throughout the day to prevent forming urine that can be irritating.
- Take your pulse twice each day, and notify your prescriber if your pulse becomes irregular, if palpitations occur, or if you become dizzy.
- Stop taking the drug and see your prescriber as soon as possible if pain or swelling in a tendon or joint occurs.
- Avoid direct sunlight, use sunscreen, and wear protective clothing (including a hat) whenever you are in the sun to prevent severe sunburn. Also avoid tanning beds and salons.
- If you have diabetes, monitor your blood glucose levels more often and keep a glucose source with you because this drug can cause your blood glucose level to become too low.
- If you are older than 75 years, have another person stay with you for several hours after taking the first doses of this drug because some people become temporarily confused or even have hallucinations.
- Report any new tingling, burning, numbness, and pain in the hands or feet while taking this drug to your prescriber as soon as possible because it can cause nerve damage.

Life span considerations for fluoroquinolones

Pediatric considerations. The use of fluoroquinolones in infants and children younger than 18 years of age is not recommended unless the infection is life threatening and not sensitive to other drugs. Fluoroquinolones can damage bones, joints, muscles, tendons, and other soft tissues when given to patients who are still growing.

Considerations for pregnancy and lactation. Fluoroquinolones have a moderate likelihood of increasing the risk for birth defects or fetal harm, especially bone, joint, and tendon defects. These drugs should not be used during pregnancy. The breastfeeding mother should use alternate methods of infant feeding during the time that she is taking fluoroquinolones.

★ Critical Point for Safety

Fluoroquinolones can only be given orally or by IV infusion. Do not give any fluoroquinolone as a bolus or by the IM or subcutaneous routes.

QSEN: Safety

! Drug Alert

Intervention Alert

Assess patients with diabetes often for hypoglycemia because fluoroquinolones can cause quick changes in blood glucose levels.

QSEN: Safety

! Drug Alert

Teaching Alert

Teach patients taking fluoroquinolones to protect themselves from sun exposure because these drugs greatly increase sun sensitivity, even among people with dark skin.

QSEN: Safety

Considerations for older adults. Tendon rupture is seen more often in older adults taking fluoroquinolones. The tendons most often affected are in the shoulder, hand, wrist, and Achilles tendon at the heel. Taking corticosteroids at the same time as a fluoroquinolone increases the risk, but tendon rupture can occur when taking fluoroquinolones alone. Tendon rupture also can occur up to 1 month after the drug has been stopped. If the patient has pain or inflammation of a tendon or around a joint, he or she should stop the drug, stop moving or exercising that joint, and see the prescriber as soon as possible.

Get Ready for the NCLEX® Examination!

Key Points

- Even a patient who has never taken an antibacterial drug can have an infection with bacteria that are resistant to antibacterial drug therapy.
- Gram-negative bacteria are harder to kill or control with antibacterial drugs because they have a protective capsule that limits the effects of drugs.
- Check the patient's vital signs (including temperature) and mental status before starting an antibacterial drug.
- The dosages listed in the drug tables are the recommended dosages for the most common infections. Specific infections may require higher or lower dosages than those listed. Always double check a prescribed dosage that is higher or lower than the average recommended dosage.
- Check to determine which solutions can be used to dilute a particular IV antibacterial drug and which solutions or drugs should be avoided with that drug.
- For drugs that are toxic to the ears and hearing (ototoxic) such as vancomycin and the aminoglycosides, check the patient's hearing before therapy begins.
- For drugs that cause heart rhythm disturbances such as macrolides and fluoroquinolones, check the patient's heart rate, rhythm and quality for a full minute before giving the first dose and regularly thereafter.
- For drugs that increase the effects of warfarin (when the patient is also taking warfarin) such as macrolides, tetracyclines, streptogramins, and fluoroquinolones, check the patient's most recent international normalized ratio (INR) before giving the first dose of the drug.
- Give antibacterial drugs on a schedule that evenly spaces them throughout 24 hours.

- Never give procaine penicillin intravenously.
- Do not give (and teach patients not to take) cephalosporins, tetracyclines, or fluoroquinolones with antacids, multiple vitamins, or iron supplements.
- For the patient taking warfarin and a macrolide, tetracycline, streptogramin, or fluoroquinolone, check the patient daily for any signs or symptoms of increased bleeding.
- Urge the patient taking any antibacterial drug to stop the drug and inform the prescriber if a rash or other skin eruption develops.
- Instruct patients to immediately call 911 if they begin to have difficulty breathing, a rapid irregular pulse, swelling of the face or neck, or the feeling of a "lump in the throat."
- Teach patients taking macrolides, tetracyclines, sulfonamides, or fluoroquinolones that these drugs can cause severe sunburn, even for patients with dark skin.
- Drug types that should be avoided during pregnancy, while breastfeeding, and with infants or children unless the infection is life threatening include aminoglycosides, tetracyclines, sulfonamides, and fluoroquinolones.
- Do not give any fluoroquinolone as a bolus or by the intramuscular or subcutaneous routes.
- Fluoroquinolones carry a black box warning for inducing mental status changes, including acute confusion, and for increasing the risk for permanent peripheral neuropathy.

Additional Learning Resources

🌐 Be sure to visit your Evolve website (http://evolve.elsevier.com/Workman/pharmacology/) for additional online resources.

SG Go to your Study Guide for additional learning activities to help you master this chapter content.

Review Questions

See *Answers to In-Text Review Questions* in the back of the book for answers to these questions.

1. **Why is the increasing development of resistant strains of bacteria a major health care concern?**

   A. More infections will be difficult to control and lead to death.
   B. Opportunistic infections are more likely to become pathogenic.
   C. New drugs are more expensive than those that have been used for many years.

   D. As bacteria become more resistant, people become more susceptible to infection.

2. **How are bactericidal drugs different from bacteriostatic drugs?**

   A. Bacteriostatic drugs are more likely to cause an allergic response than bactericidal drugs.
   B. Bacteriostatic drugs work only on bacteria, whereas bactericidal drugs are effective against other types of organisms.
   C. Bactericidal drug actions result in killing the bacteria, whereas bacteriostatic drugs only slow bacterial growth.

D. Bactericidal drugs require assistance from the patient's immune system to be effective, whereas bacteriostatic drugs are effective even when function is poor.

3. A patient with an ear infection is prescribed penicillin V potassium 500 mg to be taken orally at home four times a day. What will the nurse teach the patient about the **most effective** dosing intervals for this drug?

A. "Take the drug when you first get up and at lunch time, and then take 2 tablets with your evening meal so your sleep is not interrupted.

B. "If it is more convenient, take two doses every 12 hours instead of one tablet four times a day."

C. "Take the drug every 6 hours throughout the day and night."

D. "Take the drug every 6 hours while you are awake."

4. Which action will the nurse use to reduce the risk for vein irritation when giving a patient an irritating antibacterial drug by intravenous (IV) infusion?

A. Infusing the drug slowly over at least 30 to 60 minutes

B. Cooling the drug solution in the refrigerator before infusing it

C. Using half of the normal amount of diluent when preparing and mixing the drug

D. Keeping the patient's IV site above the level of the heart while the drug is infusing

5. Which action(s) will the nurse perform **first** when the patient has symptoms of anaphylaxis while an intravenous (IV) antibacterial drug is infusing?

A. Notifying the prescriber immediately

B. Discontinuing (removing) the IV access

C. Stopping the infusion and maintaining IV access

D. Slowing the infusion and assessing the patient's blood pressure

6. In taking the history of a patient who has just been prescribed a cephalosporin for pneumonia the nurse discovers the patient also has the following issues or health problems. For which issue or problem will the nurse notify the prescriber before the patient receives the first dose of the drug?

A. Current urinary tract infection

B. Type 2 diabetes mellitus

C. Allergy to "sulfa" drugs

D. Seizure disorder

7. A patient who has been taking oral potassium penicillin for a "strep" throat calls to report that she is now pregnant. What is the nurse's **best** response?

A. "I will notify your prescriber so the drug can be changed."

B. "No problem, this drug is safe to take during early pregnancy."

C. "If you are no longer having symptoms, just stop taking the drug."

D. "It is good you called. Continuing to take the drug could give your baby a penicillin allergy."

8. As the nurse hangs the first dose of intravenous (IV) amikacin, the patient announces that he just remembered that he is allergic to penicillin. What is the nurse's **best** action before starting the infusion?

A. Reassuring the patient that the IV drug contains no penicillin

B. Checking the patient's medical record to verify the allergy

C. Holding the dose and notifying the prescriber

D. Documenting the report as the only action

9. A patient's serious infection is only sensitive to a macrolide. This patient is also on warfarin therapy for chronic atrial fibrillation. What drug adjustment does the nurse anticipate will be needed in this situation?

A. Increasing the dosage of the macrolide

B. Decreasing the dosage of the macrolide

C. Increasing the dosage of warfarin

D. Decreasing the dosage of warfarin

10. Which precaution is **most important** to **prevent harm** for the nurse to teach a patient who is prescribed to take a combination sulfonamide/trimethoprim drug for a urinary tract infection?

A. "If you develop a skin rash with this drug, stop taking it and call your prescriber immediately."

B. "Drink a full glass of water with each dose and increase your daily fluid intake to at least 2 L."

C. "If you use an oral contraceptive, use a barrier form of contraception for the next month."

D. "Reduce your intake of salt and sodium-containing food while taking this drug."

11. A patient taking ciprofloxacin reports pain and burning on urination. What is the nurse's **best** action?

A. Notifying the prescriber that the patient's urinary tract infection is not responding to the drug

B. Reminding the patient that the pain is related to the body eliminating the infectious bacteria

C. Instructing the patient to drink a full glass of water with each drug dose and increase fluids

D. Asking the patient whether blood or pus is also present in the urine

12. A patient is prescribed to receive 1,800,000 units of penicillin G benzathine by intramuscular injection. The only available preparation of this drug is a prefilled syringe containing 2,400,000 units in 4 mL. How many mL of this drug will the nurse transfer into another syringe to administer the prescribed dose? _____mL

Clinical Judgment

1. The family member of a patient receiving intravenous (IV) vancomycin tells the nurse in a panicky voice that she thinks the patient is having an allergic reaction to the drug. When assessing the patient, the nurse notes that the patient's face, chest, and arms are very flushed and red. Which actions are most appropriate for the nurse to take at this time? **Select all that apply.**

   A. Stopping the infusion
   B. Discontinuing the IV
   C. Slowing the rate of the infusion
   D. Asking the patient if he is having any difficulty breathing
   E. Calling the rapid response team
   F. Documenting the situation
   G. Reassuring the family that this response is common but not harmful
   H. Checking the patient's urine for the presence of bright red blood
   I. Monitoring the patient every 15 minutes

2. A 22-year-old woman is prescribed sarecycline 150 mg orally daily for chronic moderate to severe acne. She is expected to take this drug for 6 months to a year. Currently, she is in college on a golfing scholarship. Other than occasional muscle soreness for which she takes ibuprofen, the patient has no other health issues and uses a low-dose estrogen oral contraceptive. The nurse is developing a teaching plan with take-home instructions/precautions about these drugs. **Use an X to indicate which instructions are Most Relevant, Not Relevant, or Potentially Harmful at this time for this patient with regard to antibacterial drug therapy with tetracycline.**

INSTRUCTION/PRECAUTION	MOST RELEVANT	NOT RELEVANT	POTENTIALLY HARMFUL
Take this drug with food or milk to prevent stomach problems.			
Drink a full glass of water with each capsule and increase your overall daily water intake.			
Avoid pickled food, red wine, soy-containing food or drinks, and sauerkraut while taking this drug.			
Whenever you golf or are outdoors, wear a hat, long sleeves, and sunscreen because you will sunburn much more easily on this drug.			
Avoid taking any vitamin supplements that contain vitamin K because they will reduce this drug's effectiveness.			
Brush your teeth and tongue thoroughly followed by rinsing with mouthwash at least 3 times daily to prevent an oral infection.			
If you notice darkening or a yellow-gray discoloration of your teeth, notify your prescriber immediately.			
If you should become pregnant while on this drug, stop taking it.			
Keep the tablets in the container that came from the pharmacy rather than using a daily pill organizer.			

Antiinfectives: Antiviral Drugs

http://evolve.elsevier.com/Workman/pharmacology/

Learning Objectives

The content presented in this chapter should help you to:

1. Explain the names, actions, usual adult dosages, possible side effects, and adverse effects of the different types of nonretroviral drug therapies.
2. Describe priority actions to take before and after giving any of the different types of nonretroviral drug therapies.
3. Prioritize essential information to teach patients taking any of the different types of nonretroviral drug therapies.
4. Explain the names, actions, usual adult dosages, possible side effects, and adverse effects of the different types of retroviral drug therapies.
5. Describe priority actions to take before and after giving any of the different types of retroviral drug therapies.
6. Prioritize essential information to teach patients taking any of the different types of retroviral drug therapies.
7. Explain appropriate life span considerations for the different types of nonretroviral and retroviral drug therapies.

Key Terms

antiretroviral drugs (ăn-tī-RĔT-rō-vī-răl DRŬGZ) (p. 122) A category of antiviral drugs that suppresses the replication (reproduction) of viruses (retroviruses) that use RNA as their primary genetic material instead of DNA.

antiviral drugs (ăn-tī-vī-răl DRŬGZ) (p. 109) Drugs that are virustatic against nonretroviruses and prevent them from either replication/reproducing or releasing their genetic material.

COVID-19 virus (KŌ-vĭd VĪ-rŭs) (p. 119) A new virulent nonretrovirus that's able to infect humans for the first time, often causing a severe influenza-like respiratory infection.

human immune deficiency virus (HIV) (HYŪ-mŭn ĭm-MYŪN dĕ-FĬSH-ĕen-sē VĪ-rŭs) (p. 121) The most common retrovirus

known to cause disease among humans. It is the organism known to cause HIV disease and AIDS.

viral load (VĪ-rŭl LŌD) (p. 123) The number of viral particles in a blood sample, which indicates the degree of viral infection.

virulence (VĬR-ŭ-lĕns) (p. 108) The measure of how well a microorganism can invade and persist in growing, even when the person's immune function is trying to destroy or eliminate it.

virus (VĪ-rŭs) (p. 107) An intracellular, submicroscopic parasite that can only reproduce by infecting a living host cell.

virustatic (vī-rŭ-STĂ-tĭk) (p. 109) Drug actions that reduce the number of viruses present by preventing them from reproducing and growing.

OVERVIEW

Viruses are intracellular, submicroscopic parasites that are unable to reproduce on their own and must infect a living host cell to replicate/reproduce (Animation 7.1). A *host* is the person infected by a virus whose cells allow replication of viral genetic material and reproduction. When viruses infect a living cell in just the right way, the resources, energy, and machinery of that living cell are used to make new viruses. Because they are so small, viruses can more easily enter the body than bacteria and funguses can. Entrance sites include mucous membranes in the nose, conjunctiva of the eye, respiratory tract, digestive tract, and genital or urinary tract. They can also enter through broken skin, and they can be injected into the body through infusion of blood or blood products.

Viral infections are common. Some, like a cold, are non-life threatening and require no drug therapy for complete resolution. Others, such as hepatitis, are more complicated and, left untreated, may cause serious damage or death.

There are two basic types of viruses that infect humans: *nonretroviruses*, which are the most common type, and *retroviruses*. Likewise, there are two basic categories of antiviral drugs: those that work against common nonretroviral infections and those that help control retroviral infections (antiretroviral drugs).

REVIEW OF RELATED PHYSIOLOGY AND PATHOPHYSIOLOGY OF COMMON NONRETROVIRUSES

Common nonretroviruses use either DNA or RNA as their genetic material and many have a relatively low efficiency of cellular infection. *Efficiency of infection* is the ease with which an organism causes disease through infection. Those that easily invade and persist in growing, even when the person's immune function is trying to destroy or eliminate it, have greater **virulence**. Virulent organisms can cause infection even when fewer viruses enter the body. Many nonretroviruses are less virulent and must invade the body in large numbers to cause disease. These viruses are responsible for common infections such as chickenpox, shingles, measles, mumps, herpes, warts, hepatitis, and the common cold. Table 7.1 lists selected diseases caused by specific viruses.

The basic anatomy of a nonretrovirus is shown in Fig. 7.1. For viruses to cause disease after they enter the body, they must actually enter human cells and use the reproductive machinery of the cell to make more viruses that then leave the cell to infect more cells. So becoming sick with a viral disease requires that many cells be infected by common nonretroviruses. Once inside the body viruses can be destroyed or removed by the immune system. A healthy person will not become ill from most nonretroviruses unless the number of invading viruses overwhelms the normal immune protections.

Viruses that enter the body and survive must enter cells and insert their genetic material into the genetic material of the host cells. Then viral genes direct the host cell to make more viruses. These new viruses fill the cell and eventually break out of it to infect more host cells (Fig. 7.2). Viral infections are not cured but are self-limiting, meaning that in a person with a healthy immune system the illness only

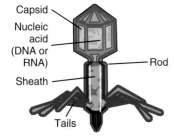

FIG. 7.1 The basic anatomy of a common virus.

Table **7.1**	Selected Diseases Caused by Specific Viruses
VIRUS	**DISEASE**
Cytomegalovirus (CMV)	Mononucleosis Serious eye infection (retinitis) in people who are immunosuppressed
Epstein-Barr virus (EBV)	Chronic fatigue syndrome Some types of lymphoma Systemic infection in newborns and people with severe immunosuppression
Hantavirus (HV)	Hantavirus pulmonary syndrome (HPS)
Hepatitis A virus (HAV)	Hepatitis A
Hepatitis B virus (HBV)	Acute hepatitis B Chronic hepatitis B Liver failure Liver cancer
Hepatitis C virus (HCV)	Chronic hepatitis C Liver failure
Herpes simplex virus type 1 (HSV1)	Cold sores Systemic infection in newborns and people with severe immunosuppression
Herpes simplex virus type 2 (HSV2)	Genital herpes infections
Respiratory syncytial virus (RSV)	Severe respiratory infection in infants, young children, and older adults
SARS-CoV-2	COVID-19
Varicella-zoster virus (VZV)	Chickenpox Shingles
West Nile virus (WNV)	Severe infection with symptoms similar to those of encephalitis or meningitis

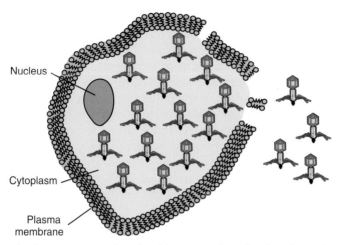

FIG. 7.2 An infected cell generates new viruses and then opens the cell and sends newly generated viruses out to infect more host cells.

lasts for so long, although the virus may never completely leave the body. If a person's immune system is working properly, the body suppresses the infection by itself. If the immune system is weak or if the body has other health problems, the person may die from the effects of the viral disease. Two of the most virulent nonretroviruses are hepatitis B virus (HBV) and hepatitis C virus (HCV). Others, such as the virus group that cause the common cold, are less virulent.

Some common nonretroviral infections are minor and can be limited by the immune system. Because more severe viral infections can cause serious harm and even death, antiviral drugs are used to prevent viruses from spreading the infection all through the body and causing severe damage.

GENERAL ISSUES IN ANTIVIRAL THERAPY

Unlike many antibacterial drugs, all antiviral drugs are **virustatic** and only reduce the number of viruses by preventing them from reproducing and growing. *They are not virucidal* and cannot kill the virus. By keeping the number of viruses low, antiviral drugs allow the natural defenses of the body to destroy, eliminate, or inactivate them.

Antiviral drugs are *virustatic* drugs that prevent viruses from either reproducing or from releasing their genetic material. Drugs that are effective against common nonretroviruses do not have specific categories and may have more than one mechanism of action. Some antiviral drugs suppress viral reproduction. Others prevent the virus from opening its coat and allowing the genetic material to be released. The exact mechanisms of action of still other antiviral drugs are not known. The dosages and lengths of therapy for these drugs depend on which virus is causing the infection, the severity of the infection, and the health of the patient's immune function.

Allergic reactions are possible with any antiviral drug. The allergy may be mild and annoying or severe and life threatening (such as anaphylaxis and angioedema). More serious reactions occur when antiviral drugs are given intravenously.

Intended Responses of Any Antiviral Drug
- The duration or intensity of an existing viral disease is shortened.
- Reactivation of a dormant viral infection is prevented.
- A viral infection is prevented from multiplying to the point that disease results.

⭐ Priority Actions to Take *Before* and *After* Giving Any Antiviral Drug
Before giving an antiviral drug, ask whether the patient has any drug allergies. If so, notify the prescriber before giving the drug.

The dosages listed in the drug tables are recommended dosages for the most common types of viral infections. Specific infections, depending on severity and

 Memory Jogger

Antiviral drugs do not kill viruses; they only suppress their reproduction and spread.

organs affected, may require higher dosages than listed. Always double check a prescribed dosage that is higher or lower than the average recommended dosage.

After giving the first dose of an intravenous (IV) antiviral drug, assess the patient every 15 minutes for signs or symptoms of an allergic reaction (hives at the IV site; low blood pressure; rapid, irregular pulse; swelling of the lips or lower face; the patient feeling a lump in the throat). If the patient is having an anaphylactic reaction, your first action is to prevent any more drug from entering him or her. Stop the drug from infusing but maintain the IV access. If the drug is infusing high into the IV tubing, change the tubing after stopping the drug and do not let any drug left in the tubing infuse into the patient.

Inspect the IV site at the beginning of the infusion, halfway through the infusion, and at the end of the infusion and document your findings. If redness is present or the patient reports discomfort at the site, slow the infusion and check for a blood return. Look for any redness or pain or the feeling of hard or cordlike veins above the site. If any of these problems occur, follow the policy of your facility for removing the IV line.

⭐ Teaching Priorities for Patients Taking Any Antiviral Drug
- Take the antiviral drug exactly as prescribed and for as long as prescribed.
- Keep in mind the need for you to take the drug long enough to ensure suppression of viral reproduction. If you stop taking the drug as soon as you feel better, symptoms of infection may recur, and resistant viruses may develop.
- If you are prescribed to take more than one dose per day, take the drug evenly throughout the 24-hour day to keep your blood drug level high enough to be effective. For example, if you are to take the drug twice daily, take it every 12 hours. For three times a day, take it every 8 hours.
- Plan an easy-to-remember schedule that keeps the drug at the best blood levels, perhaps by associating the timing with your specific important daily activities.

ANTIVIRAL DRUGS FOR NONRETROVIRAL INFECTIONS

Drugs for Herpes Simplex Infections
Antiviral drugs for herpes simplex infections most commonly are used to manage genital herpes infection but can be used when oral infections are severe. They are sometimes effective in helping to control shingles (varicella zoster virus), Epstein-Barr virus, and cytomegalovirus infections. For first-time infections, dosages are slightly higher and given for a shorter time period. For recurrent infections, dosages may be lower and given indefinitely. Other than reminding patients not to receive a live virus vaccine while taking these drugs, there are no specific actions or teaching priorities needed beyond those listed above in the general responsibilities related to antiviral therapy.

Adult Dosages for Common Antiviral Drugs to Manage Herpes Simplex Infections

Drug Names	Usual Maintenance Dose
acyclovir (Sitavig, Zovirax)	1st infection: 400 mg orally three times daily 7–10 days Recurrent infection: 400 mg orally twice daily for 5 days
famciclovir (Famvir)	1st infection: 250 mg orally three times daily 7–10 days Recurrent infection: 250 mg orally twice daily for 3-5 days
valacyclovir (Valtrex)	1st infection: 1 g orally twice daily 7–10 days Recurrent infection: 500–1000 mg once daily for 3–5 days.

How antiviral drugs for herpes simplex infections work. All three drugs suppress viral replication by forming "counterfeit" DNA bases and inhibiting the viral form of the enzyme DNA polymerase that is needed to complete the formation of viral DNA chains in virally infected cells. Acyclovir also inactivates other enzymes needed in the DNA synthesis process.

Common side effects of antiviral drugs for herpes simplex infections. Common side effects of all these drugs are headaches, dizziness, nausea, and diarrhea.

Possible adverse effects of antiviral drugs for herpes simplex infections. These drugs can reduce kidney function and lead to kidney damage and failure. This problem is caused by the drugs precipitating in the kidney tubules, which is most likely to occur when the patient is not well hydrated.

These drugs also reduce the effectiveness of some antiseizure drugs. Patients who take these antiviral drugs, especially those who may be taking them long term, need to have blood levels of antiseizure drugs checked more often and the prescriber may need to increase the dosage of the antiseizure drugs.

Pain and irritation at the injection site may occur with IV acyclovir, especially when the drug is given rapidly. The IV forms of any of these drugs have an increased risk for allergic reactions and anaphylaxis. Administer these drugs slowly over at least 60 minutes to avoid kidney problems and reduce the risk for irritation at the injection site.

Life span considerations for antiviral drugs for herpes simplex infections

Considerations for pregnancy and lactation. Antiviral drugs for herpes simplex infections have a low likelihood of increasing the risk for birth defects or fetal damage. The benefits of the use of these antiviral agents during pregnancy should be weighed against any possible risks. These drugs appear in breast milk and can enter the infant during breastfeeding. Thus, breastfeeding while taking these antiviral drugs is not recommended.

Drugs for Common Respiratory Viral Infections

Nonretrovirus-induced respiratory infections for which antiviral drugs may be prescribed include influenza and respiratory syncytial virus (RSV). Some of the drugs prescribed for influenza can be used for both prevention and for treatment of an actual infection. Antiviral drugs used to treat viral pneumonia vary depending on the infecting organism. For example, when viral pneumonia is caused by a herpes simplex virus, one of the antiviral drugs for herpes simplex infections is prescribed. When pneumonia results from influenza and does not have a bacterial infection occurring with it, influenza antiviral drugs are used.

Two older drugs once used as the mainstay of respiratory viral infections therapy, amantadine and rimantadine, are no longer recommended by the Centers for Disease Control and Prevention (CDC) for use with respiratory viral infections. Their use is associated with an increased risk for drug-resistant strains of influenza viruses.

Adult Dosages for Common Antiviral Drugs to Manage Respiratory Viral Infections

Indication	Drug Name	Usual Dosage
Influenza	baloxavir marboxil (Xofluza)	40–80 mg orally (depending on weight) as a single dose within 48 hr of symptom onset or as soon as possible after exposure
	oseltamivir (Tamiflu)	75 mg orally twice daily for 5 days or 75 mg orally twice daily for 10 days after exposure
	peramivir (Rapivab)	600 mg IV as a single dose within 48 hr of symptom onset
	zanamivir (Relenza)	10 mg by dry powder inhaler every 12 hr for 5 days
Respiratory syncytial virus (RSV)	ribavirin	*Children: 20 mg/mL for respiratory syncytial virus at 12–18 hr/day delivers an average of 190 mcg/L of air

*Adult inhalation dose not established

How antiviral drugs for respiratory viral infections work. *Baloxavir* inhibits an influenza-specific enzyme needed for viral gene transcription. The result of this inhibition is the blocking of influenza virus replication. It can be used to both prevent seasonal influenza and to treat it.

Oseltamivir, peramivir, and *zanamivir* work by binding to and inhibiting the viral enzyme neuraminidase. This enzyme is needed to spread viral particles in the respiratory tract. As a result, viral particles released from one infected cell cannot infect other cells. These drugs shorten the duration and reduce the severity of influenza. They can also prevent influenza from developing after exposure to the virus.

Ribavirin is a "counterfeit" base that suppresses viral action and reproduction by unknown mechanisms. It is effective at suppressing many viruses; however, because of its severe side effects and adverse effects, its use in respiratory viral infections is restricted to those that do not respond to other antiviral agents. It is most commonly used by inhalation to treat RSV infection in children and may also be used systemically to treat Hantavirus, hepatitis A, hepatitis C, and West Nile viruses, among other more rare viruses.

Common side effects of antiviral drugs for respiratory viral infections. Common side effects of *baloxavir, oseltamivir, peramivir,* and *zanamivir* include headache, nausea and vomiting, diarrhea, and dizziness. *Zanamivir,* as an inhaled drug, also may cause bronchoconstriction, cough, and nasal congestion. *Peramivir* also may cause hypertension and hyperglycemia.

Ribavirin is a powerful drug with many side effects, even when given by inhalation, in addition to the ones associated with other antiviral drugs for respiratory viral infections. Its additional side effects include conjunctivitis, muscle pain, fatigue, and injection site pain or irritation (parenteral form).

Possible adverse effects of antiviral drugs for respiratory viral infections. Specific adverse effects of *baloxavir, peramivir,* and *zanamivir* include acute confusion, delirium, and hallucinations. *Oseltamivir* and *peramivir* can elevate liver enzyme levels. In addition, *peramivir* can interfere with the development of antibodies in response to a live virus vaccination.

Ribavirin has many adverse effects, and its use is limited to patients who have severe viral infections for which no other drugs are effective. It is a *teratogen,* an agent that can cause birth defects, and should not be given to pregnant or breastfeeding women. It should not even be handled or inhaled by anyone who is pregnant.

Ribavirin can suppress the bone marrow production of red blood cells (RBCs) and white blood cells (WBCs). As a result, the patient can be anemic and at risk for infection.

With prolonged use, ribavirin can impair the function of the liver, kidneys, heart, and ears. In addition, it may lead to some forms of cancer.

⭐ **Priority actions to take** before *giving antiviral drugs for respiratory viral infections.* Baloxavir, oseltamivir, and zanamivir are orally or inhaled drugs that are largely prescribed for community-dwelling independent people. As a result, there are no specific actions to take before or after giving these drugs in addition to the general responsibilities and care issues related to antiviral therapy (see pp. 109-110). *Peramivir* is given intravenously only as a one-time dose. It must be diluted carefully and does not have a preservative. So, it must be given as soon as possible after mixing or stored in a refrigerator for no more than 24 hours. This drug is not to be administered with any other drugs.

Ribavirin is a powerful drug given in many settings and, even when prescribed as an inhalant, does require specific actions in addition to general responsibilities and care issues.

Keep in mind that *ribavirin* can have toxic effects on many organs. Before giving ribavirin, assess the patient's heart rate, rhythm, and pulse quality. Evaluate lung function by assessing the rate and depth of respiratory effort, breath sounds, pulse oximetry, color of skin and mucous membranes, and level of consciousness. Assess kidney function by checking the most recent 24-hour intake and output and comparing the amount of urine excreted with the amount of fluids consumed. Also review the patient's current kidney tests, especially the blood urea nitrogen (BUN) and serum creatinine levels (see Table 1.5 in Chapter 1 for a listing of normal values). If the values are higher than normal before starting the drug, the risk for kidney damage

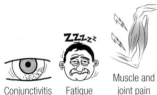

is greater. Assess liver function by examining for yellowing (*jaundice*) of the skin, palate, or whites of the eyes and by checking liver function tests (see Table 1.4 in Chapter 1 for a listing of normal values). Use these data as a baseline to detect changes that may result from adverse drug effects.

Because ribavirin often suppresses the growth of blood cells in the bone marrow, review the patient's most recent WBC and RBC counts before drug therapy begins. Use these data as a baseline in determining the presence of side effects and whether or not the drug is effective against the infection (see Table 1.6 in Chapter 1 for a listing of normal blood cell values).

Assess the patient's vital signs (including temperature and mental status) before starting ribavirin. Use this information as a baseline to determine whether any side effect or adverse effect is present and whether the drug therapy is effective against the infection.

Ribavirin can interact with many drugs, including almost all the antiretroviral drugs used in the management of human immune deficiency virus disease (HIV disease). These interactions can result in severe liver problems and death from liver failure. Be sure to obtain a complete list of all drugs the patient is currently taking before the first dose of ribavirin is given and record these in the medical record.

When administering aerosolized *ribavirin*, use only the SPAG-2 aerosol generator. Read the instruction manual before using this instrument. Prepare the aerosolized form of the drug using sterile technique and following the manufacturer's directions for preparation and dilution.

Ribavirin is a toxic drug. In its aerosolized form, ribavirin can be absorbed through the mucous membranes and respiratory passages of the person administering the treatment and by others in the room when the drug is being administered. During actual administration of aerosolized ribavirin, wear a mask to protect yourself from inhaling the drug. Ensure that visitors are not present or, if they must be present, ensure that they wear a mask.

 Priority actions to take after *giving antiviral drugs for respiratory viral infections.* In addition to the general responsibilities related to antiviral therapy (see pp. 109-110), monitor the patient receiving *ribavirin* closely for any sign of side effects or organ toxicity. Review laboratory values daily for WBC and RBC counts, bilirubin level, liver enzyme levels, and BUN and creatinine levels. Compare urine output with fluid intake. Assess hearing daily. Document all changes and notify the prescriber.

 Teaching priorities for patients taking antiviral drugs for respiratory viral infections. In addition to the general care needs and precautions related to antiviral therapy (see p. 110), teach patients taking zanamivir how to use a dry powder inhaler (see Box 18.2 in Chapter 18).

- If you take other drugs by inhalation for another breathing problem such as asthma or chronic obstructive pulmonary disease, use a bronchodilator before using the zanamivir inhaler and wait at least 5 to 10 minutes before using the zanamivir inhaler.
- If an unexpected adverse effect occurs, stop taking the drug and notify your prescriber as soon as possible.

Life span considerations for ribavirin

Considerations for pregnancy and lactation. Ribavirin has a high likelihood of increasing the risk for birth defects and fetal damage. It should never be given to a woman who is pregnant. If a woman of childbearing age who is sexually active is prescribed ribavirin, she is recommended to use two forms of contraception during the time she is receiving it and for 1 month after the drug is discontinued.

Hepatitis B Virus and Hepatitis C Virus Infections

The liver is a "clearing house" and detoxifying center for substances in the blood. It filters blood directly from the gastrointestinal system so that organisms and toxins can be removed before this blood has a chance to circulate to other body organs. As a result of this constant exposure, the liver can be infected and injured by many

 Drug Alert

Interaction Alert

Because ribavirin has many serious drug interactions, obtain a complete list of all drugs the patient is currently taking before the first dose of ribavirin is given. Check these with the pharmacist, and record the drugs in the medical record.

QSEN: Safety

 Critical Point for Safety

Keep the door to the room closed during the treatment and for 20–30 min after the treatment to prevent the aerosolized drug from coming into contact with other people.

QSEN: Safety

 Drug Alert

Teaching Alert

Teach patients who take other drugs by inhalation for another breathing problem to use the bronchodilator at least 5–10 min before using the zanamivir inhaler.

QSEN: Safety

invading organisms, including viruses. The liver is essential for life, performing dozens of different important functions. For this reason, it has the ability to restore itself after injury better than any other organ or tissue. However, chronic exposure to toxins or chronic viral infections can lead to damage and eventual liver failure.

Although almost any virus is capable of infecting the liver, a group of liver-specific viruses are responsible for viral hepatitis. These hepatitis viruses are designated as types A, B, C, D, and E (HAV, HBV, HCV, HDV, HEV), and when present in sufficient numbers, infection usually results in an acute illness that can last for weeks. For some of these viruses, when the acute phase of the disease is over, the virus has cleared and the person has no further problems. However, many people who contract infections with the virulent HBV and HCV can develop a chronic phase. These two hepatitis virus types are more virulent than other nonretroviruses and better able to evade immune system actions to clear the virus or keep them from reproducing.

HBV infection in some people has an acute phase that can rapidly progress to liver failure and death. In many others, the infection becomes chronic after the acute phase and years later may result in liver failure or liver cancer. In a few people, HBV infection does not cause *any* illness but the virus remains present and can be transmitted to others.

Unlike HBV, HCV infection seldom has an acute phase but the virus remains within the person. This virus is able to evade immune action because it constantly mutates within the infected person, so as soon as the person begins to make antibodies against it, the virus mutates its genetic material and those previously made antibodies are no longer effective.

Without an acute illness phase, the person is often unaware that he or she has been infected with HCV. However, over the course of 20 to 30 years, about 85% of people infected with HCV eventually develop chronic disease with liver cirrhosis and failure. About 20,000 patients are infected with HCV yearly in the U.S. and an estimated 3 million people are currently living with the chronic disease. The genetic variations of the virus resulting in chronic hepatitis C viral infection have been categorized into six groups known as genotypes 1, 2, 3, 4, 5, and 6.

Drugs for Chronic Hepatitis C Infection

Until recently, few drug therapies were available to manage chronic hepatitis C viral infections. New combinations of direct-acting antivirals have been so effective against HCV disease that infected individuals are now declared to have a "sustained virologic response" with a recurrence risk of only 1% after an 8- to 12-week drug treatment course. According to drug manufacturers, this sustained response can be considered a "cure." These direct-acting antiviral drugs are first-line therapy for management of chronic hepatitis C.

Before the direct-acting antiviral drugs were available, the standard drug therapy for chronic hepatitis C infection was daily oral ribavirin in conjunction with weekly subcutaneous injections of peginterferon alfa. This therapy was continued for at least 1 year. The side effects and adverse effects of the therapy were frequent and significant. For some genotypes of HCV, about 40% of patients were able to achieve a remission with the older therapy in which viral loads were significantly reduced. However, long-term sustained responses were rare. As a result of the effectiveness of newer drugs and the burden of older therapies, the use of ribavirin and peginterferon for management of chronic hepatitis C disease is no longer recommended. The drugs and dosages listed are used for patients whose liver health/function has been assessed and deemed sufficient to receive and benefit from these drugs. For those whose liver health is not sufficient, dosage adjustments and possible additional therapies may be needed or substituted.

Memory Jogger

The chronic phases of hepatitis B and hepatitis C viral infections can lead to cirrhosis and liver failure. They can also lead to the development of primary liver cancer. Virus-induced liver damage is a common reason of the need for liver transplantation.

Memory Jogger

Because HCV infection rarely has an acute phase, a patient may not realize he or she has been infected; however, about 85% of infected people develop chronic HCV infection and are at high risk for liver cirrhosis, liver failure, and liver cancer.

Memory Jogger

The direct-acting antiviral drugs are combination drugs for first-line therapy for HCV and often lead to a sustained virologic response that is considered a "cure."

Adult Dosages for Direct-Acting Antiviral Drugs to Manage Hepatitis C Viral Infections

Drug Name*	Usual Maintenance Dose
Epclusa (sofosbuvir/velpatasvir)	400 mg sofosbuvir/100 mg velpatasvir orally once daily for 12 weeks (genotypes 1, 2, 3, 4, 5, 6)
Harvoni (ledipasvir/sofosbuvir)	90 mg ledipasvir/400 mg sofosbuvir orally once daily for 12 weeks (genotypes 1, 4, 5, 6)

Drug Name*	Usual Maintenance Dose
Mavyret (glecaprevir; pibrentasvir)	3 tablets (glecaprevir 300 mg/pibrentasvir 120 mg) orally once daily for 8 weeks (genotypes 1, 2, 3, 4, 5, 6)
Vosevi (sofosbuvir/velpatasvir/ voxilaprevir)	400 mg sofosbuvir/100 mg velpatasvir/100 mg voxilaprevir orally once daily for 12 weeks (genotypes 1, 2, 3, 4, 5, 6)
ZEPATIER (elbasvir; grazoprevir)	One tablet (50 mg elbasvir/100 mg grazoprevir) orally daily for 12 weeks (genotypes 1a, 1b, 4, after appropriate testing for ns5a resistance and polymorphisms)

*The direct-acting antiviral drugs are all combination agents and the brand name of the combination is listed first.

How drugs for chronic HCV infection work. All of the direct-acting antiviral drugs for management of chronic HCV infection inhibit different viral proteins and enzymes (usually proteases) that are important to viral function and replication. The precise mechanisms are not exactly known, but both viral reproduction and possibly the ability of the virus to continue to mutate are inhibited to the extent that the person's immune system can be effective in eradicating the organism.

Because HCV is able to mutate its DNA, there are six recognized variations of the viral genotypes. Not all drugs are able to interfere with function and replication of all viral genotype variations. Thus, the drugs are only prescribed in combinations and not as single drugs. The choice of drug combination is individualized and must be made based on the results of testing that indicates which HCV genotype(s) a specific patient has as his or her dominant strain.

Common side effects of drugs for chronic HCV infection. The most common side effects for direct-acting antiviral drugs for HCV infection include headache, gastrointestinal discomfort (abdominal pain, diarrhea), rashes, and fatigue or general weakness. These side effects usually resolve within a few weeks after treatment is completed.

Possible adverse effects of drugs for chronic HCV infection. These oral drugs perform their actions within the liver and can interfere with liver function. As a result, they usually elevate liver enzymes to some degree and can increase the amount of free bilirubin in the blood, leading to jaundice. Contraindications for use of these drugs include other health problems that also affect the liver, such as liver dysfunction, cirrhosis, alcoholism, co-infection with HBV, and co-infection with HIV (human immunodeficiency virus). Other adverse effects are related to suppression of bone marrow function, especially of red blood cells (RBCs). This problem can result in anemia.

Allergic reactions that include angioedema are rare but possible. If this occurs, the drug must be stopped and other drugs from this same category are usually not prescribed either. Because these drugs interfere with liver function to some degree, they can have a profound effect on the metabolism of most other drugs, often resulting in dangerous interactions.

Although human studies of pregnant women taking direct-acting antiviral drugs for treatment of chronic hepatitis C infection have not been performed, animal studies indicate that the drugs do cross the placenta and enter fetal blood. Thus, the potential for harm to the embryo and fetus is present.

⊛ ***Priority actions to take*** *before and after* ***giving antiviral drugs for chronic HCV infection.*** In addition to the general responsibilities and care issues related to antiviral therapy (pp. 109-110), always ask about the patient's current level of alcohol use. These drugs interfere with liver function, and alcohol must be avoided for the duration of the therapy.

These drugs are highly effective when selected appropriately for the patient's viral infection genotype. Ensure that genotype testing is completed and the results known before the therapy is started. Laboratory tests for liver function and hematologic function (especially red blood cell and white blood cell counts) are important to obtain before therapy begins to use as a baseline to determine whether adverse effects are occurring.

 Critical Point for Safety

The choice of drug to treat HCV must be made based on the results of testing for each patient that indicates which hepatitis C virus genotype(s) he or she has.

QSEN: Safety

Common Side Effects
Drugs for Chronic HCV Infection

Headache

Abdominal pain, Diarrhea

Rash

Fatigue

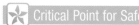 **Critical Point for Safety**

Alcohol use with direct-acting antiviral drugs greatly increases the risk for irreversible liver damage and must be avoided.

QSEN: Safety

For women of child-bearing age who are sexually active, ensure that a pregnancy test is negative before beginning the drug therapy. Instruct these women to use two reliable forms of contraception or to avoid intercourse for the duration of therapy and for 1 month after therapy is completed.

Obtain a complete list of all other prescribed and over-the-counter drugs and supplements the patient uses on a regular basis. Check with the pharmacist for which of the patient's other drugs are likely to have a negative interaction with the drug therapy for chronic hepatitis C infection and what adjustments may need to be made. Be sure the prescriber is aware of any needed adjustments.

The direct-acting antiviral drugs for chronic hepatitis C infection are used as out-patient therapy. The most important action to take is to teach patients and families exactly how to take these drugs, what signs and symptoms to monitor for, and what actions to take in different situations.

⭐ *Teaching priorities for patients taking antiviral drugs for chronic HCV infection.* In addition to the general care needs and precautions related to antiviral therapy (p. 110), teach patients taking direct-acting antiviral drugs for chronic HCV infection the following:

- Do not drink alcoholic beverages for the duration of the therapy. Only resume alcohol consumption after therapy is completed when your prescriber indicates it is safe to do so.
- If swelling of your face, lips, or tongue occurs, go to the nearest emergency department or call 911 because these may indicate a life-threatening allergic reaction.
- If you are a woman within child-bearing age and are sexually active with a male partner, either use two reliable forms of contraception during the therapy and for 1 month after therapy is completed or abstain from sexual intercourse during this time period to prevent possible birth defects.
- Take Mavyret, Vosevi, and ZEPATIER with food; Harvoni and Epclusa can be taken with or without food.
- Notify your prescriber if you develop yellowing of your skin or eyes, darkening of your urine, or lighter stools. These problems are signs of liver toxicity.
- Be sure to tell all your other health care providers that you are taking direct-acting antiviral drugs for chronic hepatitis C viral infection because of the potential for drug interactions.
- Do not take any new over-the-counter drugs or supplements unless you check with the health care provider who prescribed your hepatitis C drug therapy.

Life span considerations for drugs for chronic HCV infection

Considerations for pregnancy and lactation. Animal studies indicate that the direct-acting antiviral drugs cross the placenta and enter the embryo and fetus. Although more of the women prescribed these drugs are out of the child-bearing age range, measures to prevent birth defects, such as ensuring the woman has a negative pregnancy test before starting the drug therapy and avoiding pregnancy for the duration of therapy and for 1 month following therapy completion are strongly recommended. Breastfeeding is also not recommended during this therapy.

Drugs for Chronic Hepatitis B Infection

The management of chronic hepatitis B virus (HBV) infection has not been as successful as with HCV and there are no drug therapies that totally suppress or eliminate the virus. The available drug therapies keep the viral load lower to slow the progression of liver damage. Fortunately, the incidence of HBV infection has decreased over the last several decades as a result of widespread immunization against the virus, especially among individuals in high-risk groups.

Recommended first-line therapy for chronic hepatitis B infection includes pegylated interferon alfa-2a (*peginterferon*), *entecavir*, and the nucleoside analog reverse transcriptase inhibitor (NRTI) *tenofovir*, which is an antiretroviral drug most commonly used for HIV infection. The actions, side effects, and other issues related to tenofovir therapy are discussed later in the chapter in the antiretroviral drug therapy section NRTI. Two additional older drugs used less commonly to help manage chronic HBV infection are adefovir dipivoxil (Hepsera) and the NRTI lamivudine (Epivir).

First-line treatment for chronic HBV infection does not begin until the patient has indications of active disease, which include persistent elevation of some liver enzymes. The duration of therapy is long. The interferon injections are recommended for nearly a year and the oral drugs are taken indefinitely (and possibly life-long). The information presented here discusses first-line therapy. For the less commonly used drugs, consult a reliable drug reference for information on dosing and care issues.

Memory Jogger

Drug therapy to manage chronic HBV infection must be taken for at least 48 weeks and some of the drugs may be taken indefinitely throughout the patient's life.

Adult Dosages of First-Line Drug Therapy for Chronic Hepatitis B Infection

Drug Name	Usual Maintenance Dose
peginterferon Alfa-2a (Pegasys)	180 mcg subcutaneously once weekly for 48 weeks
entecavir (Baraclude)	0.5 mg orally daily
tenofovir (Viread)	300 mg orally once daily

How drugs for chronic HBV infection work. *Peginterferon,* a synthetic biologic agent, is an agonist to the naturally occurring interferon normally secreted by many immune system cells in response to viral infection. Interferon has many roles for health and one of its actions is to help prevent viral spread from virally infected cells to noninfected cells. The antiviral action of both natural interferon and peginterferon increases immune cell production and activation of enzymes that destroy viral genetic material (especially RNA). As a result, viral replication in infected cells is greatly decreased and viral particles are not released to infect more host cells. Additional possible antiviral actions of peginterferon include increasing the killing action of cytotoxic T cells against virally infected cells and preventing viral uncoating.

Entecavir is a "counterfeit" form of the genetic base guanine. When it is present in high concentrations it competes with natural guanine in the production of HBV RNA chains, which suppresses viral replication in infected cells. Although it has slight action against other forms of RNA, it is most effective in slowing or stopping RNA synthesis of the HBV.

Common side effects of drugs for chronic HBV infection. The most commonly reported side effects of both peginterferon and entecavir are fatigue, headache, fever, rash, and muscle aches. Additional common side effects of peginterferon include depression, injection site reactions, and alopecia. (Alopecia reverses when the drug is stopped.) Additional common side effects of entecavir include elevated blood glucose levels in patients who also have diabetes.

Common Side Effects
Drugs for Chronic HBV Infection

Fatigue   Headache   Fever

Rash

Muscle aches

Possible adverse effects of drugs for chronic HBV infection. Both drugs are known to interact with many (more than 100) other drugs and supplements. They are both contraindicated for use during lactation.

Peginterferon can worsen existing psychiatric disorders. As an injectable biologic, it is more likely to induce allergic responses. Peginterferon suppresses bone marrow activity, which increases the risk for anemia. In laboratory animals, the drug induced pregnancy loss, especially early in the pregnancy. It also appears to make autoimmune thyroid diseases, both hypothyroidism and hyperthyroidism, worse and should not be used in patients with known thyroid disorders.

Entecavir can cause liver toxicity with elevation of hepatic enzymes and serum bilirubin levels. Some patients have developed lactic acidosis with symptoms of GI discomfort; fast, shallow breathing; and unusual sleepiness, tiredness, or weakness. This problem is more severe and can be life-threatening if the patient also takes adefovir or is pregnant.

Critical Point for Safety

Peginterferon can worsen existing depression and "unmask" other psychiatric mental health issues. Be sure to warn patients to report severe mood changes, especially if they have thoughts about self-harm.

QSEN: Safety

⭐ *Priority actions to take **before** giving drugs for chronic HBV infection.* In addition to the general responsibilities and care issues related to antiviral therapy (see pp. 109-110), ensure that laboratory testing of liver function and blood cell counts are ordered and that the results are known before drug therapy is started. Use these test results to assess for possible adverse effects throughout the long duration of this therapy.

These drugs interfere with liver function and alcohol must be avoided for the duration of the therapy. Assess the patient's alcohol habits and the exact date that alcohol was last ingested.

Obtain a list of all current prescribed and over-the-counter drugs and supplements the patient takes regularly. Consult with a pharmacist for potential interactions between these drugs and the drugs for chronic HBV infection. If interactions are likely, be sure the prescriber is aware of these.

For sexually active women of child-bearing age, determine the pregnancy and lactation status. Ensure that a pregnancy test performed before drug therapy is started is negative.

Entecavir must be taken on an empty stomach. Be sure to give the drug either 2 hours before or 2 hours after a meal.

Peginterferon is available as a solution for subcutaneous injection in vials and in prefilled syringes. However, the drug concentration per mL is **not** the same. Take care to ensure you are delivering the correct dosage when switching between vials and prefilled syringes.

Check to determine whether any premedication drugs have been prescribed. Often patients may be prescribed to receive acetaminophen or ibuprofen an hour or more before the drug is injected to decrease the discomfort of fever, headache, and muscle aches.

When preparing peginterferon for injection, warm the refrigerated single-dose vial by gently rolling it between your hands. Prevent foaming by not shaking the vial. Inject air only into the airspace within the vial and not into the liquid.

Unlike some drugs for subcutaneous injection, peginterferon is harmful if given intravenously. Thus, aspirate to ensure the needle is not in a blood vessel before giving the injection.

⭐ *Priority actions to take **after** giving drugs for chronic HBV infection.* Most patients taking first-line drugs for chronic HBV infection will be doing so on an outpatient basis. However, the initial peginterferon injection must be administered by a licensed health care professional. Monitor patients closely for the first 30 minutes for indications of an allergic reaction after giving the first subcutaneous injection of peginterferon. Assess whether the patient may be an appropriate candidate to self-inject this drug weekly at home. If the patient or family is willing to perform the injections, teach them the correct techniques for safe subcutaneous injection as presented in Box 2.3 in Chapter 2.

⭐ *Teaching priorities for patients taking drugs for chronic HBV infection*
- Avoid all alcoholic beverages and drugs that may contain alcohol for the duration of your drug therapy.
- Take entecavir on an empty stomach (either 2 hours before or 2 hours after a meal).
- Use the steps taught to you for correct injection of the peginterferon, being sure to pull up on the plunger after inserting into your skin to make certain the needle is not in a vein.
- If your prescriber has ordered ibuprofen or other drugs to be taken before injecting peginterferon, be sure to take them at least 1 hour before you plan to inject the drug.
- Some patients find that injecting the peginterferon at bedtime helps them "sleep through" some of its uncomfortable side effects.
- Notify your prescriber if you develop yellowing of your skin or eyes, darkening of your urine, or lighter stools. These problems are signs of liver toxicity.
- If swelling of your face, lips, or tongue occurs, go to the nearest emergency department or call 911 because these may indicate a life-threatening allergic reaction.

- If you are a woman within child-bearing age and are sexually active with a male partner, use two reliable forms of contraception during the therapy and for 1 month after therapy is completed to prevent birth defects. If you think you may be pregnant, notify your prescriber immediately.
- Do not take any new over-the-counter drugs or supplements unless you check with the health care provider who prescribed your hepatitis B drug therapy.
- If you have diabetes, check your blood glucose levels more frequently for higher-than-normal glucose values and discuss possible alterations in diabetes drug therapy with your diabetes health care provider.
- If you notice any new feelings of depression or if you already have depression and the sensation becomes worse, notify your prescriber immediately, especially if you have thoughts of harming yourself.
- If you develop persistent abdominal and stomach discomfort; fast, shallow breathing; and unusual sleepiness, tiredness, or weakness, notify your prescriber immediately or go to the nearest emergency department.

Life span considerations for drugs for chronic HBV infection

Considerations for pregnancy and lactation. Human studies documenting the effects of first-line drugs to manage chronic HBV infection have not been performed. Animal studies indicate a strong likelihood of peginterferon inducing pregnancy loss (abortion) and is assumed to have a high risk for birth defects in humans. Both peginterferon and entecavir are contraindicated during pregnancy and lactation.

Drugs for COVID-19 Infection

The **COVID-19 virus**, also known as the SARS-CoV-2 virus, is a new nonretrovirus that is able to infect humans for the first time, often causing a severe influenza-like respiratory infection. Because this virus was previously unknown to humans, the evolutionary part of immune protection is not present in any humans, which makes this virus quite virulent. As of June 2022, this virus has infected more than 533 million people in 215 countries and territories and has resulted in more than 6.3 million deaths. In the United States at this time, about 85 million people have been infected, with more than 1.1 million deaths.

Some patients who developed COVID-19 have experienced less serious respiratory symptoms and recovered with no apparent permanent problems. More serious problems associated with this infection result from the development of a viral pneumonia and a profound inflammatory response triggered by excessive cytokine activity ("cytokine storm"). This response leads to a severe acute respiratory distress syndrome that prevents adequate gas exchange and often leads to death. Some long-term cardiac, pulmonary, and neurologic problems have been found to persist after the acute phase of the infection has passed; this is known as "long COVID."

Along with measures to avoid contact or transmission with the virus, COVID-19 prevention strategies include three approved vaccines that have shown to be effective in reducing the incidence and severity of the infection. Although no specific drugs or therapies for treatment of COVID-19 have yet been fully approved, three investigational therapies have received emergency use authorization (EUA) from the FDA for treatment of the infection. These therapies include remdesivir (Veklury), an antiviral agent, and a combination of two monoclonal antibodies casirivimab/imdevimab (REGEN-COV, formerly known as Regeneron). One oral therapy for use after symptoms appear and a COVID test is positive is Paxlovid. This drug is a combination of the antiviral drugs nirmatrelvir and ritonavir that are co-packaged and meant to be taken together. In addition, infusions of convalescent serum containing natural anti-COVID antibodies from patients who had the infection and recovered are also used to reduce the severity of the infection. Additional antibiotics such as azithromycin (discussed in Chapter 6), antiinflammatories such as dexamethasone (discussed in Chapter 10), and other drugs and supplements have provided some benefit in helping patients recover from COVID-19 infection. More new and existing antiviral drugs are in earlier phase trials to measure activity against replication of the virus.

Adult Dosages of Currently Authorized Drugs to Treat COVID-19 Viral Infection

Drug Name	Usual Dosage
remdesivir (Veklury)	200 mg IV once on day 1, followed by 100 mg IV once daily for 4–9 days
casirivimab/imdevimab (REGEN-COV)	casirivimab 600 mg/imdevimab 600 mg together as a single IV infusion as soon as possible after positive test for COVID-19 and within 10 days of symptom onset[a]
nirmatrelvir/ritonavir (Plaxlovid)	300 mg nirmatrelvir (two 150 mg tablets) with 100 mg ritonavir (one 100 mg tablet) with all three tablets taken together orally twice daily for 5 days

[a]Optimal dosing has not been established and the current dosing guidelines may change.

How drugs for COVID-19 infection work. *Remdesivir* is a "counterfeit" form of the genetic base adenine. When it is present in high concentrations it competes with natural adenine for inclusion in the virus' RNA chains. The counterfeit adenine suppresses viral replication in infected epithelial cells of the human airway tract. Remdesivir has shown good antiviral activity against other more rare viruses, including the virus responsible for Ebola infection.

Casirivimab/imdevimab are a biologic treatment composed of two synthetic human immunoglobulin G antibodies that can neutralize the COVID-19 virus. Combined together, these two antibodies bind to a specific receptor on the COVID-19 virus. Covering this receptor prevents it from binding to the human ACE2 receptor, which is present on many human epithelial cells, including those of the nose, mouth, and entire respiratory tract. As a result, infection spread from cell to cell in the airways is inhibited. In addition, binding of these monoclonal antibodies to the virus increases the chance that a variety of immune system cells will be better able to attack and eliminate or neutralize the virus.

Nirmatrelvir is the main active drug in Paxlovid and is categorized as a protease inhibitor. It works by preventing critical proteins required viral replication from being fully activated. Ritonavir, although it has some antiviral effects, its main action in Paxlovid therapy is to slow the breakdown of nirmatrelvir, allowing it to remain in the body at an effective concentration for a longer time.

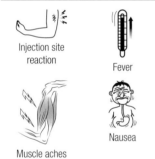

Common Side Effects

Drugs for COVID-19

Injection site reaction

Fever

Muscle aches

Nausea

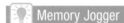

Memory Jogger

An anaphylactoid reaction is similar to anaphylaxis but the effects are mostly very uncomfortable rather than life-threatening.

Common side effects of drugs for COVID-19. The most common expected side effects for both *remdesivir* and *casirivimab/imdevimab* include injection site reactions, fever, muscle aches, and nausea. Additional side effects of *nirmatrelvir* include taste changes, diarrhea, and hypertension.

Possible adverse effects of drugs for COVID-19. Because the EUA is recent and limited numbers of patients have received these drugs, not all possible adverse effects are known at this time, including how these drugs influence pregnancy, lactation, and children under the age of 12 years. However, COVID-19 infection can be lethal and the potential benefits of these drugs in any population must be weighed for each patient individually against any potential harm.

The most likely adverse effect of *remdesivir* and *casirivimab/imdevimab* is the risk for allergic reactions and injection site reactions. In addition to true allergic reactions, such as actual anaphylaxis and angioedema, patients may have anaphylactoid reactions. These reactions resemble anaphylaxis with hypotension, cardiac dysrhythmias, and back pain, but are usually not accompanied by respiratory difficulty. Often the symptoms can be reduced by slowing the rate of infusion.

Remdesivir is renal toxic and contraindicated in patients who have renal insufficiency or renal failure. It also increases liver enzymes and has been found to induce anemia.

Ritonavir is liver toxic and should be used with caution in patients with preexisting liver problems. This drug also can induce drug resistance in people with HIV.

⭐ ***Priority actions to take*** *before and after giving drugs for COVID-19.* In addition to the general responsibilities and care issues related to antiviral therapy (see pp. 109-11), ensure that patients meet the criteria for these drugs, which includes having a positive COVID test and having symptoms.

These drugs must be administered by a licensed health care professional at a setting in which emergency equipment and support for anaphylaxis are available. *Remdesivir* is given as an IV inpatient drug over 5 to 10 days, and *casirivimab/imdevimab* is often given in clinics for patients with less severe symptoms of the infection. This drug is recommended to be administered as an IV infusion but can be given subcutaneously.

Neither drug contains a preservative. Use strict aseptic technique to prepare and administer these drugs. Follow the manufacturer instructions for reconstitution and dilution. Administer no other drugs through the IV tubing dedicated to the infusion of these drugs.

Both drugs are recommended to be given by slow IV infusion. Infuse *remdesivir* between 30 and 120 minutes. For *casirivimab/imdevimab* the infusion time varies between 20 and 50 minutes minimum.

Do not give either chloroquine or hydroxychloroquine to patients during the time they are receiving *remdesivir*. These drugs have been found to suppress the antiviral activity of remdesivir.

Both drugs can cause an allergic reaction. Monitor patients closely during the actual infusion and for a minimum of 1 hour after the infusion is completed. For *casirivimab/imdevimab*, patients are discharged to home after the monitoring period. However, allergic reactions may occur for up to 24 hours after the infusion is complete.

Remind patients receiving *casirivimab/imdevimab* not to receive any vaccinations within 90 days of receiving these monoclonal antibodies. The effectiveness of these vaccinations could be reduced.

REVIEW OF RELATED PHYSIOLOGY AND PATHOPHYSIOLOGY OF RETROVIRAL INFECTION

A *retrovirus* is a special type of virus that always uses RNA as its genetic material and carries with it the important viral enzymes *reverse transcriptase, integrase,* and *protease.* These enzymes allow high efficiency of cellular infection. As a result of a high efficiency of infection, disease may result even when low levels of retroviruses enter the body. The **human immune deficiency virus (HIV)** is a retrovirus that attacks the immune system of an infected person, eventually causing him or her to have little or no immune protection. The later stage and most severe form of immune deficiency disease caused by HIV infection is known as *HIV-III* or *acquired immune deficiency syndrome (AIDS).*

HIV has an outer layer with special "docking proteins," known as gp41 and gp120, that help the virus enter cells with receptors for these proteins (Fig. 7.3). Inside, the virus has its genetic material along with the enzymes reverse transcriptase and integrase. One of the cells that has receptors for the docking proteins is the *CD4+ cell, helper/inducer T cell,* or *T4 cell.* This cell population directs immune system

Drug Alert

Administration Alert

Both intravenous (remdesivir and casirivimab/imdevimab) drugs for COVID-19 are not to be mixed with any other drugs. Do not use the tubing to give any other drug.

QSEN: Safety

Critical Point for Safety

Before patients receiving *casirivimab/imdevimab* are permitted to leave the setting, be sure to teach them that allergic reactions can occur for up to 24 h after the infusion is completed. Instruct them to go to the nearest emergency department or call 911 if swelling of the face, lips, or tongue occur or if breathing becomes difficult.

QSEN: Safety

Memory Jogger

All people with AIDS have HIV infection but not all people with HIV infection have AIDS.

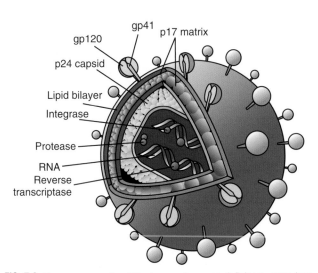

gp41 p17 matrix
gp120
p24 capsid
Lipid bilayer
Integrase
Protease
RNA
Reverse transcriptase

FIG. 7.3 The components of the human immune deficiency retrovirus.

defenses and regulates the activity of all immune system cells. If HIV enters a CD4+ T cell, it can then create more virus particles.

After entering a host cell, HIV must get its genetic material into the DNA of the human host cell. DNA is the genetic material of the human cell. The genetic material of HIV is RNA. To infect and take over a human cell, the genetic material must be the same. HIV carries the enzyme *reverse transcriptase* to convert HIV RNA into DNA. Then the enzyme *integrase* inserts this newly made viral DNA strand into the human DNA of the CD4+ T cell.

HIV particles are made in the infected CD4+ T cell using the machinery of the host cell. The new virus particle is made in the form of one long protein strand. The strand is clipped with chemical scissors, an enzyme called *HIV protease*, into several small pieces. These pieces are formed into new finished viral particles (*virions*), which then leave the infected cell to infect other CD4+ T cells (Fig. 7.4).

Over time without treatment, the number of HIV particles overwhelms the immune system, and the patient is at very high risk for pathologic and opportunistic bacterial, fungal, and viral infections and some cancers. Opportunistic infections are caused by organisms that are present as part of the normal environment and kept in check by normal immune function. In a person with AIDS the immune system is extremely suppressed. T-cell counts fall, viral load rises, and without treatment the patient dies relatively quickly of opportunistic infections or cancer.

ANTIRETROVIRAL THERAPY (ART) FOR TREATMENT OF HIV INFECTION

Antiretroviral drugs are a broad category of antiviral drugs that suppress the replication of retroviruses, which use RNA as their primary genetic material instead of DNA. The seven classes of antiretroviral drugs are nucleoside analog reverse transcriptase inhibitors (NRTIs), non-nucleoside analog reverse transcriptase inhibitors (NNRTIs), protease inhibitors (PIs), fusion inhibitors, CCR5 antagonists, integrase strand transfer inhibitors (INSTIs), and attachment inhibitors. They are classified according to how they work to suppress retroviral activity. Because the HIV retrovirus has a high efficiency of infection and uses many mechanisms to reproduce and spread, antiretroviral therapy (ART) always consists of drug regimens using at least two and often three combinations of drugs from these seven classes. Treatment with a drug from only one class is ineffective and promotes development of drug-resistant HIV strains.

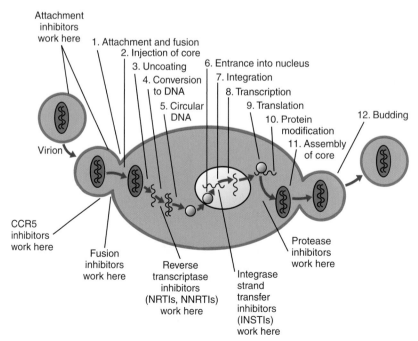

FIG. 7.4 Sites in the life cycle of the human immune deficiency virus (HIV) in which different antiretroviral drugs work. *NRTI,* Nucleoside analog reverse transcriptase inhibitor; *NNRTI,* Non-nucleoside analog reverse transcriptase inhibitor.

When resistance develops, viral replication is no longer suppressed by the drugs. The most important factor in development of drug resistance to combination ART is missing drug doses. When doses are missed, the blood concentrations become lower than that needed to inhibit viral replication, allowing the virus to replicate and produce new viruses that may be resistant to the drugs being used.

Drug therapy for HIV infection used to burden patients with taking between 20 to 30 pills daily. New combination therapy has reduced this burden to between 1 and 3 pills daily. A newly approved treatment for some patients involves extended-release combination drugs given parenterally once per month.

Combination ART begins as soon as a patient is diagnosed with HIV infection. The choice of which combination of drugs to use is based on possible side effects, how well the patient tolerates specific drugs, and what other health problems requiring drug therapy an individual patient may have.

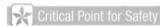

Critical Point for Safety

To help prevent development of drug-resistant strains of HIV, teach patients to not delay, skip, or reduce ART doses.

QSEN: Safety

Intended Responses of Antiretroviral Therapy
- Prevent/control retroviral reproduction and spread to uninfected cells
- Immune function and protection remain active
- Reduce symptoms of HIV disease and **viral load** (the number of viral particles in a blood sample, which indicates the degree of viral infection)
- Delay progression of HIV to later stages
- Prevent HIV infection transmission

How Antiretroviral Drugs for HIV Infection Work
The following table presents the classes, individual names (in alphabetical order), and summaries of the mechanisms of action for all currently approved antiretroviral drugs. See Fig. 7.4 for where these drugs work to disrupt HIV reproduction. Keep in mind that these drugs do **not** kill retroviruses. They are *virustatic*, not *virucidal*.

Antiretroviral Drug Classes and Actions

Drug Class	Drug Name	Mechanism of Action
Nucleoside Analog Reverse Transcriptase Inhibitors (NRTIs)	abacavir emtricitabine lamivudine tenofovir disoproxil zidovudine	Counterfeit bases similar in structure to bases that form DNA. They compete with real bases in HIV-infected cells to inhibit reverse transcriptase and reduce viral replication.
Non-Nucleoside Analog Reverse Transcriptase Inhibitors (NNRTIs)	doravirine efavirenz etravirine nevirapine rilpivirine	Inhibit the action of the enzyme reverse transcriptase by binding directly to the enzyme, preventing it from converting viral RNA to DNA. As a result, viral reproduction is suppressed.
Protease Inhibitors (PIs)	atazanavir darunavir fosamprenavir ritonavir saquinavir tipranavir	Compete with new HIV protein strands and prevent viral protease from converting the large viral proteins into active virions that, when released, can go on to infect more cells.
Fusion Inhibitors	enfuvirtide	Bind to the viral docking protein (gp41) and prevents it from fusing with the host cell membrane. Without fusion, infection of new cells does not occur.
CCR5 Antagonists	maraviroc	Bind to and blocks the CCR5 receptor on host immune system cells, preventing HIV from binding to it for entry into the host cells.
Integrase Strand Transfer Inhibitors (INSTIs)	cabotegravir dolutegravir raltegravir	Bind to the active site of the viral enzyme integrase, preventing it from inserting the newly formed viral DNA strand into the host cell's DNA. Without this insertion, the host cell cannot be used to reproduce viruses.
Attachment Inhibitors	fostemsavir ibalizumab-uiyk	Some bind to the viral gp120 docking protein and interfere with HIV entering host cells. Others block the host cell's receptor and interfere with HIV entering host cells.

General Issues with Antiretroviral Therapy

- Any antiretroviral drug can cause an allergic reaction. It may be minor, with a rash appearing days after starting the drug, or can result in anaphylaxis.
- Two common adverse effects of antiretrovirals are liver toxicity and worsening hyperglycemia.
- Most antiretroviral drugs interact with many other drugs. These interactions can cause serious adverse effects and can change the activity of drugs.
- Some antiretroviral drugs must be taken with food; others must be taken on an empty stomach.

Currently there are more than 20 different combination drugs for ART. The following table lists the combinations recommended by the expert panel of the National Institutes for Health. The listing is in alphabetical order and does not indicate a specific preference of agent. Which of these drugs, as well as whether a different combination drug, is best for an individual patient is based on the genotype of the virus, the patient's previous exposure to any HIV drugs, pregnancy status, known allergies, degree of viral load, general health, drug therapy for other health problems, and the patient's tolerance to ART. Consult a reliable drug reference for information about any of these other approved combination ART drugs (Atripla, Cimduo, Combivir, Complera, Delstrigo, Epzicom, Evotaz, Genvoya, Kaletra, Odefsey, Stribild, Symfi, Symtuza, Triumeq, Trizivir, and Truvada).

Adult Dosages of Common Combination Antiretroviral Therapy for HIV Infection

Drug Names	Usual Maintenance Dosages
Biktarvy (bictegravir/ emtricitabine/tenofovir)	1 tablet (bictegravir 50 mg, emtricitabine 200 mg, tenofovir 25 mg) once daily
Cabenuva (cabotegravir/ rilpivirine)	Pretreatment lead-in for 1 month with oral cabotegravir 30 mg and rilpivirine 25 mg to determine patient tolerance Initial parenteral therapy 600 mg cabotegravir plus 900 mg rilpivirine IM. Followed by: 400 mg cabotegravir plus 600 mg rilpivirine IM monthly or for every 2 months injection therapy 600 mg cabotegravir plus 900 mg rilpivirine IM for initial parenteral therapy and 1 month later (month 2); then the same dosage given thereafter every 2 months (starting month 4)
Dovato (dolutegravir/ lamivudine)	1 tablet 50 mg dolutegravir/300 mg lamivudine orally once daily. Tenofovir add-on recommended
JULUCA (dolutegravir/ lamivudine)	1 tablet 50 mg dolutegravir/25 mg lamivudine orally once daily
Triumeq (abacavir/ dolutagravir/lamivudine)	1 tablet 600 mg abacavir/50 mg dolutegravir/lamivudine 300 mg orally once daily. Additional dolutegravir 50 mg orally 12 hr later

Common Side Effects of Combination ART

Common side effects of combination ART drugs are rash, nausea and vomiting, abdominal pain, headache, fatigue, and weight gain (especially among black or Latina women). Additional side effects with these drugs are difficulty sleeping and vivid dreams or nightmares. *Cabenuva* also causes injection site reactions and may induce fever.

Possible Adverse Effects of Combination ART

All of the recommended combination ART drugs can elevate liver enzymes and lead to jaundice. They are not recommended for use in anyone who has chronic hepatitis or any other liver problem.

These combination drugs also have been found to increase the risk for birth defects and are to be avoided by patients who are pregnant.

Combination ART drugs have many interactions with other drugs, and some drugs are contraindicated for use with ART therapy. In particular, when patients are also taking the "statin" type of lipid-lowering drugs, muscle problems are more likely to occur.

Dovato has an increased risk for lactic acidosis. *JULUCA* can reduce glomerular filtration and is associated with hyperglycemia in patients with diabetes.

⭐ **Priority Actions to Take *Before* and *After* Giving Combination ART**

With the exception of Cabenuva, combination ART is life-long outpatient therapy for HIV disease. The most important action for nurses to perform with this therapy is to ensure appropriate, in-depth patient education regarding exactly how to take these drugs, their possible side effects and adverse effects, and when to notify the prescriber.

Before giving an antiretroviral drug, obtain a list of all other drugs that the patient takes because antiretrovirals interact with many other drugs. Check with the pharmacist for possible interactions and the need to consult the prescriber about dosage or changing the patient's other drugs.

For *Cabenuva*, the two drugs are given separately as deep intramuscular injections into the ventrogluteal site, and never mixed in the same syringe. Ensure that the injections are given in two different locations because the volume of these injections is relatively large and may be slow to be absorbed (as well as more painful). Before drawing up the solutions, allow refrigerated drugs to warm to room temperature and then shake each vial vigorously for a full 10 seconds until the suspensions look uniform. If the suspensions are not uniform, shake the vials again. Select a needle appropriate to reach the ventrogluteal muscle, which is the only site recommended for these injections. Be sure to aspirate before injecting to ensure the needle is not in a vein.

⭐ **Teaching Priorities for Patients Taking Combination ART**

- Take your antiretroviral therapy exactly as prescribed to maintain the effectiveness of ART drugs. Even a few missed doses per month can promote drug resistance.
- If swelling of your face, lips, or tongue occurs, go to the nearest emergency department or call 911 because these may indicate a life-threatening allergic reaction.
- Take JULUCA with food; Biktarvy and Dovato can be taken with or without food.
- Do not drink alcoholic beverages because these drugs reduce liver function and drinking alcohol can increase the risk for liver failure.
- Notify your prescriber if you develop yellowing of your skin or eyes, darkening of your urine, or lighter stools. These problems are signs of liver toxicity.
- Be sure to tell all your other health care providers that you are taking combination antiretroviral drugs for HIV infection because of the potential for drug interactions.
- If you also take a "statin" type of cholesterol-lowing drug, report any persistent muscle pain or weakness to the prescriber as soon as possible.
- Do not take any new over-the-counter drugs or supplements unless you check with the health care provider who prescribed your ART for HIV infection.
- Do not take an oral ART within 2 hours of taking an antacid because antacids interfere with the absorption of these drugs.
- If you become pregnant while taking a combination ART drug, notify your prescriber immediately because the drug can induce birth defects.
- If you are taking Dovato, report muscle aches; tiredness and difficulty remaining awake; abdominal pain; hypotension; and a slow, irregular heartbeat to your prescriber. These are indications of lactic acidosis, which can occur with this drug.
- If you have diabetes and take JULUCA, monitor your blood glucose levels more closely. Adjustments in diet and diabetes drug therapy may be needed.

Life Span Considerations for Combination ART

Pediatric considerations. Combination ART is not approved for use with children. Selected other types of antiretroviral drugs are prescribed for children who have HIV disease.

Considerations for pregnancy and lactation. Although HIV can be transmitted from an infected mother to her fetus during pregnancy and antiretroviral therapy can reduce this transmission, the combination ART drugs are not to be taken during pregnancy. These drugs have a higher risk for inducing birth defects, especially when taken during the first trimester. This is a situation when specific antiretroviral drugs, rather than these combination agents, are prescribed until the baby is born. HIV positive mothers are instructed not to breastfeed because HIV can be transmitted in breast milk.

❗ Drug Alert

Interaction Alert

Before giving combination antiretroviral drugs, ask the patient about all other drugs or supplements that he or she takes and then check with the pharmacist to avoid a possible drug interaction.

QSEN: Safety

 Critical Point for Safety

Inject the two drugs composing Cabenuva into two separate ventrogluteal sites. Never mix the two drugs together in the same syringe. Aspirate before injecting to prevent the possibility of IV injection.

QSEN: Safety

Considerations for older adults. Older adults are more likely to be taking other drugs, especially cardiac drugs and lipid-lowering drugs, that could interact with combination ART, although these agents may be prescribed for them. Remind older patients to tell all health care providers about all drugs they take. Also teach older adults how to take their pulse and assess it for irregularities. Remind the patient to report new irregularities to the prescriber.

ANTIRETROVIRAL THERAPY FOR PREEXPOSURE PROPHYLAXIS OF HIV INFECTION

Prevention of HIV infection by sexual transmission can be achieved by the use of drug therapy for *preexposure prophylaxis (Pr-EP)*. The use of the combination drugs Truvada and Descovy (emtricitabine and tenofovir), which contain two NRTIs, by HIV-1 negative sexual partners of known HIV-1 positive individuals effectively reduces HIV transmission. The combination of emtricitabine and tenofovir have a synergistic suppressive effect on HIV activity.

Preexposure prophylaxis does not replace the standard safer sex practices recommended to prevent HIV transmission. Also, if this type of drug therapy is used in patients who become infected with HIV-1, the risk for developing drug resistance greatly increases. Therefore, remind people prescribed Truvada or Descovy to use the traditional safer sex practices and to adhere to an every-3-month HIV testing schedule along with monitoring for side effects of this therapy.

Get Ready for the NCLEX® Examination!

Key Points

- Viruses are tiny intracellular parasites that are not capable of self-reproduction and must infect a living cell to reproduce.
- Most nonretroviruses have a relatively low efficiency of cellular infection and must invade the body in large numbers to cause disease.
- A retrovirus, specifically HIV, is virulent with a high efficiency of infection.
- Antiviral and antiretroviral drugs do not kill viruses; they only suppress viral reproduction and spread. They are virustatic rather than virucidal.
- The dosages listed in the drug tables are recommended dosages for the most common types of viral infections. Specific infections, depending on severity and organs affected, may require higher dosages than listed. Always double check a prescribed dosage that is higher or lower than the average recommended dosage.
- Teach patients taking antiviral or antiretroviral drugs to take them exactly as prescribed and for as long as prescribed and to not stop therapy just because they feel better.
- Breastfeeding is not recommended while taking an antiviral or antiretroviral drug.
- Signs and symptoms of a severe allergic reaction to an IV antiviral drug include hives at the IV site; low blood pressure; rapid, irregular pulse; swelling of the lips or lower face; and feeling of a lump in the throat.
- Ensure that patients taking antiviral drugs for herpes simplex infections drink at least 3 L of fluid daily unless another health problem requires fluid restriction.
- Antiviral drugs for herpes simplex infections reduce the effectiveness of antiseizure drugs, and dosages for seizure control may need to be increased.

- Ribavirin is highly teratogenic, which means that it can cause birth defects. Do not allow a pregnant or breastfeeding person to touch ribavirin or care for a patient taking it.
- Do not permit anyone who is pregnant or breastfeeding to administer ribavirin, handle it, care for a patient taking it, or enter the room of a patient receiving the aerosolized form.
- Keep the door to the room closed during the treatment and for 20 to 30 minutes after the treatment to prevent the aerosolized drug from coming into contact with other people.
- Teach patients who take other drugs by inhalation for another breathing problem to use the bronchodilator at least 5 to 10 minutes before using the zanamivir inhaler.
- The chronic phases of hepatitis B and hepatitis C viral infections can lead to cirrhosis and liver failure. They can also lead to the development of primary liver cancer. Virus-induced liver damage is a common reason of the need for liver transplantation.
- The choice of drug to treat HCV must be made based on the results of testing for each patient that indicates which hepatitis C virus genotype(s) he or she has.
- The direct-acting antiviral drugs for chronic hepatitis C infection interact with many (over a hundred) other drugs. It is critical to obtain a list of all other drugs and supplements the patient uses to avoid dangerous therapy complications.
- Alcohol use with direct-acting antiviral drugs for chronic HCV infection, the first-line drugs for chronic HBV infection, and combination ART for HIV disease greatly increase the risk for irreversible liver damage and must be avoided.
- Peginterferon can worsen existing depression and "unmask" other psychiatric mental health issues. Be sure to warn patients to report severe mood changes, especially if they have thoughts about self-harm.
- The concentration per mL of *peginterferon* available as a solution in a vial is different from the concentration in the prefilled

syringe. Calculate the dosage twice and check with a licensed health care professional to ensure you are preparing the correct dose.

- Before giving peginterferon, ask patients whether they have any known thyroid gland problems because hyperthyroidism and hypothyroidism are both contraindications for this drug.
- Be sure to aspirate peginterferon after inserting the needle for a subcutaneous injection because this drug is harmful if given IV.
- Both authorized (remdesivir and casirivimab/imdevimab) drugs for COVID-19 are not to be mixed with any other drugs. Do not use the IV tubing to give any other drug.
- Instruct patients receiving casirivimab/imdevimab not to receive any vaccinations within 90 days of receiving these monoclonal antibodies because the efficiency of the vaccination will be reduced.
- Antiretroviral therapy (ART) is most effective when given in multiple combinations of drugs, not as single drug therapy.
- To help prevent development of drug-resistant strains of HIV, teach patients to not delay, skip, or reduce ART doses.

- Most antiretroviral drugs have interactions with other drugs and herbals. Before giving combination antiretroviral drugs, ask patients about all other drugs or supplements they take and then check with the pharmacist to avoid a possible drug interaction.
- For therapy with Cabenuva, inject the two drugs composing Cabenuva into two separate ventrogluteal sites. Never mix the two drugs together in the same syringe. Aspirate before injecting to prevent the possibility of IV injection.
- Combination ART is not approved for children and must not be used during pregnancy or breastfeeding.

Additional Learning Resources

Be sure to visit your Evolve website (http://evolve.elsevier.com/Workman/pharmacology/) for additional online resources.

SG Go to your Study Guide for additional learning activities to help you master this chapter content.

Review Questions

See *Answers to In-Text Review Questions* in the back of the book for answers to these questions.

1. How do nonretroviral antiviral drugs assist in the management of viral infections?
   A. Attacking the outer coat of the virus to directly kill microorganism
   B. Increasing the pH of the infected cell to the point that the virus is destroyed
   C. Slowing viral replication to allow immune function to eliminate/neutralize the virus
   D. Disrupting ATP (adenosine triphosphate) production in virally infected cell so that there is not enough energy for the virus to reproduce

2. Which statement made by a patient prescribed to take an antiviral drug for influenza indicates to the nurse that more teaching is needed?
   A. "It is a good thing that my immune system is healthy to help me recover from this infection."
   B. "When I finish taking this drug, I will have full immunity against influenza in the future."
   C. "After completing this drug treatment, I will be less likely to infect other people."
   D. "Even after my symptoms go away, I will take all of the doses prescribed."

3. Which action is **most important** for the nurse to perform for a patient prescribed peramivir as prevention after exposure to a respiratory viral infection?
   A. Checking the blood return of the IV access
   B. Teaching the patient the correct technique to use with a dry powder inhaler
   C. Asking the patient about a current or previous history of a seizure disorder
   D. Ensuring the patient is neither pregnant nor breastfeeding an infant under 2 months of age

4. A patient with a herpes simplex infection is prescribed famciclovir 250 mg to be taken orally at home three times a day. What will the nurse teach the patient about the most effective dosing intervals for this drug?
   A. "Take the drug when you first get up and take 2 tablets with your evening meal so your sleep is not interrupted."
   B. "If it is more convenient, take all three doses once daily instead of one tablet three times a day."
   C. "Take the drug every 8 hours throughout the day and night."
   D. "Take the drug every 8 hours while you are awake."

5. Which precaution is **most important** for the nurse to teach a patient taking acyclovir for a recurrent herpes simplex viral infection?
   A. "Avoid caffeine-containing and alcoholic beverages until 1 month after therapy is completed."
   B. "If you become pregnant, stop taking the drug and notify your prescriber immediately."
   C. "Wear sunscreen and protective clothing when outdoors to prevent a severe sunburn."
   D. "Avoid taking a live virus vaccine until you have completed this drug therapy."

6. Which action is **most important** for the nurse to take when administering inhaled ribavirin to a patient with a respiratory syncytial virus infection?
   A. Administering the drug either 2 hours before or 2 hours after a meal
   B. Asking visitors to wear gloves while the drug is being administered
   C. Ensuring the door to the patient's room remains closed during the treatment
   D. Holding the nose of the patient during the inhalation treatment to ensure it reaches the airways

7. What problem is common among people who do not develop an acute phase illness after infection with hepatitis C virus (HCV)?

   A. The kidneys become infected in addition to the liver.
   B. Progression to the chronic phase of the disease is more rapid.
   C. Over time, the patient becomes progressively immunocompromised.
   D. Patients may not realize they have been infected until liver damage is severe.

8. A patient who has taken ZEPATIER for 6 weeks reports that his urine is coffee-colored and that his bowel movements are light gray. What is the nurse's **best** action?

   A. Reassuring the patient that this is an expected side effect
   B. Obtaining a urine specimen for culture and sensitivity
   C. Documenting the report as the only action
   D. Notifying the prescriber immediately

9. Which patient health history finding alerts the nurse to a potential problem with peginterferon therapy?

   A. Suicide attempt 4 years ago
   B. Delivered a baby 6 months ago
   C. Now 5 years sober from alcohol abuse
   D. Smoked 3 packs of cigarettes daily for 22 years

10. Which precaution is most important for the nurse to teach a patient newly prescribed Dovato?

    A. Avoid caffeinated food and beverages for the duration of this therapy.
    B. Take the drug at bedtime to avoid daytime drowsiness.
    C. Do not take within 2 hours of taking an antacid.
    D. Take this drug with meal or a substantial snack.

11. Which action or behavior the nurse teaches a patient taking antiretroviral therapy (ART) is **most likely** to result in development of drug-resistant HIV strains?

    A. Becoming pregnant
    B. Missing drug doses
    C. Taking oral antiinflammatories
    D. Having sex with multiple partners

12. Which antiretroviral drug class prevents HIV infection by stopping insertion of viral DNA into the host cells' DNA?

    A. CCR5 antagonists
    B. Fusion inhibitors
    C. Protease inhibitors
    D. Integrase strand transfer inhibitors

13. A patient is prescribed to receive 90 mcg of peginterferon. The available peginterferon is a prefilled 0.5 mL syringe that contains 180 mcg of the drug. What volume of drug will the nurse discard from the prefilled syringe to prepare the correct dose of the drug? _____mL

Clinical Judgment

1. Which assessments or actions are **most important** for the nurse to perform *before* administering the first dose of ribavirin for a respiratory viral infection? **Select all that apply.**

   A. Asking if there is any chance the patient might be pregnant
   B. Measuring the pulse rate, rhythm, and quality
   C. Determining the patient's level of consciousness
   D. Checking laboratory test results of liver and kidney function
   E. Assessing oxygen saturation by pulse oximetry
   F. Examining the color of the sclera, skin, and oral mucous membranes
   G. Listening to breath sounds and ease of breathing
   H. Checking the intake and output for the most recent 24 hours

2. The patient is a 68-year-old man who is a retired rock musician. He used injection drugs more than 30 years ago and has recently been diagnosed with hepatitis C (HCV) viral infection with genotype 1. He has been prescribed to begin direct-acting antiviral therapy with Mavyret. The nurse is developing a teaching plan with take-home instructions/precautions about this drug. Use an X to indicate which patient statements indicate Correct Understanding of therapy with Mavyret and which statements indicate that More Instruction Is Needed.

PATIENT STATEMENT	CORRECT UNDERSTANDING	MORE INSTRUCTION NEEDED
"If I forget a dose on one day, I will take two doses the next day."		
"In addition to avoiding alcohol during this treatment phase, I will do my liver a favor and quit drinking altogether."		
"To prevent a drug interaction, I will stop my blood pressure drug just until this therapy is over."		
"When my therapy is completed, I will be immune to being infected with this virus again."		
"I will avoid sexual intercourse until 1 month after this therapy is completed."		
"If I take this drug at night, I can be sure my stomach is empty."		

Antiinfectives: Antitubercular and Antifungal Drugs

Learning Objectives

The content presented in this chapter should help you to:

1. Explain the names, actions, usual adult dosages, possible side effects, and adverse effects of antituberculosis drugs.
2. Describe priority actions to take before and after giving any of the antituberculosis drugs.
3. Prioritize essential information to teach patients taking any of the antituberculosis drugs.
4. Explain the names, actions, usual adult dosages, possible side effects, and adverse effects of antifungal drugs.
5. Describe priority actions to take before and after giving antifungal drugs.
6. Prioritize essential information to teach patients taking antifungal drugs.
7. Explain appropriate life span considerations for antituberculosis drugs and antifungal drugs.

Key Terms

fungicidal (fŭn-jĭ-Sĭ-dŭl) (p. 138) Having the ability to kill a fungus.

fungistatic (fŭn-jĭ-STĂT-ĭk) (p. 138) Having the ability to suppress fungal reproduction and growth.

fungus (FŬN-gĭs) (p. 137) A simple organism with one or more cells (e.g., yeasts, molds, and mushrooms) that reproduces by

spores, has walled cells, and can live peacefully with humans or infect humans and cause disease.

tuberculosis (TB) (tū-bŭr-kyū-LŌ-sĭs) (p. 129) A highly communicable disease caused by infection with *Mycobacterium tuberculosis*.

REVIEW OF RELATED PHYSIOLOGY AND PATHOPHYSIOLOGY OF TUBERCULOSIS

Tuberculosis (TB) is a highly communicable disease caused by *Mycobacterium tuberculosis*. This bacterial infection usually starts in the respiratory tract as pulmonary TB, but the organism is capable of infecting almost any body organ. Although *M. tuberculosis* is a bacterium, it has many features that allow it to evade nearly all antibacterial drugs and requires special drug therapy to eradicate. In addition, more strains of the bacterium are becoming drug resistant.

TB is the most common bacterial infection worldwide and spreads by aerosol transmission, which transfers bacteria-filled droplets through the air when a person with active TB coughs, laughs, sneezes, whistles, or sings. These droplets may then be inhaled by others (Fig. 8.1). Far more people are infected with the bacteria and overcome the infection than actually develop active TB.

Once inhaled, the bacteria multiply freely when they reach a susceptible site in the lungs (usually in the upper lobes) and form a primary TB lesion, which is a small, inflamed pocket of bacteria, white blood cells (WBCs), and exudate. The lesion is surrounded by more WBCs that cause a response known as *pneumonitis*. During this time, people who have an intact immune system develop immunity to the TB organism, and further growth of bacteria is controlled by confining it to the primary lesions (see Fig. 8.1). These lesions usually resolve, leaving few residual bacteria, and may show on chest x-ray as a scar.

Only a small percentage of people initially infected with the bacteria ever develop active TB. Immune responses develop 2 to 10 weeks after the first infection with a TB organism and can be detected by a positive reaction to an intradermal TB skin test (Fig. 8.2). A skin test is positive when a reddened area of 10 mm or more that is much harder than the surrounding soft tissue *(induration)* forms around the injection site. Most people who are exposed to TB will have a positive TB skin test but never fully

 Memory Jogger

A positive TB skin test means only that the person has been infected with the bacteria at some point in his or her life but does **not** mean that he or she is infectious with active disease that can be spread to others.

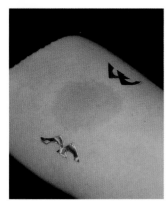

FIG. 8.2 A positive tuberculosis skin test. The markings on either side of the test area are used to identify the skin test site and to assess the size of the reaction. (From Forbes, C. D. [2003]. *Color atlas and text of clinical medicine* [3rd ed.]. St. Louis: Mosby.)

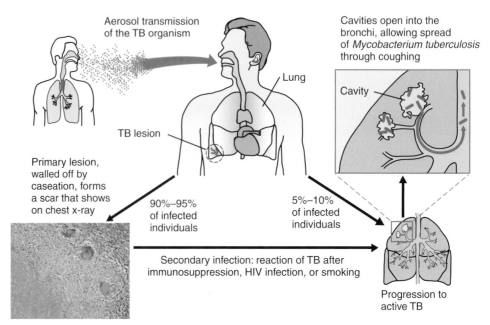

Aerosol transmission of the TB organism

Cavities open into the bronchi, allowing spread of *Mycobacterium tuberculosis* through coughing

Lung

Cavity

TB lesion

Primary lesion, walled off by caseation, forms a scar that shows on chest x-ray

90%–95% of infected individuals

5%–10% of infected individuals

Secondary infection: reaction of TB after immunosuppression, HIV infection, or smoking

Progression to active TB

FIG. 8.1 Primary TB infection with progression to secondary infection and active disease. *HIV,* Human immune deficiency virus; *TB,* tuberculosis. (Photo from Kumar, V., Abbas, A., Fausto, N., & Aster, J. [2009]. *Robbins and Cotran pathologic basis of disease* [8th ed.]. Philadelphia: Saunders. Photo courtesy Dominick Cavuoti, D.O., Dallas, Texas.)

Memory Jogger

Symptoms of active TB include a persistent productive cough, weight loss, poor appetite, night sweats, bloody sputum, shortness of breath, fever, aching chest pain that occurs with the cough, and chills.

Critical Point for Safety

Drug therapy will not control TB unless it is strictly followed as prescribed and continued for at least 6 months.

QSEN: Safety

develop the disease (the organism is alive but contained in a dormant state). Remember that once a TB skin test is positive, it will always be positive unless the immune system is very suppressed.

When a person is heavily exposed to the organism and has any type of reduced immunity, the infection process may progress. Then bacteria in the primary lesions multiply and start to kill off cells in the center of the lesion, turning it into a *necrotic* (dead tissue) mass. The mass and the area around it liquefy and are destroyed, forming a cavity (see Fig. 8.1). Bacteria continue to grow in the cavity and spread into new lung areas. Unchecked, the TB organism may enter the bloodstream and eventually spread throughout the body and damage many organs (a disorder known as *miliary TB*).

TB is slow growing, and it may take years for symptoms to develop. A person infected with TB that is progressing beyond the initial stage cannot spread the disease to others until active symptoms occur. Active TB is diagnosed by chest x-ray, blood assay to test for the TB organism, and sputum culture.

Secondary TB is reactivation of the disease in a previously infected person. This process is most likely to occur when immune defenses are weak, such as when a person has HIV/AIDS, is very old, or is taking immunosuppressive drugs on a regular basis. Without treatment, active TB can destroy so much lung tissue that death occurs.

TYPES OF DRUG THERAPY FOR TUBERCULOSIS

First-Line Antitubercular Drugs for Drug-Susceptible Tuberculosis

The risk for TB transmission is reduced after an infectious person has received first-line anti-TB drug therapy for 2 to 3 weeks and clinical improvement occurs. However, even with initial improvement, drug therapy must continue for at least 6 months to control the disease.

The slow growth of the TB organism is the reason most common antibacterial drugs are not effective in controlling or killing it. Combination drug therapy is needed to treat TB and prevent its transmission. Therapy continues until the disease is under control. Current first-line therapy for TB uses isoniazid, rifampin, pyrazinamide, and ethambutol in different combinations and schedules. Some are available in two- or three-drug combination tablets to reduce the burden of taking so many pills daily. TB control depends on strict adherence to drug therapy.

How first-line antitubercular drugs work. Fig. 8.3 shows where each of the first-line TB drugs works. With the exception of ethambutol, these drugs can be either *bactericidal* (kills the bacteria) or *bacteriostatic* (only suppresses bacterial growth), depending on the drug concentration within an infected site and the susceptibility of the organism.

Isoniazid works by inhibiting several enzymes important to mycobacteria metabolism and reproduction. It is able to inhibit these enzymes even when TB is dormant (inactive). It is most often given orally but can be given as an IV or IM injection.

Rifampin prevents reproduction of the TB organism by binding to the enzyme that allows RNA to be transcribed from DNA. As a result, TB cannot make the proteins needed to reproduce.

Pyrazinamide has an unknown mechanism of action but does reduce the pH of the intracellular fluid of WBCs in which the TB bacillus resides. The lower pH inhibits TB reproduction, especially in the early stages of the disease.

Ethambutol suppresses the reproduction of TB bacteria by an unknown mechanism. It is only bacteriostatic and must be used in combination with other TB drugs.

Usual Adult Dosages for First-Line Antitubercular Drugs

Drug Name	Usual Maintenance Dose
ethambutol (EMB) (Myambutol)	15 mg/kg orally once daily (max: 1.5 g)
isoniazid (INH) (Nydrazid)	5 mg/kg orally once daily or 5 days/week (max 300 mg) or 15 mg/kg orally twice or three times weekly (max 900 mg)
pyrazinamide (PZA)	15–30 mg/kg orally once daily (max: 3 g/day) or 50–75 mg/kg orally twice weekly
rifampin (RIF) (Rifadin, Rimactane)	10 mg/kg orally once daily (max: 600 mg) or 5 days/week, or 3 days/week or twice weekly

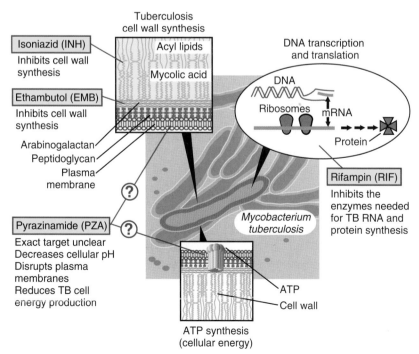

FIG. 8.3 Probable sites of drug activity against the TB organism. *ATP,* Adenosine triphosphate; *TB,* tuberculosis.

Intended responses of first-line antitubercular drugs
- Control of active TB disease
- Reduction or absence of active TB symptoms (reduced cough, less sputum, weight gain, less fatigue)
- Sputum cultures are negative for TB organisms

Common side effects of first-line antitubercular drugs. Because the first-line drugs are taken either as combination tablets or are taken individually every day, certain side effects are associated with all of these drugs together. These side effects are diarrhea, headache, nausea, vomiting, and difficulty sleeping.

Isoniazid's additional side effects include breast tenderness or enlargement (in men), loss of appetite, difficulty concentrating, and sore throat.

Rifampin's additional side effects include abdominal pain and urinary retention. This drug stains the skin, urine, tears, and all other secretions a reddish-orange color.

Pyrazinamide's additional side effects include muscle aches and pains, acne, and increased sensitivity to sun or ultraviolet light.

Pyrazinamide and *ethambutol* increase the formation of uric acid, which can cause gout or make it worse.

Possible adverse effects of first-line antitubercular drugs. The most common adverse effect of all first-line drug therapy for TB is liver toxicity, with possible progression to permanent liver damage and failure. This risk is greatly increased if the patient drinks alcoholic beverages or uses acetaminophen while taking the TB drugs.

First-line therapy has the potential to interact with many other drugs and herbal supplements. The interactions can be complex and serious. Consult a reliable drug reference for a complete list of possible interactions.

Isoniazid can cause peripheral neuropathy with loss of sensation, especially in the hands and feet. This effect occurs most often in malnourished patients, those with diabetes, and alcoholics.

Rifampin often causes anemia. *Ethambutol* at high doses can cause optic neuritis with vision changes that include reduced color vision, blurred vision, and reduced visual fields. This problem can lead to blindness. When the problem is discovered early, the eye problems are usually reversed when the drug is stopped.

⭐ **Priority actions to take** before *giving first-line antitubercular drugs.* *All the first-line drugs for TB can lead to liver toxicity.* It is important to make sure that the patient has no liver problems before starting this therapy. Check the patient's most recent laboratory values for evidence of liver problems, such as elevated liver enzymes (Refer to Table 1.4 in Chapter 1 for a listing of normal values.)

Ask male patients whether they have an enlarged prostate. Ask all patients whether they have any problem that causes urine retention. If so, report this problem to the prescriber before giving TB drugs.

Because *rifampin* can lead to anemia, assess for anemia before starting this drug. Check the patient's most recent laboratory values for anemia (low red blood cell [RBC] count, low hemoglobin level). (Refer to Table 1.6 in Chapter 1 for a listing of normal values.)

Before giving *pyrazinamide* or *ethambutol*, ask whether the patient has ever had gout. If so, other precautions need to be taken. For example, the patient should drink a full glass of water with the drug and drink at least 3000 mL of water daily.

Before giving the first dose of *ethambutol*, assess the patient's vision and document your findings in the medical record. Use this information to determine whether vision changes are occurring during therapy.

Patients who have memory or compliance problems and those who are homeless may benefit from *directly observed therapy (DOT)*, in which the nurse or other health care provider watches the patient swallow the drugs. This practice contributes to more treatment successes, fewer relapses, and less drug resistance. DOT can be done remotely using a video format (VDOT) in which patients use a phone or other

---

Common Side Effects

First-Line Antitubercular Drugs

| Diarrhea, Nausea/ Vomiting | Headache | Insomnia |

 Memory Jogger

Peripheral neuropathy from isoniazid therapy is caused by a deficiency of the B complex vitamins and can be prevented by increasing the intake of these vitamins during drug therapy.

 Drug Alert

Interaction Alert

First-line anti-TB drugs interact with many drugs and herbal supplements. Before giving a TB drug, ask the patient about all other drugs or supplements that he or she takes; then check with the pharmacist to avoid a possible drug interaction.

QSEN: Safety

Drug Alert

Administration Alert

When giving *pyrazinamide* or *ethambutol*, have the patient drink a full glass of water to help excrete uric acid crystals faster and prevent them from precipitating in joints or the kidneys.

QSEN: Safety

real-time electronic device to demonstrate compliance with the drug regimen. This method helps patients "live their lives" without having to physically come to a place for DOT. Drawbacks to this method include whether the patient is willing and able to use such a device and how good the connectivity is for both the patient's device and the nurse's access to the video.

⭐ *Priority actions to take **after** giving first-line antitubercular drugs.* For IV drug forms, assess the patient's vital signs and respiratory status at least every 15 minutes for the first hour. Tell the patient to immediately report any shortness of breath or change in breathing.

Assess the patient daily for yellowing *(jaundice)* of the skin or sclera, which is a symptom of liver problems. The best places to check are the whites of the eyes closest to the iris, the roof of the mouth, and the chest. Review the results of liver function tests for abnormalities.

If a patient has diabetes, check blood glucose levels more frequently and assess fasting blood glucose levels or levels of hemoglobin A1C whenever they are ordered. Report higher than normal levels to the prescriber for adjustments in the dosages of antidiabetic drugs.

At each clinic visit, ask the patient about any numbness, tingling, or pain in the hands and feet. Use monofilaments to check for peripheral neuropathy.

Assess intake and output. If output is 1000 mL less than the patient is drinking or if other symptoms of urinary retention are present (enlarged bladder, lower abdominal discomfort), notify the prescriber.

Urge patients to drink plenty of water throughout the day and night. Ask about any pain in the joints (especially the big toe, foot, or ankle), and check for any joint swelling. These are all indications of gout from precipitation of uric acid crystals.

⭐ *Teaching priorities for patients taking first-line antitubercular drugs.* Teach patients the following care needs and precautions:

- Keep a supply of the prescribed drugs on hand at all times.
- You are usually no longer contagious after drugs have been taken for 2 to 3 consecutive weeks and symptoms improve or disappear. However, **you must continue taking the drugs for 6 months or longer, exactly as prescribed.**
- Avoid alcoholic beverages and drugs containing acetaminophen for the entire drug therapy period because, when combined with the TB drugs, serious liver complications can occur. In addition, if you are under the influence of alcohol, you may not remember to take your drugs.
- Notify your prescriber if you develop yellowing of your skin or eyes, darkening of your urine, or lighter stools. These problems are signs of liver toxicity.
- If these drugs cause nausea, take your daily dose at bedtime.
- If you have diabetes, check your blood glucose level as often as prescribed and notify your prescriber if the level is consistently out of the target range. Your prescriber may need to change the antidiabetic drug dosage, schedule, or drug type.
- If you have high blood pressure, avoid coffee, tea (including green tea), chocolate, colas, and any other forms of caffeinated drinks or "stay-awake" pills because isoniazid, when combined with caffeine, can raise your blood pressure to dangerous levels.
- Rifampin will stain the skin, urine, and all other secretions a reddish-orange tinge but will be clear to normal within a few weeks after you stop taking the drug. Soft contact lenses used at this time will become permanently stained.
- Drink at least 8 oz of water when taking these drugs and increase your fluid intake to at least 3 L of water daily. It is best to drink water throughout the day and at least one full glass of water during the night.
- These drugs increase your skin's sensitivity to the sun and can cause a severe sunburn, even if you have dark skin. Wear protective clothing, a hat, and sunscreen when going outdoors in the sunlight.

 Drug Alert

Teaching Alert

Teach all patients on TB drug therapy to avoid alcoholic beverages and acetaminophen for the entire therapy period.

QSEN: Safety

 Drug Alert

Teaching Alert

Teach patients taking isoniazid to avoid coffee, tea (including green tea), chocolate, colas, and any other forms of caffeinated drinks or "stay-awake" pills because isoniazid and caffeine together can raise blood pressure to dangerous levels.

QSEN: Safety

Drug Alert

Teaching Alert

Tell patients taking ethambutol to notify their prescriber immediately if any change in vision occurs.

QSEN: Safety

Drug Alert

Teaching Alert

Teach patients taking TB drugs to avoid taking any other type of drugs (prescribed or over the counter) or supplements without first checking with the TB drug prescriber.

QSEN: Safety

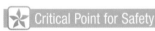

Critical Point for Safety

The most common cause of MDR TB and XDR TB is mismanagement of drug therapy or nonadherence to prescribed drug therapy. *Patients who contract TB from a person with a resistant strain will also have a resistant strain of TB.* So, teaching patients to strictly adhere to TB drug therapy helps to prevent the development and spread of MDR TB and XDR TB.

QSEN: Safety

- If you take ethambutol, notify your prescriber immediately if any change in vision develops. In addition, if you have glaucoma or cataract, see your ophthalmologist during ethambutol therapy.
- Be sure to tell all your other health care providers that you are taking first-line drugs for TB, because of the potential for drug interactions.
- Do not take any over-the-counter drugs or herbal preparations without checking with the prescriber of the TB drugs.

Life span considerations for first-line antitubercular drugs

Pediatric considerations. With the exception of ethambutol, infants and children of any age who have active TB should take first-line anti-TB drugs.

Considerations for pregnancy and lactation. First-line anti-TB drugs are approved for treatment of active TB in pregnant women. The risk for liver toxicity is higher when taking TB drug therapy during pregnancy, and close monitoring of liver function is needed. In addition, the pregnant woman needs higher doses of a B-complex vitamin supplement when taking isoniazid.

First-line anti-TB drugs appear in breast milk. When possible, breastfeeding should be avoided. If breastfeeding cannot be stopped, the breastfed infant should receive supplementation with B-complex vitamins.

Considerations for older adults. The risk for liver toxicity is higher among older adults taking drugs for TB. Gout is more common among older adults and may be aggravated in the older adult who has to use fluid restrictions because of other health problems.

Older adults may have some degree of cataract formation in one or both eyes. This condition makes visual assessment for optic neuritis more difficult. Older adults taking ethambutol should be followed monthly by an ophthalmologist during therapy.

Antitubercular Drug Therapy for Drug-Resistant Tuberculosis

Some TB strains are resistant to isoniazid and rifampin. These strains are known as *multidrug-resistant TB* (MDR TB) strains. For MDR TB, other powerful antibacterial drugs are usually prescribed as second-line antibiotics, particularly the fluoroquinolones and at least one of the aminoglycosides (discussed in Chapter 6). Some MDR TB strains now have become extensively drug-resistant TB (XDR TB). These infections are resistant not only to the first-line anti-TB drugs but also to the second-line antibiotics. The most common cause of MDR TB and XDR TB is mismanagement of drug therapy or nonadherence to prescribed drug therapy. *Patients who contract TB from a person with a resistant strain will also have a resistant strain of TB.* Resistant strains more frequently lead to death.

Drug therapy for MDR TB and XDR TB is limited and requires some very powerful and dangerous drugs to prevent TB progression and death. Currently, a three drug-regimen with bedaquiline, pretomanid, and the oxazolidinone protein synthesis antibacterial drug linezolid (discussed in Chapter 6) is specifically targeted to MDR TB or XDR TB. Side effects and adverse effects of this drug combination can be life threatening, so it is not used when other drugs will work. This combination therapy is strongly recommended to be given through DOT.

Adult Dosages for Multidrug-Resistant and Extensively Drug-Resistant Tuberculosis

Drug Name	Recommended Dose
bedaquiline ❶ (Sirturo)	400 mg orally once daily for 2 weeks, then 200 mg orally three times weekly for 24 weeks
pretomanid	200 mg orally once daily for 26 weeks
linezolid (Zyvox)	1200 mg orally once daily for 26 weeks

❶ High-alert drug.

How combination therapy for drug-resistant tuberculosis works. With MDR and XDR forms of TB, drug therapy with a single drug is usually not effective in stopping the progression of the disease or eradicating the organism. The three drugs have very different mechanisms of action, and all three are needed to increase the likelihood that therapy will be effective.

Bedaquiline stops production of the high-energy substance ATP (adenosine triphosphate) in the TB organism, making it unable to complete its critical metabolic functions or reproduce. This drug appears to be bactericidal even when the TB organism is dormant.

Pretomanid inhibits the synthesis of a substance important for building cell walls in actively dividing TB organisms. This action is bactericidal.

Linezolid is a protein synthesis inhibitor. The drug can be bacteriostatic or bactericidal.

Common side effects of combination therapy for drug-resistant tuberculosis. Because the drugs are given as combination therapy, determining which drug actually causes specific side effects and adverse effects is not precise. The most common side effects for the combination are hypertension, abdominal pain, headache, nausea, joint pain, and rash.

Possible adverse effects of combination therapy for drug-resistant tuberculosis. All three drugs in this combination are liver toxic. They all also interact with more than a hundred other drugs and botanicals.

Both *bediquiline* and *linezolid* often induce cardiac changes including a prolonged QT interval on electrocardiogram (ECG) even after the drug is stopped. This problem is worse in patients who already have a prolonged QT interval and in those who are also taking other drugs that prolong the QT interval, such as the fluoroquinolones. The risk is also increased for development of other life-threatening dysrhythmias.

Both *pretomanid* and *linezolid* are associated with blurred vision and damage to the optic nerve. *Pretomanid* has adverse effects on the nervous system, including peripheral neuropathy and seizures. *Linezolid* is kidney toxic and reduces blood cell counts, especially RBCs (red blood cells) and platelets.

This combination therapy has been found to reduce sperm production in males. It is not known if this fertility issue resolves when therapy is complete or has longer-lasting negative effects on male reproductive potential.

 Priority actions to take before *giving combination therapy for drug-resistant tuberculosis.* Assess the patient's understanding about the need for this important therapy and his or her likelihood of adherence. Make arrangements for the patient to participate in a directly observed program for the duration of the therapy period.

Ask the patient about what other drugs, botanicals, and nutritional supplements he or she takes on a regular basis. This drug combination interacts with more than one hundred other drugs and will require significant adjustments in general drug therapy.

Assess the patient's blood pressure as a baseline and take his or her pulse for a full minute, noting rate and rhythm. Document this in the medical record. If an ECG has been ordered, be sure that is obtained before the first dose.

Ensure that blood work for liver function tests, complete blood counts, and renal function tests is ordered and performed before the patient starts this combination of drugs. The combination is toxic to the liver and kidneys and is known to suppress bone marrow production of RBCs and platelets. Use this information to compare with tests performed later in the therapy period to determine whether liver or kidney adverse effects are present, along with anemia and increased bleeding or bruising.

Ask the patient about his or her usual vision and perform a baseline visual assessment with a hand-held pocket eye chart. Record this assessment to use for comparison after treatment begins.

 Priority actions to take after *giving combination therapy for drug-resistant tuberculosis.* Ensure the patient drinks a full glass of water with the tablets and that he or she does not crush or chew them. Check under the tongue and in the area

---

Combination Therapy for Drug-Resistant Tuberculosis

Hypertension   Abdominal   Headache
                    pain, Nausea/
                    Vomiting

                    Rash

Joint pain

 Critical Point for Safety

Untreated multidrug-resistant and extensively drug-resistant TB infections are highly likely to be fatal. Because of this and the fact that being poorly adherent to therapy increases the development of even more drug-resistant strains, combination therapy for drug-resistant TB must be given as directly observed therapy.

QSEN: Safety

 Critical Point for Safety

Baseline information on kidney function, liver function, cardiac function, vision, and blood cell counts are essential to obtain and document to identify changes that could indicate toxicities from the drug therapy before serious or irreversible harm develops.

QSEN: Safety

between the teeth and the gums to be certain the tablets have actually been swallowed.

This drug therapy regimen can cause many side effects and adverse reactions. Teaching the patient about what to check and notice daily is critical.

 Teaching priorities for patients receiving combination therapy for drug-resistant tuberculosis

- Keep your daily appointment to receive these drugs. Missing even a few days can make this therapy less effective and worsen your TB infection.
- Keep all your appointments for laboratory work. The results of these tests can help to identify an adverse effect early and help prevent problems.
- Do not chew these drugs. They can be taken on a full or an empty stomach.
- Avoid drinking grapefruit juice or eating grapefruit, because these interfere with the drugs' metabolism.
- Drink a full glass of water when taking these drugs, and increase your intake of fluids, especially water throughout the day, to prevent kidney problems.
- Do not drink alcohol or take acetaminophen, because both these substances contribute to liver damage.
- Do not take any over-the-counter drugs, herbal supplements, or vitamins without first checking with your prescriber. Your TB drugs interact with many other substances, which could either make your drugs less effective or increase the risk for harmful side effects.
- These drugs can have harmful effects on your liver. Inspect yourself daily for signs of liver problems, including yellowing of the skin or whites of your eyes, darkening of your urine, having light or clay-colored stools, having constant pain or discomfort on your right side around the bottom of the rib cage, chronically feeling tired, and having worsening nausea. Report any of these changes to your prescriber immediately.
- These drugs can harm your kidneys. Keep a general sense of whether the amount you urinate each day is close to the amount of fluids you drink each day. If you are urinating much less than you are drinking, report this to your prescriber immediately.
- These drugs can interfere with production of certain blood cells and cause both anemia and an increased risk for bleeding. If you appear paler than usual, have a pale appearance to the insides of your lower eyelids, are increasingly tired, or have increased bruising and bleeding, report these changes to your prescriber immediately.
- These drugs can interfere with your heart's electrical conduction and cause changes in your heart rate and rhythm. Check your pulse at least twice daily, and report any consistent irregular beats to your prescriber.
- Two of the three drugs can have harmful effects on your eyes and vision. If you notice your vision is becoming blurry or your vision decreases in any way, notify your prescriber immediately.
- Report any changes of sensation in your hands or feet, such as tingling, burning, or numbness, to your prescriber. These are signs of peripheral neuropathy. Although the drugs may not have to be stopped for this, other precautions will be needed.

Life span considerations for combination therapy for drug-resistant tuberculosis. The drugs for combination therapy to treat drug-resistant TB are powerful and have many side effects and adverse effects on people of all ages and developmental stages. *However, without treatment, drug-resistant TB is usually fatal.* Therefore the use of this combination therapy in children, pregnant women, and older adults must be balanced by the detrimental problem of delaying or not treating a disease that usually has a fatal outcome. Breastfeeding while taking combination therapy for drug-resistant TB is not recommended.

 Drug Alert

Teaching Alert

Teach patients to assess themselves daily for indications of liver toxicity, including jaundice of the skin or sclera, dark urine, light-colored stools, right upper quadrant pain, chronic fatigue, and persistent nausea.

QSEN: Safety

 Drug Alert

Teaching Alert

Teach patients to take their pulse at least twice daily and to check for irregularities or persistent changes in rate. Instruct the patient to report any such changes to his or her prescriber immediately.

QSEN: Safety

Drug Alert

Teaching Alert

Teach patients to assess their vision daily for new onset blurriness or a decrease in visual acuity. Instruct the patient to report any such changes to his or her prescriber immediately.

QSEN: Safety

REVIEW OF RELATED PHYSIOLOGY AND PATHOPHYSIOLOGY OF FUNGAL INFECTIONS

OVERVIEW

Fungi are common microorganisms in our environment. A **fungus** is a simple organism with one or more cells (e.g., yeasts, molds, and mushrooms) that reproduces by spores, has walled cells, and can either live peacefully with humans or infect humans and cause disease. They have a thick, tough cell wall and a plasma membrane that is made of materials different from bacterial cell walls (Fig. 8.4). Some of the internal features of fungi more closely resemble human cells than the cells of other microorganisms.

Fungi live in places that are moist and dark. There are more than 100,000 different types of fungi, some of which are harmless and others that can cause infection and disease. Because of their tough cell walls, fungi can live easily on human skin and mucous membrane surfaces and are not completely removed by usual bathing. Some types such as *Candida* are part of normal skin flora that do not cause problems unless they overgrow or enter the body. Without treatment, fungal infections remain and can become widespread, especially in people whose immune systems are not functioning well. Superficial fungal infections are uncomfortable and change the appearance and function of the infected skin area. When fungal infections enter the body by inhalation or through breaks in the skin, deep fungal infections can result. With deep fungal infection, function in the affected organ is reduced and the organ can be destroyed.

TYPES OF ANTIFUNGAL DRUGS

The thick fungal cell walls make fungi resistant to most standard antibacterial antiinfective drugs. Currently, some fungi also are becoming resistant to antifungal drugs. In addition, fungal DNA is similar to human DNA, causing antifungal drugs to often have more side effects than other types of antiinfective drugs.

Drugs for Superficial Fungal Infections

Treatment for superficial fungal infections of the skin or mucous membranes involves topical application of antifungal drugs. These are usually the same types of drugs used to treat deeper fungal infections but are prepared as creams, lotions, ointments, shampoos, powders, oral lozenges, inhalants, and vaginal suppositories. Topical drugs are successful at clearing fungal infections that are not severe in patients with healthy immune systems. An exception is fungal infection of the

> **Memory Jogger**
>
> Deep fungal infections require systemic therapy. Superficial fungal infections may be cured with topical antifungal therapy, although, if persistent, these infections also may require systemic therapy.

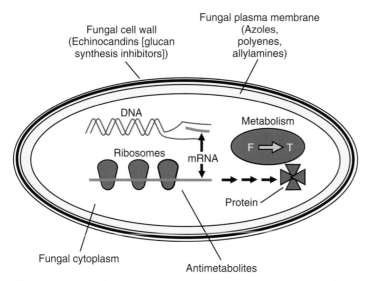

FIG. 8.4 Sites of antifungal drug activity. $F \rightarrow T$, Metabolic conversion of folic acid to thymine.

fingernails or toenails. Because the fungus is under the nail, topical application is not usually successful. Box 8.1 lists points and precautions to teach patients using topical antifungal therapy.

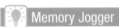

Memory Jogger

- Allylamines
- Antifungal antibiotics
- Antimetabolites
- Azoles
- Echinocandins
- Polyenes

Drugs for Deep or Systemic Fungal Infections

When fungal infections are deep or extensive, systemic drugs are needed to kill the fungi (**fungicidal** action) or slow their reproduction (**fungistatic** action). The classes of antifungal drugs are the allylamines, antifungal antibiotics, antimetabolites, azoles, echinocandins, and polyenes. (See Fig. 8.4 for where specific types of antifungal drugs work to kill or disrupt the growth of fungi.) *All systemic antifungal drugs have more side effects and adverse effects than most antibacterial drugs.*

How antifungal drugs work. To reproduce and live, fungal cells must keep their plasma membranes and cell walls intact. Membranes are made up of phospholipids and ergosterol, as shown in Fig. 8.5. Ergosterol is a fat (lipid) similar to the cholesterol that is part of human cell plasma membranes. The *azoles*, *polyenes*, and *allylamines* either prevent the fungus from making ergosterol or bind to the ergosterol and prevent it from being properly placed in the fungal membrane. As a result, the fungal membranes are leaky and allow damage to the fungus to occur. This action can prevent fungal reproduction (**fungistatic**) and may kill some fungi (**fungicidal**).

Antifungal antibiotics work by inhibiting the formation of spindle fibers, which stops the process of fungal cell division and reproduction.

Antimetabolites work by entering the fungal cell and acting as a "counterfeit" DNA base. When flucytosine is part of fungal cell DNA, it prevents fungal proteins needed for reproduction and growth from being made.

Box 8.1　Patient Teaching Tips and Precautions for Topical Antifungal Agents

GENERAL

- Report any indication of an allergic reaction (new redness, swelling, blisters, or drainage) to the prescriber.
- Immediately after applying the drug, wash your hands to remove all traces of it.
- If another person applies the drug for you, ensure that he or she wears disposable gloves to reduce his or her risk for absorbing the drug.
- Avoid getting any antifungal drug in your eye. If the drug does get into your eye, wash the eye with large amounts of warm, running tap water and notify the prescriber.
- Use the drug exactly as prescribed and for as long as prescribed to ensure that the infection is cured.

POWDERS

- Ensure that the skin area is clean and completely dry before applying the powder.
- Hold your breath while applying to prevent inhaling the drug.
- For the foot area, be sure to apply the powder between and under your toes. Wear clean cotton socks (night and day). Change the socks at least twice daily.
- For the groin area, wear clean, close-fitting (but not tight) cotton underwear (briefs or panties).

SKIN CREAMS, LOTIONS, OINTMENTS

- Ensure that the skin area is clean and dry before applying the drug.
- Be careful to apply it only to the skin that has the infection. Keep it away from the surrounding skin.
- Apply a thin coating as often as prescribed.
- Wash and dry the area right before reapplying the next dose.

- Loosely cover the area to prevent spreading the drug to other body areas, clothing, or furniture.

ORAL LOZENGES

- Brush your teeth and tongue before using the tablet or troche.
- Let the tablet or troche completely dissolve in your mouth.
- Clean your toothbrush daily by running it through the dishwasher or soaking it in a solution of one part household bleach with nine parts water. After using bleach, rinse the toothbrush thoroughly.

VAGINAL CREAMS OR SUPPOSITORIES

- Place creams or suppositories just before going to bed to help keep them within the vagina longer.
- Wash your hands before inserting the drug.
- Insert the suppository (rounded end first) into the vagina as far as you can with your finger.
- Insert a full applicator of the cream as far into the vagina as is comfortable.
- Wash the applicator and your hands with warm, soapy water; rinse well; and dry.
- A sanitary napkin can be worn to protect your clothing and the bed from drug leakage.
- Avoid sexual intercourse during the treatment period. If you do have intercourse, the drug can create holes in a condom or damage a diaphragm and increase your risk for an unplanned pregnancy. In addition, you could spread the infection or become reinfected.
- Use the drug on consecutive days for as long as prescribed.

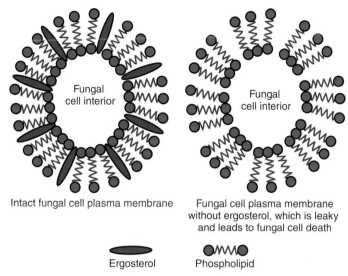

Intact fungal cell plasma membrane   Fungal cell plasma membrane
without ergosterol, which is leaky
and leads to fungal cell death

Ergosterol   Phospholipid

FIG. 8.5 Intact fungal cell plasma membrane *(left)* and the effects of azoles, polyenes, and allylamines on fungal cell membranes *(right)*.

The *echinocandins* are also called *glucan synthesis inhibitors*. Fungi have a tough cell wall for protection (see Fig. 8.4) that is different from and in addition to the plasma membrane. This wall is made up of many substances that serve as "bricks" in the cell wall; glucan, which serves as "mortar" in the cell wall, holds the bricks tightly in place. Echinocandins stop fungal production of glucan so the mortar is thin and weak. This makes the entire fungal cell wall weak and unable to protect the fungal cell.

Drug dosages and length of therapy vary, depending on the specific organism and infection severity. Some therapy schedules may be as short as 7 days; others may last 6 to 12 months. The most common drugs in each class are discussed in this chapter. Consult a reliable drug reference for fungal type indications and for other specific antifungal drugs.

Adult Dosages for Common Systemic Antifungal Drugs

Drug Type	Drug Name	Usual Maintenance Dose
Azoles	fluconazole (Diflucan)	200–400 mg orally or 200–800 mg IV daily
	ketoconazole (Nizoral)	200–400 mg orally once daily
	itraconazole (ONMEL, Sporanox, TULSURA)	130–200 mg orally once or twice daily
	posaconazole (Noxafil)	100–400 mg orally twice daily for 1 day, then 100–400 mg orally once daily 300 mg IV twice daily for 1 day, then 300 mg IV once daily
	voriconazole (VFEND)	200–400 mg orally every 12 hr
Allylamines	terbinafine (Lamisil, Terbinex)	250 mg orally daily 6 mg/kg IV every 12 hr on day 1, then 3–4 mg/kg IV every 12 hr
Antifungal Antibiotics	griseofulvin (Fulvicin, Grifulvin, Grisactin, Gris-Peg)	varies by size (microsize; ultramicrosize) 300–1000 orally once daily or in 2–4 divided doses daily
Antimetabolites	flucytosine (Ancobon)	50–150 mg/kg orally daily in divided doses every 6 hr in combination with amphotericin B
Echinochandins	anidulafungin (Eraxis)	200 mg IV loading dose; then 100 mg IV daily
	caspofungin (Cancidas)	70 mg IV loading dose, then 50 mg IV daily
Polyenes	amphotericin B ❶ (Amphocin, Fungizone)	0.25–1 mg/kg IV every 24 hr (max dose 1.5 mg/kg daily)

❶ High-alert drug.

Do Not Confuse

Lamisil *with* Lamictal

An order for Lamisil can be confused with Lamictal. Lamisil is an antifungal drug, whereas Lamictal is an anticonvulsant prescribed for seizure disorders and certain psychiatric problems.

QSEN: Safety

Common Side Effects

Antifungal Drugs

Nausea/Vomiting,   Headache   Hair loss
Diarrhea

Injection site
reaction   Photosensitivity   Taste
changes

 Memory Jogger

Antifungal drugs are used with caution in patients who have kidney failure, liver disease, heart failure, or severe dysrhythmias.

 Memory Jogger

Amphotericin B causes renal insufficiency in all patients receiving it. For people who had normal renal function before therapy, many can recover normal renal function. For those who had some degree of renal impairment before therapy, renal impairment is worse and may be permanent.

 Memory Jogger

All patients receiving amphotericin B develop side effects, and most develop serious adverse effects. Monitor these patients very carefully because they are very sick.

 Drug Alert

Interaction Alert

Before giving an antifungal drug, ask the patient about all other drugs or supplements that he or she takes. Then check with the pharmacist to avoid a possible drug interaction.

QSEN: Safety

Intended responses of antifungal drugs. The intended responses of successful antifungal drug therapy are the eradication of the infection and normal function of all tissues and organs.

Common side effects of antifungal drugs. Common side effects of most antifungal drugs are changes in how food tastes, diarrhea, headache, nausea, and vomiting. Many patients taking a drug for several weeks report hair thinning. Drugs given intravenously may cause pain and redness at the injection site. *Ketoconazole, voriconazole,* and *griseofulvin* increase sun sensitivity and can lead to a severe sunburn.

Possible adverse effects of antifungal drugs. Antifungal drugs have many possible adverse effects, including anemia, liver toxicity, low serum potassium levels *(hypokalemia),* severe rashes, abnormal heart rhythms, and reduced kidney function. Most occur only at high doses or in patients with other health problems.

Skin irritation and rashes can occur with systemic antifungal therapy. Rashes may be severe with many types of lesions (Stevens-Johnson syndrome) (see Chapter 1). If the rashes become widespread with crusting, fever, and tissue necrosis, the condition can be life threatening.

Antifungal drugs have the potential to interact with many other drugs and herbal supplements. These interactions can be complex and serious.

Terbinafine (Lamisil) and *flucytosine* (Ancobon) can reduce WBC counts and increase the risk for infection.

The *azoles* and *amphotericin B* and can cause renal insufficiency. When renal insufficiency is present, the drugs are retained longer and are then more likely to cause additional severe side effects and adverse effects. If the patient is also being treated with an additional drug that also impairs the kidney, the risk for kidney damage increases greatly.

Griseofulvin, which is usually taken for 2 to 6 months to treat fungal infections of the fingernails and toenails, is associated with liver toxicity and paresthesia of the hands and feet. (Paresthesias are areas of numbness and tingling.)

Flucytosine (Ancobon) and the *echinocandins* can cause peripheral neuropathy with loss of sensation. The degree of sensation loss is related to how long the nerve-damaging drugs are used.

At very high doses the *azoles* may cause cardiac dysrhythmias, especially prolonged QT and *torsades de pointes,* a condition of unusual ventricular tachycardia. In addition, the drugs can interfere with cardiac drugs that are prescribed to control abnormal heart rhythms.

The *echinocandins* can increase the rate of clot formation, which increases the risk for deep vein thrombosis (DVT). DVT is most likely to occur in veins of the lower legs and pelvis. *Amphotericin B* has more adverse reactions than other antifungal drugs. For this reason, systemic therapy with amphotericin B is used only for serious, life-threatening fungal infections. Common adverse effects of systemic amphotericin B include fever and severe chills. The drug dilates blood vessels, causing widespread skin flushing *(red man syndrome).* Hypotension and shock may occur as a result of blood vessel dilation. In addition, allergic reactions are possible, including anaphylaxis. Amphotericin B has a long half-life (15 days), and adverse effects may be present for weeks to months after the drug has been stopped.

⭐ *Priority actions to take before giving antifungal drugs.* Because antifungal drugs may cause anemia and liver toxicity, make sure that the patient is not anemic and has no liver problems before starting these drugs. Check the patient's most recent laboratory values for anemia (low RBC count, low hemoglobin level) and liver problems (elevated liver enzyme levels). (Refer to Table 1.6 and Table 1.4 in Chapter 1 for a listing of normal values.)

Check the patient's current laboratory work, especially blood urea nitrogen (BUN) and serum creatinine levels, because these drugs can cause kidney impairment. (Refer to Table 1.5 in Chapter 1 for a listing of normal values.) Use these values as a baseline to determine whether the patient develops any kidney problems while taking an antifungal drug.

Some of the antifungal drugs should be taken with meals, whereas others should be taken on an empty stomach. Carefully plan the dosing schedule around meals. Do not give an azole with grapefruit or grapefruit juice because the activity of *azole* antifungal drugs can be reduced by these. In addition, *ketoconazole* should not be given with drugs that reduce gastric acid, such as proton pump inhibitors or histamine blockers, because the drug is activated by stomach acids.

For amphotericin B, hypersensitivity is common. Check and recheck the exact dose each time the drug is given. At times the first dose of amphotericin B is much smaller than the daily maintenance doses. Dosages vary considerably from one patient to another.

Many health care providers order premedication with specific drugs to counteract the side effects of amphotericin B. These drugs may include acetaminophen or ibuprofen to prevent or reduce fever, antihistamines (e.g., diphenhydramine), IV corticosteroids (e.g., cortisol) to reduce blood vessel dilation, and meperidine to reduce or prevent excessive chills and shaking *(rigors)*. Check the order to determine whether these drugs should be given in advance, and administer them at the appropriate time.

Parenteral *amphotericin B* must be used as soon as it is mixed. Administer the drug slowly, regardless of the dose.

 Priority actions to take after *giving antifungal drugs.* When giving the first IV dose of an antifungal drug, assess the patient every 15 minutes for any signs or symptoms of an allergic reaction (hives at the IV site, low blood pressure, rapid, irregular pulse, swelling of the lips or lower face, the patient feeling a lump in the throat). If the patient is having an anaphylactic reaction, your first action is to prevent any more drug from entering the body. Stop the drug from infusing, but maintain the IV access.

Assess the patient's skin every shift for rash, blisters, or other skin eruption that may indicate a reaction to the drug. Ask the patient about any itching or skin changes. Also assess daily for yellowing *(jaundice)* of the skin or sclera, which is a symptom of liver problems.

Assess the patient's apical pulse for a full minute at least twice daily. Check whether there is a change in heart rate or regularity, document any changes, and notify the prescriber.

Check the patient's laboratory values, especially WBC counts, RBC counts, platelets, blood hematocrit, hemoglobin, BUN, creatinine, and potassium levels, every time they are taken. Compare these values with those obtained before drug therapy was started. If the potassium level is less than 3.5 mEq/L or if kidney function test values (BUN, creatinine) are increasing, notify the prescriber. Examine the patient's intake and output record daily to determine if urine output is within 500 mL of the total fluid intake. Notify the prescriber if any blood counts are low.

With *terbinafine* or *flucytosine*, assess the patient every shift for any signs of a new infection (e.g., the presence of fever, drainage, foul-smelling urine, productive cough, or redness around an open skin area) because these drugs suppress the immune response. Report any symptoms to the prescriber.

With *echinocandins*, assess the patient's calves daily for signs of DVT (swelling, warmth, and pain or discomfort). If present, check and compare the opposite calf and notify the prescriber.

With *amphotericin B*, assess blood pressure at least every hour while the drug is infusing because the drug causes blood vessel dilation with hypotension. This can become severe enough to induce shock. Check for other symptoms of shock (pulse oximetry reading less than 90%, rapid heart rate, rapid and shallow respirations, decreased urine output, change in level of consciousness). If shock symptoms are present or if blood pressure drops more than 15 mm Hg below the patient's normal level, call the Rapid Response Team and notify the prescriber immediately.

 Drug Alert

Administration Alert

Infuse the IV form of any *azole* slowly, no faster than 200 mg/hr. Flush the line only with sterile normal saline that does not contain a preservative.

QSEN: Safety

 Drug Alert

Administration Alert

Check and recheck the exact dose each time *amphotericin B* is given. The dose may not be the same any 2 days the drug is prescribed. It also may be different from one patient to another.

QSEN: Safety

 Drug Alert

Administration Alert

Administer parenteral *amphotericin B* and the *echinocandins* slowly, over at least 6 hr.

QSEN: Safety

Drug Alert

Action/Intervention Alert

If the patient appears to be having anaphylaxis from an IV drug, prevent any more drug from entering the body, but maintain the IV access.

QSEN: Safety

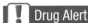

Drug Alert

Administration Alert

Examine the IV site during amphotericin B administration at least every 2 hours for a change in blood return, any redness or pain, or the feeling of hard or "cordlike" veins above the site. If such problems occur, follow the policy of your facility about removing that IV access.

QSEN: Safety

Drug Alert

Teaching Alert

Teach patients taking an azole to check their pulse daily and to report new irregularities, rates faster than 100 beats/min, or rates lower than 50 to the prescriber.

QSEN: Safety

Drug Alert

Teaching Alert

Warn patients taking terbinafine or flucytosine for more than 1 week that they are at an increased risk for infection and should avoid crowds and people who are ill.

QSEN: Safety

Drug Alert

Teaching Alert

Teach parents of children taking terbinafine sprinkles to avoid mixing the drug with applesauce or any acid-containing fruit or food.

QSEN: Safety

Expected side effects that usually occur during (or shortly after) the infusion with IV *amphotericin B* include headache, chills, fever, rigors, flushing, hypotension, nausea, and vomiting. Unlike other parenteral drugs, further slowing of the IV rate does **not** prevent these effects. Assess the patient hourly for these side effects. Administer drugs as prescribed to reduce side effects. Even if these effects occur, it is important to attempt to administer the entire prescribed dose of amphotericin B because the infection is often life threatening.

★ *Teaching priorities for patients taking antifungal drugs*
- Be sure to tell all other health care providers that you are taking an antifungal drug, because of the potential for drug interactions.
- Do not take any over-the-counter drugs without consulting your prescriber.
- If you are taking an "azole" drug, avoid or minimize drinking grapefruit juice or eating grapefruit because these substances change the drug's metabolism.
- Check your pulse for a full minute twice daily for irregularities. Report new irregularities, rates faster than 100 beats/min at rest, or rates slower than 50 beats/min to your prescriber.
- Immediately notify your prescriber if you develop yellowing of the skin or eyes, darkening of the urine, or lightening of the stools because these are signs of liver toxicity.
- If you notice increased fatigue, paleness, and increased heart rate or shortness of breath, report these symptoms to your prescriber because you may be anemic.
- Examine or have your partner examine your entire skin surface at least once daily for any rashes, blisters, or other skin changes. If skin changes occur, notify your prescriber immediately.
- If you are taking ketoconazole or voriconazole or griseofulvin, avoid direct sunlight, use sunscreen, and wear protective clothing (including a hat) whenever you are in the sun, to prevent a severe sunburn. Also avoid tanning beds and salons.
- If you are taking terbinafine or flucytosine for longer than 1 week, avoid crowds and people who are ill, because your resistance to infection is now decreased.
- Notify your prescriber at the first sign of an infection.

Life span considerations for antifungal drugs
   Pediatric considerations. The safety and effectiveness of many systemic antifungal drugs have not been established. However, they are used cautiously in infants and children who have severe fungal infections.
   Children are prescribed terbinafine for ringworm of the scalp (tinea capitis). Terbinafine is provided as granules to be sprinkled on a spoonful of pudding or other soft, nonacidic food. Tell the child to swallow the entire spoonful without chewing.
   Considerations for pregnancy and lactation. Antifungal drugs are not recommended during pregnancy unless the fungal infection is serious or life threatening. *Griseofulvin* has a high likelihood of increasing the risk for birth defects or fetal damage and should **never** be given during pregnancy. Breastfeeding is not recommended during antifungal therapy.
   Considerations for older adults. With *amphotericin B*, older adults may develop neurologic reactions more often. These reactions include abnormal thinking, agitation, anxiety, cerebral vascular accident, coma, confusion, depression, blurred vision, dizziness, drowsiness, hallucinations, hearing loss, and peripheral neuropathy. Assess older adults every shift for the presence of any of these changes.
   With *echinocandins*, older adults are at greater risk for DVT. Use prescribed DVT prevention strategies. Assess patients daily for swelling, pain, or tenderness in the lower legs. Document positive findings and notify the prescriber.

Get Ready for the NCLEX® Examination!

Key Points

- TB is spread by the airborne route, which allows droplets containing the bacteria to be exhaled when a person with active TB coughs, laughs, sneezes, whistles, or sings.
- For active TB to be controlled, the patient must adhere to combination anti-TB therapy for at least 6 months, even when symptoms are no longer present.
- A person who has a positive TB skin test will never have a negative test in the future, even after treatment has successfully controlled or eradicated the TB organism (unless he or she is profoundly immunosuppressed).
- All first-line drugs for TB can cause liver toxicity.
- Without treatment, drug-resistant TB is usually fatal. For many reasons, the combination therapy to manage drug-resistant TB is usually given as DOT (directly observed therapy).
- Patients who contract TB from a person with a drug-resistant strain of the organism will also have a drug-resistant strain of TB.
- Combination therapy for drug-resistant TB is liver toxic, and these drugs also interact with more than a hundred other drugs and botanicals.
- Teach patients taking combination therapy for drug-resistant TB to assess themselves daily for indications of liver toxicity, including jaundice of the skin or sclera, dark urine, light-colored stools, right upper quadrant pain, chronic fatigue, and persistent nausea.
- Teach patients to take their pulse at least twice daily and check for irregularities or persistent changes in rate, and report any such changes to the prescriber immediately.

- Teach patients to assess their vision daily for new onset blurriness or a decrease in visual acuity and to report any such changes to the prescriber immediately.
- All systemic antifungal drugs have more side effects and adverse effects than most antibacterial drugs.
- The most common adverse effect of antifungal therapy is anemia.
- Amphotericin B and the echinocandins are IV drugs that are usually given only in the in-patient setting. Patients receiving these drugs are usually very ill.
- Teach patients to avoid drinking grapefruit juice while taking an azole.
- Treatment with systemic amphotericin B is reserved for severe or life-threatening fungal infections.
- Amphotericin B has a long half-life (15 days), which means that side effects and adverse effects may be present for days to weeks after the drug has been stopped.
- Premedication may be prescribed before administration of amphotericin B to counteract the uncomfortable side effects of the drug.
- Do not administer amphotericin B at the same time as any blood product because the expected side effects of the drug may mask a transfusion reaction.

Additional Learning Resources

⊕ Be sure to visit your Evolve website (http://evolve.elsevier.com/Workman/pharmacology/) for additional online resources.

SG Go to your Study Guide for additional learning activities to help you master this chapter content.

Review Questions

See *Answers to In-Text Review Questions* in the back of the book for answers to these questions.

1. Why are there many more people infected with the *Mycobacterium tuberculosis* organism than there are people who develop the actual infectious tuberculosis (TB) disease?

   A. There are many strains of the bacterium, and most are not pathogenic.
   B. Most people infected with the organism quickly develop immunity to it.
   C. In this country, most people are immunized against *M. tuberculosis* in infancy.
   D. Most people are usually infected with TB and a virus at the same time, so that the virus kills off the TB organism.

2. A patient admitted for a compound fracture of the femur is found to have a positive tuberculosis (TB) skin test. What is the **best** explanation a nurse will provide this patient about the test results?

   A. "Active TB infection is present, but you are not yet infectious to others."
   B. "Active TB infection is present, and you need to start drug therapy immediately."
   C. "You have been infected at some time in your life, but this does not mean an active infection is present."
   D. "A repeat skin test is necessary because this TB test is associated with many false-positive results."

3. A patient diagnosed with active tuberculosis (TB) asks what is most likely to happen if the disease is not treated. What is the nurse's **best** response?

   A. "Your disease could become resistant to most or all of the effective anti-TB drugs."
   B. "Eventually, this disease will convert from being an infection to becoming lung cancer."
   C. "The disease now confined to your lungs will worsen to the point that you will be unable to breathe effectively and die."
   D. "Prolonged TB infection will result in the loss of normal immune function leading to greatly increased risk for you to develop other serious infections."

4. Which patient with drug-susceptible tuberculosis (TB) will the nurse recommend to receive first-line anti-TB drug therapy using directly observed therapy (DOT)?

   A. 25-year-old man with an opioid addiction who is homeless
   B. 35-year-old woman who delivered her first baby 3 months ago
   C. 58-year-old man who has been blind since birth and lives independently
   D. 76-year-old woman who lives alone and works full-time as an accountant

5. Which action to **prevent harm** is **most important** for a nurse to include when teaching a patient with tuberculosis (TB) about the prescribed first-line drug therapy?

   A. "Take these drugs at bed time to reduce the chances for nausea."
   B. "Do not drink alcohol in any quantity while taking these drugs."
   C. "Avoid grapefruit and grapefruit juice while taking these drugs."
   D. "Restrict fluid intake to 2 quarts of liquid a day."

6. Which antitubercular drug does the nurse anticipate will be excluded from first-line therapy for a 3-year-old patient who has active drug-susceptible tuberculosis?

   A. Isoniazid (INH)
   B. Rifampin (RIF)
   C. Pyrazinamide (PAS)
   D. Ethambutol (EMB)

7. Which patient change noted 2 months after starting first-line therapy for drug-susceptible tuberculosis (TB) indicates to the nurse that the therapy is most likely effective?

   A. Blood pressure consistently within the normal range
   B. White blood cell count (WBC) of 8000 mm³
   C. Negative TB skin test
   D. Weight gain of 8 lb

8. Which assessment is **most important** for the nurse to perform 2 weeks after the patient with extensively drug-resistant tuberculosis (XDR TB) begins receiving the recommended combination therapy for XDR TB?

   A. Heart rate and rhythm
   B. Range of joint motion
   C. Respiratory rate and rhythm
   D. Whole body skin inspection

9. What is the **most important** precaution for the nurse to teach the spouse who will be applying an antifungal lotion to the patient's back?

   A. Hold your breath while applying the drug
   B. Wear disposable gloves to apply the drug
   C. Wash your hands before applying the drug
   D. Check the expiration date before applying the drug

10. A patient prescribed a systemic antifungal drug reports a change in how food tastes. What is the nurse's **best** action?

    A. Documenting the report as the only action
    B. Holding the dose and notifying the prescriber immediately
    C. Cautioning the patient to wear sunglasses and a hat when outside
    D. Reassuring the patient that this is a common side effect of the drug

11. Which laboratory value in a 76-year-old woman taking systemic fluconazole will the nurse report immediately to the prescriber?

    A. Hematocrit of 38%
    B. Bilirubin of 0.4 mg/dL
    C. Potassium of 2.2 mEq/L
    D. Blood urea nitrogen (BUN) of 12.2 mg/dL

12. A patient is prescribed 50 mg of amphotericin B by intravenous infusion in 500 mL of dextrose 5% in water (D_5W) over 6 hours. How many milliliters (mL) per minute will the nurse set the pump to infuse?

    A. 1.4 mL
    B. 2.2 mL
    C. 4.2 mL
    D. 6.2 mL

Clinical Judgment

1. Which precautions are **most important** for the nurse to teach a woman using a vaginal cream form of an antifungal drug? **Select all that apply.**

   A. Wear gloves to insert the cream.
   B. Wash the applicator with soap and water.
   C. Do not tub bathe until treatment is completed.
   D. Avoid sexual intercourse during the treatment period.
   E. The cream can make holes in a condom or diaphragm.
   F. Stop the drug immediately if you think you are pregnant.
   G. Avoid wearing jeans, slacks, or panties as long as you are taking this drug.
   H. Stop the drug when symptoms have disappeared to avoid unnecessary exposure to it.

2. The patient is a 55-year-old Latino who has recently been diagnosed with drug-susceptible tuberculosis (TB). He also is 20 lbs overweight and has type 2 diabetes. He was born in Mexico and has lived for the past 25 years in Texas as a full American citizen. He is a chef who owns his own food truck and manages two other employees. His English language skills are very good, and he serves as an interpreter for newly arrived Spanish-speaking immigrants. The patient tells the nurse that when he was a young boy in Mexico, his maternal grandfather died of TB. He remarks that he is not ready to die. The nurse is developing a teaching plan with take-home instructions/precautions about these drugs. **Use an X to indicate which instructions are Most Relevant, Not Relevant, or Potentially Harmful at this time for this patient with regard to all four drugs for first-line anti-TB therapy.**

INSTRUCTION/PRECAUTION	MOST RELEVANT	NOT RELEVANT	POTENTIALLY HARMFUL
With a family history of TB and the fact that English is not your first language, you will need to be enrolled in a directly observed therapy program.			
Drink a full glass of water with each days' doses, and increase your overall daily water intake.			
Fortunately, there is no need to modify your dietary or alcohol consumption habits with this drug therapy.			
Try to take the drugs at the same time every day so that you do not forget any doses.			
You will need to eat more carbohydrates daily and decrease the dosage of your antidiabetic drug because these drugs increase the risk for hypoglycemia greatly.			
Do not worry about a change in urine color to a reddish orange; this is a harmless side effect.			
If you notice any numbness or tingling in your hands or feet, notify your prescriber immediately.			
Even if your symptoms go away after a month or so, it is critical that you continue taking the drugs.			
Keep the tablets in the container that came from the pharmacy rather than using a daily pill organizer.			
Keep all appointments for laboratory tests and follow-up because these drugs can have harmful effects on your liver, kidneys, and eyes, and close monitoring is important.			

9 Drugs for Pain Control, Migraines, and Skeletal Muscle Spasms

Learning Objectives

The content presented in this chapter should help you to:

1. Explain the physiology, pathophysiology, origins, and transmission patterns for different types of pain.
2. Describe the names, actions, usual adult dosages, possible side effects, and adverse effects of opioid and nonopioid drug therapy for general pain management.
3. Describe the priority actions to take before and after giving drug therapy for general pain management.
4. Prioritize essential information to teach patients taking drug therapy for general pain management.
5. Explain the names, actions, usual adult dosages, possible side effects, and adverse effects of drugs for migraine headache.
6. Describe priority actions to take before and after giving drugs for migraine headache.
7. Prioritize essential information to teach patients taking drugs for migraine headache.
8. List the names, actions, usual adult dosages, possible side effects, and adverse effects of drugs to manage skeletal muscle spasms.
9. Describe the priority actions to take before and after giving drugs for skeletal muscle spasms.
10. Prioritize essential information to teach patients taking drugs to manage skeletal muscle spasms.
11. Explain appropriate life span considerations for drug therapy to manage general pain, migraine headache, and muscle spasms.

Key Terms

addiction (ă-DĬK-shŭn) (p. 152) The psychological need or craving for the "high" feeling that results from using opioid agonists when pain is either not present or minimally present.

analgesics (ăn-ăl-JĒ-zē-ŭ) (p. 149) Drugs of any class that provide pain relief either by changing the perception of pain or by reducing its source.

biologics (bīō LÄ jik) (p. 157) A class of complex antiinflammatory drugs derived from living sources that target specific inflammatory cells, components, or products to modify chronic disorders associated with inflammation and tissue damage.

dependence (dē-PĔN-dĕns) (p. 152) Physical changes in autonomic nervous system function that can occur when opioid agonists are used long term and are not needed for pain control.

migraine (MĪ-grān) (p. 156) A special type of severe, throbbing headache pain often occurring with nausea, vomiting, and extreme sensitivity to light and sound that is not caused by inflammation or tissue injury.

nonopioid analgesics (NŎN-Ō-pē-ōyd ăn-ăl-JĒZ-ĭk) (p. 154) Drugs that reduce a person's perception of pain; it is not similar to opium and has little potential for psychological or physical dependence.

opioid agonist analgesic (Ō-pē-ōyd ăn-ăl-JĒZ-ĭk) (p. 150) A drug containing any ingredient derived from the poppy plant (or a similar synthetic chemical) that changes a person's perception of pain and has potential for psychological or physical dependence.

pain (PĂN) (p. 147) An unpleasant sensory and emotional experience associated with tissue injury; pain is whatever a patient says it is and exists whenever a patient says it does.

skeletal muscle relaxants (SKĒL-ĭ-tăl MŪS-ăl rē-LĂK-sănts) (p. 161) A class of drugs that generally act by depressing the central nervous system (CNS), resulting in a reduction of skeletal muscle spasms and reduction of pain perception.

tolerance (TŎL-ŭr-ĕns) (p. 150) The adjustment of the body to long-term opioid agonist use that increases the rate at which a drug is eliminated and reduces the main effects (pain relief) and side effects of the drug.

withdrawal (wĭth-DRŎ-ĕl) (p. 152) Autonomic nervous system symptoms occurring when long-term opioid agonist therapy is stopped suddenly after physical dependence is present.

REVIEW OF RELATED PHYSIOLOGY AND PATHOPHYSIOLOGY FOR GENERAL PAIN

General pain is a common sensation most often caused by tissue injury and inflammation. Types of pain that are not associated with tissue injury include migraine headache pain and skeletal muscle spasms. These types of pain are discussed later in this chapter.

General pain is the most common reason people consult with a health care professional. **Pain** is defined as an unpleasant sensory and emotional experience usually associated with tissue injury. Every person experiences it in a different way with all his or her senses, including any previous experiences with pain. As a result, pain is best described using the patient's own report, making pain whatever the patient says it is, occurring whenever he or she says it does. A patient's reaction to pain also depends on his or her emotional makeup.

PAIN ORIGIN AND TRANSMISSION

Acute pain, although uncomfortable, can be a helpful response because it tells us that something is wrong and often where it is wrong. The brain is the place where pain is actually "felt" (Fig. 9.1). If you stub your toe, the tissue injury and inflammation stimulate nerve endings that send messages along a sensory nerve to the place in your brain where that particular nerve stops. The message triggers your brain to know that your toe hurts. So, even though the tissue injury causing the pain occurs in the toe, it is your brain that *perceives* the pain. If the sensory nerves between your injured toe and your brain were severed, you would not feel pain in your toe. In addition, if the area of your brain that is connected to the sensory nerve of the toe were damaged or destroyed, you would not feel pain as a result of injuring your toe.

Nociceptors are sensory nerve endings that, when activated, trigger the message sent to the brain that allows the perception of pain (Fig. 9.2). Nociceptors can be activated when body chemicals called *mediators* bind to them. The mediators for pain include substance P ("P" is for "pain") and many of the same mediators that cause the symptoms of inflammation, especially bradykinin (see Chapter 10). When mediators are released from injured tissue (e.g., when you stub your toe), they bind to the nociceptors and activate them (see Fig. 9.2). Activated receptors start electrical signals that send the message along the nerve to the brain. Other ways that the receptors can be triggered include changing their shapes (by stretching or applying pressure), exposing them to extreme heat or cold, and reducing the oxygen level in the tissue surrounding them. Different types of nerve fibers transmit pain messages to the brain. These fibers differ in how fast they transmit the message, where they are located, and what type of pain sensation is transmitted. This is one reason why not all pain drugs work in the same way and why some drugs are effective in relieving one type of pain and not effective at all for another pain type.

PAIN PERCEPTION

Different nerve fibers end in different areas of the brain. This means that the brain perceives pain on different levels. Some fibers pass through areas of the brain where emotions and memories are stored, allowing emotions, memories, and behavior to affect pain perception. Because nerve fibers pass through many body areas on the way to the brain and interact with other nerves, the perception of pain location is not always direct. When a painful stimulus is present and we perceive it, all of our senses are activated. How we feel and react to any painful event depend on our emotional makeup along with our previous experiences with pain.

Personal factors make each person's perception of pain different. The smallest amount of tissue damage that makes a specific person aware of having pain is known as his or her *pain threshold*, or the point at which pain is first felt. The pain threshold is different for every person and varies from one body site to another. Most drugs used for pain control raise the patient's pain threshold.

The severity of how much pain the patient feels is called *pain intensity*. There are several ways to work with the patient to determine the intensity of his or her pain. Fig. 9.3 shows an example of a common pain scale that is useful for an alert patient to rate his or her pain. When the patient cannot speak or when working with young children, a nonverbal scale called FACES may be used (Fig. 9.4). The patient picks the face on the scale that best represents how he or she is feeling. Another scale, the FLACC (Face, Legs, Activity, Cry, Consolability) scale, is used for infants, very young

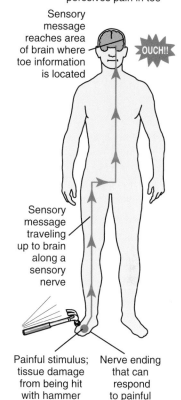

Person is aware of damage to toe and perceives pain in toe

Sensory message reaches area of brain where toe information is located

OUCH!!

Sensory message traveling up to brain along a sensory nerve

Painful stimulus; tissue damage from being hit with hammer

Nerve ending that can respond to painful stimulation

FIG. 9.1 A sensory pathway for pain perception.

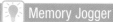
Memory Jogger

Pain is whatever the patient says it is and exists whenever he or she says it does.

Memory Jogger

Although the stimulus for pain, usually injury and inflammation, occurs outside of the brain, we actually perceive the pain in the specific area of the sensory cortex of the brain that receives the signal generated by the sensory nerve at the site of injury.

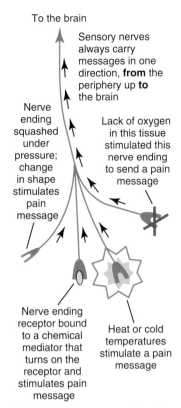

FIG. 9.2 Sensory nerve endings (nociceptors) triggered by different types of stimuli to send pain messages to the brain.

To the brain

Sensory nerves always carry messages in one direction, **from** the periphery up **to** the brain

Nerve ending squashed under pressure; change in shape stimulates pain message

Lack of oxygen in this tissue stimulated this nerve ending to send a pain message

Nerve ending receptor bound to a chemical mediator that turns on the receptor and stimulates pain message

Heat or cold temperatures stimulate a pain message

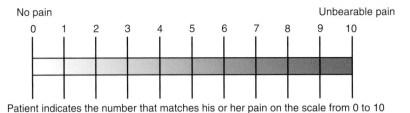

FIG. 9.3 A common numeric pain distress scale.

Patient indicates the number that matches his or her pain on the scale from 0 to 10

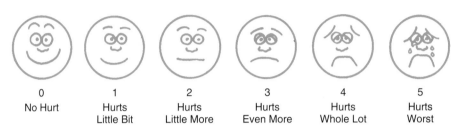

0	1	2	3	4	5
No Hurt	Hurts Little Bit	Hurts Little More	Hurts Even More	Hurts Whole Lot	Hurts Worst

FIG. 9.4 The Wong-Baker FACES Pain Rating Scale for children and nonverbal adults. (From Hockenberry, M. J., & Wilson, D. [2015]. *Wong's nursing care of infants and children* [10th ed.]. St. Louis: Mosby. Used with permission. Copyright © 2015 Mosby.)

Category	Score		
	0	**1**	**2**
Face	No particular expression or smile	Occasional grimace or frown, withdrawn, disinterested	Frequent-to-constant quivering chin, clenched jaw
Legs	Normal position or relaxed	Uneasy, restless, tense	Kicking, or legs drawn up
Activity	Lying quietly, normal position, moves easily	Squirming, shifting back and forth, tense	Arched, rigid, or jerking
Cry	No cry (awake or asleep)	Moans or whimpers, occasional complaint	Crying steadily, screams or sobs, or frequent complaints
Consolability	Content, relaxed	Reassured by occasional touching, hugging, or being talked to, distractible	Difficult to console or comfort

Each of the five categories–(F) Face, (L) Legs, (A) Activity, (C) Cry, (C) Consolability– is scored from 0-2, which results in a total score between 0 and 10.

FIG. 9.5 The Face, Legs, Activity, Cry, Consolability (FLACC) pain rating scale for infants and patients who are not alert.

 Memory Jogger

Always assess behaviors for pain in patients who cannot point or express pain in words.

 Critical Point for Safety

Never assume that a patient who is tolerating pain well is comfortable or that his or her condition has not worsened. Reassess a patient's pain, especially by asking him or her to rate it at regular intervals, not only to determine therapy effectiveness but also to identify possible complications earlier.

QSEN: Safety

children, and any patient who cannot express pain in words or point to a face (Fig. 9.5). It uses the observation and scoring of behaviors to establish a pain intensity level.

Pain tolerance is any one person's ability to endure or "stand" his or her perception of the pain intensity. Behavioral and emotional factors as well as physical factors affect a person's pain tolerance. This makes pain tolerance unique to each person. Pain tolerance is so personal that you cannot assess a person's level of pain on the basis of behavior alone. Always ask patients about their pain. Just because a person tolerates pain does not mean that he or she is not suffering!

TYPES OF PAIN

General pain is broadly categorized into types on the basis of its cause, how long it lasts, and whether it is present continuously or comes and goes (*intermittent*). The three main types of pain are acute, chronic, and cancer. All are associated with external or internal tissue injury.

Acute pain is the most common type. It has a sudden onset, an identifiable cause, and a limited duration and improves with time even when it is not treated. It is often caused by trauma, surgery, heart attack, inflammation, and burns. Acute pain usually triggers the physical stress responses of elevated heart rate, respiratory rate, and blood pressure. Skin becomes cool and clammy with increased sweating of the hands and feet. The mouth becomes dry, and usually the pupils of the eyes dilate. A person's behavioral responses to acute pain often include restlessness, inability to concentrate, general distress, and a sense that something bad is happening (a sense of impending doom).

Chronic pain is present daily for at least 3 to 6 months. It persists or increases with time, may not have an identifiable cause, and no longer triggers the physiologic responses associated with the stress response. This means that a person with chronic pain can have severe pain without changes from the normal ranges for heart rate, breathing rate, or blood pressure. As a result, changes in vital signs are not useful in assessing the intensity of chronic pain. Chronic pain may hurt less on some days than others but is always present. Causes may be difficult to find, and the area of pain is often more generalized rather than localized.

Cancer pain has many causes and is complex. This means that more than one pain strategy and often more than one type of drug for pain control are needed. The patient with cancer often receives traditional pain-control drugs but at much higher doses than those prescribed for other types of pain. The drug therapy plan may include every type of pain-control drug given in combination to ensure adequate pain relief. Drug therapy for cancer pain must be tailored to each patient for the most effective pain control.

GENERAL ISSUES RELATED TO ANALGESIC DRUG THERAPY

General pain interferes with every aspect of a person's life and often decreases the quality of life. Pain control involves many different approaches, and drug therapy is just one approach. Nondrug therapies for pain control often are used along with drug therapy and, for some types of pain, may either replace traditional opioid agonist therapy or reduce the dosages needed to make pain as tolerable as possible. The goal of drug therapy for acute pain is not to make the person completely unaware of the pain but to relieve the pain to a level that is acceptable to the patient. Ideally, at this level the patient is comfortable, remains cognitively intact, can interact with others, can sleep as needed, and is able to participate in self-care to the extent that cause of the pain permits (e.g., knee replacement surgery requires activity restrictions beyond pain issues).

Analgesics are drugs of any class that control pain either by changing the perception or by reducing the source of pain. Different types of drugs are used for pain control based on how they work. These include opioid agonists and nonopioid miscellaneous drugs. Different types of pain respond differently to each drug type.

All analgesic drugs provide some degree of pain relief, but some drugs are stronger than others. It may take a greater amount of a weaker drug or have the weaker analgesic prescribed along with other drug types (e.g., antiinflammatories) to provide the same amount of pain relief that a stronger drug provides.

When drug therapy is prescribed for control of acute pain, best results are achieved when doses are given on a schedule around the clock to prevent complete elimination of the drug before the next dose, or the patient is given a machine to "punch in" a small intravenous (IV) dose whenever the need arises (*patient-controlled analgesia*). Sometimes these two techniques are used at the same time for personalized and effective pain control.

Many drugs for pain control have ingredients that may be addictive. In the United States any drug that contains ingredients known to be addictive is classified and regulated by the federal government as a *controlled substance*. Table 1.1 in Chapter 1 describes five schedules of controlled substances and lists examples of drugs in each category.

 Memory Jogger

Acute pain is usually accompanied by common physiologic changes triggered by the stress response, including elevated heart rate, blood pressure, and respiratory rate; cool, clammy skin; dry mouth; restlessness; and an inability to concentrate.

 Critical Point for Safety

Changes in vital signs do **not** indicate the intensity of chronic pain. Relying on this information alone often results in poor assessment/management of chronic pain and increased patient suffering.

QSEN: Safety

 Memory Jogger

The goal of drug therapy for acute pain is **not** to make the person completely unaware of the pain but to relieve the pain to a level that is acceptable to the patient.

(★) *Priority actions to take* before *and* after *giving any type of drug for general pain control.* Many drug types can be used as analgesia for pain control. Each type has both different and common actions and effects. The intended response of all pain-control drugs is to reduce pain to a level that is acceptable to the patient. Responsibilities, precautions, and issues before administering pain-control drugs include:

* Assessing the patient's pain intensity using the pain scale preferred by your work-place.
* Checking to see when the patient last received the drug for pain control. Giving doses too close together can lead to more side effects or toxic levels. Giving doses too far apart can lead to more suffering for the patient.
* If the patient is to receive a drug on a regular schedule rather than as needed (PRN), maintain the schedule even if the patient is sleeping or is not reporting pain.
* Teach the patient taking a pain-control drug that the best pain relief occurs when drugs are taken on a regular schedule rather than PRN. If the patient thinks that the pain is improving and less drug is needed, tell him or her first to reduce the dose but to maintain the schedule. If the pain continues to improve, the time between doses may be increased.
* About 30 minutes after giving an oral pain-control drug (less time after a parenteral drug), ask how much pain relief the patient has received as a result of the drug to determine whether the drug is right for the patient's pain, if the dose needs to be changed, or if the pain-control strategy must be adjusted.

Drug Alert

Action/Intervention Alert

Assess the patient's pain level 30 min after giving a pain-control drug and then hourly.

QSEN: Safety

TYPES OF DRUGS FOR GENERAL PAIN CONTROL

Opioid Agonists (Narcotics)

Opioid agonist analgesics, also called *narcotics*, are drugs that contain any ingredient derived from the poppy plant (or a similar synthetic chemical) that change a person's perception of pain and have the potential for psychological or physical dependence. All opioid agonists work in the same way and have similar side effects. The main difference among various types of opioids is the strength of the drug.

All prescribed opioid agonists can be addictive and are classified as controlled substances because they have a high potential for abuse that can lead to psychological or physical dependence. In addition, *opioids are high-alert drugs that have an increased risk for causing patient harm if used in error*. The error may be giving too high a dose, giving too low a dose, giving a dose to a patient for whom it was not prescribed, and not giving it to a patient for whom it was prescribed.

Although most opioid agonists are prescribed for pain control, there are other uses. These uses include controlling coughing, reducing diarrhea, and reducing respiratory difficulties at the end of life and with end-stage chronic respiratory diseases. Very potent opioid agonists may be used for anesthetic purposes.

An issue that can occur with longer-term opioid agonist use is drug tolerance. **Tolerance** is the adjustment of the body to long-term opioid agonist use that increases the rate of drug elimination and reduces the main effect (pain relief) and side effects of the drug. It occurs with anyone who is taking opioid agonists for a long period of time. More drug is needed to achieve the same degree of pain relief. Thus, although there are recommended dosages for acute pain and short-term opioid agonist use, dosages for long-term use can be many times more than the "standard" short-term dose as the person becomes drug tolerant. For this reason, there is no true cap or ceiling on opioid agonist drug doses with long-term use, such as with prolonged cancer pain.

The following table lists usual adult dosages for the opioid agonists most commonly used for short-term control of acute pain. The dosages used for other pain types may be much higher. Opioid agonists given parenterally are usually single-agent drugs. When given orally, opioid tablets, capsules, or liquids may contain other drugs such as acetaminophen, ibuprofen, aspirin, or other nonsteroidal antiinflammatory drugs (NSAIDs). Be sure to consult a reliable drug reference for more information about less commonly prescribed opioids agonists and for those combined with other drug types.

Memory Jogger

Although individuals who are addicted to opioid agonists may also have tolerance, the development of tolerance can occur separately from addiction as a normal physiologic response to longer-term opioid agonist use.

Adult Dosages for Commonly Prescribed Opioid Agonist Drugs

Drug Names	Usual Maintenance Dosage
morphine sulfate ❶ (Astramorph, Avinza, Duramorph PF, MS Contin, Roxanol)	15–30 mg orally every 4 hr 2–10 mg IV, IM, or subcutaneously every 3–4 hr
codeine ❶	15–60 mg orally every 4 hr
fentanyl ❶ (ABSTRAL, Actiq, Duragesic, Fentora, IONSYS, Lazanda, Onsolis, Sublimaze, SUBSYS)	50–100 mcg IM or slow IV over 1–2 min, dose may be repeated in 1–2 hr Drug is available as a sublingual (transmucosal) lozenge, spray, or liquid; transdermal patch; intranasal spray **Dosages differ by delivery method, pain intensity, and patient experience with the drug. Also may be used as an anesthetic**
hydrocodone ❶ (Hysingla ER, VANTRELA ER, Zohydro)	10 mg orally every 12 hr
hydromorphone ❶ (Dilaudid, Exalgo, Palladone)	2–4 mg orally every 4–6 hr 0.2–1 mg IV slowly over 2–3 min, every 2–3 hr
oxycodone ❶ (Dazidox, Endocodone, Oxaydo, OXECTA, OxyContin, Oxydose, Percolone, Roxicodone, Roxybond)	Immediate-release dosing: 5–15 mg orally every 4–6 hr Extended-release dosing: 10 mg orally every 12 hr
tramadol ❶ (Ultram)	Immediate-release dosing: 25–100 mg every 4–6 hr Extended-release dosing: 100 mg orally once daily

❶ High-alert drug.

How opioid agonists work. The brain has opioid receptors because you make your own internal opioids to provide some pain relief and an increased sense of well-being when you are physically stressed. These internal morphine-like chemicals produced in the brain are *endorphins, enkephalins,* and *dynorphins.* These substances bind to specific opioid receptors in the brain and activate the receptor to change your perception from discomfort and pain to comfort. So these internal opioids are *opioid agonists* because they "turn on" (activate) the opioid receptors to change your perception of discomfort. External opioids that are given for pain relief also bind to opioid receptors as *agonists* to activate the opioid receptors.

The classic opioid agonist is morphine. Morphine and all opioid agonists work by binding to opioid receptor sites in the brain and other areas. The main opioid receptors are mu (OP3), kappa (OP2), and delta (OP1). When a drug binds to and acts as an agonist at mu receptors, the responses include pain relief, some degree of respiratory depression with slower breathing, some sleepiness or sedation, decreased intestinal motility with constipation, pupil constriction, lower blood pressure, and *euphoria* (a feeling of emotional happiness). When a drug binds to and acts as an agonist at kappa receptors, the responses include some pain relief, sedation, pupil constriction, and *dysphoria* (a state of feeling emotional or mental discomfort, restlessness, and anxiety). When a drug binds to and acts as an agonist at delta receptors, the responses include some pain relief, dysphoria, and hallucinations.

Morphine binds most tightly and best to the mu receptor, acting as an agonist. This activates the mu receptors, and the person's perception of pain is changed. Some drugs act as an agonist at one type of opioid receptor site and, at the same time, act as an antagonist at other opioid receptor sites, providing mixed responses. The opioids that provide the best pain relief bind most strongly (tightly) to the mu receptors. Pain drugs that are strong morphine agonists include morphine, hydromorphone, oxymorphone, and fentanyl. Those that bind moderately well to the mu receptors and provide some degree of pain relief include codeine, hydrocodone, and oxycodone.

Drugs that are opioid agonist-antagonists have mixed responses, acting as agonists at kappa and delta and as antagonists at mu. As a result, they provide less pain relief than pure opioid agonists and more hallucinations and dysphoria. For these reasons, they are less commonly used for pain control. These drugs include pantazocine (Talwin), butorphanol (Stadol), and nalbuphine (Nubain).

 Memory Jogger

Opioid agonists change only the perception of pain; they do nothing at the site of injured tissue to reduce the cause of pain. Those that most selectively bind to mu receptors provide the most pain relief.

 Memory Jogger

Strong opioid agonist analgesics include:
- morphine
- hydromorphone
- oxymorphone
- fentanyl

Common Side Effects

Opioid Agonists

Constipation,   Drowsiness   Flushing
Nausea/
Vomiting

Itchiness

Genetic/genomic variation in metabolism of codeine. When codeine, a weak opioid agonist, is first ingested, it is inactive and provides no pain relief. To be an effective pain drug, codeine must be converted to morphine by specific metabolizing enzymes. Variation in gene sequences for these enzymes change how well (or if) codeine is converted to morphine. About 80% of people have enzymes that convert codeine to morphine at the expected rate and do obtain pain relief from it without excessive complications. However, genetic variation of these enzymes, which changes drug effectiveness and its risks for side effects, occurs in about 20% of people.

Some people have metabolizing enzymes with genetic variations that allow codeine to be converted to morphine very rapidly and completely. These people are known as *ultrarapid metabolizers*. When ultrarapid metabolizers receive codeine at usual dosages, the rapid conversion causes blood concentrations of morphine to be higher than expected, greatly increasing the risk for toxicity, especially respiratory depression.

Some people have metabolizing enzymes with genetic variations that barely convert codeine to morphine at all (blood morphine levels reach less than 3% of what is expected). These people are known as *poor metabolizers* and essentially derive no pain relief from codeine.

Common side effects of opioid agonists. The most common side effects of opioid agonists are constipation and drowsiness. Some patients may have nausea and vomiting if intestinal motility is affected. Flushing and skin itching also may occur as blood vessels dilate.

Possible adverse effects of opioid agonists. Respiratory depression is possible with opioid agonists, especially at higher doses and when the drugs are given intravenously. Most patients have only mild respiratory depression, with respirations dropping to 9 to 12 breaths/min. If severe (less than 8 breaths/min), action must be taken to prevent hypoxia (low tissue oxygen levels). Respiratory depression is more common among patients who have never received an opioid agonist in the past (are *opioid naïve*).

Addiction, dependence, and withdrawal can occur with opioid agonist use. **Dependence** is the physical changes in autonomic nervous system function that can occur when opioid agonists are used long term (more than a few weeks, especially after pain is reduced or no longer present). **Addiction** is the psychological need or craving for the "high" feeling resulting from the use of opioid agonists when pain is either not present or minimally present.

Withdrawal is the occurrence of autonomic nervous system symptoms when long-term opioid agonist therapy is stopped suddenly after physical dependence is present. Symptoms include nausea, vomiting, abdominal cramping, sweating, delirium, and seizures. This reaction seldom occurs in a patient who is taking opioid agonists for pain. It is common among people who are not in pain but who take opioid agonists for the psychological "high" that they can produce.

When opioid agonists are needed strictly for severe pain, their use seldom causes either dependence or addiction. However, because of the recent response to the philosophy that no one should ever be in pain, many opioid agonist drugs were overprescribed both at higher dosages and for longer periods of time. This action increased the availability of prescription opioid agonists, which ultimately has resulted in an *opioid epidemic*, and a greatly increased level of addiction. When patients could no longer obtain prescription drugs for their addiction, many people turned to illicit opioids, which has resulted in a crisis of overdose deaths.

⊛ ***Priority actions to take*** **before** *giving opioid agonists.* In addition to the general responsibilities related to analgesic therapy for pain (p. 150), check the dose and the specific drug name carefully. Opioid agonists are not interchangeable because the strength of the drugs varies. Only the prescriber can change the drug order. Drug doses must be recalculated by the prescriber when one opioid agonist is switched to another.

When giving the first dose of an opioid agonist to a patient who is opioid naïve, assess the patient's respiratory rate and oxygen saturation. Opioid agonists can cause some degree of respiratory depression.

⭐ *Priority actions to take after giving opioid agonists.* In addition to the general responsibilities related to analgesic therapy for pain (p. 150), be sure to monitor the patient's respiratory rate and oxygen saturation for indications of respiratory depression. This is especially important when the patient is receiving an opioid agonist for the first time or when the drug dosage has been increased. If the respiratory rate is 8 or less and the patient is sleeping, try to wake him or her. First call the patient's name. If there is no response, gently shake an arm. Shake more firmly if needed. If the patient does not respond to these actions, use a slightly stronger trigger (without using enough force to cause harm), such as:
- Squeezing the trapezius muscle (located at the angle of the shoulder and neck muscle)
- Applying pressure to the nail bed

If the patient cannot be aroused, immediately call for help. If the patient's oxygen saturation is below 95% or is five percentage points lower than his or her normal saturation, arouse the patient and check the saturation when fully awake. If the saturation does not improve when fully awake, apply supplemental oxygen and notify the prescriber.

When respiratory depression is severe, the opioid agonist effects may need to be reversed by giving an opioid blocker (antagonist) such as *naloxone* (Narcan) or *naltrexone* (Depade, ReVia, Trexan). When an IV opioid antagonist is given, it displaces opioid agonists on the opioid receptors (Animation 9.1). When the opioid agonist is off the receptors, all its effects are reversed, usually within 1 minute, including respiratory depression. Unfortunately, the pain control effects are also reversed. Watch the patient who has received an opioid receptor blocker (antagonist) for respiratory depression closely for several hours in case respiratory depression recurs.

Patients receiving opioid agonists may become drowsy and are at risk for falling. Be sure to raise the side rails, instruct the patient to call for help, and place the call light button within easy reach for the patient.

When a patient is receiving opioid agonists for several days, assess for constipation daily. Most patients taking opioids for 2 days or longer have constipation. Be sure to give any prescribed stool softeners or laxatives.

Opioid agonists can cause a sudden lowering of blood pressure, especially when the patient changes position (orthostatic hypotension). Instruct the patient change position slowly.

⭐ *Teaching priorities for patients taking opioid agonists.* In addition to the general precautions related to analgesic therapy for pain (p. 150), teach patients these precautions and care issues:
- Take opioids with food rather than on an empty stomach to reduce the risk for nausea.
- If you are prescribed to take an extended-release (ER) form of an oral opioid drug, swallow the capsule or tablet whole because chewing it or opening the capsule allows too much of the drug to be absorbed all at once and an overdose can occur.
- Do not drive, operate heavy machinery, or make critical decisions when taking these drugs, because they induce drowsiness.
- Move slowly when rising or changing positions, because these drugs can cause a sudden drop in blood pressure that may make you feel dizzy or light-headed.
- Remember that constipation is a common side effect of these drugs. If your prescriber has ordered a stool softener or laxative, start using these agents **before** constipation occurs.

Life span considerations for opioid agonists
Pediatric considerations. Opioid agonists are high-alert drugs that are used for pain control in children of all ages. Dosages are calculated for each child on the basis of

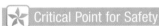
⭐ **Critical Point for Safety**

The half-life of the opioid antagonist is not as long as opioid agonists. Thus the effects of the antagonist can wear off faster than the opioid agonist is eliminated. More than one dose of an opioid antagonist may be needed to prevent recurrence of respiratory depression.

QSEN: Safety

 Drug Alert

Teaching Alert

Teach patients taking an extended-release (ER) form of an oral opioid drug to swallow the capsule or tablet whole because chewing it or opening the capsule allows too much of the drug to be absorbed all at once and an overdose can occur.

QSEN: Safety

Memory Jogger

What is painful for an adult also is painful for a child. Children's pain must be taken seriously, and interventions to relieve it are needed.

Drug Alert

Action/Intervention Alert

If a mother receives an opioid during labor, watch her newborn closely for at least 4 hours after birth for any sign of respiratory depression.

QSEN: Safety

the child's age, size (weight in kilograms), health, and pain severity. Identifying pain intensity with a young child can be difficult but is still needed. For a child who is old enough to talk, use the FACES pain scale (see Fig 9.4) to help determine pain severity. For an infant or child too young to talk, rely on behavior to help determine pain severity such as the behaviors described in the FLACC scale (see Fig. 9.5). Infants in pain cry frequently with great intensity. They do not smile, laugh, or show interest in toys and are not comforted by holding, cuddling, rocking, or a pacifier.

A child can have the same side effects as an adult when taking opioid agonists. Constipation is a problem for a child, and the same steps must be taken to avoid it.

Respiratory depression can be a dangerous problem for infants or young children. When opioid agonists are used with an infant or a small child, it is best to use an apnea monitor and/or pulse oximeter. When these devices are not available, check the child's rate and depth of respiration at least every 15 minutes. Remember that infants and small children may have a normal respiratory rate between 30 and 40 breaths/min. A respiratory rate of less than 20 in an infant or small child is cause for concern.

Considerations for pregnancy and lactation. Opioid agonists may be prescribed to women during pregnancy. These drugs do cross the placenta and enter the fetus. The fetus can become addicted to opioids and go through withdrawal after birth. If the mother receives long-term opioid therapy or abuses other opioid agonists during pregnancy and the drug is discontinued several weeks before birth, the newborn should not have any symptoms of withdrawal. However, if the mother is still receiving opioid agonists when the baby is born, the newborn will need special care for withdrawal.

When opioid agonists are given to a woman in labor, the baby may have respiratory depression after delivery. If an opioid is given intravenously within an hour of delivery, the baby may need a dose of an opioid antagonist such as *naloxone* (Narcan) after delivery.

Breastfeeding is best avoided when a woman is taking an opioid agonist for more than a couple of days. If the mother is unable to stop breastfeeding while taking the drug, teach her the strategies listed in Box 1.1 in Chapter 1, to reduce infant exposure to these drugs.

Considerations for older adults. In addition to the usual effects of opioid agonists, an older adult is at risk for falls because of low vision. The pupil of the older adult does not dilate fully, and less light enters the eye, reducing vision. When the older patient takes an opioid agonist, the pupil is even smaller than usual, reducing vision even more. This problem increases the risk for falling. Teach the older adult to increase room lighting to make reading easier and reduce the risk for tripping and falling over objects.

Opioid agonists can make the chest muscles of older adults tighter, which makes breathing and coughing more difficult. Thus the risk for pneumonia and hypoxia is greater for them. Assess the respiratory rate and depth and the oxygen saturation at least every 2 hours.

Nonopioid Pain-Control Drugs

A variety of nonopioid drugs can be used alone or with other pain-control drugs to manage special types of pain. **Nonopioid analgesics** are drugs that reduce a person's perception of pain but are not similar to opium and have little potential for psychological or physical dependence. These additional drugs are sometimes termed *adjuvant* drugs because they enhance the pain-control features of other pain drugs. Most have other main uses and are discussed in more detail elsewhere in this text.

Acetaminophen. Acetaminophen alone (e.g., Panadol, Tylenol, and many others) can be effective for pain relief. It works in the brain to change the perception of pain and reduces the sensitivity of pain receptors.

Acetaminophen is given orally in tablets, capsules, or liquids and can also be given as a rectal suppository. It is available over the counter as a single drug or combined with other substances such as caffeine and aspirin (Excedrin). It also is combined with other pain-control drugs, especially opioid agonists. The usual adult dose is 325 to 650 mg every 4 to 6 hours and should not exceed 3 g/day. For children the usual dose is 7 to 15 mg/kg every 4 hours.

One formulation of acetaminophen can be given intravenously by intermittent infusion only and never as a bolus. Recommended adult dosages are either 1000 mg IV every 6 hours or 650 mg IV every 4 hours as needed infused over 15 minutes.

Important issues with acetaminophen include that because it is available without a prescription, many people believe that it has no side effects or adverse effects. However, one of its metabolites can be toxic when taken at high doses or too often, especially to the liver, which can be damaged or destroyed. With higher dosages or overdose, kidney damage also can occur. Taking this drug with alcohol greatly increases the risk for permanent liver damage.

Warn patients that many over-the-counter drugs for colds, headache, allergies, and sleep aids also contain acetaminophen, as do a variety of drugs prescribed for pain. The acetaminophen in these drugs must be figured into the maximum daily dose of 3 g along with any separate acetaminophen. Remind patients not to drink alcoholic beverages on days when they take acetaminophen or any drug containing acetaminophen.

Pediatric considerations with acetaminophen are related to its liver toxicity at higher dosages. A young child should never receive an adult dose of acetaminophen. Because acetaminophen comes in liquid forms with different strengths, it is critically important to teach parents to read labels carefully and not assume that the doses are the same for all liquids. Some liquid forms contain as few as 16 mg/mL, and others may contain as much as 70 mg/mL.

Nonsteroidal antiinflammatory drugs. Nonsteroidal antiinflammatory drugs (NSAIDs) are one type of nonopioid analgesic that can help to manage pain associated with inflammation, bone pain, cancer pain, and soft tissue trauma. These drugs act at the tissue where pain starts and do not change a person's perception of pain. Chapter 10 provides a complete discussion of the actions and uses of NSAIDs and the patient care responsibilities.

Antidepressants. Some antidepressants have been found to reduce some types of chronic pain and cancer pain. The most common antidepressant drugs used for pain control are *amitriptyline* (Elavil), *nortriptyline* (Pamelor), *paroxetine* (Paxil), and *sertraline* (Zoloft). They are usually given orally, and the doses for pain control can be different from those used to treat depression. Antidepressants help increase the amount of natural opioids (endorphins and enkephalins) in the brain and also reduce the depression that can occur with chronic pain. Usually, the patient must take one of these drugs for 1 or 2 weeks before he or she feels any relief from pain. Chapter 25 provides a complete discussion of the actions and uses of antidepressant drugs and the patient care responsibilities.

Antiepileptic drugs. Certain antiepileptic drugs (drugs that reduce seizure activity) have been found to reduce some types of chronic pain and cancer pain, especially neuropathic pain (nerve pain with tingling and burning) and migraine headaches. The two most common antiepileptic drugs used for pain control are *gabapentin* (Neurontin) and *pregabalin* (Lyrica). They appear to work by reducing the rate of electrical transmission along sensory nerves and may also affect pain perception. The doses for pain control are often higher than those used to control seizures. Chapter 23 provides a complete discussion of the actions and uses of antiepileptic drugs and the patient care responsibilities.

Muscle relaxants. Skeletal muscle relaxants are another class of drugs that act by depressing the central nervous system (CNS), resulting in a reduction of skeletal muscle spasms and reduction of pain perception when part of the pain experience

 Critical Point for Safety

Acetaminophen can be toxic to the liver and should not be taken by anyone with liver health problems. Teach patients to avoid alcohol and other liver-toxic drugs on days when they take acetaminophen.

QSEN: Safety

 Drug Alert

Teaching Alert

Teach parents to read the label on liquid acetaminophen bottles for infants and small children carefully and ensure that the correct dose is given for the child's size. Teach parents to telephone the nearest pharmacy and talk with the pharmacist to ensure that the dose is correct if they are not confident in their own calculations.

QSEN: Safety

 Memory Jogger

Antidepressants used for certain types of pain relief usually require 2–3 weeks for a change in pain perception to be noticed.

includes muscle spasms. A complete discussion of the actions, dosages, and side effects of muscle relaxants is presented later in this chapter.

Medical marijuana (cannabinoids). Medical marijuana (cannabinoids) is now legal in some states and is used for management of pain, especially chronic pain, along with other chronic medical conditions such as seizure disorders, Parkinson disease, and chemotherapy-induced nausea and vomiting. Cannabis is the plant from which cannabinoids are derived. Two common cannabinoids are tetrahydrocannabinol (THC) and cannabidiol (CBD). THC is the cannabinoid responsible for many of the psychoactive side effects of marijuana. CBD does not contain the psychoactive properties, and this is the cannabinoid most commonly used for pain control. It is available in oral and topical forms.

The mechanism of action for relief of pain from cannabinoids appears to be activation of cannabinoid-specific receptors (CB_1Rs and CB_2Rs) within pain pathways of the brain and spinal cord. Once activated, these receptors can block transmission of pain from the periphery into the brain. They also inhibit the release of pain-specific neurotransmitters within sensory pathways. Another mechanism thought to relieve pain sensation is by cannabinoid reduction of CNS inflammation and irritation (which may be one of the ways cannabinoids also can modify seizure activity).

An interesting feature of all cannabinoids is that there are many different varieties of marijuana plants and the cannabinoids produced from them have different effects. Some have greater analgesic properties than others. Some induce sleep, whereas others increase alertness. In addition, patient responses to a specific cannabinoid vary from person to person. One person with arthritis pain may obtain significant relief with a specific cannabinoid, whereas another person with arthritis pain may take the exact same cannabinoid and derive no relief.

At the present time, cannabinoid processing is not regulated by the US Food and Drug Administration. Therefore, like botanicals, the concentration of CBD in any product is not certified to be uniform. Although the use of this product for pain control holds promise, well-controlled, randomized, clinical trials are needed to establish effective dosing, consistent side effects and adverse effects, common patient teaching issues, and best practices for nursing care.

REVIEW OF RELATED PHYSIOLOGY AND PATHOPHYSIOLOGY FOR MIGRAINE HEADACHE

OVERVIEW

Migraines are a special type of severe, throbbing headache pain often occurring with nausea, vomiting, and extreme sensitivity to light and sound that is not caused by inflammation or tissue injury. They are very common and affect at least 10% of the US population. Some people may only have one or two migraines in a year, and others may experience as many as 20 migraine days each month. These headache episodes are very disabling and can last from hours to days, with the patient unable to think clearly or perform physical actions.

The origin of migraine headache is not completely understood but involves changes in the sensitivity and constriction of arteries in the head and neck in a local area known as the *trigeminovascular system*. The development of the headache appears to occur in two stages. During the first stage, arteries are triggered to constrict tightly and continuously. This constriction may occur in one area, on one side of the head or neck, or over the entire head, face, and neck. The constrictive stage usually lasts at least 2 hours. For many people, this stage may be associated with "auras" that include visual disturbances (flashing lights, zig-zags, blind spots), nausea, numbness in the head or neck, dizziness, confusion, and difficulty speaking.

In the second stage, instead of constriction, arteries become very dilated and cause the classic "throbbing" and "pounding" of a typical migraine headache. These symptoms may last from hours to days and are very debilitating. The arteries appear to be unable to respond by constricting, even when exposed to substances that normally

Memory Jogger

Medical marijuana is not legal in all states. An important issue is that, as a botanical, the strength, purity, and additives of cannabinoids are not certified by the US Food and Drug Administration.

Memory Jogger

Migraine headaches are a vascular response in which a period of intense vasoconstriction is followed by a prolonged and massive vasodilation in the trigeminovascular system of the head and neck. This vasodilation is responsible for the throbbing and pounding sensations of migraine headaches.

cause constriction, probably because the prolonged and intense constriction in the first stage made the tissues less responsive. During this time, any stimuli can increase the intensity of the pain. Thus people need a dark and quiet environment in which they can remain still and avoid other stimuli.

The events that cause the excessive vasoconstriction during the first stage (prodromal stage) of a migraine are not known but may include irritation and inflammation. However, recently a specific protein has been found that appears to play a big role in causing the second stage of migraine headaches. This protein, calcitonin gene–related peptide (CGRP), is released as a result of the excessive and tight vasoconstriction. When it binds to its receptors in the blood vessels in the head and neck, it causes a prolonged vasodilation of these arteries, leading to the severe throbbing headache of a migraine. It is primarily found in the trigeminovascular system and does not appear to be part of any other body system.

DRUG THERAPY FOR MIGRAINE HEADACHE

Older Migraine Drugs

For decades, drug therapy for migraine headaches has consisted of combinations of agents to induce vasoconstriction and reduce inflammation. The main agents include triptans, nonsteroidal antiinflammatory drugs (NSAIDs), and ergotamine. NSAIDs help to reduce the irritation and inflammation around the affected arteries. The triptans, which are serotonin agonists, can act directly on vascular smooth muscle to induce vasoconstriction and help reduce the release of CGRP. Ergotamine induces some degree of vasoconstriction. This treatment plan has had some success in reducing the duration of the migraine in people with less severe symptoms who have relatively few headache days per month (3 or less). All of these drugs cause systemic side effects, including hypertension, and interactions with many other drugs that limit their usefulness. NSAIDs are discussed in Chapter 10. The following table lists adult dosages for ergotamine and the most commonly prescribed new-generation triptans.

 Critical Point for Safety

When used systemically, ergotamine derivatives and triptans cause general arterial constriction, which can cause severe hypertension, angina, myocardial ischemia, and stroke. Monitor patients closely for these problems, especially if they have any preexisting hypertension.

QSEN: Safety

Adult Dosages for New-Generation Triptans and Ergotamine

Drug Class	Drug Name	Usual Dosages
Ergotamine	dihydroergotamine (Migranal, TRUDHESA)	1 mg IV once, may repeat dose up to 2 mg/day 1 mg IM or subcutaneously once, may repeat dose up to 3 mg/day Migranal: 0.5 mg in each nostril, followed by 0.5 mg in each nostril 15 min later for total of 2 mg TRUHESA: 0.725 mg in each nostril once, may repeat dose after at least 1 hr to a maximum of 2.9 mg/day
Triptans	lasmiditan (REYVOW) sumatriptan (Alsuma, Imitrex, ONZETRA, Sumavel, ZEMBRAC)	50, 100, or 200 mg orally as a single dose 25, 50, or 100 mg orally once, may repeat dose once after at least 2 hr for a maximum of 200 mg/day 3–6 mg subcutaneously once, may repeat dose after at least 1 hr to a maximum of 12 mg/day Some brands available as a nasal spray

Biologic Agents for Migraine Headache: Onobotulinumtoxin A

Biologics or biologic agents are a class of complex antiinflammatory drugs, usually antibodies, derived from living sources that target specific inflammatory cells, components, or products to modify chronic disorders associated with inflammation and tissue damage. Often these agents are antibodies that are specifically targeted to a body chemical or receptor. Although most commonly used for inflammatory problems, antibodies are now being generated to specific body tissues and receptors for purposes beyond control of inflammation. When biologics bind to their target, these agents usually act as antagonists to disrupt a specific action.

The first biologic agent approved for migraine headache prevention was *onobotulinumtoxin A (Botox)*. The action of Botox is to inhibit the release of the neurotransmitter acetylcholine from motor neurons, thereby causing a chemical paralysis of the skeletal muscles controlled by the affected motor neurons. This action leads to a prolonged relaxation of those muscles (weeks to months).

When used for migraine headache prevention, onobotulinumtoxin A is injected intramuscularly into 31 sites within seven different head and neck muscles. The treatment is repeated every 12 weeks. The muscles in the areas injected have a greatly decreased ability to contract, which appears to be the major mechanism for reducing migraine pain. This muscle relaxation may also help reduce irritation of nerves in the area.

The source of onobotulinumtoxin A is donated human serum. This means that transfer of bloodborne pathogens is possible. The drug can spread beyond the injection site, and some may be absorbed systemically, causing spread of muscle weakness elsewhere in the body, including the muscles that are used for breathing. More of the many side effects and adverse effects are noticed in the head and neck area where the injections occur. These include injection site reactions, eye inflammation and reduced eye movement, excessive tearing or too little tearing, visual impairment, and nasal congestion, among many others.

Biologic Agents for Migraine Headache: Calcitonin Gene-Related Peptide Antibodies

Drugs that are biologic agents for CGRP were developed specifically to prevent or treat migraine headaches. They are antibodies that are laboratory produced initially using mice to generate the immune response with B lymphocytes. When the correct antibody is produced by one cell, that cell is selectively grown and all of its descendants produce many molecules of just the one specific antibody. This is known as *monoclonal antibody production*, and all the antibodies produced by this group of cells are identical to each other. The mouse proteins from the antibodies have been removed, so it is "fully humanized" and will not cause people who receive it to develop a mouse protein allergy. The following table lists all current biologic drugs that are CGRP monoclonal antibodies.

Adult Dosages for Calcitonin Gene-Related Peptide Antibodies

Drug Name	Usual Maintenance Dose
atogepant (QULIPTA)	10, 30, or 60 mg orally once daily for prevention of migraine headaches
eptinezumab (Vyepti)	100–300 mg IV infusion (over 30 min) every 3 months
erenumab (Aimovig)	70–140 mg subcutaneously once monthly for prevention of migraine headaches
galcanezumab-gnlm (Emgality)	240 mg subcutaneously once as a loading dose, followed by 120 mg subcutaneously once monthly for prevention of migraine headaches 300 mg subcutaneously at the onset of a headache for treatment
rimegepant (NURTEC ODT)	75 mg orally as a single dose for treatment of migraine headache 75 mg orally once every other day for prevention of migraine headache
ubrogepant (Ubrelvy)	50–100 mg orally as a single dose, may repeat once after at least 2 hr to a maximum of 200 mg/day. Not to be used more than eight times per month

How CGRP antibodies work. The CGRP monoclonal antibodies are directed either against the CGRP receptors of the blood vessels in the local trigeminovascular system or to a part of the actual CGRP molecule. By binding to these targets, the drug acts as an antagonist and prevents CGRP from binding to its receptors on the blood vessels, especially arteries. Thus massive vasodilation of these vessels does not occur.

Intended responses of CGRP antibodies
- Reduced frequency and intensity of migraine headaches
- Increased ability to participate in activities of daily living
- Improved quality of life

Common side effects of CGRP antibodies. With the CGRP antibodies exerting their main effects within the local trigeminovascular system, the drugs have fewer systemic side effects than other antimigraine drugs. The most common side effects of all these drugs include constipation, fatigue, nausea, weight loss, and hair loss. The injectable drugs *eptinezumab*, *erenumab*, and *galcanezumab* can cause injection site reactions. *Eptinezumab* is associated with flushing and itchiness.

Possible adverse effects of CGRP antibodies. The CGRP antibody drugs have been in common use to prevent or treat migraine headaches for a relatively short time. Although some adverse effects have been reported, it is likely that additional ones will emerge over time as they become more widely prescribed.

Hypersensitivity reactions are possible with any monoclonal antibody–based drugs because they are foreign proteins that initially were developed in nonhuman cells. Such reactions tend to increase in intensity over time. Similarly, because these antibodies are foreign proteins, the person taking one of these drugs may begin to develop their own antibodies directed against the drugs. When this occurs, the effectiveness of the drug is decreased because the antibodies directed against the drug ultimately may destroy it or inactivate it.

All of the CGRP antibodies can elevate liver enzymes and may impair liver function. In addition, the oral drugs interact with many other drugs, especially ones used to manage tuberculosis and human immunodeficiency virus (HIV) disease.

⭐ **Priority actions to take** *before and* **after** *giving CGRP antibodies.* The oral drugs *(atogepant, rimegepant, ubrogepant)* usually are taken at home by the patient either on a scheduled basis to prevent the migraine or to halt the progression of a migraine after symptoms have begun. The drugs given subcutaneously *(erenumab* and *galcanezumab)* are available in prefilled syringes for patients to self-inject. For drugs that are taken at home, the priority action is to educate patients about these drugs for safe administration and to know when to contact the prescriber or seek medical help.

Before infusing *eptinezumab*, dilute the drug only with normal saline. Gently mix the solution in the container by inverting it, **not shaking it**. Infuse the solution over at least 30 minutes and observe the patient for any indications of hypersensitivity for at least 1 hour after the infusion is completed. Single-use containers do not have a preservative, any unused portion must be discarded. Flush the line with 20 mL of 0.9% sodium chloride injection after the infusion is complete. Do not give other IV drugs with eptinezumab or through the same infusion set.

⭐ *Teaching priorities for patients taking CGRP antibodies*
- Take or inject the drugs exactly as prescribed and no more frequently than prescribed, to avoid serious adverse reactions.
- For the subcutaneous drugs, use the injection techniques taught to you to prevent complications from the injection.
- Oral drugs can be taken with or without food.
- Avoid drinking grapefruit juice with the oral drugs because grapefruit juice increases the activity of the migraine drug and increases the risk for side effects and adverse effects.
- Do not drive or operate heavy machinery when taking these drugs because they induce drowsiness.
- Remember that constipation is a common side effect of these drugs. If your prescriber has ordered a stool softener or laxative, start using these agents before constipation occurs.

Common Side Effects

Calcitonin Gene–Related Peptide Antibodies

Constipation, Nausea

Fatigue

Weight loss

Hair loss

- Notify your prescriber if you develop yellowing of your skin or eyes, darkening of your urine, or lighter stools. These problems are signs of liver toxicity.
- Be sure to tell all your other health care providers that you are taking an oral drug for migraine headaches because of the potential for drug interactions, especially if you are being treated for HIV or tuberculosis.
- Do not take any new over-the-counter drugs or supplements unless you check with the health care provider who prescribed your migraine drug.

Life span considerations for CGRP antibodies

Considerations for pregnancy and lactation. Currently, no specific risks for adverse pregnancy outcomes have been reported for any of the CGRP antibody drugs. However, manufacturers recommend these drugs be avoided during any stage of pregnancy unless benefits outweigh any unknown risks. For the same reason, breastfeeding is not recommended while taking these drugs, especially the oral drugs.

REVIEW OF RELATED PHYSIOLOGY AND PATHOPHYSIOLOGY OF MUSCLE SPASM

The skeletal muscles and their associated structures (tendons and ligaments) allow movement of specific bones for mobility. Muscles are attached as opposing groups around joints in a way that when one muscle group contracts (shortens), the joint flexes so that the two connecting bones move toward each other by pulling motions (Fig. 9.6A). To straighten the bones around a joint, the flexor muscles relax (stretch) and the opposing muscles (extensors) contract so that the bones are pulled back into their original positions (see Fig. 9.6B).

Skeletal muscles do not normally contract on their own. They require stimulation from the nervous system. Thus smooth, coordinated motion requires the input of the nervous system to alternately stimulate the opposing muscle groups that cause joints to bend and then straighten. For example, when you want to scratch your nose, you first consciously think about scratching your nose. The motor area of the brain triggers the nerves that specifically control the muscles of one arm and hand so that only those muscles are depolarized and you just scratch your nose without having a whole-body muscle response. If, for some reason, the nerves connecting your brain to your arm and hand's skeletal muscles are not working, the muscles will not contract and no movement occurs.

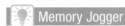
Memory Jogger

Skeletal muscles always "pull" bones in response to contraction. They never "push."

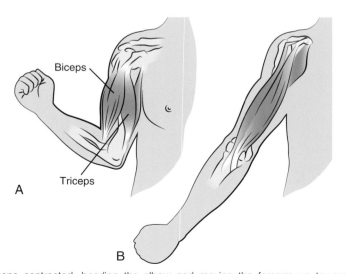

FIG. 9.6 (A) Biceps contracted, bending the elbow and moving the forearm up toward the shoulders. (B) Triceps contracted, pulling the forearm down, straightening the elbow.

A *skeletal muscle spasm* is the involuntary contraction of a single muscle, group of related muscles, or just a part of a muscle. This most often occurs when a nerve or nerves controlling contraction to that muscle depolarizes spontaneously or inappropriately. Common causes of inappropriate nerve depolarization include pressure on the nerve, inflammation and swelling along the nerve path, and electrolyte imbalances, especially low blood calcium and magnesium levels. Spasms can also occur when a muscle is irritated or injured. When a large muscle has a spasm, rather than just an isolated twitch, the contraction can be so tight that no blood flows through the muscle. Then, intense pain from a lack of oxygen *(anoxia)* getting to the muscle can result. (Think about how it feels to have a "Charlie horse" in your calf muscle.) In some instances, skeletal muscle spasms are continuously repeating muscle twitches (fasciculations) that are less painful but very annoying. In either case, muscle function is reduced during spasms and twitches.

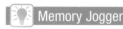 **Memory Jogger**

The pain of skeletal muscle spasms is caused by local lactic acidosis in response to tissue anoxia.

SKELETAL MUSCLE RELAXANTS

Skeletal muscle relaxants are drugs that often act by depressing the central nervous system (CNS), which reduces motor nerve depolarization and results in a reduction of skeletal muscle spasms and increased mobility of affected skeletal muscles. They are used for pain and insomnia when excessive skeletal muscle contractions or spasms contribute to these problems. The following table lists the adult dosages of the five most commonly prescribed skeletal muscle relaxants. For the less commonly prescribed skeletal muscle relaxants, consult a reliable drug reference. In addition, a benzodiazepine may be the first drug prescribed for a patient experiencing painful or bothersome temporary skeletal muscle spasms. Benzodiazepines have other uses and are fully described in Chapter 26.

Adult Dosages of the Common Skeletal Muscle Relaxants

Drug Names	Usual Maintenance Dosages
baclofen (Enova, Equipto, Gablofen, Lioresal, Ozobax)	Initially: 5 mg orally every 8 hr. Dosages can be increased slowly every 3 days by 5 mg orally three to four times daily up to a total daily dose of 40–80 mg
carisoprolol (Soma, Vanadum)	250–350 mg orally three times daily and at bedtime
cyclobenzaprine (Amrix, Fexmid, Flexeril)	5–10 mg orally three times daily
methocarbamol (Robaxin)	Initially: 1.5–2 g orally every 6 hr for 2–3 days Maintenance: 4–4.5 g total daily, orally given in 3–6 divided doses 1–2 g intravenously at a rate of 300 mg/min
tizanidine (Zanaflex)	Initially: 2 mg orally every 8 hr, can increase over time to 4 mg orally every 6–8 hr

How Skeletal Muscle Relaxants Work

None of the skeletal muscle relaxants work directly on the muscles themselves. Instead, they interfere with transmission of nerve impulses that stimulate the muscles. *Cyclobenzaprine* and *methocarbamol* appear to inhibit nerve transmission in the brain, depressing CNS function and altering the perception of pain. *Baclofen* and *carisoprolol* interfere with nerve transmission at the level of the spinal cord. In addition, *baclofen* is chemically similar to the inhibitory neurotransmitter gamma-amino butyric acid (GABA) and binds to GABA receptors in the motor inhibitory pathways. The mechanism of *tizanidine* is different. It is an alpha$_2$ adrenergic agonist in the CNS. When tizanidine binds to these CNS receptors, the release of excitatory neurotransmitters is inhibited and spinal motor neurons are less active.

Intended Responses of Skeletal Muscle Relaxants

- Reduced muscle spasms and pain
- Increased mobility/function of affected muscles
- Improved sleep and rest

Common Side Effects of Skeletal Muscle Relaxants

Although each drug has some unique side effects, the most common side effects of all the skeletal muscle relaxants include drowsiness/sedation, headache, hypotension, nausea, dry mouth, and dizziness.

Unique side effects of *baclofen* include muscle weakness, constipation, and frequent urination. *Cyclobenzaprine* has additional side effects of blurred vision, increased photosensitivity, dry eyes, and urinary retention. Both *methocarbamol* and *cyclobenzaprine* induce a more profound sedation than do the other drugs. In addition, *methocarbamol* and *tizanidine* can induce hallucinations.

Possible Adverse Effects of Skeletal Muscle Relaxants

All of these drugs induce some degree of sedation and drowsiness. This effect is much more intense if the patient drinks alcohol or takes another CNS depressant. Another major adverse effect of all the skeletal muscle relaxants is that they interact with more than 100 other drugs. It is important that patients understand the need to avoid taking any other prescribed or over-the-counter drugs without the knowledge of the health care provider who prescribed the skeletal muscle relaxants.

Baclofen increases the risk for worsening any preexisting psychiatric disorders. It also lowers the seizure threshold in people who have a seizure disorder and potentiates the effects of anticoagulants. If baclofen is discontinued abruptly, a syndrome of withdrawal may occur with symptoms of increased muscle spasms, hallucinations, and seizures. Thus baclofen therapy should be withdrawn slowly.

Carisoprolol has adverse effects that include a risk for bronchospasms and sinus tachycardia. Decreased bone marrow function with reduced blood counts of all types, including white blood cells (WBCs), has been reported. With reduced WBCs, the patient is at increased risk for infection.

Cyclobenzaprine can trigger cardiac dysrhythmias and prolonged cardiac conduction. This drug is not to be used in a patient who is recovering from a myocardial infarction or who has any preexisting, persistent heart rhythm problems. In addition, cyclobenzaprine should never be prescribed for a patient who is taking certain drugs for psychiatric problems, especially monoamine oxidase inhibitors (MAOIs) or selective serotonin reuptake inhibitors (SSRIs), because of the risk for severe hypertension and serotonin syndrome (see Chapter 25). Cyclobenzaprine also lowers the seizure threshold and should never be used for patients who have a seizure disorder. The anticholinergic effects of cyclobenzaprine can increase intraocular pressure and should not be used by anyone who has glaucoma.

Methocarbamol may cause amnesia and angioedema. The drug should be used cautiously, if at all, in patients who have a seizure disorder because it can lower the seizure threshold. When methocarbamol is given intravenously and *infiltration* or *extravasation* (leakage of fluid into the tissues) occurs, pain, phlebitis, and sloughing at the injection site may occur.

Tizanidine may worsen any preexisting psychiatric disorder and is contraindicated for use in anyone being managed for a known psychiatric disorder. Although the drug induces hypotension, when is drug is stopped abruptly, a rebound hypertension can occur and be dangerously high.

⭐ Priority Actions to Take *Before* Giving Skeletal Muscle Relaxants

Before giving a skeletal muscle relaxant to patients for the first time, assess the level of consciousness, cognition, and skeletal muscle reactivity. Also ask whether they have a seizure disorder or have ever had a seizure in the past, because many of these drugs lower the seizure threshold.

All skeletal muscle relaxants interact with a hundred or more other drugs. Obtain a list of all other drugs the patient takes on a regular basis, and consult with a pharmacist to determine whether any adjustments are needed in the patient's drug therapy regimen. Notify the prescriber of the need to make adjustments if this is indicated.

Before giving the first dose of *cyclobenzaprine*, assess the patient's blood pressure and radial and apical pulses for any skipped beats, extra beats, or any other type of irregular heartbeat. If you find any persistent heart beat irregularity, notify the prescriber before administering the drug.

Although these drugs may be taken with or without food or milk, the manufacturers recommend that they be given with food or milk to reduce gastric side effects.

⭐ Priority Actions to Take *After* Giving Skeletal Muscle Relaxants

Assess for level of consciousness and degree of skeletal muscle relaxation or muscle weakness after giving any skeletal muscle relaxant. Patients may become very drowsy and are at risk for falling. Raise the side rails, and remind them to call for help to get out of bed for any reason.

Muscle relaxants can cause a sudden lowering of blood pressure, especially when the patient changes position (orthostatic hypotension). Help the patient change position slowly. When getting out of bed, he or she should sit for a few minutes on the side of the bed before attempting to get up. Help him or her during walking to prevent falling.

Cyclobenzaprine and *methocarbamol* can cause urinary retention. If a patient receiving one of these drugs has an enlarged prostate gland, assess for symptoms of urinary retention.

For patients receiving IV doses (by bolus or continuous infusion) of *methocarbamol*, assess the site immediately after giving a bolus dose or every 2 hours during a continuous infusion. Assess for pain, redness, swelling, and a cordlike feel over the vein. If any signs of infiltration are present, stop the infusion, remove the IV, and notify the prescriber.

After giving the first dose of *cyclobenzaprine*, assess the patient's radial and apical pulses hourly for any skipped beats, extra beats, or any other type of irregular heartbeat. If you find persistent irregularity, notify the prescriber.

⭐ Teaching Priorities for Patients Taking Skeletal Muscle Relaxants

- A skeletal muscle relaxant is to be taken only on a short-term basis because drugs of this type do have a risk for dependence and abuse.
- Avoid operating any dangerous equipment, driving a car, or making critical decisions while under the influence of these drugs.
- Do not drink alcohol or take any other drug that causes drowsiness while taking a skeletal muscle relaxant because drowsiness is made worse and you can fall, become confused, or have hallucinations.
- It is recommended that any oral skeletal muscle relaxant be taken with food or milk to reduce your risk for gastrointestinal problems.
- All of these drugs can have serious interactions with other drugs. Tell your prescriber about all other drugs (prescribed or over the counter) you take on a regular basis, and do not start taking other drugs unless your prescriber has indicated that this is not a problem.
- If you take cyclobenzaprine, take your pulse at least twice daily. If you notice that your pulse becomes persistently irregular, notify your prescriber. If you develop shortness of breath or chest pain, call 911 or go to the nearest emergency department.
- Skeletal muscle relaxants can lower your blood pressure and make you dizzy, especially when changing positions. Be sure to get up slowly and to use the hand rail when going up or down steps.
- Because cyclobenzaprine increases sun sensitivity and can lead to severe sunburn, be sure to use sunscreen and wear hats and protective clothing during sun exposure.

Life Span Considerations for Skeletal Muscle Relaxants

Considerations for pregnancy and lactation. *Methocarbamol* and *cyclobenzaprine* have a low to moderate likelihood of increasing the risk for birth defects or fetal harm. They can be used during pregnancy. The risk for adverse pregnancy outcomes is not known for the other skeletal muscle relaxants. Thus, for any of these drugs, it is recommended that the drugs be used only if clearly needed and the benefits are believed to outweigh potential risks.

Drug Alert

Action/Intervention Alert

When giving an IV dose of *methocarbamol*, assess for pain, redness, swelling, and a cordlike feel over the vein, which indicate an infiltration or extravasation.

QSEN: Safety

Some of the drugs are known to be excreted in breast milk; for others, it is not known whether they enter breast milk. Therefore manufacturers recommend that breastfeeding be avoided for the duration of skeletal muscle relaxant therapy.

Considerations for older adults. None of the skeletal muscle relaxants are recommended to be used with older adults because of the sedation and anticholinergic effects, especially confusion, hallucinations, and urinary retention. The muscle relaxant effect also causes muscle weakness and increases the risk for falls in this population.

Get Ready for the NCLEX® Examination!

Key Points

- Pain is whatever the patient says it is and exists whenever he or she says it does.
- Never assume patients who are tolerating pain well are comfortable or that their condition has not worsened. Reassess patients' pain, especially by asking them to rate it, at regular intervals, not only to determine therapy effectiveness but also to identify possible complications earlier.
- Acute pain is usually accompanied by common physiologic changes triggered by the stress response, including elevated heart rate, blood pressure, and respiratory rate; cool, clammy skin; dry mouth; restlessness; and an inability to concentrate.
- Changes in vital signs do **not** indicate the intensity of chronic pain. Relying on this information alone often results in poor assessment/management of chronic pain and increased patient suffering.
- The goal of drug therapy for acute pain is **not** to make the person completely unaware of the pain but to relieve the pain to a level that is acceptable to the patient and permit him or her to participate in activities of daily living.
- Assess the patient's pain level 30 minutes after giving a pain-control drug and then reassess hourly.
- Although individuals who are addicted to opioid agonists may also have tolerance, the development of tolerance can occur separately from addiction as a normal physiologic response to longer-term opioid agonist use.
- Opioid drugs that provide the best pain relief bind most strongly (tightly) to mu receptors.
- Never substitute one opioid agonist for another without an order from the prescriber that includes a recalculation of the dose. Strengths vary.
- The half-life of the opioid antagonist is not as long as for opioid agonists. Thus the effects of the antagonist can wear off faster than the opioid agonist is eliminated. More than one dose of an opioid antagonist may be needed to prevent recurrence of respiratory depression.
- Teach patients taking an extended release (ER) form of an oral opioid agonist to swallow the capsule or tablet whole because chewing it or opening the capsule allows too much of the drug to be absorbed all at once and an overdose can occur.
- What is painful for an adult also is painful for a child. Children's pain must be taken seriously, and interventions to relieve pain are needed.
- Use an apnea monitor and pulse oximeter to monitor the breathing effectiveness of an infant or small child receiving an opioid agonist.

- Acetaminophen can be toxic to the liver and should not be taken by anyone with liver health problems. Teach patients to avoid alcohol and other liver-toxic drugs on days when they take acetaminophen.
- Teach parents to read the label on liquid acetaminophen bottles for infants and small children carefully and ensure that the correct dose is given for the child's size. Teach parents to telephone the pharmacy and talk with the pharmacist to ensure that the dose is correct if they are not confident in their own calculations.
- When used systemically, ergotamine derivatives and triptans cause general arterial constriction, which can cause severe hypertension, angina, myocardial ischemia, and stroke. Monitor patients closely for these problems, especially if they have any preexisting hypertension.
- The actions of onobotulinumtoxin A can spread beyond the areas of injection and cause problems related to the inability of other muscles to respond to stimuli. Teach patients to report immediately any change in muscle responses beyond the injection area.
- All skeletal muscle relaxants cause some degree of drowsiness and sedation that is made worse if the patient either drinks alcohol with these drugs or takes other drugs that cause central nervous system (CNS) depression.
- Baclofen, cyclobenzaprine, and methocarbamol should not be given to anyone who has a seizure disorder because these drugs lower the seizure threshold.
- When giving an IV dose of methocarbamol, assess for pain, redness, swelling, and a cordlike feel over the vein, which indicate an infiltration or extravasation.
- Warn patients taking any skeletal muscle relaxant to avoid driving, operating any heavy equipment, and making critical decisions while under the influence of these drugs.
- Neither *baclofen* nor *tizanidine* should be discontinued abruptly. Discontinuing baclofen suddenly without tapering can trigger a syndrome of withdrawal with symptoms of increased muscle spasms, hallucinations, and seizures. Discontinuing tizanidine abruptly can cause a dangerous rebound hypertension.

Additional Learning Resources

🌐 Be sure to visit your Evolve website (http://evolve.elsevier.com/Workman/pharmacology/) for additional online resources.

[SG] Go to your Study Guide for additional learning activities to help you master this chapter content.

Review Questions

See *Answers to In-Text Review Questions* in the back of the book for answers to these questions.

1. How are drug tolerance and drug addiction different?

   A. Addiction occurs first and much more quickly to opioid agonist therapy than does tolerance.
   B. Tolerance requires lower opioid agonist doses for effective pain relief, and addiction requires higher doses for effective pain relief.
   C. Tolerance is an expected, and normal physiologic response to opioid agonist therapy lasting 10 days or longer and addiction is a psychological response to opioid agonist therapy.
   D. Addiction is an expected, and normal physiologic response to opioid agonist therapy lasting 10 days or longer and tolerance is a psychological response to opioid agonist therapy.

2. Which assessment question is important for the nurse to ask a patient who has been taking an opioid agonist every 6 hours for the past 3 days for acute pain?

   A. "Have you noticed a craving for the drug before it is time to take it again?"
   B. "Are you having any hallucinations or unusual dreams?"
   C. "Have your bowel habits changed in any way?"
   D. "Do you seem to be thirstier than usual?"

3. Which outcome indicates to the assessing nurse that a patient's pain control medication is effective 45 minutes after receiving pain medication for pain intensity rated as the "worst possible"?

   A. Reports a pain level of 4/10
   B. Tightly constricted pupils
   C. Tolerates the dressing change without grimacing.
   D. Nausea and drowsiness have increased.

4. How many milliliters (mL) of morphine will the nurse administer by IV push to a patient who is prescribed to receive 3 mg when the drug is available in a solution of 5 mg/mL?

   A. 0.2 mL
   B. 0.4 mL
   C. 0.6 mL
   D. 0.8 mL

5. Which precaution is **most important** for the nurse to teach a patient who has been prescribed codeine with acetaminophen for pain to prevent harm?

   A. "Avoid alcoholic beverages while taking this drug."
   B. "Avoid caffeinated drinks or food while taking this drug."
   C. "Notify your prescriber if this drug makes you drowsy or sleepy."
   D. "Use a stool softener or laxative to prevent constipation while taking this drug."

6. With which patient does the nurse expect to administer gabapentin?

   A. Older patient who is 1 day postoperative from knee replacement surgery
   B. 60-year-old patient who expresses fear, anxiety, and uncertainty related to episodes of chest pain
   C. Middle-aged patient who has persistent burning and tingling sensation in the lower extremities
   D. Young male patient who reports a gnawing and burning discomfort in the epigastric area between meals

7. How does ubrogepant help to prevent or reduce the severity of migraine headaches?

   A. Preventing calcitonin gene–related peptide (CGRP) from causing excessive vasoconstriction
   B. Preventing calcitonin gene–related peptide (CGRP) from causing excessive vasodilation
   C. Acting as an antagonist at mu and kappa opioid receptors to alter the perception of pain
   D. Acting as an agonist at mu and kappa opioid receptors to alter the perception of pain

8. For which patient does the nurse question a prescription for ergotamine?

   A. 25-year-old man with anemia
   B. 36-year-old woman with type 1 diabetes
   C. 42-year-old woman with hypertension
   D. 55-year-old man with an enlarged prostate gland

9. A patient who received onobotulinumtoxin A injections 2 days ago calls to tell the nurse that now her mouth and lips are numb. What is the nurse's **best** advice or action?

   A. Go to the nearest emergency department.
   B. Ask her to rate her current migraine headache pain.
   C. Avoid hot beverages until the drug effects wear off.
   D. Apply a heating pad on the lowest heat setting to the affected area.

10. Which assessment is **most important** for the nurse to perform before giving a patient the first dose of any prescribed skeletal muscle relaxant?

   A. Measuring blood pressure
   B. Asking the patient to rate his or her pain on a 0 to 10 scale
   C. Checking arm strength and deep tendon reflexes on both sides
   D. Asking about all other prescribed and over-the-counter drugs the patient takes

11. A patient taking methocarbamol for skeletal muscle cramping reports facial flushing. What is the nurse's **best** action?

A. Asking the patient whether he or she is taking any other drugs

B. Reassuring the patient that this is a mild side effect of the drug

C. Instructing the patient to go to the nearest emergency department

D. Notifying the prescriber to obtain a prescription for a different drug

12. A patient whose pain from skeletal muscle spasms has now resolved asks the nurse why he must slowly reduce the tizanidine rather than just stopping the drug because it is no longer needed. What is the nurse's **best** response?

A. "This drug lowers blood pressure, and stopping it suddenly can result in dangerously high blood pressure."

B. "Tizanidine lowers the seizure threshold, and suddenly stopping it increases your risk for a seizure."

C. "Slowly reducing the drug prevents you from having the drug-craving sensation associated with suddenly stopping this controlled substance."

D. "The drug is similar to natural adrenal hormones, and tapering it down rather than stopping it suddenly keeps your blood hormone levels normal."

Clinical Judgment

1. Which physiologic responses indicate to the nurse that a patient is experiencing acute pain? **Select all that apply.**

A. Diaphoresis
B. Somnolence
C. Bradypnea
D. Hypotension
E. Tachycardia
F. Dilated pupils
H. Diarrhea

2. The patient is a 28-year-old woman who has an average of 20 days per month with migraine headache pain. Her only other health problem is asthma, for which she uses a prevention inhaler (Advair) twice daily. She tries to swim for an hour three times weekly for exercise. She is now prescribed to use rimegepant 75 mg orally every other day to prevent or reduce her incidence of migraine headaches. The nurse is developing a teaching plan with take-home instructions/precautions about this drug. **Use an X to indicate which patient statements indicate Correct Understanding of therapy with rimegepant and which statements indicate that More Instruction Is Needed.**

PATIENT STATEMENTS	CORRECT UNDERSTANDING	MORE INSTRUCTION NEEDED
If I develop a migraine on a day when I have already taken a dose for prevention, I will wait 2 hours to repeat the dose.		
If I lose more than 2 lb in a week, I will notify my prescriber.		
Even though I love grapefruit juice, I will not take it on the days I take the drug.		
If I have nausea and am unable to keep an oral dose of the drug down, I will go to the prescriber to get an injection of the drug.		
I will test my facial muscles daily, especially around my eyes, to make sure they are not weaker or will not work.		
I will drink plenty of water and take a stool softener daily to prevent constipation.		

Learning Objectives

The content presented in this chapter should help you to:

1. Describe the names, actions, usual adult dosages, possible side effects, and adverse effects of commonly prescribed corticosteroids and nonsteroidal antiinflammatory drugs (NSAIDs).
2. Describe priority actions to take before and after giving corticosteroids and NSAIDs.
3. Prioritize essential information to teach patients taking corticosteroids and NSAIDs.
4. Describe the names, actions, usual adult dosages, possible side effects, and adverse reactions of commonly prescribed

drugs for allergic inflammation and general disease-modifying antirheumatic drugs (DMARDs).
5. Describe priority actions to take before and after giving drugs for allergic inflammation and general DMARDs.
6. Prioritize essential information to teach patients taking drugs for allergic inflammation and general DMARDs.
7. Describe appropriate life span considerations for corticosteroids, NSAIDs, drugs for allergic inflammation, and general DMARDs.

Key Terms

antihistamines (ăn-tē-HĬS-tĕ-mēnz) (p. 177) Drugs that reduce general inflammation by preventing the inflammatory mediator histamine from binding to its receptor site; same as histamine blockers or histamine antagonists.

antiinflammatory drugs (ăn-tī-ĭn-FLĂM-ĕ-tōr-ē DRŬGZ) (p. 169) Drugs that prevent or limit general inflammatory responses to injury or invasion.

biologics (bīō LÄ jik) (p. 169) A class of complex antiinflammatory drugs derived from living sources that target specific inflammatory cells, components, or products to modify chronic disorders associated with inflammation and tissue damage.

corticosteroids (kōr-tĭ-kō-STĔR-ōydz) (p. 170) Drugs similar to natural cortisol that prevent or limit general inflammation by slowing or stopping inflammatory mediator production.

disease-modifying antirheumatic drugs (dĭ-zēz MŎD-ĭ-fī-ĭng ăn-tĭ-ROO-mă-tĭk DRŬGZ) (p. 179) Drugs that reduce the progression and tissue destruction of the general inflammatory

disease processes by a variety of mechanisms against inflammatory and immune system cells.

histamine (HĬS-tĕ-mēn) (p. 176) A chemical mediator made by the body that binds to its receptor sites and causes inflammatory responses, especially allergic inflammatory responses.

inflammation (ĭn-flă-MĀ-shŭn) (p. 167) A set of normal reactions of tissues and blood vessels in general responses to injury or invasion.

leukotriene (LŪ-kō-trēn) (p. 174) A chemical mediator made by the body that works with histamine to enhance and prolong allergic inflammatory responses.

nonsteroidal antiinflammatory drugs (NSAIDs) (non-stĕr-ŌY-dŭl ăn-tī-ĭn-FLĂM-ĕ-tōr-ē DRŬGZ) (p. 173) Antiinflammatory drugs that are not similar to cortisol but prevent or limit the tissue and blood vessel general responses to injury or invasion by slowing the production of one or more inflammatory mediators.

RELATED PHYSIOLOGY AND PATHOPHYSIOLOGY OF INFLAMMATION

Inflammation, or the *inflammatory response*, is a set of normal reactions of tissues and blood vessels in general response to injury or invasion. This response is a *syndrome* because it occurs in a predictable series of steps and stages. Overall, it is a helpful and protective response that also causes temporary pain and some loss of function in tissues and organs experiencing it.

Because inflammation is a general and nonspecific response, the same tissue responses occur with any type of injury or invasion, regardless of the location on the body or what caused the response to start. This means that inflammation triggered by a scald burn to the hand is the same as inflammation triggered by bacteria in the middle ear. The size and severity of the inflammatory response depend on the intensity, severity, duration, and extent of the injury. For example, a splinter in the finger

 Memory Jogger

The inflammatory response can be small and localized or may involve the whole body depending on the intensity, severity, duration, and extent of the injury. Regardless of the size of the response, the same actions are occurring at the tissue level.

triggers inflammation only at the splinter site. A burn injuring 60% of the skin surface triggers inflammation involving the entire body.

Inflammatory responses start tissue actions that cause visible and uncomfortable symptoms. Despite the discomfort, these actions are important in ridding the body of harmful organisms and helping repair damaged tissue. However, if the inflammatory response is excessive or prolonged, tissue damage may result.

The inflammatory response occurs both as a result of tissue injury and as a result of infection by invading organisms. Although infection usually occurs with inflammation, inflammation can occur without infection. Examples of inflammation without infection include sprained joints, blisters, and allergic reactions. Inflammation with infection includes appendicitis, otitis media (ear infection), and bacterial pneumonia, among many others. So, inflammation does not always mean that an infection is present.

The syndrome of inflammation has the same responses, regardless of the triggering event. These responses at the tissue level cause the five signs and symptoms of inflammation: warmth, redness, swelling, pain, and decreased function (Animation 10.1). Inflammation occurs in three stages, some of which overlap.

INFLAMMATION STAGE I: VASCULAR

Stage I involves white blood cells (WBCs) and changes in blood vessels. Injured tissues and WBCs in the area release *mediators*, which are body chemicals such as histamine, leukotriene, prostaglandins, kinins, tumor necrosis factor (TNF), and cytokines that cause and sustain the tissue responses. Some mediators act on blood vessels in the area of injury or invasion, causing dilation of the blood vessels and *capillary leak syndrome*. These responses cause the symptoms of swelling, redness, and warmth of the tissues. The increased blood flow brings oxygen, nutrients, and more WBCs to injured tissues. Some mediators, such as bradykinin and substance P, cause pain. Other mediators, such as leukotriene and tumor necrosis factor (TNF), work on WBCs to enhance and prolong the inflammatory response.

INFLAMMATION STAGE II: EXUDATE

In stage II, large numbers of WBCs are created, and an *exudate* (tissue drainage) known as *pus* is formed. At this stage, the total number of WBCs in the blood can increase up to five times above normal and indicates that an inflammatory response is taking place (see Table 1.6 in Chapter 1 for normal WBC counts).

During this phase, a cascade reaction starts to increase the inflammatory response (Figure 10.1). This action begins by converting fat from broken cell membranes into arachidonic acid, which then enters the cyclo-oxygenase (COX) pathway. Cyclo-oxygenase (COX), especially COX-2, is an enzyme important in converting body chemicals into mediators of inflammation that continue the inflammatory response in the tissues. Many antiinflammatory drugs stop this cascade by preventing COX-2 from converting arachidonic acid into mediators.

INFLAMMATION STAGE III: TISSUE REPAIR

Although stage III is completed last, it begins at the time of injury, and is very important in helping the injured tissue regain function. WBCs secrete chemicals that trigger the remaining healthy cells to divide, when the damaged tissue is able to divide. For damaged tissues such as the heart that are unable to divide, WBCs trigger new blood vessel growth and scar tissue formation. When scar tissue replaces normal tissue, some permanent loss of function occurs.

This stage can be harmful if it lasts too long. For example, some diseases cause inflammation in the lungs and trigger scar tissue growth there. If too much scar tissue forms in the lungs, not enough oxygen enters the blood, and the person dies of respiratory failure. When large amounts of TNF are released, such as in many chronic inflammatory diseases, tissues, especially bone and cartilage cells, are destroyed.

Although inflammation is an important protective response, it is uncomfortable, reduces function while it is occurring, and can cause tissue damage if it is prolonged.

Memory Jogger

Infection usually is accompanied by inflammation, but inflammation can occur without infection.

Memory Jogger

The five signs and symptoms of inflammation are warmth, redness, swelling, pain, and decreased function.

Memory Jogger

Excess scar tissue formation from prolonged inflammation is more harmful than helpful.

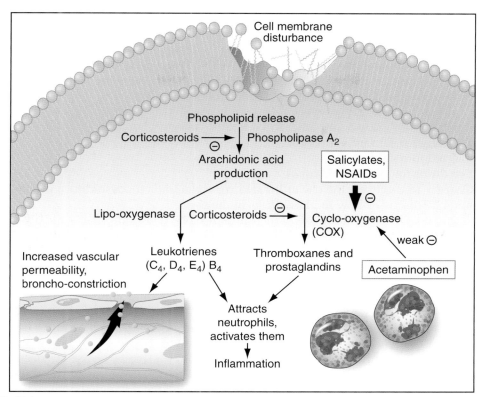

FIG. 10.1 Arachidonic acid cascade and mediator production. *NSAIDs,* Nonsteroidal antiinflammatory drugs. (From Bluth, M. H., Pincus, M. R., & Abraham, N. Z. [2022]. Toxicology and therapeutic drug monitoring. In R. A. McPherson & M. R. Pincus (Eds.), *Henry's clinical diagnosis and management by laboratory methods* [24th ed.]. Philadelphia: Elsevier.)

Antiinflammatory drugs that prevent or limit general inflammatory responses to injury or invasion are prescribed to increase comfort and prevent tissue-damaging complications. These drugs are used as therapy for many common acute problems such as asthma, allergic reactions, and local or systemic irritation.

In addition to managing acute inflammatory problems, antiinflammatory drugs can help manage some aspects of autoimmune health problems. Autoimmunity is caused by inappropriate inflammatory and immune responses when WBC actions and products are directed against healthy normal cells and tissues. These responses are similar to normal inflammatory responses, but these reactions are now directed against normal body cells.

General antiinflammatory drugs can help provide some relief for autoimmune disorders; however, biologic drugs are now recommended as first-line therapy for control of many of these disorders. **Biologics** are a class of complex antiinflammatory drugs derived from living sources that target *specific* inflammatory cells, components, or products to modify chronic disorders associated with inflammation and tissue damage. Examples of autoimmune diseases that can be helped with biologics include rheumatoid arthritis, psoriasis, ankylosing spondylitis, and ulcerative colitis, among many others. Chapter 11 discusses mechanisms of actions and care issues related to biologics.

THERAPY WITH GENERAL ANTIINFLAMMATORY DRUGS

TYPES OF GENERAL ANTIINFLAMMATORY DRUGS

There are many general antiinflammatory drugs. Some must be prescribed, and others are available over the counter. The five main categories of antiinflammatory drugs include corticosteroids, nonsteroidal antiinflammatory drugs (NSAIDs), antihistamines, leukotriene inhibitors, and general disease-modifying antirheumatic drugs (DMARDs).

 Memory Jogger

Classes of general antiinflammatory drugs
- Corticosteroids
- NSAIDs
- Antihistamines and leukotriene inhibitors
- General DMARDs

Systemic Corticosteroids

Corticosteroids are drugs similar to natural cortisol and prevent or limit general inflammation by slowing or stopping all known pathways of inflammatory mediator production, including the cyclo-oxygenase-1 (COX-1) and cyclo-oxygenase-2 (COX-2) pathways. These drugs are the most powerful of all the drugs used for general inflammation and may be taken or used in the following ways.

- Orally or parenterally
- Inhalation for asthma and other inflammatory airway problems
- Topically for skin inflammation
- Injected into joints
- Eye drops for eye inflammation

Chapter 18 discusses the use of inhaled corticosteroids for respiratory problems. Chapter 27 discusses how to place drugs in the eye.

Systemic (oral and parenteral) corticosteroids have many side effects and adverse effects. For this reason, corticosteroids are usually prescribed for only a short period of time. However, if the inflammation cannot be controlled with less powerful drugs, they may need to be taken for weeks, months, or indefinitely. When needed for long periods of time, the goal is for the patient to take the lowest dose of corticosteroids that will control the inflammation so drug side effects and complications can be minimized.

In addition to controlling inflammation, corticosteroids are used as hormone replacement therapy for adrenal gland hypofunction (see Chapter 22) and as part of chemotherapy treatment, especially for leukemia. They also may be used to decrease cranial swelling from trauma or cranial surgery. The dosages used for these other health problems may be very different than those used for inflammation.

Adult dosages for the most commonly used systemic corticosteroids to manage general inflammatory disorders are listed in the following table. Consult a reliable drug reference for information about less common corticosteroids and for when they are used for other purposes. Inhalation corticosteroid therapy is discussed in Chapter 18.

Usual Adult Dosages for Common Systemic Corticosteroids

Drug Name	Usual Maintenance Dose
betamethasone (Adbeon, Celestone)	0.6–7.2 mg orally daily, given as a single dose or in divided doses 0.5–9 mg IM or IV daily
cortisone (Cortone)	12.5–50 mg/day orally or IM. Dosage highly variable depending on the health problem and patient response
dexamethasone (Baycadron, Decadron, Solurex)	0.5–9 mg/day orally, IV, or IM, in 2–4 divided doses. Adjusted based on patient response
hydrocortisone (Solu-Cortef)	20–240 mg/day orally given in 2–4 divided doses 100–500 mg IM or IV. Repeat doses at 2, 4, or 6 hr intervals
methylprednisolone (Duralone, Medalone, Solu-Medrol)	10–60 mg IM or IV, two to four times daily, depending on disorder
prednisolone	5–40 mg orally daily
prednisone	5–60 mg orally daily in two doses (or as prescribed) depending on disorder

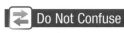 **Do Not Confuse**

prednisoLONE *with* **predniSONE** **or methylprednisolone**

An order for prednisolone can be confused with prednisone or methylprednisolone. All three drugs are corticosteroids, but methylprednisolone is more potent and can be given parenterally. Prednisone is an oral drug only. Oral prednisolone is more potent than prednisone.

QSEN: Safety

How systemic corticosteroids work. Corticosteroids decrease the production of all known body chemical mediators that trigger inflammation. They also slow the production of WBCs in the bone marrow. Because WBCs are the source of the mediators that trigger inflammation, this action also helps reduce inflammation. *Corticosteroids have main effects and side effects in all cells and tissues.*

Intended responses of systemic corticosteroids
- Swelling and excessive warmth at the site of inflammation are reduced.
- Redness and pain at the site of inflammation are reduced.
- The body area affected by inflammation resumes normal function.

Common side effects of systemic corticosteroids. Because systemic corticosteroids enter and affect every type of body cell, they have many side effects. The most common are listed in Box 10.1 and shown in Figure 10.2. Most side effects do not occur with just one dose of corticosteroids but may be present as soon as 5 to 7 days after starting drug therapy. Other side effects may not be present for up to a month or more of therapy. The higher the dose of corticosteroids, the sooner the side effects appear, and the more severe they are. Many side effects change the patient's appearance ("Cushingoid appearance" as shown in Fig. 10.2), which may cause distress. The good news is that most of these side effects and body changes return to normal after therapy stops, although it may take a year or longer. Stretch marks fade and shrink but are permanent. This is because they result from damage and actual structural changes within the skin.

Possible adverse effects of systemic corticosteroids. Three important adverse effects of systemic corticosteroids are adrenal gland suppression, reduced immune function, and delayed wound healing. These can occur in anyone taking systemic corticosteroids for a long period of time. For this reason, systemic corticosteroids are taken for inflammation only if the inflammation is severe and cannot be controlled in other ways.

As explained in Chapter 22, the adrenal glands normally make the corticosteroid cortisol. How much cortisol is made each day is determined by how much cortisol is already circulating in the blood. If there are less than normal amounts of cortisol in the blood, the adrenal glands produce and release more cortisol. If there are higher than normal levels of cortisol in the blood, the adrenal glands reduce production of cortisol. When blood levels of cortisol are very high, the adrenal glands stop producing it, and the cells of the adrenal glands atrophy (shrink).

Corticosteroid drugs closely resemble cortisol. When a person is taking corticosteroids, the blood levels of the drug are high. This high level fools the adrenal glands into stopping their production of cortisol and shrinking (Figure 10.3). The atrophied adrenal glands become a problem if the person suddenly stops taking corticosteroids. The adrenal glands will begin making cortisol again, but this process takes weeks to months. As a result, the person who suddenly stops taking systemic corticosteroids has no circulating cortisol, which is necessary for life, and could die from the effects of acute adrenal insufficiency. (Box 10.2 lists the signs and symptoms of acute adrenal insufficiency.) Instead of stopping corticosteroid drugs suddenly when therapy is no longer needed, the patient must slowly decrease the doses over time. This process is *tapering,* and it allows the adrenal gland cells to gradually resume the

Common Side Effects

Systemic Corticosteroids

Hypertension   Weight gain   Acne

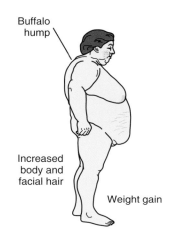
Nervousness   Insomnia   Hypernatremia

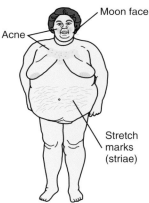

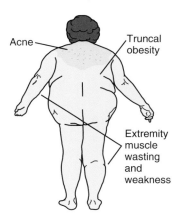

FIG. 10.2 Physical changes from long-term corticosteroid therapy, known as a "Cushingoid" appearance.

Box 10.1 | **Common Side Effects of Systemic Corticosteroids**

AFTER 1 WEEK OF THERAPY
- Acne
- Sodium and fluid retention
- Elevated blood pressure
- Sensation of "nervousness"
- Difficulty sleeping
- Emotional changes, crying easily

WITHIN A MONTH AFTER THERAPY
- Weight gain
- Fat redistribution (moon face and "buffalo hump" between the shoulders)

- Increased risk for gastrointestinal ulcers and bleeding
- Fragile, thin skin that bruises and tears easily
- Loss of muscle mass and strength
- Thinning scalp hair
- Increased facial and body hair
- Increased susceptibility to colds and other infections
- Stretch marks

Box 10.2	Signs and Symptoms of Acute Adrenal Insufficiency

- Acute confusion
- Profound muscle weakness
- Slow, irregular pulse
- Hypotension
- Abdominal pain
- Nausea and vomiting
- Salt craving
- Weight loss
- Low blood glucose levels (hypoglycemia, less than 70 mg/dL)
- Low serum sodium levels (hyponatremia, less than 130 mEq/L)
- High serum potassium levels (hyperkalemia, more than 5.5 mEq/L)

---

process of making cortisol. In addition, some loss of adrenal function occurs whenever corticosteroids are taken long term. Because more cortisol is needed during periods of stress or illness and the adrenal gland may not be able to release more, most patients will require a higher daily dose during these times.

Because systemic corticosteroids reduce WBC numbers and the inflammatory response, the person taking these drugs is at greater risk for infection. When inflammation is reduced, the symptoms of infection may not be obvious. Infection symptoms (fever, redness, pain, pus, or drainage) are caused by the same mediators that cause inflammation. When corticosteroids block their production, an infection may be present but not produce obvious symptoms.

Because inflammation begins the process of wound healing, reducing inflammation with corticosteroids reduces wound healing and slows cell growth. These actions delay wound healing, which also increases the risk for infection.

⭐ *Priority actions to take **before** giving systemic corticosteroids.* Check the dose and the specific drug name carefully. *Different types of corticosteroids are **not** interchangeable because the strength of the drugs varies.* For this reason, drug doses must be recalculated by the prescriber if it is necessary to switch from one type of systemic corticosteroid to another.

Assess for symptoms of infection (e.g., fever, drainage, foul-smelling urine, productive cough, or redness around an open skin area) and report any symptoms to the prescriber. Systemic corticosteroids may make an existing infection worse.

Assess the patient's blood pressure and weight. Corticosteroids cause sodium and water retention that can lead to high blood pressure (*hypertension*) and weight gain.

⭐ *Priority actions to take **after** giving systemic corticosteroids.* Assess vital signs at least once per shift for changes in blood pressure or temperature elevation. Examine the skin for bruises or tears that indicate the skin is becoming more fragile. Minimize the use of tape and be gentle when handling the patient to avoid skin trauma and bleeding. Weigh the patient at least weekly to monitor for fluid retention.

⭐ *Teaching priorities for patients taking systemic corticosteroids*
- Never stop taking the drug suddenly. Doing so can cause serious and sometimes life-threatening complications of the adrenal glands.
- If you are ill and unable to keep the drug down, call your prescriber so the drug can be given by injection.
- Take the drug exactly as prescribed. Do not increase or decrease the dose unless you have been taught how to do so safely and are monitored by your prescriber.
- Take corticosteroids with food to help prevent stomach ulcers.
- Obtain and wear a medical alert bracelet or carry a card stating that you are taking corticosteroids daily. This allows health care personnel to take steps to prevent adrenal insufficiency if you should suddenly become ill or hurt and are unable to communicate.
- Avoid crowds and people who are ill because resistance to infection is decreased and you are more susceptible to infectious illnesses.

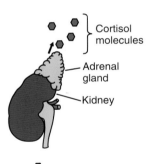
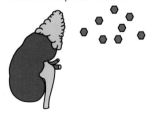
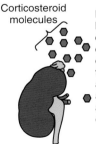

Cortisol molecules — Adrenal gland — Kidney

Low blood levels of cortisol cause a series of reactions that increase adrenal output of cortisol

Corticosteroid molecules

High blood levels of corticosteroids cause a series of reactions that shrink the adrenal gland and reduce adrenal output of cortisol

FIG. 10.3 Corticosteroid influence on adrenal production of cortisol.

- Notify your prescriber if you experience high stress or are ill because you may need a higher dose of the drug during these times.

Life span considerations for systemic corticosteroids

Pediatric considerations. Corticosteroids are prescribed for children who have severe or chronic inflammatory problems. Children are at risk for the same corticosteroid side effects and adverse effects as adults, even stomach ulcers. Remind parents to follow the same instructions for giving the drug to their child as are listed in the Teaching Priorities section.

Considerations for pregnancy and lactation. Severe inflammatory responses during pregnancy can be treated with corticosteroids, although the drug does cross the placenta. Babies born to mothers taking these drugs through the last 3 months of pregnancy tend to be smaller than normal. Because these drugs cross into breast milk, mothers who must take corticosteroids long term should stop breastfeeding because the baby will have the same side effects as the mother.

Considerations for older adults. The increased risk for infection can be very serious in older adults, who may have age-related reduced immune function. The older patient taking systemic corticosteroids must take extra precautions to avoid infection.

Another side effect of systemic corticosteroid therapy is an increase in blood glucose level. Because the older adult is more likely to have diabetes than a younger adult, this side effect may make controlling diabetes in an older adult much more difficult. For an older adult who is prescribed a systemic corticosteroid and who has diabetes, both diet and diabetic drug therapy may need to be adjusted while the patient is on corticosteroid therapy.

Nonsteroidal Antiinflammatory Drugs (NSAIDs)

Nonsteroidal antiinflammatory drugs (NSAIDs) are antiinflammatory drugs that are not similar in chemical structure to cortisol but prevent or limit the tissue and blood vessel general responses to injury or invasion by slowing the production of one or more inflammatory mediators. Some of these drugs are available only by prescription; others are available over the counter. NSAIDs most commonly are taken for pain and inflammation. They are used to treat many health problems, including fever, arthritis and other rheumatologic disorders, gout, systemic lupus erythematosus, pain after surgery, menstrual cramps, and blood clots.

There are many different NSAIDs. They can first be placed into a class on the basis of whether they nonselectively inhibit both the COX-1 and COX-2 forms of the cyclo-oxygenate enzymes or whether they are more selective for inhibiting the COX-2 form. Then they are further separated into groups on the basis of specific chemical makeup. All NSAIDs work in similar ways but vary in some side effects. The listings in the following table describe only the most common drugs in each group. Be sure to consult a reliable drug reference for more information about less commonly prescribed NSAIDs.

> **Critical Point for Safety**
>
> It is possible for an infection to be present without the usual symptoms of fever, pus formation, or redness when a person is taking systemic corticosteroids. Carefully examine the patient daily for other, less obvious symptoms, especially a sudden change in personality or a decrease in the sense of well-being.
>
> QSEN: Safety

> **Critical Point for Safety**
>
> Never substitute one corticosteroid for another because strengths vary. Too much drug can increase the side effects. Too low a dose can lead to adrenal insufficiency in addition to not managing the patient's inflammation problems.
>
> QSEN: Safety

Usual Adult Dosages for Common Nonsteroidal Antiinflammatory Drugs (NSAIDs)

Drug Class	Drug Name	Usual Maintenance Dosage
Nonselective Inhibitors of Cyclo-Oxygenase-1 and -2 (COX-1 and COX-2)		
Salicylates	aspirin (Anacin, Bayer, Bufferin, Ecotrin, Genacote, St. Joseph Aspirin, VAZALORE)	325–650 mg orally—three to four times daily
	diclofenac (Cambia, Cataflam, Licart, Voltaren)	50 mg orally two to three times daily 4 g (4.5 inches) topical gel for each knee, ankle, or foot four times daily
	diflunisal (Dolobid)	250–500 mg orally twice daily
	salsalate (Amigesic, Argesic-SA, Disalcid, MonoGesic, Salflex)	1500 mg orally twice daily or 1000 mg orally three times per day

Continued

Usual Adult Dosages for Common Nonsteroidal Antiinflammatory Drugs (NSAIDs)—cont'd

Drug Class	Drug Name	Usual Maintenance Dosage
Propionic Acid	flurbiprofen (Ansaid)	50–100 mg orally two to four times daily
	ibuprofen (Advil, Motrin)	300 mg orally four times daily or 400–800 mg orally three to four times daily
	naproxen (Aleve, Anaprox, Naprosyn)	250–500 mg orally twice daily
Acetic Acid	oxaprozin (Daypro)	600–1800 mg orally once daily
	indomethacin (Indocin, TIVORBEX)	25–75 mg orally two to three times daily
	nabumetone (Relafen)	500–1000 mg orally once or twice daily
Enolic Acid	piroxicam (Feldene)	20 mg orally once daily
Selective Inhibitors of Cyclo-Oxygenase-2 (COX-2)		
Pyrazole	celecoxib (Celebrex, ELYXYB)	200 mg orally once daily or 100 mg orally twice daily
Enolic Acid	meloxicam (Anjeso, Mobic, Qmiiz, Vivlodex)	7.5–15 mg orally once daily

 Do Not Confuse

Celebrex *with* **Celexa**

An order for Celebrex can be confused with Celexa. Celebrex is an antiinflammatory drug. Celexa is an antidepressant.

QSEN: Safety

Common Side Effects

Nonsteroidal Antiinflammatory Drugs

GI upset/ GI pain

Bleeding problems

Fluid retention

Hypertension

How NSAIDs work. The main action of NSAIDs is to inhibit the action of the COX enzyme that helps to make many of the different types of prostaglandins inside each cell (see Figure 10.1). Prostaglandins are a family of chemicals made by the body. Some prostaglandins have "housekeeping" cell jobs, helping cells and tissues remain healthy and functional. COX-2 is an enzyme found mostly in inflammatory cells. Its purpose is to help make all the mediators of the inflammatory response, including prostaglandins, leukotriene, and kinins. **Leukotriene** is a chemical made by the body that binds to its receptors and maintains an inflammatory response. Kinins are a group of chemicals made by the body that cause some of the signs and symptoms of inflammation, especially pain. The most common one is *bradykinin*. These mediators are responsible for creating all of the uncomfortable signs and symptoms of inflammation.

Most NSAIDs are nonselective and suppress both the COX-1 and COX-2 forms of the enzyme, so production of the helpful housekeeping mediators along with the inflammatory mediators is slowed. This means that these drugs cause side effects that are related to a reduction in the housekeeping mediators. Selective NSAIDs primarily suppress the COX-2 form of the enzyme and have fewer side effects from reducing the housekeeping mediators. *However, when taken at higher dosages or more frequently than prescribed, the selective NSAIDs also suppress the COX-1 form of the enzyme and have as many side effects as the nonselective NSAIDs.*

Intended responses of NSAIDs
- Redness and pain at the site of inflammation are reduced.
- Swelling and warmth at the site of inflammation are reduced.
- Body function in the area affected by inflammation is increased.
- Fever is reduced.

Common side effects of NSAIDs. Because COX-1 NSAIDs reduce the activity of the COX-1 and COX-2 enzymes, some normal healthy cell functions are affected. For example, all nonselective NSAIDs reduce platelet clumping and blood clotting. In fact, aspirin is often prescribed just for this action. However, just one dose of aspirin can reduce blood clotting for up to a week. Other NSAIDs reduce blood clotting only for the duration of the drug therapy. Blood clotting returns to normal within 24 to 48 hours after stopping the drug. Because anyone taking a nonselective NSAID is at increased risk for bleeding in response to slight injuries, surgery, or dental work, these drugs are discontinued before planned invasive procedures.

Nonselective NSAIDs can irritate the stomach lining and the rest of the gastrointestinal (GI) tract. The stomach is irritated when the drug touches it directly and again when the drugs are absorbed into the blood. This can lead to development of serious bleeding ulcers and pain in the GI tract.

All the NSAIDs except aspirin can reduce blood flow to the kidney and slow urine output. This action can lead to high blood pressure and kidney damage. In addition, the action of the nonselective NSAIDs on the kidney is exactly the opposite of the angiotensin-converting enzyme (ACE) inhibitor drugs for high blood pressure and can make them less effective (see Chapter 13).

Because selective NSAIDs mostly suppress the COX-2 pathway (see Figure 10.1), which allows the normal housekeeping functions of the COX-1 pathway to continue, they have fewer side effects than nonselective NSAIDs. However, if a patient takes more than the prescribed dose, the side effects are the same as for nonselective NSAIDs. These drugs do not reduce platelet action and blood clotting, so bruising and gum bleeding are not expected side effects.

Possible adverse effects of NSAIDs. In addition to possible kidney damage, common adverse effects of NSAIDs are the induction of asthma and allergic reactions. People who are sensitive to one NSAID are likely to be sensitive to all of them. In addition, taking two or more different NSAIDs at the same time increases the side effects and the risk for adverse effects.

Celecoxib (Celebrex) is made from a chemical similar to the sulfa drug type of antibiotic. A patient who is allergic to sulfa drugs is likely to also be allergic to celecoxib.

Another adverse reaction that was responsible for removing other selective NSAIDs from the market was an increase in heart attacks and strokes among patients taking these drugs. These drugs can increase clot formation in the small arteries of the heart and brain, especially when these arteries are narrowed by atherosclerosis or cigarette smoking. These drugs should be avoided by any patient who has angina, smokes, or has undergone coronary artery bypass graft surgery (CABG).

The higher the dose of NSAIDs and the longer they are taken, the more likely they are to trigger an adverse effect. Except for low-dose aspirin, most NSAIDs should not be taken daily for longer than 1 week for common aches and pains. For chronic diseases such as arthritis, the drugs may need to be taken much longer. When NSAIDs are needed long term, the patient is urged to find the lowest dose that still reduces his or her inflammation and pain.

The nonselective and selective NSAIDs can cause a reversible liver toxicity that may cause abdominal pain, elevated liver enzymes, and jaundice. This toxicity usually resolves when the patient stops taking the drug.

 Priority actions to take **before** ***giving NSAIDs.*** Before giving *celecoxib*, ask whether the patient has an allergy to sulfa antibiotics. A patient who is allergic to sulfa drugs is likely also to be allergic to celecoxib.

Always ask the patient whether he or she has had any problems with aspirin or any other over-the-counter NSAID. If the patient reports a previous problem with NSAIDs, do not give this drug without checking with the prescriber.

Give the drug at the time the patient is eating or shortly after a meal. When possible, have the patient drink a full glass of water or milk with the drug.

Tell the patient not to chew an NSAID capsule or an enteric-coated tablet because it will ruin its stomach-protective properties.

Assess the patient's blood pressure because NSAIDs can cause the patient to retain sodium and water, leading to higher blood pressure. If the patient is taking an ACE inhibitor for high blood pressure, NSAIDs can reduce its effectiveness and make heart failure and hypertension worse.

All NSAIDs interact with a hundred or more other drugs. Obtain a list of all other drugs the patient takes on a regular basis and consult with a pharmacist to determine whether any adjustments are needed in the patient's drug therapy regimen. Notify the prescriber of the need to make adjustments if this is indicated.

 Critical Point for Safety

Teach patients **not** to increase the dose of *celecoxib* or *meloxicam* because the risk for side effects, especially GI problems, is greatly increased and similar to those of the nonselective NSAIDs.

QSEN: Safety

 Critical Point for Safety

Do not give celecoxib (Celebrex) to a patient who is allergic to the sulfa drug type of antibiotics because celecoxib has a sulfa component.

QSEN: Safety

Drug Alert

Teaching Alert

Teach the patient to avoid chewing or crushing an NSAID capsule or enteric-coated tablet.

QSEN: Safety

⭐ *Priority actions to take after giving NSAIDs.* Bleeding risk increases within several hours after a dose of a COX-1 NSAID. Assess the patient's gums, mucous membranes, and open skin areas (around IV sites) during each shift for bleeding. Look for bruises and for pinpoint purple-red spots *(petechiae)*. Check urine, stool, and emesis for bright red blood, coffee-ground material, or other indications of bleeding.

When giving an NSAID to a patient who has never taken a drug from this family before, assess his or her blood pressure, breathing pattern, and pulse oximetry hourly after the first dose of an NSAID in case he or she is sensitive to it. Immediately report any breathing difficulty, drop in blood pressure, or decrease of 5% or more in oxygen saturation. Any of these signs and symptoms may indicate hypersensitivity to the drug.

⭐ *Teaching priorities for patients taking NSAIDs*
- To avoid GI side effects, always take an NSAID with food or on a full stomach.
- Do not chew an NSAID capsule or an enteric-coated tablet because doing so will ruin its stomach-protective properties.
- Check your bowel movements for the presence of bright red blood or dark, tarry-looking material that would indicate bleeding somewhere in the GI tract. Immediately report such symptoms to your prescriber.
- Because many NSAIDs reduce blood clotting, examine your gums daily while taking the drug for bleeding, especially after toothbrushing or flossing.
- Be sure and tell your dentist that you take NSAIDs before any dental procedure is performed.
- Inform all other health care providers and prescribers that you take NSAIDs to avoid a possible adverse interaction.
- If you are prescribed warfarin (Coumadin), do not take aspirin and other NSAIDs. These two drug types reduce blood clotting in different ways, so you would be at extreme risk for excessive bleeding and stroke.
- If you take celecoxib (Celebrex) or meloxicam (Mobic), take the drug exactly as prescribed. At higher doses, these drugs also cause the same side effects and problems as other NSAIDs.
- Weigh yourself at least twice each week in the morning before eating or drinking anything. Wear similar clothes each time so the weight is not changed by different types of clothing. Keep a record of your weight and tell your prescriber about a weight gain of more than 3 lb in a week. Also check your ankles for swelling (which could mean heart failure, especially if it is present in the morning).

Life span considerations for NSAIDs
Pediatric considerations. With the exception of ibuprofen, NSAIDs are not recommended for children except for selected chronic inflammatory disorders. In particular, aspirin and COX-2 NSAIDs are avoided because these drugs are associated with the development of Reye syndrome in children who also have a viral infection. Reye syndrome is a liver disease that can lead to coma, brain damage, and death.

Considerations for pregnancy and lactation. The stronger NSAIDs, particularly indomethacin and celecoxib, are avoided during the last 3 months of pregnancy because they may cause early closure of a blood vessel (the ductus arteriosus) important to fetal circulation and oxygenation.

Considerations for older adults. The older adult is at higher risk for cardiac problems when taking NSAIDs. Except for aspirin, these drugs cause salt and water retention that can lead to fluid overload and high blood pressure. Both of these problems increase the risk for heart attack and heart failure. Teach older adults taking NSAIDs to carefully monitor their weight, pulse, and urine output. Teach them the signs and symptoms of heart failure (weight gain; ankle swelling; and shortness of breath, especially when lying down).

Drugs for Allergic Inflammation
The two major mediators that are released during allergic reactions and lead to noninfectious inflammation are histamine and leukotriene. **Histamine** is a chemical mediator made by the body that binds to its receptor sites and often initiates changes

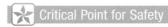

Critical Point for Safety

Nonselective NSAIDs, especially aspirin, should not be taken with warfarin (Coumadin) because they potentiate the effects of warfarin and greatly increase the risk for uncontrollable bleeding and hemorrhagic stroke.

QSEN: Safety

Critical Point for Safety

Do not give and teach parents not to give aspirin to children to prevent the development of Reye syndrome.

QSEN: Safety

that lead to inflammatory responses. It is the main mediator initiating allergic inflammation and capillary leak. The type of histamine receptors involved in allergic inflammation are the H_1 receptors located in blood vessels and respiratory mucous membranes. When histamine binds to H_1 receptors, tissue changes occur, causing blood vessel dilation, swelling, decreased blood pressure, poor heart contractions, narrowed airways, increased mucus production, and the formation of hives on the skin. When histamine binds to H_2 receptors, stomach acid production increases, and the risk for stomach ulcers is greatly increased. Drugs that specifically block H_2 receptors are discussed in Chapter 20.

Leukotriene, another inflammatory mediator that binds to a receptor, works with histamine to keep the inflammatory response going once it has started. The drugs used to slow or stop an inflammatory reaction once it has started or to prevent one from starting are the *antihistamines* (histamine antagonists) and *leukotriene inhibitors*. Both are most commonly used for symptoms of inflammation triggered by allergic reactions such as hives, watery eyes, and runny nose. Adult dosages of common drugs for allergic inflammation are listed in the following table. Consult a reliable drug reference for information about less common drugs for allergic inflammation.

Memory Jogger

Histamine and leukotriene are major mediators of inflammation and are responsible for many of the uncomfortable symptoms associated with allergic inflammation.

Usual Adult Dosages of Common Drugs for Allergic Inflammation

Drug Name	Usual Maintenance Dosages
Antihistamines (Histamine Antagonists)	
cetirizine (Zyrtec)	5–10 mg orally once daily
diphenhydramine (Benadryl)	12.5–50 mg orally or IV every 6 hr
fexofenadine (Allegra)	60 mg orally twice daily or 180 mg orally once daily
loratadine (Alavert, Claritin)	10 mg orally once daily
Leukotriene Inhibitors	
montelukast sodium (Singulair)	10 mg orally once daily in the evening
zafirlukast (Accolate)	20 mg orally twice daily
zileuton (Zyflo CR)	1200 mg orally twice daily within 1 hr after morning and evening meals

Do Not Confuse

Zyrtec *with* Zyban or Zyflo

An order for Zyrtec can be confused with Zyban or Zyflo. Zyrtec is an antihistamine. Zyban (bupropion) is an antidepressant used to help people stop smoking. Zyflo is a leukotriene inhibitor.

QSEN: Safety

How drugs for allergic inflammation work. Antihistamines (histamine antagonists) bind to H_1 histamine receptor sites in mucous membranes of the respiratory tract and in blood vessels, heart muscle, and the skin. This binding prevents the histamine produced by the body from binding to its receptors, thus slowing or stopping the tissue effects of inflammation (Figure 10.4).

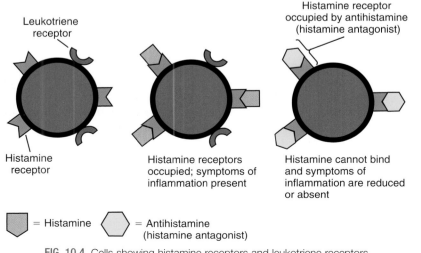

FIG. 10.4 Cells showing histamine receptors and leukotriene receptors.

Leukotriene inhibitors work in several ways to limit or prevent an allergy episode. Zileuton (Zyflo) prevents leukotriene production within WBCs. Montelukast (Singulair) and zafirlukast (Accolate) block the leukotriene receptors on cells. As a result of these drugs, a person with allergies has less of an inflammatory response.

Intended responses of drugs for allergic inflammation
- Blood vessels do not dilate and swelling is reduced.
- Mucus and other nasal, eye, and respiratory secretions are reduced.
- Narrowed airways widen.
- Hives decrease in size and itchiness.

Common side effects of drugs for allergic inflammation. Many *antihistamines* cause some degree of drowsiness. Each one varies in this side effect, and every person reacts differently. For some people, even a low dose causes severe drowsiness; for others, little or none occurs. Drinking alcohol when taking an antihistamine worsens the side effect of drowsiness.

Most *antihistamines* cause some degree of anticholinergic side effects of dry mouth, increased heart rate, increased blood pressure, dilated pupils, and urinary retention. The severity depends on which drug is used or prescribed and how the person responds.

The most common side effects of leukotriene inhibitors are headache and abdominal pain.

Possible adverse effects of drugs for allergic inflammation. *Leukotriene inhibitors* can cause allergic reactions, including hives and anaphylaxis. Both of these responses are rare.

Antihistamines may cause the pressure inside the eye (intraocular pressure [IOP]) to become too high for some people, especially those who already have glaucoma. The increased IOP can make glaucoma worse or even lead to blindness.

Antihistamines that induce sedation should not be given during an acute asthma attack. This is not because the drug causes asthma but because it can make the patient so drowsy that he or she may not be alert enough to work at breathing.

⭐ **Priority actions to take before *giving drugs for allergic inflammation*.** Ask if the patient is being treated for glaucoma, high blood pressure, or prostate enlargement. *Antihistamines* are contraindicated for a patient with any of these problems because these drugs could make these conditions worse.

Check to see what other drugs are prescribed for the patient. Opioids, sedatives, muscle relaxants, and barbiturates all increase the drowsy effect of *antihistamines*. If it is necessary to give an antihistamine to a patient who is taking any of these drug types, it should not be given within 4 hours of these drugs.

Because *leukotriene inhibitors*, especially zileuton, can cause liver impairment, ask the patient about any previous liver problems or jaundice (yellowing of the skin, sclera, or mucous membranes), tenderness in the liver area of the abdomen (right upper quadrant), nausea, or fatigue. Review baseline liver function tests for comparison after the patient has been taking the drug for several months. Table 1.4 in Chapter 1 lists normal liver function tests.

⭐ **Priority actions to take after *giving drugs for allergic inflammation*.** Assess the patient's pulse, blood pressure, and respiratory rate at least every 4 hours for the first 8 hours after giving the first dose an antihistamine. Notify the prescriber if heart rate becomes irregular, blood pressure changes significantly from the patient's baseline, or respiratory rate falls below 10 breaths/min and stays low.

For patients taking any leukotriene inhibitor, regularly assess the patient for signs and symptoms of decreased liver function, including constant fatigue, itchy skin, and yellowing of the skin or sclera.

Common Side Effects
Drugs for Allergic Inflammation

Headache Drowsiness

Blurred vision

Tachycardia Urinary retention

⭐ **Critical Point for Safety**

Do not give antihistamines to a patient who has glaucoma, prostate enlargement, hypertension, or urinary retention because these drugs have anticholinergic effects that worsen all of these problems.

QSEN: Safety

⭐ **Critical Point for Safety**

Do not give an antihistamine that causes drowsiness to a patient who is having an acute asthma attack to avoid interfering with the patient's respiratory efforts that require concentration.

QSEN: Safety

❗ **Drug Alert!**

Interaction Alert

When giving an antihistamine, especially one known to cause drowsiness, to a patient who is also taking opioids, sedatives, muscle relaxants, or barbiturates, avoid giving the antihistamine within 4 hr of these drugs.

QSEN: Safety

Teaching priorities for patients taking drugs for allergic inflammation

- Do not drink alcoholic beverages when taking antihistamines because the interaction can make you very sleepy.
- Avoid driving or operating dangerous or heavy machinery within 6 hours of taking these drugs.
- Contact your prescriber immediately if you develop vision changes or pain over the eyebrows, which could mean an increase in intraocular pressure.
- If you have prostate problems, remember to make sure you are urinating close to the same amount of fluid that you drink each day because urinary retention can be made worse by antihistamines. If you notice a sudden decrease in urine output or feel an urgent need to urinate and are unable to, contact your prescriber.
- If you have asthma, do not take antihistamines during an acute asthma attack at home because the drug could cause enough sleepiness to impair your ability to breathe.
- When taking a leukotriene inhibitor including montelukast (Singulair), zafirlukast (Accolate), or zileuton (Zyflo) report any skin yellowing, pain over the liver area, or darkening of the urine to your prescriber immediately because these drugs can reduce liver function.
- If you take montelukast (Singulair), report any depression or thoughts of suicide immediately to your prescriber.

> ⭐ **Critical Point for Safety**
>
> Assess the patient taking montelukast (Singulair) for mood changes, especially depression and suicidal thoughts, because this drug may intensify depression and other psychiatric disorders.
>
> QSEN: Safety

General Disease-Modifying Antirheumatic Drugs (DMARDs)

General disease-modifying antirheumatic drugs (DMARDs) or traditional DMARDs are drugs that reduce the progression and tissue destruction of the inflammatory disease processes. These oral drugs are somewhat more specific for the mediator they target than are NSAIDs. They are used to treat many types of chronic inflammatory disorders, including autoimmune disorders, such as rheumatoid arthritis, ankylosing spondylitis, psoriasis, psoriatic arthritis, Crohn disease, and ulcerative colitis. Most of these diseases involve excessive amounts of cytokines and other inflammatory mediators, which cause severe tissue damage and destruction. Very specific DMARDs are given parenterally and are considered *biologics* for targeted therapy. These specific DMARDs are presented in Chapter 11.

The general DMARDs are oral agents. The listings in the following table describe only the most commonly used DMARDs. Many of these drugs have uses beyond controlling inflammation. The dosages, as well as routes of drug delivery, for these other uses are different. Be sure to consult a reliable drug reference for more information about any less common DMARDs.

Adult Dosages of Common General Disease-Modifying Antirheumatic Drugs (DMARDs)

Drug Name	Usual Maintenance Dosages
azathioprine ❶ (Azasan, Imuran)	25 mg or 50 mg orally once daily, depending on patient response
hydroxychloroquine ❶ (Plaquenil, Quineprox)	200–400 mg orally once daily or in 2 divided doses
leflunomide ❶ (Arava)	20 mg orally once daily
methotrexate ❶ (Rheumatrex, Trexall)	7.5 mg orally once **weekly**, increased gradually to 20 mg orally once **weekly**[a]
sulfasalazine ❶ (Azulfidine, Sulfazine)	500–1000 mg orally per day for the first week. Increase the daily dose by 500 mg each week up to a maintenance dose of 2 g/day, given in 2–3 divided doses

[a]Methotrexate is given/taken once weekly, not daily.
❶ High-alert drug.

How general DMARDs work. *Azathioprine* is an immunosuppressive agent that interferes with DNA and RNA synthesis, especially in white blood cells (WBCs). This action reduces the number of inflammatory cells present and greatly reduces WBC production of inflammatory mediators.

> ⭐ **Critical Point for Safety**
>
> Methotrexate is administered or taken once *weekly*, not daily. Giving this drug daily is an overdose and would result in serious side effects and adverse effects.
>
> QSEN: Safety

Hydroxychloroquine, by unknown exact mechanisms, helps reduce inflammation by decreasing cell production of cytokines and inflammatory mediators. It is believed that this response is caused by interference with oxygen-dependent cellular metabolism in more rapidly dividing cells, including WBCs.

Leflunomide appears to inhibit one or more enzymes important for energy production in the mitochondria of some WBCs. The results of this inhibition are reduced WBC reproduction and reduced synthesis/release of inflammatory mediators, especially histamine and cytokines in joints. The drug also appears to slow osteoclast (bone destroying) activity to reduce bone damage and loss in arthritic joints.

Methotrexate is an antimetabolite drug often used in the treatment of many types of cancer. It suppresses an enzyme responsible for making the genetic base thymine. When thymine levels are low, DNA synthesis and replication in rapidly dividing cells, including WBCs, greatly reduce cell division and release of inflammatory mediators. Lower levels of mediators result in less inflammation.

Sulfasalazine is metabolized in the GI tract to its active forms (sulfapyridine and mesalamine). These agents inhibit the enzyme cyclo-oxygenase, resulting in less synthesis of most inflammatory mediators. In addition, mesalamine directly inhibits the synthesis of leukotriene in WBCs involved in the inflammatory responses.

Intended responses of general DMARDs
- Redness and pain at the site of inflammation are reduced.
- Swelling and warmth at the site of inflammation are reduced.
- Body function in the area affected by inflammation is increased.

Common side effects of general DMARDs. All general DMARDs have the side effects of nausea and vomiting, rash and other skin reactions, headache, thinning hair, and weight loss. *Hydroxychloroquine* and *sulfasalazine* also cause photosensitivity with a greatly increased risk for burns associated with sun exposure and other exposures to ultraviolet light. *Leflunomide* and *methotrexate* often cause hypertension and muscle aches and pains.

Possible adverse effects of general DMARDs. All of the general DMARDs are high-alert drugs and have many possible adverse effects. These drugs suppress bone marrow activity, leading to anemia and increased risk for infection. Additionally, all of these drugs are somewhat cytotoxic and increase the risk for development of malignancy. This risk is greater when higher dosages are taken over the course of years.

These drugs are liver toxic and can result in liver impairment with elevated liver enzymes and development of jaundice. Usually, the liver problems are reversed once the drug therapy is stopped. However, the liver problems are worsened if the patient also drinks alcohol or takes other liver toxic drugs (e.g., acetaminophen, drugs to treat hepatitis C, antitubercular drugs).

With the immunosuppression caused by the general DMARDs, vaccinations taken during therapy or within 2 weeks of starting therapy are less effective. Another adverse effect of all general DMARDs is the huge number of interactions these drugs can have with other drugs and supplements.

Azathioprine is broken down by two specific enzymes, thiopurine S-methyltransferase (TPMT) and nucleotide diphosphatase (NUDT15). In patients who have a genetic deficiency for the active forms of either of these enzymes, even normal doses of the drug accumulate, resulting in severe toxicities including profound bone marrow suppression and even death. Patient testing for such deficiencies is highly recommended before treatment with azathioprine is started. Most males taking azathioprine have greatly reduced sperm production and infertility. Usually, this problem is reversed after the drug is stopped.

Hydroxychloroquine has several possible additional but not common adverse effects. It can cause ocular toxicities, such as making the cornea opaque and inducing retinal damage that result in permanent vision loss. The drug may suppress red blood cell (RBC) formation, leading to anemia. In people who are deficient in the

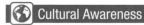

Common Side Effects
General DMARDs

Nausea and   Rash   Headache
Vomiting

Thinning   Weight loss
hair

Cultural Awareness

Before hydroxychloroquine is prescribed for a man of Mediterranean heritage, he should be tested for a G6PD deficiency. If he has a deficiency of this enzyme, the drug will trigger a severe hemolytic anemia.

enzyme glucose-6-phosphate dehydrogenase (G6PD), hydroxychloroquine triggers a hemolytic anemia. (This enzyme deficiency is most common among men of Mediterranean heritage.)

At higher dosages, severe cardiac problems, including a variety of dysrhythmias, heart failure, and prolonged QT syndrome, have been reported. This drug should be avoided in patients who have preexisting cardiac problems. Hydroxychloroquine is associated with severe hypoglycemia, even among patients who are not taking anti-diabetic drugs.

The severe skin reaction of Stevens-Johnson syndrome has also been reported with this drug. Patients with preexisting depression have an increased risk for suicide ideation. Both *hydroxychloroquine* and *sulfasalazine* may cause tinnitus (ringing in the ears) and hearing loss.

Leflunomide has a very long half-life. Side effects and adverse effects may continue to be present weeks after the drug is discontinued. This drug is known to cause birth defects and must be avoided during pregnancy. Serious pulmonary disease, including interstitial pulmonary problems, has developed among people taking the drug long term, and the drug is not recommended for use in people with preexisting pulmonary problems. In addition, the hyperglycemia of diabetes is intensified with leflunomide. Both *leflunomide* and *sulfasalazine* have induced some degree of peripheral neuropathy with numbness, tingling, burning, and decreased sensory perception in the feet and hands.

Methotrexate can cause pulmonary problems including pulmonary fibrosis, and should not be used in patients with preexisting pulmonary problems. Ocular toxicities, even with the lower doses used as once weekly drug administration, have occurred with methotrexate. Most of the more severe neurologic and kidney adverse reactions do not occur with the dosages of methotrexate used as general DMARD therapy.

Sulfasalazine's mechanism of action to reduce thymine synthesis can result in a folic acid deficiency. Patients taking this drug often need vitamin supplements containing folic acid. Most males taking this drug have greatly reduced sperm production and infertility. Usually, this problem is reversed after the drug is stopped. The drug has a sulfa component. Any patient with an allergy to a sulfonamide drug is likely to have an allergy to sulfasalazine. Because the drug has a sulfa component and can form crystals in the urine, there is a risk for kidney injury with sulfasalazine. The drug also turns the urine an orange color.

 Priority actions to take before *giving general DMARDs.* Review the patient's laboratory test results for bone marrow function (see Table 1.6 in Chapter 1) and liver function (see Table 1.4 in Chapter 1). Use these results to assess the patient's baseline hematologic status and liver function before therapy begins and to determine possible side effects of therapy. If these tests are abnormal, therapy with DMARDs may be delayed.

Assess the patient for any active infection. If an infection is present, therapy is delayed until the infection is gone.

For women of child-bearing age who are sexually active, ensure that a pregnancy test is negative before beginning the drug therapy with *azathioprine, leflunomide,* or *methotrexate.* Instruct these women to use two reliable forms of contraception or to avoid intercourse for the duration of therapy and for 1 month after therapy is completed.

Obtain a complete list of all other prescribed and over-the-counter drugs and supplements the patient uses on a regular basis. Check with the pharmacist for which of the patient's other drugs are likely to have a negative interaction with general DMARD therapy and what adjustments may need to be made. Be sure the prescriber is aware of any needed adjustments.

Before giving the first dose of sulfasalazine, ask the patient whether he or she has ever had an allergic reaction to sulfa antibiotics. A patient who is allergic to sulfa drugs is likely also to have an allergic reaction to sulfasalazine.

For patients prescribed *hydroxychloroquine* or *methotrexate,* assess the patient's vision before therapy begins.

 Memory Jogger

The long half-life of *leflunomide* results in the persistence of side effects and adverse effects for weeks after the drug is discontinued.

Memory Jogger

All of the general DMARDs have the potential to interact with a large number of other drugs. Always ask the patient what other drugs or supplements he or she takes on a regular basis and check with the pharmacist for potential interactions.

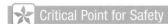
Critical Point for Safety

Both hydroxychloroquine and methotrexate can cause serious eye damage that can lead to permanent loss of vision. Assess the patient's vision before therapy begins and teach him or her to see an ophthalmologist regularly. If a patient notices any persistent blurring or other vision changes, he or she needs to notify the prescriber immediately.

QSEN: Safety

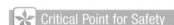
Critical Point for Safety

Assess the patient taking *methotrexate* for mood changes, especially depression and suicidal thoughts, because this drug may intensify depression and other psychiatric disorders.

QSEN: Safety

When preparing to give any general DMARD, use gloves or a "no-touch" technique because these drugs are highly toxic and can be absorbed through the skin of anyone coming into direct contact with them. Only the patient should touch these drugs.

⭐ *Priority actions to take* **after** *giving general DMARDs.* Most people prescribed a general DMARD for an inflammatory autoimmune disorder will be taking the drug on an outpatient basis. However, when these patients are hospitalized for other issues, they will need to continue the prescribed general DMARD therapy.

For patients taking any general DMARD, regularly assess the patient for signs and symptoms of decreased liver function, including constant fatigue, itchy skin, and yellowing of the skin or sclera. Review and compare liver function tests for elevated enzyme and bilirubin levels.

Ensure that the patient drinks a full glass of water when taking *sulfasalazine* and understands the need to drink more fluids throughout the 24-hour day.

Assess for symptoms of infection (e.g., fever, drainage, foul-smelling urine, productive cough, or redness around an open skin area) and report any symptoms to the prescriber. General DMARDs may make an existing infection worse.

⭐ *Teaching priorities for patients taking general DMARDs*
- Do not allow other people to touch the drug directly. These drugs are toxic and can be absorbed through the skin. They can affect people who come into direct contact with them.
- Check yourself daily for signs and symptoms of infection (e.g., fever, cough, malaise, foul-smelling drainage, pain or burning on urination). If any of these are present, notify your prescriber immediately.
- Avoid crowds and people who are ill because resistance to infection is decreased and you are more susceptible to infectious illnesses.
- If you are a sexually active woman of child-bearing age and your partner is a fertile male, use two reliable methods of birth control while taking azathioprine, leflunomide, or methotrexate and for at least 1 month after therapy is stopped. If you think you have become pregnant, stop the drug and notify your prescriber immediately.
- This therapy can damage your liver and you should avoid drinking alcohol or using any other drugs that can also damage your liver.
- Notify your prescriber if you develop yellowing of your skin or eyes, darkening of your urine, or lighter-colored stools. These problems are signs of liver toxicity.
- If you notice a rash or other skin changes, be sure to have your prescriber check the skin change because some rashes are expected and not serious, whereas other changes can indicate a dangerous condition.
- Whenever you notice a new change or persistent side effect, notify your prescriber to determine whether it is safe to continue taking the drug or if the problem is serious.
- Remember that methotrexate is taken only once per week and not daily.
- While taking methotrexate, if you notice some new feelings of depression or if you already have depression and the sensation becomes worse, notify your prescriber immediately, especially if you have thoughts of harming yourself.
- If you take hydroxychloroquine or methotrexate, report any changes in your vision immediately to your prescriber. Keep all appointments with your ophthalmologist.
- If you take hydroxychloroquine, take your pulse at least twice daily. If you notice a persistent irregular pulse or if your pulse is consistently below 60 beats/min, notify your prescriber immediately.
- If you take hydroxychloroquine or sulfasalazine, be sure to wear a hat, protective clothing, and sunscreen whenever you are outdoors. These drugs increase your sensitivity to the sun and can cause severe sunburn even with minimal exposure.
- If you take leflunomide or methotrexate, report any new persistent episodes of coughing or other breathing changes to your prescriber immediately.

- When taking sulfasalazine, drink at least 3 liters of fluid, especially water, daily to prevent kidney problems. A change in urine color to an orange appearance is expected and does not indicate a problem.

Life span considerations for general DMARDs

Pediatric considerations. Although all general DMARDs can be highly toxic, they are used for severe pediatric inflammatory autoimmune disorders. It is important to ensure that parents know the specific side effects and adverse effects associated with their child's therapy and understand how to monitor for them. These drugs must be kept out of reach of children because accidental overdosages can be fatal.

Considerations for pregnancy and lactation. *Azathioprine, leflunomide,* and *methotrexate* are known to cause severe birth defects and are to be avoided during pregnancy. If taken during the first trimester, the risk for embryonic or fetal loss is high. Teach women of childbearing age who are sexually active with a male partner to use two reliable methods of contraception. Also instruct women who suspect that they have become pregnant to stop the drug immediately and contact their prescriber.

Hydroxychloroquine and *sulfasalazine* are not known to cause birth defects and may be used during pregnancy when the benefits of the therapy have been determined to outweigh possible harm. Breastfeeding is not recommended during therapy with any of the general DMARDs.

 Critical Point for Safety

Teach women of childbearing age who are sexually active with a male partner and taking *azathioprine, leflunomide,* or *methotrexate* to use two reliable methods of contraception. Also instruct women who suspect that they have become pregnant to stop the drug immediately and contact their prescriber.

QSEN: Safety

Get Ready for the NCLEX® Examination!

Key Points

- Teach the patient taking systemic corticosteroids for a week or longer to never suddenly stop taking the drug to prevent adrenal insufficiency. These patients may also need higher dosages of corticosteroids during periods of high stress or illness to prevent adrenal insufficiency.
- Do not substitute one type of corticosteroid for another because strengths vary. Too much drug can increase the side effects. Too low a dose can lead to adrenal insufficiency in addition to not managing the patient's inflammation problems.
- Remind patients taking systemic corticosteroids to avoid crowds and people who are ill because the effects of corticosteroids reduce a patient's immunity and resistance to infection.
- It is possible for an infection to be present without the usual symptoms of fever, pus formation, or redness when a person is taking systemic corticosteroids. Carefully examine the patient daily for other, less obvious symptoms, especially a sudden change in personality or sense of well-being.
- Teach patients to always take an NSAID with food or on a full stomach.
- Teach patients to never take aspirin if they are also taking warfarin (Coumadin).
- Teach patients **not** to increase the dose of *celecoxib* or *meloxicam* because the risk for side effects, especially GI problems, is greatly increased and similar to those of the nonselective NSAIDs.
- Do not give celecoxib (Celebrex) to a patient who is allergic to the sulfa drug type of antibiotics because celecoxib also contains a sulfa component.
- Do not give and teach parents not to give aspirin to children to prevent the development of Reye syndrome.

- Do not give an antihistamine known to cause drowsiness to a patient having an acute asthma attack.
- Do not give antihistamines to a patient who has glaucoma, prostate enlargement, hypertension, or urinary retention because these drugs have anticholinergic effects that worsen all of these problems.
- Warn patients who are taking antihistamines at home not to drink alcohol, drive, or operate heavy machinery within 6 hours of taking these drugs because of the risk for excessive drowsiness.
- Avoid giving an antihistamine within 4 hours of the time when an opioid, sedative, muscle relaxant, or barbiturate was given to the patient.
- Assess the patient taking montelukast (Singulair) for mood changes, especially depression and suicidal thoughts, because this drug may intensify depression and other psychiatric disorders.
- All general DMARDs are high-alert drugs and increase the risk for development of malignancy (cancer).
- Methotrexate is administered or taken once *weekly*, not daily. Giving this drug daily is an overdose and would result in serious side effects and adverse effects.
- Before *hydroxychloroquine* is prescribed for a man of Mediterranean heritage, he should be tested for a G6PD deficiency. If he has a deficiency of this enzyme, the drug will trigger a severe hemolytic anemia.
- *Azathioprine, leflunomide,* and *methotrexate* are teratogens known to cause birth defects. Teach women of childbearing age who are sexually active with a male partner and taking one of these drugs to use two reliable methods of contraception. Also instruct women who suspect that they have become pregnant to stop the drug immediately and contact their prescriber.

- Assess the patient taking *methotrexate* for mood changes, especially depression and suicidal thoughts, because this drug may intensify depression and other psychiatric disorders.
- Assess the patient's vision before therapy with either hydroxychloroquine or methotrexate begins and teach him or her to see an ophthalmologist regularly. If a patient notices any persistent blurring or other vision changes, he or she needs to notify the prescriber immediately.

Additional Learning Resources

🌐 Be sure to visit your Evolve website (http://evolve.elsevier.com/Workman/pharmacology/) for additional online resources.

SG Go to your Study Guide for additional learning activities to help you master this chapter content.

Review Questions

See *Answers to In-Text Review Questions* in the back of the book for answers to these questions.

1. **Which statement regarding inflammation or the inflammatory response is true?**

   A. Inflammation is either accompanied by infection or causes infection.
   B. The responses of inflammation occur only in tissues and organs of the immune system.
   C. The tissue responses caused by inflammation provide immediate protective and repair processes.
   D. Because inflammation can lead to tissue damage, suppressing this response as soon as possible after its onset is critical for maintaining health.

2. **Which side effect of corticosteroid therapy will the nurse warn a patient is a permanent change even after the drug is stopped?**

   A. Difficulty sleeping
   B. Stretch marks
   C. Weight gain
   D. Moon face

3. **Which clinical symptom(s) will the nurse expect to find in a patient who has a release of histamines by white blood cells (WBC)?**

   A. Excessive bleeding
   B. Foul-smelling urine
   C. Swelling and edema
   D. Diarrhea and abdominal cramping

4. **A patient who is to be discharged with a prescription for prednisone asks the nurse why it is necessary to report any illness to the health care provider. What is the nurse's best response?**

   A. "The usual daily dosage may not be adequate during periods of illness or severe stress."
   B. "You will need to have your dosage tapered to safely come off of this drug."
   C. "The drug will increase your risk for nausea and vomiting when you are ill."
   D. "You may need an increased drug dose to protect you from infection."

5. **A patient is prescribed to receive 20 mg of oral prednisone right now. The drug received from the pharmacy is prednisolone 40 mg tablet. What is the nurse's best first action?**

   A. Calculating the equivalent dose of prednisolone for the prescribed prednisone dose
   B. Notifying the prescriber and requesting a prescription for an equivalent prednisolone dose
   C. Cutting the prednisolone in half and administering the dose
   D. Notifying the pharmacy and requesting the prescribed drug

6. **How are selective and nonselective nonsteroidal antiinflammatory drugs (NSAIDs) different?**

   A. Nonselective NSAIDs are available over the counter because they have few side effects and selective NSAIDs are only available by prescription.
   B. Nonselective NSAIDs disrupt cyclo-oxygenase enzymes type 1 and 2 equally and selective NSAIDs primarily disrupt only type 2.
   C. Selective NSAIDs can be taken or administered orally or parenterally, whereas nonselective NSAIDs can only be given orally.
   D. Selective NSAIDs are less habit-forming than are nonselective NSAIDs.

7. **Which patient history information alerts the nurse to an increased risk for a possible adverse effect for celecoxib?**

   A. Smokes two packs of cigarettes daily
   B. Received an influenza vaccination 4 days ago
   C. Usually drinks a glass of beer every night
   D. Has a serious penicillin allergy

8. **Why is the use of the antihistamine diphenhydramine avoided during an allergic asthma attack?**

   A. The drowsiness side effect can reduce the patient's conscious efforts to breathe.
   B. It is of little use because most asthma attacks are not caused by excessive histamine release.
   C. Major adverse effects of this drug are bronchoconstriction and increased mucous production.
   D. Diphenhydramine competes with adrenal cortisol for its receptors and can reduce the antiinflammatory action of this natural hormone.

9. **A 2-year-old child is prescribed to receive 2.5 mg of loratadine syrup. The available drug is loratadine 5 mg/5 mL. How many mL will the nurse prepare are the correct dose for this patient?**

   A. 10 mL
   B. 7.5 mL
   C. 5 mL
   D. 2.5 mL

10. **A patient who is prescribed to take oral naproxen daily is scheduled to have oral surgery in 2 weeks. How far in advance of the oral surgery does the nurse advise the patient to stop taking the drug to ensure that the risk for excessive bleeding from the procedure is reduced?**

    A. 1 hour
    B. 12 hours
    C. 24 to 48 hours
    D. 7 days

11. What is the **most important** question for the nurse to ask a patient who is to start taking the drug sulfasalazine for rheumatoid arthritis?

   A. "Are you pregnant or breastfeeding?"
   B. "When was your last test for tuberculosis?"
   C. "Have you ever had a reaction to a 'sulfa' drug?"
   D. "Have you had a vaccination within the last 30 days?"

12. What is the most **important precaution** for the nurse to teach a patient taking hydroxychloroquine to **prevent harm**?

   A. "Avoid crowds and people who are ill."
   B. "Remember to take this drug only once weekly, not daily."
   C. "If you gain more than 2 lb in 1 week, report this to your prescriber immediately."
   D. "If your vision becomes persistently blurred, report this to your prescriber immediately."

Clinical Judgment

1. The patient is a 44-year-old woman who has a serious inflammatory respiratory problem of 4 months duration that requires high-dose corticosteroid therapy daily. She is currently hospitalized for an acute exacerbation of the problem and her dose of corticosteroids has been increased. Indicate which actions are **most important** for the nurse to specifically instruct any assistive personnel (AP) assigned to this patient to perform to **prevent harm. Select all that apply.**

   A. Using a lift sheet to move the patient in bed
   B. Taking blood pressure measurements only in the right arm
   C. Wearing gloves while providing personal care
   D. Padding elbows and heels
   E. Offering fluids every 2 hours while awake
   F. Applying a gait belt when ambulating with the patient
   G. Weighing the patient daily
   H. Carefully measuring intake and output

2. The patient is a 38-year-old woman who was diagnosed with rheumatoid arthritis 2 years ago. She is a nursing assistant on an inpatient oncology unit. During the past 6 months, her mobility has decreased and her pain has increased. She takes 10 mg of prednisone daily and is now prescribed to start taking methotrexate. The nurse is developing a teaching plan with take-home instructions/precautions about this drug. **Use an X to indicate which patient statements indicate Correct Understanding of therapy with methotrexate, which statements indicate that More Instruction Is Needed, and which statements are Neither Correct nor Incorrect (not directly relevant to the proposed drug therapy).**

PATIENT STATEMENT	CORRECT UNDERSTANDING	MORE INSTRUCTION NEEDED	NEITHER CORRECT NOR INCORRECT
I have watched nurses give a lot of injections and am sure I can learn to give them to myself.			
My husband had a vasectomy 3 years ago, so I don't have to worry about getting pregnant while taking this drug.			
I understand that I should see my dentist and ophthalmologist regularly while I am taking this drug.			
I plan to take the methotrexate at the same time daily so I won't forget to take it.			
My daughter gave me a large hat to protect me when I am out in the sun.			
Wearing gloves when I prepare my dose of methotrexate will protect me from absorbing it.			
Luckily, I am not allergic to sulfa types of antibiotics.			
Last month I took my "flu shot" so I won't need another one until next year.			

Immunizations and Immunosuppressant Drugs

Learning Objectives

The content presented in this chapter should help you to:

1. Explain the differences between active immunity and passive immunity and between natural and artificial immunity.
2. Explain how vaccination affects immunity.
3. Explain the names, actions, usual adult dosages, possible side effects, and adverse effects of biologic immunosuppressive drugs to manage autoimmune disorders.
4. Describe priority actions to take before and after giving biologic immunosuppressive drugs.
5. Prioritize essential information to teach patients taking biologic immunosuppressive drugs.
6. Explain the actions of selective immunosuppressant drugs used to prevent transplant rejection.
7. Describe priority actions to take before and after giving selective immunosuppressant drugs to prevent transplant rejection.
8. Prioritize essential information to teach patients taking selective immunosuppressant drugs to prevent transplant rejection.
9. Describe appropriate life span considerations for vaccination, biologic immunosuppressive drugs, and selective immunosuppressant drugs.

Key Terms

acquired immunity (ă-KWĬRD ĭ-MŪ-nĭ-tē) (p. 187) An adaptive (learned) internal protection that results in long-term resistance to the effects of invading microorganisms.

active immunity (ĂK-tĭv ĭ-MŪ-nĭ-tē) (p. 190) The antibody-mediated immunity you acquire when your body actually learns to make specific antibodies in response to the presence of specific antigens.

antibody (ĂN-tĭ-bŏd-ē) (p. 188) A Y-shaped protein with areas on its "arms" that bind directly and tightly to anything that has the same specific code that triggered the B cell to respond by making specific antibodies. Also called immune globulins or immunoglobulins.

antigen (ĂN-tĭ-jĕn) (p. 188) Any cell, product, or protein with a code different from your own that enters your body and is recognized by your immune system as "foreign" and that will trigger your B cells to produce specific antibodies against it.

antirejection drugs (ĂN-tĭ-rē-jĕk-shŭn DRŬGZ) (p. 201) Drugs that suppress the components of the immune system responsible for rejection of transplanted tissues and organs.

artificially acquired active immunity (ăr-tĭ-FĬSH-ăl-ē ă-KWĬRD ĂK-tĭv ĭ-MŪ-nĭ-tē) (p. 190) The type of antibody-mediated immunity that is started when an antigen is placed purposefully into your body to force your B cells to make a specific antibody against it.

artificially acquired passive immunity (ăr-tĭ-FĬSH-ăl-ē ă-KWĬRD PĂ-sĭv ĭ-MŪ-nĭ-tē) (p. 193) The type of antibody-mediated immunity you would have if antibodies made by another person, animal, or a laboratory against an antigen were injected into your body.

autoimmune disorder (ŏ-tō-ĭ-MŪN dĭs-ŌR-dŭr) (p. 194) A pathologic condition in which a person's immune system sees his or her own cells and tissues as foreign and develops inappropriate immune responses that attack these body cells or tissues.

biologics (bīō LÄ jik) (p. 196) A class of complex antiinflammatory drugs derived from living sources that target specific inflammatory cells, components, or products to modify chronic disorders associated with inflammation and tissue damage.

immunization (ĭ-MŪ-nĭ-ZĂ-shŭn) (p. 191) The desired outcome or response of successful vaccination in which the person actually develops immunity to the substance in the vaccine. Often used interchangeably with the term vaccination.

immunosuppressant drugs (ĬM-ū-nō-sŭ-PRĔS-ĕnt DRŬGZ) (p. 195) Drugs that inhibit or prevent the optimal or excessive functioning of immune system.

innate immunity (ĭn-ĀT ĭ-MŪ-nĭ-tē) (p. 187) The natural native resistance to infection provided by the general responses of inflammation. Innate immunity is nonspecific and does not require white blood cell training.

monoclonal antibodies (mŏn-ō-KLŌ-năl ăn-tĭ-BŌD-ēs) (p. 196) A type of biologic drug composed of antibodies produced by mouse cells or a combination of mouse and human antibody-producing cells targeted against specific proteins that cause tissue damage.

naturally acquired active immunity (NĂ-chŭr-ăl-ē ă-KWĬRD ĂK-tĭv ĭ-MŪ-nĭ-tē) (p. 190) The type of antibody-mediated immunity that is started when your body is invaded by a foreign organism without assistance and your B cells learn to make antibodies against the invaders.

naturally acquired passive immunity (NĂ-chŭr-ăl-ē ă-KWĬRD PĂ-sĭv ĭ-MŪ-nĭ-tē) (p. 190) The type of antibody-mediated immunity you acquired as a result of antibodies transferred to you as a fetus or infant from your mother through the placenta and through breast milk.

polyclonal antibodies (pŏl-ē-KLŌ-năl ăn-tĭ-BŌD-ēs) (p. 204) Antibodies produced by other animals (usually horses and rabbits) in response to the administration of human white blood cells, especially T cells.

vaccination (văk-sĭn-Ā-shŭn) (p. 191) The deliberate injection or ingestion of an organism or other antigen for the intended purpose of stimulating B cells into producing antibodies specific to the antigen, resulting in immunologic resistance to any disease caused by the antigen.

vaccine (văk-SĒN) (p. 191) A biologic preparation containing the universal product code of a specific disease-causing microorganism. It can be composed of the organism itself, a part of the organism that retains its unique code, or a protein the organism produces that also contains the unique code.

OVERVIEW OF THE IMMUNE SYSTEM AND IMMUNITY

As discussed in Chapter 10, inflammation and the inflammatory responses provide day-to-day, nonspecific protection against invasion of disease-causing (*pathogenic*) organisms. These nonspecific responses recognize when an invading organism enters the body through the skin, mucous membranes, respiratory tract, or the gastrointestinal tract and take general steps to remove or destroy the invaders. Because these protective inflammatory responses are general and can be triggered by any invasion, they are considered **innate immunity** (native immunity) providing resistance to infection that your body performs without training. It is called *innate* or *native* because you were born with it and it is one of the reasons that humans do not get some types of animal disorders, such as distemper or mange. These general protective responses are helpful but can be overwhelmed when organisms invade in great numbers. In addition, these general protective responses do not prevent us from getting sick over and over again every time our bodies are heavily invaded by the same organisms. General inflammatory responses are protective but do not provide true immunity to a specific invader. However, these general responses are essential in working with the immune system to provide true immunity.

True immunity is the ability of the body to recognize a specific organism when it re-invades a person and to take steps to remove, inactivate, or destroy the invading organisms before illness can occur. The immune system is critical to developing true immunity. Parts of the immune system are located throughout the body and are more heavily concentrated in areas where invasion and injury are more likely to occur. The main tissues of the immune system are the white blood cells (WBCs) or *leukocytes*, the substances these cells produce, and tissues containing colonies of WBCs, such as lymph nodes, tonsils, the intestinal tract, and the spleen. The bone marrow is the original source of WBCs, many of which then circulate throughout the body. The WBCs involved in inflammation are the neutrophils, macrophages, eosinophils, and basophils, along with a tissue-based cell called a mast cell. These are the cells that provide the general innate protection against invasion.

The B lymphocytes (B cells) and T lymphocytes (T cells) together are responsible for providing long-lasting true immunity so that with many types of diseases caused by infectious organisms, you actually develop the disease only once. For example, if you had chickenpox (caused by the *varicella zoster* virus [VZV]) as a child, it is unlikely that you will develop chickenpox again even when you are tremendously re-exposed to VZV. This is because the lymphocytes that were exposed to VZV when you originally got sick with the chickenpox learned to recognize VZV and began making specific immunity in the form of antibodies to that virus. Because the immune system has to learn to make antibodies, this type of immunity is *acquired* rather than innate.

Acquired immunity is an *adaptive* or learned internal protection that results in long-term resistance to the effects of invading microorganisms. These protective responses are not automatic. Much of acquired immunity occurs through the processes of antibody formation by B cells and antibody actions.

ANTIBODY PRODUCTION

Antibody production is an adaptive process performed by B cells after they learn to recognize a specific invader. All WBCs can recognize an invader, and the WBCs

 Memory Jogger

Inflammation (innate immunity) helps protect the body but cannot provide true immunity to any specific disease-causing microorganism.

 Memory Jogger

The lymphocyte types (T cells and B cells) of WBCs are the ones that provide long-lasting true immunity but require the assistance of WBCs of general inflammation to do so.

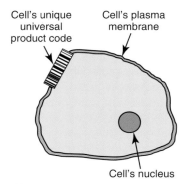

FIG. 11.1 Human cell with unique universal product code.

Cell's unique universal product code

Cell's plasma membrane

Cell's nucleus

---

involved in inflammation are best at it. All cells in your body have a universal product code specific to you (and any identical siblings you may have) (Figure 11.1). This code, which is your *tissue type,* is genetically determined by genes you inherit from your parents. So these codes are similar among family members but only exactly the same in identical siblings (e.g., identical twins or triplets). Your immune system cells, which also have this unique "you" code, have the special ability to compare the code of any cell or protein it encounters to determine whether it is one of your cells. If the code is identical to your code, the encountered cell is considered "self," and the normal immune system takes no action against it. If the code of the encountered cell or protein is not a perfect match to your code, the immune system cells consider it an invader that is "foreign" to you (Figure 11.2). Once a foreign or invading cell is recognized, the general inflammatory cells take steps to eliminate, neutralize, or destroy it. If you are heavily invaded by infectious organisms and get sick, the general inflammation cells help the lymphocytes also recognize the organisms as foreign so that they can start specific antibody production to develop immunity to them.

Any cell, product, or protein with a code different from your own that enters your body and is recognized by your immune system as foreign is an **antigen** to you. Usually, the general WBCs first recognize the antigen as foreign. Some of these WBCs bring the invading antigen into contact with fresh, newly made "unsensitized" lymphocytes. The T cell helps the B cell learn exactly how the invading antigen's code is different from your code and sensitizes the B cell against the specific invader as an antigen (Animation 11.1). Then, the sensitized B cell starts making and releasing antibodies that will bind only to cells or products that carry that specific invader's code. An **antibody** is a "Y"-shaped protein with areas on its "arms" that bind directly and tightly to anything that has the same specific code that triggered the B cell to make the antibody to begin with. (Another name for antibodies is *immunoglobulins.*) Each B cell learns to make only one specific type of antibody that can only recognize and bind to one specific antigen. Figure 11.3 outlines this process.

When you are invaded by so many influenza A viruses that you actually develop influenza, many fresh unsensitized B cells in your body start learning to make anti-influenza antibodies. Not a lot of anti-influenza antibodies are made at this time, but the ones that are made are important in helping you get well in a week to 10 days so that your influenza does not last for several months. The most important part about B cells becoming sensitized against an antigen and learning to make a specific antibody is that they always remember how to make those antibodies (Animation 11.2). Also, all future cells produced by these sensitized B cells (known as plasma cells) are not really "fresh" or unsensitized. They are born sensitized and already know how to make the specific antibody. So with time, you have millions of B cells sensitized against the specific influenza A virus you caught. When you are re-exposed to the same strain of influenza A virus later, even when the exposure is huge, you will not

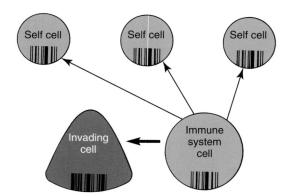

FIG. 11.2 Immune system cell recognizing an invading or foreign cell by differences in its universal product code. (Modified from Ignatavicius, D. D., & Workman, M. L. [2016]. *Medical-surgical nursing: Patient-centered collaborative care* [8th ed.]. St. Louis: Saunders.)

1. Invasion of the body by new antigens in sufficient numbers to stimulate an immune response.

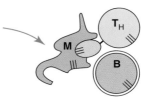

2. Interaction of macrophage (M) and helper/inducer T cell (T$_H$) in the processing and presenting of the antigen to the unsensitized "virgin" B lymphocyte (B).

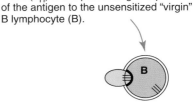

7. On reexposure to the same antigen, the sensitized lymphocytes and their progeny produce large quantities of the antibody specific to the antigen. In addition, new "virgin" B lymphocytes become sensitized to the antigen and also begin antibody production.

3. Sensitization of the virgin B lymphocyte to the new antigen.

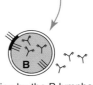

6. Antibody binding causes cellular events and attracts other leukocytes to the complex. The interaction of other leukocytes along with the cellular events results in the neutralization, destruction, or elimination of the antigen.

4. Antibody production by the B lymphocyte. These antibodies are directed specifically against the initiating antigen. The antibodies are released from the B lymphocyte and float freely in the blood and some other fluids.

5. Antibodies bind to the antigen, forming an immune complex.

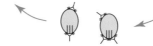

FIG. 11.3 The steps involved in making antibodies for immunity. (From Ignatavicius, D. D., & Workman, M. L. [2016]. *Medical-surgical nursing: Patient-centered collaborative care* [8th ed.]. St. Louis: Saunders.)

get sick with that influenza because all those sensitized B cells produce enormous amounts of anti-influenza A antibodies. These antibodies bind to the invading viruses and act to destroy, eliminate, or neutralize them so that you do not actually get sick again with influenza A and you now have antibody-mediated immunity to influenza. In fact, with every re-exposure to the influenza A virus, you become more and more immune to it. This great protection continues until your immune system is damaged (by drugs, diseases, or environmental agents) or just plain wears out as you age.

A special feature about antibody-mediated immunity is that the antibodies made by B cells are released into the blood and other body fluids. This means that the antibodies can go where they are needed most in the body, such as sites of invasion. Also, because the antibodies are released into the blood, they can be taken from the blood of one person and injected into another person's body. In addition to the blood and body fluids, B cells are heavily concentrated in the spleen, parts of lymph nodes, tonsils, and the mucosa of the intestinal tract.

ANTIBODY PROTECTION

True immunity provided by antibodies has several subtypes. These include *naturally acquired immunity* and *artificially acquired immunity*. Both types of acquired immunity can be divided into *active immunity* and *passive immunity*. Although all subtypes are helpful and provide some protection, they differ in how well they protect and how long that protection lasts. Figure 11.4 shows how the various types of immunity develop.

Memory Jogger

All future B cells produced from sensitized B cells are also sensitized against the same specific antigen and can make antibodies very quickly against that antigen.

Memory Jogger

Unlike inflammation and other types of immunity, antibody-mediated immunity can be transferred from one person to another.

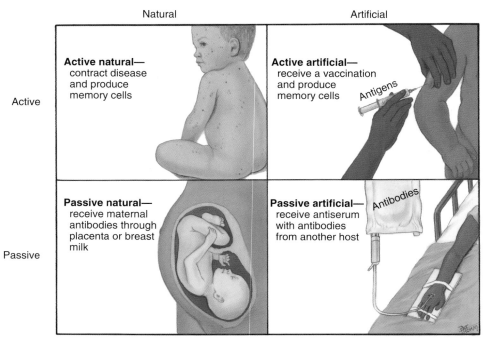

FIG. 11.4 Examples demonstrating how different types of immunity develop. (From Applegate, E. J. [2011]. *The anatomy and physiology learning system* [4th ed.]. St. Louis: Saunders.)

Naturally Acquired Immunity

Naturally acquired immunity starts to develop when a person's body is invaded by a foreign organism. So, when you are invaded by any common cold virus, an influenza virus, or an infectious type of bacteria as a result of being exposed to someone who is sick with any of these organisms, the exposure is unintentional and "natural." Your immune system has the opportunity to develop immunity against the organism even though you also may get sick with this exposure. So, naturally acquired refers to how the exposure to an invader occurs. This type of immunity can be active or passive. **Active immunity** means that your own body developed the antibodies. **Naturally acquired active immunity** starts when you are invaded by a foreign organism without assistance and your B cells then learn to make antibodies against the invaders. This type of immunity is the strongest and most long lasting. It can provide good protection for many decades.

Naturally acquired passive immunity is the type of antibody-mediated immunity you acquired as an antibody transfer from your mother through the placenta and through breast milk. Your body did not make these antibodies. This type of immunity is very important in helping to keep young infants healthy but provides protection for only a matter of months, not years.

Artificially Acquired Active Immunity

Although naturally acquired active immunity is the best type, sometimes having a person actually become ill with infectious organisms to make his or her own antibodies is not a good idea. For example, when a person catches diphtheria, he or she develops long-lasting immunity to it and will not get sick with diphtheria again. However, diphtheria has a high mortality rate, and some people who get the disease die from it. So artificially acquired active immunity is used to assist the body to learn to make antidiphtheria antibodies without having to first get sick with the disease. **Artificially acquired active immunity** is an antibody-mediated immunity that starts when an antigen is placed purposefully into your body to force your B cells to make a specific antibody against it. This type of immunity is commonly developed in most countries with the widespread use of vaccination, starting in early childhood.

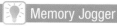

Memory Jogger

Naturally acquired active immunity is the most effective and long-lasting type of immunologic protection. Naturally acquired passive immunity is temporary because the antibodies were made elsewhere and decrease over time.

Memory Jogger

Artificially acquired active immunity is used to help people develop immunity to a dangerous disease without the risks associated with becoming sick first.

Vaccination. **Vaccination** is the deliberate injection or ingestion of an organism or other antigen for the intended purpose of stimulating B cells into producing antibodies specific to the antigen, resulting in immunologic resistance and protection against any disease caused by the antigen. Most often, vaccination involves the injection of a vaccine (Animation 11.3). A **vaccine** is a biologic preparation containing the universal product code of a specific disease-causing microorganism. The preparation can be composed of the organism itself, a part of the organism that retains its unique code, or a protein the organism produces that also contains the unique code. Although vaccination results in the person's B cells becoming sensitized and making the desired antibodies, this method of stimulating antibody production is less efficient than naturally acquired active immunity. Often, more than one vaccination with the same vaccine may be required and protection is not permanent. The person requires periodic "boosting" with revaccination to recruit more B cells to produce the antibodies and to remind existing sensitized B cells to continue to make antibodies. Vaccination and immunization are often used as interchangeable terms; however, **immunization** is the desired response of successful vaccination when the person actually develops immune resistance to the substance in the vaccine.

 Memory Jogger

Successful vaccination results in immunization with the development of immunologic resistance and protection against the organism in the vaccine.

Types of vaccines. Different substances are used in the vaccine preparations. These include inactivated (killed) organisms, attenuated live organisms, toxoids, biosynthetic substances, and mRNA. *Inactivated vaccines* contain organisms that could cause diseases but have been killed or inactivated, which prevents them from reproducing and causing disease. Examples of inactivated vaccines include those for immunity against influenza, cholera, and hepatitis A.

Attenuated vaccines contain live organisms (e.g., live-virus vaccine) that have been modified so that they are no longer capable of reproducing or causing disease, but still retain their unique code. Examples of attenuated vaccines include those for immunity against measles, mumps, rubella, and polio.

Toxoids are vaccines that contain either a modified toxin that an organism produces or an actual part of the organism. In either case, the toxoid has the unique code to stimulate antibody production against it. Examples of toxoid vaccines are those for immunity against tetanus, diphtheria, whooping cough, and human papilloma virus (HPV).

Biosynthetic vaccines contain science-made substances that are similar to the parts of an organism that cause disease. Examples of these vaccines are those for immunity against *Haemophilus influenzae* type B (Hib).

mRNA vaccines are laboratory-generated pieces of genetic material that code for making a specific part of an organism (in COVID-19, the part is the "spike" of the knobs present on the outside of the virus). The mRNA is taken up by human cells, which begin to make just that part of the virus (and that part is not capable of causing infection by itself). Then, the person's immune system cells make antibodies to the spike protein that also attack the entire virus. At the present time, this type of vaccine has been developed only against the COVID-19 virus.

Vaccination and boosting schedules. Vaccines for artificially acquired active immunity usually require more than one injection on a specific schedule to ensure that adequate numbers of B cells become sensitized to the antigen and begin making antibodies. These boosting vaccinations contain smaller doses of the original antigens and are needed to retain protection. For example, infants are usually vaccinated against diphtheria, tetanus, and pertussis (DTaP) with a single injection containing all three antigens at ages 2 months, 4 months, and 6 months for a total of three separate injections (doses). The vaccination is repeated as a fourth dose between the ages of 15 and 18 months, and again as a fifth dose between the ages of 4 and 6 years. Different formulations of these same three antigens are recommended as boosters between the ages of 11 and 12 years, during pregnancy, and for all adults every 10 years. Additional childhood vaccinations include hepatitis B (HVB), *Haemophilus influenzae* type B (Hib), pneumonia, polio, measles, mumps, rubella, hepatitis A

 Memory Jogger

Vaccinations for artificial acquired active immunity must be re-administered periodically as a "booster" to maintain immunity.

(HVA), varicella, rotavirus, human papilloma virus (HPV), and meningitis. For current recommended pediatric vaccine schedules, go to the Centers for Disease Control and Prevention website at: https://www.cdc/gov/vaccines/schedules/hcp/imz/child-adolescent.html

Vaccinations and boosters are recommended for adults, especially older adults and those with a chronic health problem, to stimulate immune protection for adults against common adult infectious diseases that can have serious or fatal consequences, and to maintain previously acquired immunity. Recommended vaccinations include seasonal influenza, pneumonia, shingles (*varicella*), hepatitis A, and hepatitis B Box 11.1 outlines responsibilities associated with the administration of vaccines. For current recommended adult vaccine schedules, go to the Centers for Disease Control and Prevention website at: https://www.cdc/gov/vaccines/schedules/hcp/imz/adult.html

---

Memory Jogger

Adults need initial vaccination and "booster" vaccination for continued active immunity.

Box 11.1   **Responsibilities When Administering Vaccines**

Storage

Upon receiving vaccines from the manufacturer:
- Immediately unpack and store in a designated area or with a designated refrigeration device that is separate from other drugs or food.
- Ensure refrigerator is plugged into an outlet that is serviced with emergency power and that the refrigerator is labeled "Do Not Unplug."
- Keep all vials (opened and unopened) in their original boxes.
- Do not store vaccine vials on the door of the refrigerator or in the freezer compartment.
- Check the vials on a weekly basis for expired vaccines or diluents, and discard those that are expired.
- Check the recommended schedule for whether the vaccination is appropriate for the patient.
- Check the expiration date on the vaccine vial and, if a diluent is to be used, also check the expiration date on the diluent vial.
- Read the package insert to determine all components of the vaccine (including preservatives), the recommended dosage, appropriate techniques and solutions for dilution, and any special instructions for administration.
- Ask whether the patient has ever had a reaction to the vaccine or any component of the vaccine.
- Ask when the patient last received this or any other vaccine.
- Ask the patient (or the parent/guardian of the patient) about any known allergies.
- Determine whether the patient is ill or has been ill within the previous 24 hours (some vaccines should NOT be given to a patient who has a fever or any type of infection).
- Using aseptic technique, draw up the appropriate dose into the syringe type recommended by the manufacturer and adjusted for patient size.
- Administer the drug using the recommended technique and site.

After Administration

- Document the vaccination in the patient's medical record or permanent vaccination log, including:
  - Name and age of the patient
  - Name of the vaccine
  - Manufacturer, lot number, and expiration date of the vaccine
  - Dosage of the vaccine
  - Site of vaccination
  - Condition of the site
- Provide a copy of the specific vaccine's Vaccine Information Statement (VIS) developed by the Centers for Disease Control and Prevention (CDC) to the patient or parents/guardians.
- Document which version of the VIS was provided.
- Observe the patient as recommended by the manufacturer for any immediate reaction to the vaccination.
- Teach the patient what side effects to expect and which ones require immediate medical attention.

Seasonal influenza vaccination. So, why are adults and children recommended to receive seasonal influenza vaccination every year? Doesn't the protection last longer than a year? Yes, the protection does last longer than a year. The big problem is that there are many strains of influenza. Each strain has a different unique code. If you get sick with one specific strain this year, you will develop long-lasting naturally acquired active immunity to that strain. However, if next year a different strain comes to your community, you do not have any immunity against it and, if sufficiently infected, you will get sick with the new strain of influenza. This is also true for "flu shots." When you receive an annual flu shot, the vaccination contains antigens for several influenza virus codes that are predicted as the ones most likely to be prevalent this year. Receiving this vaccination allows you to develop artificially acquired active immunity to these selected influenza strains that will protect you against these strains for many years. However, next year the most likely strains predicted to be prevalent may not be the ones you were vaccinated against this year. So, if you skip next year's vaccination you will be susceptible to the different strains of influenza and may get sick if heavily exposed.

Artificially Acquired Passive Immunity

Artificially acquired passive immunity is antibody-mediated immunity from the infusion of antibodies made by another person (or animal) or in a laboratory and injected into your body. Because these antibodies are foreign to you, your immune system recognizes them as foreign and eliminates them quickly. For this reason, passive immunity provides only immediate and short-term protection against a specific antigen. It is mainly used when a person is exposed to a serious disease for which he or she has little or no actively acquired immunity. The injected antibodies are expected to inactivate the invading organism or antigen. An example of laboratory-generated antibodies for this purpose is a combination of two laboratory-generated monoclonal antibodies casirivimab/imdevimab (REGEN-COV, formerly known as Regeneron) used for COVID-19, as described in Chapter 7. In addition, artificial acquired passive immunity to COVID-19 can occur with infusions of convalescent serum containing natural anti-COVID antibodies from patients who had the infection and recovered from it. Early after they have recovered from COVID-19, their serum contains high concentrations of anti-COVID antibodies that they have learned to make. This form of immunity was also used to improve survival rates for people infected with the Ebola virus. This type of temporary immunity may reduce the severity of an infectious disease or, depending on when and how much antibody is received, may prevent it completely. Disorders for which artificial acquired immunity are most commonly used to prevent severe disease or death include tetanus, rabies, and poisonous toxins from snakebites.

Artificially acquired passive immunity can also be used to prevent problems that are not related to infections. The primary example of this use is the administration of RhoGAM (Rho D immunoglobulin) to a woman who is Rh-negative and has just given birth to an Rh-positive baby. In addition to the A, B, and O blood types, there is another protein type on some people's red blood cells (RBCs). This is the rhesus ("Rh") factor. People who have the gene for this factor have RBCs that are Rh-positive. People who do not have the gene for this factor do not have the Rh protein on their RBCs and are Rh-negative. If a person who is Rh-negative is exposed to RBCs that are Rh-positive, his or her immune system will start making anti-Rh antibodies to get rid of any Rh-positive cells.

Although maternal blood and fetal blood do not mix heavily during pregnancy, some of the fetus's RBCs do enter maternal circulation, especially during labor and delivery. If the mother is Rh-negative and the fetus is Rh-positive, the mother then starts to make anti-Rh antibodies. The first pregnancy usually does not result in many of these antibodies, and the first child usually is not affected. However, if the mother becomes pregnant again with another Rh-positive fetus, she makes many more anti-Rh antibodies that can cross the placenta and destroy that fetus's RBCs, which can cause major problems and death for the fetus or newborn (Figure 11.5).

Memory Jogger

For some infectious organisms, such as influenza, there are many strains, each of which requires vaccination for immunologic protection.

Memory Jogger

Artificially acquired passive immunity through the transfer of antibodies from another person or animal, or from laboratory-generated antibodies provides only very short-term immunologic protection. This "immunity" may prevent the disorder or may reduce the disease severity.

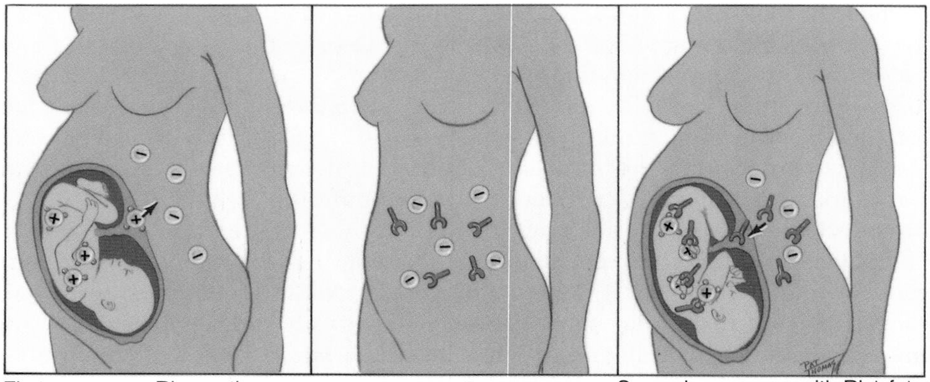

First pregnancy Rh– mother exposed to Rh+ agglutinogens.

After exposure, Rh– mother produces anti-Rh agglutinins.

Second pregnancy with Rh+ fetus. Anti-Rh agglutinins cause agglutination of fetal red blood cells.

FIG. 11.5 How anti-Rh antibodies are generated during pregnancy with an Rh-negative mother and an Rh-positive fetus. (From Applegate, E. J. [2011]. *The anatomy and physiology learning system* [4th ed.]. St. Louis: Saunders.)

To prevent an Rh-negative mother's immune system from making large amounts of anti-Rh antibodies, she is given a heavy dose very soon after delivery of these anti-Rh antibodies that were made in other people. These preformed injected anti-Rh antibodies attack any remaining Rh-positive cells still circulating in the mother's blood so that her immune system cells do not have a chance to become sensitized to them and make anti-Rh antibodies. Without the stimulation, there are few if any anti-Rh antibodies in the mother's blood during the next pregnancy and that fetus is safe from having its RBCs destroyed. To be effective, RhoGAM must be given to the Rh-negative *mother* as soon as possible after delivery of every Rh-positive baby.

Life span considerations for vaccination

Pediatric considerations. Although childhood is a time for extensive vaccination, it is also when the recommended schedules must be closely followed for best effect. A consideration is that a child who is sick with a viral or bacterial infection should not be vaccinated until he or she is well. This is because the child's immune system is making antibodies to the organism causing the sickness, and may not be capable of sensitizing enough B cells and to make sufficient antibodies in response to the vaccine.

Considerations for pregnancy and lactation. Live-virus vaccines are recommended to be given at least 1 month before pregnancy and avoided during pregnancy. These include measles, mumps, rubella, polio, and chickenpox. Seasonal influenza vaccination is highly recommended during any stage of pregnancy. It is also recommended that during each pregnancy, women receive the Tdap (tetanus, diphtheria, acellular pertussis) vaccination.

Considerations for older adults. As a person ages, the efficiency of the immune system slowly declines. The function of already sensitized B cells is diminished and the person often does not have as many antibodies even to organisms that actually stimulated their naturally acquired active immunity. Thus, older adults can become ill with diseases to which they once had either natural or artificial immunologic protection. Revaccination (boosting) becomes more important with age, especially in people over 90 years of age.

RELATED PHYSIOLOGY AND PATHOPHYSIOLOGY OF AUTOIMMUNE DISORDERS

An **autoimmune disorder** is a pathologic condition in which a person's immune system sees his or her own cells and tissues as foreign and develops inappropriate immune responses that attack these body cells or tissues. Thus, even though the immune system is protective most of the time, some of its cells and products can overreact

---

★ Critical Point for Safety

Be sure to teach parents the importance of following the recommended schedule for all childhood vaccinations for optimum development of immunity and protection.

QSEN: Safety

and cause inappropriate tissue-damaging excessive responses. In an autoimmune response, the body's antibodies or lymphocytes are directed against the body's own healthy normal cells and tissues, not just against invaders. (Antibodies directed against self-tissues or cells are known as *autoantibodies*.) The immune system loses some ability to tolerate self-cells and tissues.

Although inappropriate immune reactions may be triggered by infection or inflammation in the area, the actual cause of autoimmune disease is not known. Immune system cells and products, such as antibodies, can form against one type of cells and cause problems only for specific tissue, organ, or system, or can have more widespread effects. Regardless of whether the continuing autoimmune attack occurs against only one specific tissue or against many different tissues, autoimmune disorders are chronic, tissue destructive, progressive, and cannot be cured. Common autoimmune diseases include psoriasis, rheumatoid arthritis (RA), polyarteritis nodosa, and Hashimoto thyroiditis. Other diseases, such as type 1 diabetes mellitus, may have multiple causes, one of which is autoimmune. Without appropriate therapy, these disorders are destructive.

Management of autoimmune disorders depends on the organ or organs affected. For example, in type 1 diabetes, the person uses insulin to manage the disease and its complications, not drugs that alter the immune system. For other autoimmune diseases in which controlling the immune response is the best way to manage the disorder (e.g., RA, psoriasis), antiinflammatory drugs and drugs that more specifically suppress the excessive and inappropriate immune responses are used. **Immuno-suppressants drugs** are a class of drugs that inhibit or prevent the optimal or excessive function of the immune system.

RHEUMATOID ARTHRITIS

A classic example of an autoimmune disorder is *rheumatoid arthritis (RA)*. General osteoarthritis (OA) is a "wear and tear" problem in which joint injury, from trauma or even just excessive use, first damages the tissues within joints, especially cartilage and bone (Animation 11.4). The injury results in chronic inflammation as described in Chapter 10. Long-term chronic inflammation of the joints causes pain, scar tissue formation, and loss of function. OA is more common in weight-bearing joints (e.g., hips, knees, ankles) and in those joints involved in repetitive motions. Unlike OA, with RA, immune system components *first* attack different parts of the joint causing inflammation, which then induces changes that damage the joint. Also unlike OA, the areas most often affected first in RA are the small joints of the hands, fingers, and feet.

Although the trigger(s) for the inappropriate immune responses responsible for RA is not known, the key cell type beginning the attack on self-tissues is a T-lymphocyte "helper" cell (helper T-cell). These cells then stimulate B-lymphocytes to produce auto-antibodies directed against cartilage and other joint connective tissues. In addition, the attacking T-lymphocytes increase production of a variety of mediators *(cytokines)* that continually attack joint tissues, causing progressive changes in joint anatomy and destruction of these tissues. The mediator or cytokine most often involved in RA joint destruction is *tumor necrosis factor (TNF)*. The mediators directly damage bone and cartilage, increase blood vessel growth in the area, and activate enzymes that continue the tissue destruction. Attacked joints become swollen, reddened, spongy in texture, and painful with reduced function.

TRADITIONAL ANTIINFLAMMATORY THERAPY FOR AUTOIMMUNE DISORDERS

Traditional antiinflammatory therapy to help manage RA and most other autoimmune disorders are the general antiinflammatory drugs presented in Chapter 10. These include systemic corticosteroids, nonsteroidal antiinflammatory drugs (NSAIDs), and general disease-modifying anti-rheumatic drugs (DMARDs). Systemic corticosteroids and NSAIDs are helpful in reducing some of the pain and inflammation associated with RA and other autoimmune disorders but do not

Memory Jogger

Autoimmune disorders represent a failure of the immune system to recognize a person's normal cells as "self" and attacks these cells as if they were foreign invaders.

Memory Jogger

In osteoarthritis, a joint injury or excessive use first triggers inflammation; however, in rheumatoid arthritis, inappropriate immune responses with inflammation occur first and these responses cause progressive joint injury.

control the abnormal immune system responses and do not prevent progressive tissue destruction. DMARDs have effects that temporarily slow progressive destruction somewhat by generally suppressing cell division of bone marrow cells (the origin of lymphocytes). However, DMARDs are high-alert drugs with many serious systemic side effects. Any or all of these drug categories may still be used for management of autoimmune disorders, depending on the severity of the disorder and the patient's response to the drug therapy. An in-depth presentation of the actions, side effects, adverse effects, and care issues for DMARDs can be found in Chapter 10.

BIOLOGIC IMMUNOSUPPRESSIVE THERAPY FOR AUTOIMMUNE DISORDERS

Biologic immunosuppressive therapy using "biologics" is now often the first-line therapy for control of autoimmune disorders. **Biologics** are a class of complex anti-inflammatory drugs derived from living sources that target specific inflammatory cells, components, or products to modify chronic disorders associated with inflammation and tissue damage. Not only are these agents able to reduce the pain and inflammation associated with these disorders, but they also significantly delay the progression of damage by acting on the specific parts of the immune system causing the continual inappropriate attack on normal tissues. Thus, biologic therapy is very specific in its actions with fewer changes in systemic immune function. Although the cell types and mediators (cytokines), which are the "targets" of these agents, are very specific, their influence occurs in many tissues. Thus, any given biologic drug is often effective in reducing the effects of more than one autoimmune disorder (Animation 11.5).

Drugs in this category are antibodies, mostly monoclonal antibodies. Some of these antibodies directly target specific mediator (cytokine) molecules or their receptors. Another antibody type targets an intracellular enzyme (Janus kinase [JAK]), which functions to promote signaling systems that increase the growth and function of almost all immune system cells and their products.

Direct-Acting Monoclonal Antibody Therapy

Monoclonal antibodies are a type of biologic drug composed of antibodies produced by mouse cells or a combination of mouse and human antibody-producing cells targeted against specific proteins that cause tissue damage. When the correct antibody is produced by one cell, that cell is selectively grown and all of its descendants produce large amounts of just the one specific antibody. This is known as *monoclonal antibody production*, and all the antibodies produced by this group of cells are identical to each other. The mouse proteins from the antibodies have been removed so it is "fully humanized" and will not cause people who receive it to develop a mouse protein allergy. In addition, through recombinant DNA technology, some monoclonal antibodies generated in laboratories come from sensitized human cells rather than mouse cells.

All direct-acting monoclonal antibody biologics used as drug therapy for autoimmune disorders are parenteral drugs. These antibodies are poorly absorbed by the gastrointestinal system and are inactivated by gastric enzymes. Most are injected subcutaneously at specified intervals and a few must be given as intravenous infusions. Two drugs have been in use for autoimmune disorders for more than 20 years (*adalimumab* and *etanercept*). Many more have been developed and approved within the past 5 years. So, less is known about the newer direct-acting monoclonal antibody biologics. The following table lists the names of the direct-acting monoclonal antibody biologics, routes of administration, specific mediator/cytokine targets, and the approved autoimmune disorder for which they are used. Dosages vary by disorder, patient size, and patient responses. Consult a reliable drug reference for less common drugs in this class, for any newer approved uses, and for disorder-specific dosages and dosing schedules.

Common Direct-Acting Monoclonal Antibody Biologics

Drug Names	Drug Routes	Antibody Targets	Approved Uses
abatacept (Orencia)	IV	CTLA4 receptors	RA, PA
adalimumab (Abrilada, AMJEVITA, CYLTEZO, Humira)	SC	TNF	AS, CD, PA, RA, UC
certolizumab (Cimzia)	SC	TNF	AS, CD, PA, RA,
dupilumab (Dupixent)	SC	IL-4, IL-13	A, atopic dermatitis
etanercept (Enbrel, ERELZI, Eticovo)	SC	TNF	AS, PA, PP, RA
golimumab (Simponi)	SC, IV	TNF	AS, PA, RA
guselkumab (Tremfya)	SC	IL-23	PA, PP
infliximab (Avsola, INFLECTRA, Remicade)	IV	TNF	AS, CD, PA, PP, RA, UC
ixekizumab (Taltz)	SC	IL-23	PA, PP
risankizumab (Skyrizi)	SC	IL-23	PP

A, Asthma; *AS,* Ankylosing spondylitis; *CD,* Crohn disease; *CTLA4,* cytotoxic T-lymphocyte-associated protein 4; *IL,* interleukin; *IV,* intravenous; *PA,* psoriatic arthritis; *PP,* Plaque psoriasis; *RA,* rheumatoid arthritis; *SC,* subcutaneous; *TNF,* tumor necrosis factor; *UC,* ulcerative colitis.

How direct-acting monoclonal antibodies work. Generally, these antibodies bind to a specific pro-inflammatory mediator or cytokine and prevent them from binding to their receptors and performing their usual functions.

TNF inhibitors, which include adalimumab, certolizumab, etanercept, golimumab, and infliximab, bind to and prevent TNF from triggering cell and tissue destruction. In addition, the release of other pro-inflammatory cytokines such as IL-1 (IL-1) and IL-6 is also inhibited. All of these actions greatly reduce inflammation and immune functions that trigger the production of autoantibodies.

Interleukin-23 (IL-23) inhibitors, which include guselkumab, ixekizumab, and risankizumab, bind to IL-23 and prevent it from binding to its receptors. Activated IL-23 receptors are important in promoting certain types of helper T cells to increase inflammatory responses. With reduced activation of these helper T cells, less autoantibodies are synthesized and the concentrations of pro-inflammatory cytokines IL-6, IL-17, and IL-22 are reduced.

Dupilumab binds to IL-4 and IL-13. These interleukins stimulate allergic responses, increased mucous production, and activate many inflammatory cells within the skin and mucous membranes. The monoclonal antibodies against IL-4 and IL-13 are especially effective at reducing inflammation in mucous membranes and the skin.

Abatacept is a monoclonal antibody to the CTLA4 receptor and works differently from other monoclonal antibodies used to manage autoimmune disorders. CTLA4 is cytotoxic T-lymphocyte-associated protein 4, which is a regulatory protein that, when it binds to its receptors on lymphocytes and other WBCs, helps *prevent* immune overreactions. CTLA4 antibodies bind to CTLA4 receptors on lymphocytes and act as an agonist. This action increases immunosuppressive actions that reduce autoantibody production and inflammatory attacks on normal body cells and tissues.

 Memory Jogger

The monoclonal antibodies composing *abatacept* act as an agonist as the CTLA4 receptor, which enhances the action of CTLA4 in preventing immune system excessive reactions.

Intended responses of direct-acting monoclonal antibodies
- Reduced general inflammation
- Reduced production of autoantibodies
- Reduced symptoms of autoimmune disorders
- Delayed or reduced tissue destruction
- Improved quality of life

Common side effects of direct-acting monoclonal antibodies. These drugs are all given parenterally. The most common side effect is injection site reactions. Because all of these drugs reduce inflammation and immunity, the risk for infection is increased. Such infections include new infections, as well as reactivation of dormant bacteria or viruses. Other common side effects include headache, fatigue, flu-like body aches, and fever. Some people also experience a variety of gastrointestinal side effects.

Possible adverse effects of direct-acting monoclonal antibodies. The most common adverse effect is the greatly increased risk for infection, especially reactivation of dormant tuberculosis (TB) bacteria and hepatitis viruses. A previous history of either of these infections requires close monitoring of these patients and, in some cases, is considered a contraindication for direct-acting monoclonal antibody therapy.

Because these drugs can reduce the body's normal production of new antibodies, vaccination may not result in immunization. This effect also increases the patient's risk for development of infection.

The injected antibodies may be considered "foreign" by the patient's own immune system and trigger antibodies directed against the drugs. If sufficient antibodies are directed against the drugs, their effectiveness may be reduced over time. Patient development of antibodies against the drugs also can trigger hypersensitivity reactions including angioedema and anaphylaxis.

Patients receiving these drugs long term have an increased risk for developing a malignancy. This adverse reaction is most common for drugs that inhibit TNF and those that reduce helper T-cell functions.

These drugs can worsen heart failure and should be used with caution in patients who have a history of cardiac issues, including heart failure.

 Priority actions to take **before** ***and*** **after** ***giving direct-acting monoclonal antibodies.*** In addition to the usual actions before giving any drug as described in Chapter 2, be sure to implement these actions:

Ask whether the patient has ever had a positive TB test or is known to have had viral hepatitis. Be sure the patient has a negative TB test before giving the first dose of any of these drugs. Also ensure that TB tests are routinely performed throughout the therapy period. If the TB test becomes positive, therapy is immediately stopped.

Regardless of whether the drug doses are given as an intravenous infusion or subcutaneously, the first dose must be given by a registered nurse or physician in a setting equipped to manage an allergic adverse reaction. IV doses must be infused over at least 30 minutes. Observe the patient for any adverse reactions for 30 minutes to 1 hour after the injection is performed or the IV drug infused.

Most of the drugs to be administered subcutaneously are available in prefilled syringes for self-injection. Use the teaching guide for self-administration of subcutaneous injections presented in Box 2.3 in Chapter 2 to ensure the patient can safely manage his or her own therapy.

For women who are of child-bearing age, ask whether they are pregnant or using a reliable method of contraception. The older drugs in this class appear to cause immune suppression of the fetus in later (the last 2 months) pregnancy. The effects of the newer drugs on pregnancy are not known.

Obtain and monitor laboratory tests for liver function and bone marrow function. The direct-acting monoclonal antibodies do induce some degree of reduced immune function and anemia. Changes in liver function have also been reported.

Rotate subcutaneous injection sites to prevent tissue injury. Also, aspirate after inserting the needle to ensure the solution will not enter a blood vessel. If using prefilled syringes or single-use vials and two injections are needed for a complete dose, inject the doses into two separate sites.

 Teaching priorities for patients taking direct-acting monoclonal antibodies
- Avoid crowds and people who are ill because these drugs reduce your immunity and increase your risk for infection.
- Check yourself daily for symptoms of infection, including fever, cough, feeling slow and tired, foul-smelling drainage, and pain or burning on urination. If any of these are present, notify your prescriber immediately.
- If you are performing self-injection of this drug, follow the directions taught to you. If two injections are required for a full dose, inject at two completely separate sites.

Common Side Effects

Direct-Acting Monoclonal Antibodies

Injection site reaction   Headache   Fatigue

Muscle aches   Fever

 Critical Point for Safety

The patient must have a negative TB test before initiating direct-acting monoclonal antibody therapy because the immune suppression caused by these drugs can reactivate dormant TB organisms and cause the patient to have an active TB infection.

QSEN: Safety

Critical Point for Safety

The first dose of any subcutaneously administered direct-acting monoclonal antibody and all doses of IV antibodies must be given by a licensed professional nurse or physician and the patient must be monitored for 30 min to an hour after for any adverse reactions.

QSEN: Safety

Critical Point for Safety

If using prefilled syringes or single-use vials and two injections are needed for a complete dose, inject the doses into two separate sites. Aspirate after inserting each needle to ensure the solution will not be injected into a blood vessel.

QSEN: Safety

- If you develop swelling of the lips, throat, or tongue after an injection or have difficulty breathing and are dizzy, call 911 immediately.
- Keep all appointments for laboratory tests to make sure these drugs are not causing problems in other organs.
- Be sure to participate in regular cancer screenings because your risk for cancer development is higher when your immune system is suppressed.
- If you notice a worsening of any other health problem you also have, notify your prescriber immediately.
- Report any persistent body change or new symptom to your prescriber so that he or she can assess its significance.
- Vaccinations may not work as well for you while you are taking these drugs. Consult with your prescriber about when in your dosing schedule a vaccination should be received.

Life span considerations for direct-acting monoclonal antibodies

Considerations for pregnancy and lactation. Monoclonal antibodies are mostly composed of immunoglobulin G (IgG). IgG in maternal blood does cross the placenta and does enter breast milk. These drugs are not known to induce birth defects when taken early in pregnancy. However, some immunosuppression has been seen in infants whose mothers received these drugs in the last 2 months of pregnancy. Thus, the drugs are not recommended for use in late pregnancy.

IgG does enter breast milk. The effects of this on the infant are not known; however, it is thought that the infant's digestive system may inactivate the antibodies. At this time, manufacturers recommend against breastfeeding by mothers receiving these drugs. However, the benefits of breastfeeding a particular infant must be weighed against possible unknown harm.

Indirect-Acting Monoclonal Antibody Therapy: Janus Kinase Inhibitors

A newer class of monoclonal antibodies for autoimmune disorders is the Janus kinase inhibitors. Janus kinases (JAKs) are a family of intracellular enzymes present in regulatory immune system cells, especially lymphocytes. When mediators and cytokines bind to lymphocyte receptors, JAKs transmit the activation signals from the lymphocyte's membrane to its nucleus, which then turns on the genes to synthesize many cytokines that will increase the growth and activity of nearly all white blood cells. As a result of this action, JAK activation increases all pro-inflammatory pathways and mediators, including TNF and autoantibodies, and increases immune attacks.

How Janus kinase inhibitors work. JAK inhibitors are monoclonal antibodies that bind to some of the many types of JAKs in the JAK family of enzymes. When the antibodies bind to JAKs, they cannot transmit as many signals to the nucleus of immune system cells. As a result, fewer pro-inflammatory mediators and cytokines are available to maintain and enhance autoimmune responses.

The JAK inhibitors are all oral drugs and prescribed after other drugs, including the direct-acting monoclonal antibodies, have not provided sufficient relief from the symptoms and damage of autoimmune disorders. These drugs are also classified as "target specific" disease-modifying antirheumatic drugs (DMARDs). They are most commonly used in patients with rheumatoid arthritis. The table below lists the usual adult dosages for common JAK inhibitors. Consult a reliable drug reference for less common drugs in this class.

Adult Dosages of Common Janus Kinase Inhibitors

Drug Names	Usual Maintenance Dosages
baricitinib (OLUMIANT)	2 mg orally once daily
tofacitinib (Xeljanz)	Immediate-release: 5 mg orally twice daily Extended-release: 11 mg orally once daily
upadacitinib (RINVOQ)	15 mg orally once daily

Common Side Effects
Janus Kinase Inhibitors

GI problems Headache Hypertension

Fatigue Rash

Common side effects of Janus kinase inhibitors. The most common side effects of JAK inhibitors include nausea and other GI problems, headache, hypertension, fatigue, and rash. In addition, upper respiratory infections and elevated blood cholesterol levels are common.

Possible adverse effects of Janus kinase inhibitors. Like other drugs to manage autoimmune disorders, JAK inhibitors reduce immunity and increase the risk for infection, including reactivation of dormant TB organisms and hepatitis viruses. They are not to be used in patients who have a neutrophil white blood cell count (WBC) of less than 1000 cells/mm^3.

JAK inhibitors increase platelet counts and greatly increase the risk for thromboembolic events including pulmonary embolism, heart attacks, and strokes. The drugs should not be prescribed for patients who have a history of previous thromboembolic events or who have other risk factors for inappropriate clot formation. This risk is further increased if the patient also smokes.

Patients receiving these drugs long term have an increased risk for developing any type of malignancy, including lymphoma.

Vaccinations are less likely to provide immunization for patients taking JAK inhibitors. Live-virus vaccines are contraindicated while taking these drugs because of the risk for disease development.

JAK inhibitors may be given while receiving immunosuppressive therapy with methotrexate or other non-biologic DMARDs. They are not to be used along with direct-acting monoclonal antibodies or other inhibitors of TNF because of the likelihood of severe immunosuppression.

Bowel perforation has occurred in patients receiving JAK inhibitors. A patient history of diverticulitis is a contraindication for therapy with these drugs.

These drugs elevate serum cholesterol levels and can be liver toxic.

⭐ ***Priority actions to take*** *before* ***and*** *after* ***giving Janus kinase inhibitors.*** Ensure that the patient has a negative TB test and that female patients of child-bearing age who are sexually active have a negative pregnancy test.

Assess the patient for any symptoms of active infection, including the results of a complete blood count (CBC). If an infection is present or if the white blood cell (WBC) count is too low, therapy is delayed until the infection is gone and WBC counts are high enough. Use CBC results as a baseline to determine whether the drug is causing any adverse effects on platelet and WBC counts.

Make sure immunizations are up to date *before* JAK inhibitor therapy is started, especially for live-virus vaccines.

Ensure that laboratory tests for blood counts and liver function are performed before therapy begins and at regular intervals after the patient starts taking a JAK inhibitor. Compare later findings with the baseline results to determine whether the drug is adversely affecting liver function, increasing platelet numbers, or making WBC counts too low.

Ask about all prescribed and over-the-counter drugs and supplements the patient takes regularly because JAK inhibitors can interact with a large number of other drugs. Consult with a pharmacist for potential interactions with the patient's usual drugs. If interactions are possible, inform the prescriber so that appropriate drug therapy adjustments can be made. Although these drugs can be taken along with methotrexate and other DMARDs, they are not to be taken with direct-acting monoclonal antibodies, other TNF inhibitors, or another JAK inhibitor.

Ask about any current abdominal pain or chronic abdominal discomfort. Reassess this issue at every appointment and instruct patients to notify their prescribers rather than ignoring any severe or persistent abdominal pain because these drugs can cause bowel perforation.

⭐ *Teaching priorities for patients taking Janus kinase inhibitors*
- You may take the drug with or without meals. However, be sure to take it as close as possible to the same time every day for the best effects.

- Avoid eating grapefruit or drinking grapefruit juice with this drug because grapefruit increases blood levels of this drug, which can increase your risk for serious side effects.
- This drug can cause a severe intestinal problem. If you begin having sharp, intense abdominal pain, do not ignore these or attempt to treat this on your own. Instead, notify your prescriber immediately.
- Keep all your appointments for laboratory blood tests to make sure these drugs are not causing serious problems with your blood counts or liver.
- Check with your prescriber before receiving any vaccination. Those containing live viruses cannot be taken while you are on these drugs and other vaccinations may be less effective.
- Assess yourself weekly and report any skin yellowing, pain over the liver area, or darkening of the urine to your prescriber immediately because these drugs can reduce liver function.
- Avoid crowds and people who are ill because resistance to infection is decreased and you are more susceptible to infectious illnesses.
- Check yourself daily for signs and symptoms of infection (e.g., fever, cough, feeling slow and tired, foul-smelling drainage, pain or burning on urination). If any of these are present, notify your prescriber immediately.
- If you are a sexually active woman of child-bearing age and your partner is a fertile male, use two reliable methods of birth control while taking this drug. If you think you have become pregnant, stop the drug and notify your prescriber immediately.
- This drug increases your risk for blood clots. If you notice a persistent pain in your calves, any veins that start feeling hard or "cord-like," or you have a sudden change in breathing, notify your prescriber immediately.

Life span considerations for Janus kinase inhibitors

Considerations for pregnancy and lactation. No formal studies have been performed that indicate whether JAK inhibitors are safe to use during human pregnancy and/or lactation. Manufacturers recommend that these drugs be avoided during pregnancy and lactation unless drug benefits are considered to outweigh potential adverse pregnancy outcomes or adverse effects to the breastfed infant. Sexually active women of child-bearing age are encouraged to use two reliable forms of contraception to prevent pregnancy during this therapy.

RELATED PHYSIOLOGY AND PATHOPHYSIOLOGY OF TRANSPLANTATION

Modern medical therapy has made it possible to surgically replace a diseased or nonfunctioning organ of one patient *(recipient)* with a healthy organ from another person *(donor)*. The success of this type of therapy depends on preventing the recipient's immune system from recognizing the newly transplanted organ as "foreign."

GENERAL REJECTION

Most solid organ transplants occur between people who are not a perfect tissue type match. This means that the recipient's immune system is continually attempting to rid the body of this foreign tissue. For organ transplantation to be successful, either the transplanted organ must be a tissue type match between the donor and recipient, or the recipient must take general immunosuppressive and antirejection drugs daily to prevent the recipient's immune system from attempting to reject the donor organ. **Antirejection drugs** suppress the components of the immune system most responsible for the rejection of transplanted organs and tissues. The T-cell lymphocytes are mainly responsible for attacking and destroying transplanted organs. Current general antirejection drugs work by selective immunosuppression, suppressing only the immune system cells most responsible for transplant rejection, placing the recipient at less risk for developing overwhelming infection.

Critical Point for Safety

JAK inhibitor use has resulted in intestinal perforations, especially among people who have or have had diverticulosis or diverticulitis. Teach patients to not ignore or self-medicate if severe or persistent abdominal pain develops and to immediately notify their prescriber.

QSEN: Safety

Memory Jogger

General antirejection drugs are needed for the recipient whenever the donor is not a perfect tissue type match with the recipient.

General Antirejection Drug Therapy

General drug therapy to prevent day-to-day solid organ immunologic rejection is life-long and includes corticosteroids, disease-modifying antirheumatic drugs (DMARDs), and selective immunosuppressants. These drugs do suppress the immune system to some degree, and the dosage must be adjusted to the immune response of each patient. Antirejection drugs are used to suppress the components of the immune system responsible for rejection of transplanted tissues and organs. The most commonly transplanted organ is the kidney. Usually, a combination of three of the drugs listed in the following table is used to prevent rejection of a transplanted kidney. Usual adult dosages are listed; however, drug dosages vary based on the patient's responses to these drugs, whether the therapy is for acute or chronic rejection, and on which organ is transplanted.

Adult Dosages for General Antirejection Drugs

Drug Category	Drug Names	Usual Maintenance Dosages
Corticosteroids	prednisone	5 mg–30 mg orally once daily
Calcineurin inhibitors	cyclosporine (Neoral)	15 mg/kg orally as a single dose 4–12 hr before transplantation followed by 7 mg/kg orally every 12 hr. Gradually titrated down to 2 mg orally once daily
	tacrolimus (Prograf)	Initially 0.03–0.05 mg/kg/day as a continuous IV infusion followed by 0.1 mg/kg orally every 12 hr or 0.2 mg/kg orally once daily
Semi-selective immuno-suppressants	azathioprine (Azasan, Imuran)	Initially 3–5 mg/kg orally once daily before transplantation, then 1–3 mg/kg orally once daily
Selective immunosup-pressants	everolimus (Zortress)	Initially, 0.75 mg orally every 12 hours or 1.5 mg orally once daily then adjusted every 5 days depending on responses
	mycophenolate (CellCept, Myfortic)	1 g orally or IV twice daily
	sirolimus (Rapamune)	6 mg orally loading dose followed by 2 mg orally daily

How general antirejection drugs work. *Corticosteroids*, as described in Chapter 10, suppress bone marrow production of all white blood cells (WBCs) and inhibit immune responses as well as inflammation. Prednisone is a common drug taken daily to prevent transplant rejection. See Chapter 10 for a full discussion of the actions, side effects, and other issues related to immunosuppressive therapy with corticosteroids.

Calcineurin inhibitors work to prevent the first phase of T-cell activation by binding to protein and forming a complex that inhibits calcineurin present in some immune system cells. Calcineurin normally promotes the expression of genes that allow T cells both to divide and to be activated. With less calcineurin around, T-cell activation and cell division are significantly reduced, resulting in less damage to transplanted tissues and organs.

Azathioprine, as a semiselective immunosuppressive drug, is an immunosuppressive agent that interferes with DNA and RNA synthesis, especially in white blood cells (WBCs). This action reduces the amount of inflammatory cells present and greatly reduces WBC production of inflammatory mediators, including those directed at transplanted solid organs. See Chapter 10 for a full discussion of the actions, side effects, and other issues related to immunosuppressive therapy with azathioprine.

Selective immunosuppressants are drugs that more selectively target the immune system cells and products responsible for transplant rejection. They are less likely to cause profound generalized immune suppression. *Mycophenolate* reversibly inhibits an enzyme needed for lymphocyte reproduction. It also prevents T cells already present in tissues from being activated. Both actions selectively suppress the immune responses most associated with transplant rejection. *Sirolimus* and *everolimus* selectively inhibit T-cell activation and reproduction by blocking the signal transduction pathways, especially the mTOR pathway, that promotes movement of T cells through the cell cycle for cell division. They also interfere with the ability of B cells to mature into antibody-producing cells. The overall amount of antibodies produced, including the ones that attack transplanted organs, is reduced.

Intended responses of general antirejection drugs
- Transplanted organs continue normal function
- The patient retains enough immune function to prevent serious infections

Common side effects of general antirejection drugs. The most common side effects for all of these drugs are gastrointestinal disturbances of all types and a variety of skin rashes. *Sirolimus* and *everolimus* elevate serum cholesterol levels. The most common side effects of the *calcineurin inhibitors* are hypertension, elevated serum cholesterol levels, and hyperglycemia. *Cyclosporine* also causes many patients to have gingival (gum) hyperplasia.

Possible adverse effects of general antirejection drugs. In addition to the risk for serious bacterial and fungal infections, all antirejection drugs increase the risk for cancer development. This problem is thought to be related to reduced immunosurveillance by loss of immune system cell recognition when normal cells transform to cancer cells.

Adverse effects of these drugs vary by their mechanism of action. *Azathioprine* and the *calcineurin inhibitors* can cause liver toxicity and liver failure. Intravenous drugs increase the risk for phlebitis and thrombosis at the administration site. The *calcineurin inhibitors* are associated with electrolyte imbalances, especially of potassium, phosphorus, and magnesium.

⭐ **Priority actions to take** before **and** after *giving general antirejection drugs.* Obtain a list of all other drugs that the patient takes because most selective immunosuppressants interact with many other drugs. Check with the pharmacist for possible interactions and the need to consult the prescriber about dosage or changing the patient's other drugs.

Because many general antirejection drugs can lead to liver toxicity, make sure that the patient does not have a liver problem before starting these drugs. Check the patient's most recent laboratory values for liver problems (elevated liver enzyme levels). (See Table 1.4 in Chapter 1 for a listing of normal values.)

Ensure that all patients taking or receiving any general antirejection drugs have close regular monitoring of blood cell counts with a complete blood cell count (CBC). Assess CBCs and report abnormalities to the prescriber.

Assess the patient daily for yellowing of the skin or sclera (jaundice), which is a symptom of liver problems. The best places to check are the whites of the eyes closest to the iris, the roof of the mouth, and the skin of the chest.

Monitor electrolyte values, especially potassium, phosphorus, and magnesium. Report abnormal electrolytes to the prescriber.

⭐ Teaching priorities for patients taking antirejection drugs
- Avoid crowds and people who are ill because your resistance to infection is decreased and you are more susceptible to infectious illnesses.
- Check yourself daily for signs and symptoms of infection (e.g., fever, cough, feeling slow and tired, foul-smelling drainage, pain or burning on urination). If any of these are present, notify your prescriber immediately.
- Check with your prescriber for which types of vaccinations you should receive.
- Be sure to keep all appointments for monitoring of blood counts and other laboratory tests.

Common Side Effects
General Antirejection Drugs

GI problems

Rash

⚠ Drug Alert

Interaction Alert

Before giving general antirejection drugs, ask the patient about all other drugs or supplements that he or she takes and then check with the pharmacist to avoid a possible drug interaction.

QSEN: Safety

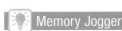
- Remember to take these drugs exactly as prescribed to maintain their effectiveness in preventing transplant rejection. Even a few missed doses can lead to transplant rejection episodes.
- These drugs can cause liver toxicity. Check yourself at least weekly for yellowing of your skin or eyes, darkening of the urine, or lightening of the stools. If any of these symptoms are present, notify your prescriber immediately. Avoid drinking alcohol or using acetaminophen while taking these drugs.
- Swallow the capsules whole, and do not crush or open them. Drink a full glass of water every time you take the drugs.
- If you take oral sirolimus or tacrolimus, avoid eating grapefruit or drinking grapefruit juice.
- Do not take any over-the-counter drugs or supplements without checking with your prescriber because antirejection drugs can interact with many other drugs.

Life span considerations for general antirejection drugs

Considerations for pregnancy and lactation. Antirejection drugs are associated with poor pregnancy outcomes. It is recommended that sexually active women in childbearing years use two reliable methods of contraception during therapy with these drugs. Breastfeeding while on these drugs is also contraindicated.

ACUTE TRANSPLANT REJECTION

Despite daily therapy with general antirejection drugs, periods of increased immune attack, known as *acute rejection*, on the transplanted organ may occur intermittently throughout the life span of the donated organ. Two pathologic mechanisms are responsible. The first mechanism is antibody mediated and results in vasculitis and blood vessel necrosis within the transplanted organ and leads to organ destruction. In the second mechanism, some of the recipient's T cells enter the new organ and start inflammatory responses that, without temporary increased immunosuppressive therapy, can destroy the organ.

An episode of acute rejection after solid organ transplantation does not automatically mean that the patient will lose the new organ. Timely drug management of the recipient's immune responses at this time helps limit organ damage and allows it to continue to function.

Therapy for Acute Episodes of Transplant Rejection

Acute episodes of transplant rejection can occur at any time. These episodes can be managed so that the transplanted organ is not destroyed by immunologic attack. Often, when acute rejection is recognized, the same general antirejection drugs used daily are used at temporary higher dosages. Some may be given through the episode intravenously. In some cases, monoclonal and polyclonal antibodies may be used temporarily for 10 to 14 days to provide additional antirejection actions to save the transplanted organ.

How drugs for acute transplant rejection work. Monoclonal antibodies are antibodies produced by mouse cells or a combination of mouse and human antibody-producing cells against a protein found on the surface of all human T cells. Once these antibodies have bound to their target, they stop all T-cell functions, including those that attack transplanted tissues and organs. These drugs do not have any effect on other types of immune system cells. They must be administered intravenously. For the drugs that are made as a result of recombinant technology using mouse/human cell hybrids, the drug targets only a receptor on activated T cells. Thus, these are the most specific immunosuppressants and are very effective at initially stopping an acute transplant rejection once it starts.

Polyclonal antibodies are antibodies directed against human T cells. These antibodies are produced by other animals (horses and rabbits) in response to the administration of human WBCs, especially T cells. They are very effective in attacking and eliminating human T cells and can lead to a profound immunosuppression. Their use is now confined to times when a person is having an acute rejection episode after kidney transplantation that does not respond to other types of immunosuppressive therapy.

Possible adverse effects of drugs for acute transplant rejection. The monoclonal and polyclonal antibodies used to reduce acute transplant rejection episodes are given only in specialized acute care settings. These drugs have dangerous side effects and must be administered by health care professionals who are knowledgeable about the drugs and capable of recognizing and managing adverse effects.

Electrolyte imbalances are common during administration of these agents. The electrolytes most affected are potassium, phosphorus, and magnesium.

Serious allergic responses and anaphylaxis are possible for patients receiving monoclonal antibodies and very high for patients receiving polyclonal antibodies. Proteins from other species (e.g., mouse, horse, rabbit) are present in these formulations and can trigger severe reactions. Emergency equipment and medications are kept close at hand in case of severe allergic reactions or anaphylaxis.

Many patients have severe reactions during and after infusion of these drugs, including fever, shaking, muscle aches and pains, and other uncomfortable flu-like symptoms. Drugs to reduce these reactions may be prescribed as premedication before giving either monoclonal antibodies or polyclonal antibodies.

Get Ready for the NCLEX® Examination!

Key Points

- Inflammation helps protect the body from infection but cannot provide true immunity to any specific disease-causing microorganism.
- Antibody-mediated immunity can be transferred from one person or animal to another and, when transferred, has only a short-term effect.
- The five types of vaccines currently available are inactivated vaccines, attenuated vaccines, toxoids, biosynthetic vaccines, and mRNA vaccines.
- Natural, active immunity is the most beneficial and long-lasting type of immunity.
- Vaccinations cause artificial active immunity and require "boosting" for best long-term effects.
- For some infectious organisms, such as influenza, there are many strains, each of which requires vaccination for immunologic protection.
- Artificially acquired passive immunity is indicated when people are known to have been exposed to deadly diseases and their vaccination status is not known or insufficient for protection.
- Urge pregnant women to receive seasonal influenza vaccination and the Tdap vaccination during every pregnancy.
- Artificially acquired active immunity is used to help people develop immunity to a dangerous disease without the risk for becoming sick first.
- Any long-term immunosuppressive therapy, regardless of the reason it was prescribed, reduces the patient's immune responses and increases his or her risk for both new infections and reactivation of dormant organisms from previous infections.
- Autoimmune disorders represent a failure of the immune system to recognize a person's normal cells as "self" and the system attacks these cells as if they were foreign invaders.

- The patient must have a negative TB test before initiating direct-acting monoclonal antibody therapy because the immune suppression caused by these drugs can reactivate dormant TB organisms and cause the patient to have an active TB infection.
- The first dose of any subcutaneously administered direct-acting monoclonal antibody and all doses of IV antibodies must be given by a licensed professional nurse or physician and the patient must be monitored for 30 minutes to an hour after for any adverse reactions.
- If using prefilled syringes or single-use vials and two injections are needed for a complete dose, inject the doses into two separate sites. Aspirate after inserting each needle to ensure the solution will not be injected into a blood vessel.
- Transplant rejection is a normal response of the immune system that can damage or destroy the transplanted organ.
- Patients who receive transplanted organs (unless from an identical sibling) need to take general antirejection drugs that are immunosuppressive daily to prevent transplant rejection.
- Patients who take immunosuppressive drugs have an increased risk for cancer development.
- Monoclonal and polyclonal antibodies contain some proteins from other animal species and are more likely to cause severe allergic reactions and anaphylaxis.
- Before giving any immunosuppressant drug, ask the patient about all other drugs or supplements that he or she takes and then check with the pharmacist to avoid a possible drug interaction.
- Always use personal protective equipment when mixing or administering immunosuppressant drugs to prevent accidental exposure.
- Teach sexually active women in childbearing years taking drugs for autoimmune disorders to use two reliable methods of contraception during therapy with these drugs and for 12 weeks after they are discontinued.

Additional Learning Resources

🌐 Be sure to visit your Evolve website (http://evolve.elsevier.com/Workman/pharmacology/) for additional online resources.

SG Go to your Study Guide for additional learning activities to help you master this chapter content.

Review Questions

See *Answers to In-Text Review Questions* in the back of the book for answers to these questions.

1. **How do sensitized B cells provide immune protection?**

   A. Actively secreting immunoglobulins against specific antigens
   B. Stimulating increased bone marrow production of other leukocytes
   C. Attacking and eliminating unhealthy self-cells such as infected cells or cancer cells
   D. Balancing helper T-cell activity to prevent overactive immune responses that can result in autoimmune disorder

2. **Which type of immunity does the nurse expect will develop in a patient who has received two vaccinations and a "booster" with the COVID-19 mRNA vaccine?**

   A. Naturally acquired passive immunity
   B. Naturally acquired active immunity
   C. Artificially acquired passive immunity
   D. Artificially acquired active immunity

3. **Which precaution is most important for the nurse to teach a patient taking *any* immunosuppressant drug or agent?**

   A Report an increase in urine output to your prescriber immediately.
   B. Eat a diet that is high in fruits and vegetables.
   C. Drink at least 4 L of liquids every day.
   D. Avoid crowds and people who are ill.

4. **What outcome does the nurse expect to occur in response to administering RhoGAM to an Rh-negative mother who gave birth to an Rh-positive infant 12 hours ago?**

   A. The mother will develop anti-Rh antibodies
   B. The mother will **not** develop anti-Rh antibodies
   C. The infant will develop anti-Rh antibodies
   D. The infant will **not** develop anti-Rh antibodies

5. **Which problem is characteristic of a patient who has an autoimmune disorder?**

   A. Greatly elevated total white blood cell counts
   B. Greatly decreased total white blood cell counts
   C. Development of immune responses that destroy normal tissues
   D. Significant immunosuppression and an inability to form new antibodies

6. **What is the most important question for the nurse to ask a patient prescribed to receive a direct-acting monoclonal antibody before giving the first dose of the drug?**

   A. Have you ever had tuberculosis or hepatitis?
   B. Have you ever had an allergic reaction to a "sulfa" drug?
   C. Do you eat grapefruit or drink grapefruit juice on a regular basis?
   D. Would you like to learn how to perform self-injections of a subcutaneous drug?

7. **For which patient will the nurse question a prescription for a Janus kinase (JAK) inhibitor?**

   A. 24-year-old woman with low blood pressure
   B. 34-year-old man with type 1 diabetes
   C. 44-year-old woman with rheumatoid arthritis
   D. 54-year-old man with diverticulosis

8. **Which statement regarding rejection of transplanted solid organs is true?**

   A. Rejection actions are part of normal immune function.
   B. Risk for transplant rejection is highest among people with reduced immune function.
   C. Once an episode of acute rejection starts, the damaged organ must be removed immediately.
   D. Nonsteroidal antiinflammatory drugs (NSAIDs) are a critical part of daily antirejection therapy.

9. **A patient taking cyclosporine for 1 month reports that his gums are thicker and larger than before he started taking the drug. What is the nurse's best action?**

   A. Asking whether he is performing good oral hygiene, including flossing, at least twice daily
   B. Reassuring him that this is a harmless and expected side effect of the drug
   C. Obtaining a culture of the gums to rule out an oral infectious process
   D. Notifying the prescriber immediately

10. **A patient is prescribed to receive 520 mg of cyclosporine orally. The drug on hand is cyclosporine suspension of 50 mg/mL. How many mL will the nurse prepare to administer for the correct dose of this drug?**

    A. 2.4 mL
    B. 5.2 mL
    C. 10.4 mL
    D. 15.6 mL

Clinical Judgment

1. Which information is most important for the nurse to document after injecting a patient with seasonal influenza vaccine?

   A. Age of the patient
   B. Color of the vaccine
   C. Condition of the site
   D. Expiration date on the vaccine vial
   E. Insurance type
   F. Name of the patient
   G. Needle length and diameter
   H. Site of vaccination

2. The patient is a 60-year-old woman who was diagnosed with rheumatoid arthritis (RA) when she was 34. For many years, oral methotrexate and prednisone helped to control her joint pain and swelling and also allowed her to maintain her mobility enough to keep her position as a librarian at a small college. For the past 8 months her pain, swelling, and joint stiffness have become worse and she is having a difficult time writing legibly. She is prescribed adalimumab as an addition and received the first dose 2 weeks ago. She has expressed a strong interest in self-injection of this drug. The nurse is developing a teaching plan with take-home instructions/precautions about this drug. **Use an X to indicate which instructions are Most Relevant, Not Relevant, or Potentially Harmful at this time for this patient with regard to adalimumab therapy.**

INSTRUCTION/PRECAUTION	MOST RELEVANT	NOT RELEVANT	POTENTIALLY HARMFUL
Use two reliable forms of birth control because this drug is known to cause birth defects and fetal death.			
The weeks you take this drug, stop taking your other drugs for rheumatoid arthritis to avoid any possible serious drug interactions.			
Wear nonsterile gloves when preparing your dose of adalimumab to prevent absorbing it through the skin.			
Rotate the sites so that you do not inject within 8 inches of the most recently used site.			
Pull back on the plunger after placing the needle in the skin and check to see if blood enters the syringe. If it does, do not inject that dose and prepare another dose to be injected at a different site.			
If you develop swelling of the face, lips, or tongue after injecting the drug, apply cold packs to the sites to reduce the swelling and avoid drinking anything until your lips can comfortably form a seal around a straw.			

12 | Drugs That Affect Urine Output

Learning Objectives

The content presented in this chapter should help you to:

1. Describe the names, actions, usual adult dosages, possible side effects, and adverse effects of commonly prescribed diuretics.
2. Discuss the priority actions to take before and after giving commonly prescribed diuretics.
3. Prioritize essential information to teach patients about commonly prescribed diuretics.
4. Explain appropriate life span considerations for commonly prescribed diuretics.
5. Describe the names, actions, usual adult dosages, possible side effects, and adverse effects of drug therapy to manage overactive bladder.
6. Discuss the priority actions to take before and after giving commonly prescribed drugs for overactive bladder.
7. Prioritize essential information to teach patients about commonly prescribed drugs for the management of overactive bladder.
8. Explain appropriate life span considerations for commonly prescribed drugs for overactive bladder.

Key Terms

antispasmodics (ăn-tī-spăz-MŎD-ĭks) (p. 217) Drugs used to relieve the spasm of involuntary muscle (e.g., bladder detrusor muscle).

diuretics (dī-ŭr-ĔT-ĭks) (p. 209) Drugs that help rid the body of excess water and salt (sodium).

loop diuretic (LŪP dī-ŭr-ĔT-ĭk) (p. 213) Powerful diuretic class of drugs that act on the ascending loop of Henle in the kidney. It is used primarily to treat hypertension and edema often caused by heart failure or renal insufficiency.

natriuretic diuretic (nă-trē-yū-RĔ-tĭk dī-ŭr-ĔT-ĭk) (p. 210) Diuretic that causes the excretion of sodium and water in the urine.

overactive bladder (OAB) (ŏ-vŭr-ĂK-tĭv BLĂ-dŭr (p. 217) A problem with bladder function that causes a sudden urge to

urinate and can even lead to the involuntary loss of urine (incontinence).

potassium-sparing diuretic (pō-TĂS-ē-ŭm SPĀR-ĭng dī-ŭr-ĔT-ĭk) (p. 215) A drug that blocks the exchange of sodium for potassium and hydrogen ions in the distal tubule, leading to increased sodium and chloride excretion without increased potassium excretion.

thiazide diuretic (THĪ-ŭ-zīd dī-ŭr-ĔT-ĭk) (p. 211) A diuretic drug class that slows down or turns off the sodium pumps in the nephron tube farthest away from the capillaries and causes more sodium, potassium, and water to stay in the urine and leave the body through urination. It is used primarily in the treatment of hypertension.

REVIEW OF RELATED PHYSIOLOGY AND PATHOPHYSIOLOGY

The bloodstream is the major body fluid from which the kidneys produce and excrete urine to maintain body water and electrolyte balance. Blood travels to the kidneys where there are millions of small tubes called *nephrons*, which are the filtering units of the kidneys (Figure 12.1) that create urine (Animation 12.1). Each nephron has a collection of capillaries at the beginning of the nephron. Whole blood flows into these capillaries, which are leaky to water and small particles such as sugar, sodium, potassium, and chloride but not leaky to blood cells, proteins, and large particles. When whole blood goes through capillaries, the water and small particles leave the capillaries and go into the nephrons. The blood cells, proteins, and large particles go directly back into the blood.

The purpose of the nephrons is to act like a "washing machine" and take out all the waste products (e.g., urea and ammonia), extra water, sodium, and potassium to keep the blood "clean." In healthy kidneys, about 100 mL (3 to 4 oz) of water (and

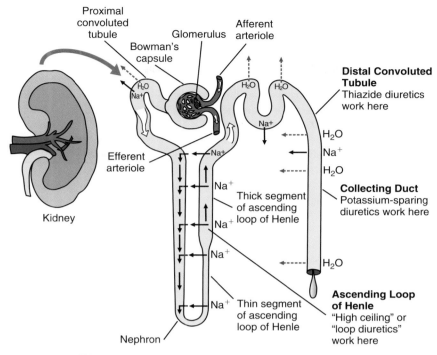

FIG. 12.1 Sites of diuretic action on the kidney and nephrons.

small particles) enters the nephron tubules each minute. If nothing happened to this 100 mL of water, everyone would have a urine output of 6000 mL (6 qt or 6 L) every hour, which is too much water for the body to lose and would lead to dehydration. To prevent this much water from being lost along with the waste products, sites along the nephron tubes *(renal tubules)* draw out most of the water and helpful particles but keep the waste products in the urine. The cleaned water and helpful particles are put back into the blood by *reabsorption.* The waste products and excess sodium and potassium stay in the urine, along with just enough water to allow them to be removed by urination out of the body *(excretion).* In this way, a person loses waste products and excess particles without losing too much water.

The places in the nephron tubes that allow water, sodium, and potassium to be pulled out from the urine and put back into the blood have special "pumps" that remove the sodium and potassium. Because of the rule "where sodium goes, water follows," the pulling of sodium from the urine pulls water along with it. This process allows each person to make only about 1 mL of urine each minute. The urine collects in the bladder until it is ready to be eliminated through urination. Most people have a urine output of about 2400 mL (nearly 2.5 quarts) each day. The amount of urine output increases when a person's fluid intake increases and decreases when fluid intake decreases.

DIURETICS

OVERVIEW OF DIURETICS

Often called "water pills," diuretic drugs cause the body to lose water. **Diuretics** are drugs that help rid the body of excess water and sodium by increasing a person's urine output. They may work on the kidneys directly, or they may increase blood flow to the kidney. Either way, these drugs cause a patient to urinate more and lose water from the body.

Most often, diuretics are used to treat problems when the body retains too much water, too much sodium, or too much potassium. They are often prescribed for patients who have the following health problems:

• High blood pressure (hypertension)

 Memory Jogger

Total-body water and electrolyte balance is maintained by the ability of the kidneys to selectively retain or eliminate fluids and small molecules.

 Memory Jogger

The rule "where sodium goes, water follows" works with sodium-excreting diuretics in the kidney. When sodium moves into the nephron tubules, water follows and is excreted in the urine.

> **Box 12.1 Indications of Dehydration with Diuretic Therapy**
>
> - Increased pulse rate with a "thready" pulse that may be hard to feel
> - Low blood pressure (hypotension)
> - Thirst
> - Sunken appearance to the eyeballs
> - Dry mouth with a thick, sticky coating on the tongue
> - Skin "tenting" on the forehead or chest (gently pinch up a section of skin on the forehead or chest, release it, and see how long it takes for the "tent" you made to go away)
> - Constipation
> - Decreased urine output (less than 30 mL/hr) with urine that is dark and strong-smelling

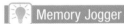

Memory Jogger

Diuretics do **not** cure health problems, and patients may need to take them daily for the rest of their life.

Memory Jogger

The three most commonly used types of diuretics are called natriuretic diuretics and include thiazide, loop, and potassium-sparing diuretics.

- Heart failure
- Kidney disease
- Liver disease (cirrhosis)

Because the action of diuretics leads to increased urine output, patients taking these drugs are at increased risk for *dehydration*, a condition caused by the loss of too much water from the body. Signs and symptoms of dehydration to watch for with diuretic therapy are listed in Box 12.1.

TYPES OF DIURETICS

The five classes of diuretics include thiazides and thiazide-like diuretics, loop diuretics, carbonic anhydrase inhibitors, potassium-sparing diuretics, and osmotic diuretics. The three most commonly used classes of diuretics are called **natriuretic diuretics**, which usually are taken daily for chronic conditions. These drugs slow down or turn off the sodium pumps in the nephrons and make a person excrete more sodium and water. They are discussed in more detail separately and include:

- Thiazide diuretics
- Loop diuretics
- Potassium-sparing diuretics

Two additional non-natriuretic types of diuretics, osmotic diuretics and carbonic anhydrase inhibitors, are used less frequently and most often for short-term management of a few specific health problems. *Osmotic diuretics,* such as mannitol (Osmitrol), increase the blood flow to the kidneys and are used only in critical situations (e.g., reduction of intracranial or intraocular pressure, promotion of excretion of toxins in cases of drug poisoning). Consult a critical care source for a discussion of the use of osmotic diuretics.

Carbonic anhydrase inhibitors, such as acetazolamide (Diamox), are another class of drugs that are sometimes used for diuresis. These drugs are primarily used for treatment of glaucoma (e.g., to lower intraocular pressure) and are discussed in Chapter 27.

GENERAL ISSUES WITH DIURETIC THERAPY

Most common diuretic drugs have unique, as well as common, actions and effects. In addition to the practices for drug administration discussed in Chapter 27, general responsibilities for safe administration of **any** diuretic drug are listed in the following paragraphs. Older adults are more sensitive to all diuretics, with an increased risk for side effects and often require lower dosages. Specific responsibilities are presented with each class of diuretics.

⭐ *Priority actions to take* before *giving any diuretic.* Obtain a complete list of drugs that the patient is currently taking, including over-the-counter and herbal preparations. Check baselines for weight, blood pressure, and heart rate and rhythm for comparison after giving a diuretic drug. If blood pressure is low (less than 90/60 mm Hg.), ask the prescriber if the patient should receive the drug. Also, check the latest set of blood electrolyte levels and notify the prescriber of any abnormal values. Ask patients about their usual urine output pattern.

Check to be certain that the patient does not have a problem with blockage in any area of the urinary system (e.g., an enlarged prostate that interferes with urine flow out of the bladder, narrowed ureters that block or slow urine flow from kidneys to the bladder). Giving diuretics to a person with a blockage can cause backflow of urine into the kidneys and damage them.

Give scheduled doses in the morning to avoid the loss of sleep because of the patient's need to urinate. Make sure that the patient has a urinal or other collection device to measure urine output.

⭐ *Priority actions to take* **after** *giving any diuretic.* Be sure to recheck and continue to monitor blood pressure and heart rate at least once every 8 hours because rapid water loss decreases blood volume and lowers blood pressure. Monitor for signs of orthostatic hypotension, such as dizziness or light-headedness. Ensure that the call light is within easy reach and instruct patients to call for help getting out of bed. Assist patients to change positions slowly. Have them sit on the side of the bed for 1 to 2 minutes before getting up, and then stand up slowly.

Keep a record of urine output because increased urine output is an expected response to all diuretic drugs. Obtain daily weights at the same time each day, using the same scale and with the patient wearing the same or similar clothing.

Continue to monitor blood electrolyte levels for any changes that may result from the diuretic drug. The most important electrolytes to monitor are potassium and sodium. Although dosages may vary depending on the patient's response to diuretic therapy—and sometimes drugs are started at lower doses than the patient will eventually take daily—the drug tables indicate the most common adult maintenance dosages prescribed.

⭐ *Teaching priorities for patients taking any diuretic*
- Make a schedule that interferes the least with your daily activities, such as taking the drug early in the morning to prevent needing to get up at night to urinate.
- Take drugs exactly as prescribed.
- If you take more than one dose daily, take the last dose by 6:00 pm.
- If a daily dose is missed, take it when you remember it.
- Do not double the next day's dose if you forgot the dose the day before.
- Because the drugs change your blood pressure and make you feel light-headed or dizzy if you change positions quickly, get up from a lying or sitting position slowly, and wait a minute before walking.
- If you check your blood pressure daily, notify your prescriber if it is lower than 90/60, or if you are frequently light-headed.
- Notify your prescriber if your heartbeat becomes irregular, consistently lower than 60 beats per minute, or higher than 100 beats per minute.
- Weigh yourself daily at the same time of day, on the same scale, and wearing the same amount of clothing, and keep a record of your weights.
- If you gain more than 2 lb in 1 day or 3 lb in a week, notify your prescriber.
- Drink about the same amount of fluid each day that you urinate to keep from becoming dehydrated.

Thiazide Diuretics

How thiazide diuretics work. Thiazide diuretics slow down or turn off the sodium pumps in the nephron tubes farthest away from the capillaries (see Figure 12.1). They cause more sodium, potassium, and water to stay in the urine and leave the body through urination. This action reduces blood volume and lowers blood pressure. Commonly prescribed thiazide diuretics are listed in the following table. Be sure to consult a valid drug reference source for more information about specific thiazide diuretics.

⚠ Drug Alert

Monitoring Alert

After giving any diuretic drug, monitor blood pressure at least once every 8 hr. Rapid water loss decreases blood volume and lowers blood pressure and can lead to hypotension.

QSEN: Safety

Adult Dosages for Commonly Prescribed Thiazide Diuretic Drugs

Drug Category	Drug Name	Usual Maintenance Dose
Natriuretics: Thiazide	chlorothiazide (Diuril)	500–1000 mg orally once or twice daily 500–1,000 mg IV once or twice daily
	hydrochlorothiazide (Aquazide H, Microzide, Esidrix, Oretic)	12.5–25 mg orally once daily.
	metolazone (Zaroxolyn)	2.5–5 mg orally once daily
	chlorthalidone (Thalitone)	15–25 mg orally once daily Max: 100 mg/day

Intended responses of thiazide diuretics
- Urine output is increased.
- Urine is lighter in color.
- Blood pressure is lower.

Common side effects of thiazide diuretics. At lower doses, side effects of thiazide diuretics are less common—however, side effects increase with higher blood levels of these drugs. Potential side effects of thiazide diuretics include fluid and electrolyte imbalances, such as decreased blood volume, and changes in electrolytes, such as lowered potassium (hypokalemia), sodium (hyponatremia), chloride (hypochloremia), and magnesium (hypomagnesemia), and increased calcium (hypercalcemia) and urea (hyperuremia). Because of decreased blood volume, blood pressure drops faster when the patient moves from a sitting or lying position to a standing position, causing some dizziness or light-headedness *(postural hypotension)*. When postural hypotension is severe, the patient could faint and fall.

Decreased potassium levels may result in dry mouth, increased thirst, irregular heartbeat, mood changes, muscle cramps, nausea, vomiting, fatigue or weakness, and weak pulses.

Decreased sodium levels may lead to confusion, convulsions, decreased mental activity, irritability, muscle cramps, and unusual fatigue or weakness.

Possible adverse effects of thiazide diuretics. Adverse effects of thiazide diuretics include "passing out" or falling when changing positions, muscle weakness, and blurred vision. Metolazone can cause impaired glucose tolerance, glucosuria, and hyperglycemia in patients with diabetes. Recently, thiazide diuretic use has been associated with the development of skin cancer.

⭐ *Priority actions to take before giving thiazide diuretics.* In addition to the general priority actions to take before giving any diuretic drug therapy (p. 210), check the most recent serum potassium levels. If it is below 3.5 mEq/L or 3.5 mmol/L, inform the prescriber. Patients who have low blood potassium levels may develop life-threatening abnormal heart rhythms.

Ask patients about prior allergic reactions to thiazide diuretics. Ask women in their childbearing years if they are pregnant, plan to become pregnant, or are breastfeeding because thiazide diuretics should not be used during pregnancy or breastfeeding.

⭐ *Priority actions to take after giving thiazide diuretics.* In addition to the general priority actions to take after giving any diuretic drug therapy (p. 211), keep track of the patient's blood electrolyte levels, including potassium. Watch for signs of decreased potassium, such as abnormal heart rhythms, muscle cramps, constipation,

---

Common Side Effects

Thiazide Diuretics

Hypotension

Hypokalemia

Hyponatremia

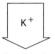
Nausea and Vomiting

⭐ **Critical Point for Safety**

Check the apical pulse of patients receiving a thiazide diuretic for a full minute to determine whether or not the rhythm is regular.

QSEN: Safety

and changes in reflexes. Table 1.4 in Chapter 1 provides a summary of normal electrolyte values.

 Teaching priorities for patients taking thiazide diuretics. In addition to the general priority teaching for patients taking diuretic drug therapy (p. 211), include these teaching points and precautions:

- The normal range for blood potassium is 3.5 to 5 mEq/L. Report side effects of low potassium (e.g. muscle weakness or cramps, sudden decrease in urination, and irregular heartbeat) to your prescriber.
- Take all prescribed potassium pills or liquids as instructed by your prescriber.
- If upset stomach occurs when taking your prescribed potassium pills or liquids, take the medication with food.
- If you forget to take your thiazide diuretic, do **not** take a double dose the next day.

Life span considerations for thiazide diuretics

Pediatric considerations. The dosage of diuretic drugs is based on weight for children. Thiazide diuretics are used with caution when infants have jaundice because the drugs worsen the condition.

Considerations for pregnancy and lactation. Thiazide diuretics have a moderate likelihood of increasing the risk for birth defects or fetal damage. They should be avoided during pregnancy because they may cause side effects in the newborn, including jaundice and low potassium levels. These drugs have been shown to cause birth defects (are teratogenic) in animals. They should also be avoided during breastfeeding because they pass into breast milk. The action of diuretics also may decrease the flow of breast milk.

Considerations for older adults. Dizziness or light-headedness and signs of low potassium levels are more likely in older adults because they are more sensitive to the effects of thiazide diuretics. This greatly increases the older adult's risk for falls. Teach these patients to change positions slowly, and always use the handrails when going up or down stairs.

Loop Diuretics

How loop diuretics work. Loop diuretics are the most powerful diuretics. Although this power can be helpful, it also means that the *side effects are more severe* because there is greater water, sodium, and potassium loss. Also called "high-ceiling" diuretics, these drugs slow down or turn off the sodium pumps in the nephron tube in a place different from thiazide diuretic action. They cause more sodium, potassium, and water to stay in the urine and leave the body through urination (see Figure. 12.1). Another difference between loop diuretics and thiazide diuretics is that loop diuretics cause patients to lose calcium in the urine.

Commonly prescribed loop diuretics are listed in the following table. Be sure to consult a reliable source for more information about a specific loop diuretic.

Adult Dosages for Commonly Prescribed Loop Diuretic Drugs

Drug Category	Drug Name	Usual Maintenance Dose
Natriuretics: Loop	furosemide (Delone, Lasix)	20–80 mg orally as a single dose. May be given in 2 or 4 divided doses Max: 600 mg/day 20–40 mg IV or IM. Max: 600–800 mg/day *Special Considerations:* **Given IV slowly, no more than 20 mg/min**
	bumetanide (Bumex)	0.5–1 mg orally once daily
	ethacrynic acid (Edecrin)	50–100 mg orally once or twice daily. Max: 400 mg/day (200 mg twice a day) 0.5–1 mg/kg IV
	torsemide (Demadex)	10–20 mg orally or IV once daily

 Critical Point for Safety

If a patient forgets to take a thiazide diuretic, a double dose should **not** be taken the next day.

QSEN: Safety

Critical Point for Safety

Thiazide diuretics should not be given during pregnancy or to breastfeeding mothers because they cause side effects, pass into breast milk, and may cause a decrease in the flow of breast milk.

QSEN: Safety

 Critical Point for Safety

An order for Lasix can be mistaken for Luvox. Lasix is a loop diuretic; Luvox is an antidepressant.

QSEN: Safety

Intended responses of loop diuretics
- Urine output is increased.
- Urine is lighter in color.
- Blood pressure is lower.

Common side effects of loop diuretics. Common side effects of loop diuretics include dizziness or light-headedness when the patient moves from a sitting or lying position to a standing position. This occurs because blood pressure drops in response to the loss of fluid from the blood vessels *(orthostatic hypotension; also called postural hypotension).*

Blood levels of potassium and sodium decrease *(hypokalemia, hyponatremia)* with loop diuretics. Signs and symptoms of low potassium include dry mouth, increased thirst, irregular heartbeat, mental and mood changes, muscle cramps or muscle pain, nausea, vomiting, fatigue, weakness, and weak pulses. Signs and symptoms of low sodium include confusion, convulsions, decreased mental activity, irritability, muscle cramps, and unusual fatigue or weakness.

An additional side effect of furosemide is increased sensitivity of the skin to sunlight *(photosensitivity)*, possibly with skin rash, itching, redness, or severe sunburn. Ethacrynic acid may cause confusion, diarrhea, loss of appetite, and nervousness. Blurred vision, chest pain, premature ejaculation, or difficulty maintaining an erection may occur with bumetanide.

Possible adverse effects of loop diuretics. Fainting or falling when changing positions, muscle weakness, and irregular heart rhythms can occur.

Loop diuretics can be *ototoxic* (cause hearing loss from damage to the auditory [ear] tissues). Ototoxicity is reversible when the drug is discontinued, and it becomes worse when the patient is taking other ototoxic drugs, such as aminoglycoside antibiotics, while taking a loop diuretic. Hearing loss can occur when these drugs are given too rapidly intravenously (IV) and/or in very high doses. This hearing loss is usually temporary.

High blood glucose (hyperglycemia) levels can also occur. Patients with diabetes must check their blood sugar (glucose) levels regularly.

⭐ *Priority actions to take* **before** *giving loop diuretics.* In addition to the general priority actions to take before giving diuretic therapy (p. 210), check the most recent serum potassium level. If it is below 3.5 mEq/L or 3.5 mmol/L, be sure to inform the prescriber. Check to see whether the patient is scheduled to receive a potassium supplement. If the potassium level is low, the prescriber may order an extra dose of potassium. Check the serum sodium level. If it is below 135 mEq/L or 135 mmol/L, inform the prescriber.

Check the patient's prescribed drugs to determine whether another drug is also ototoxic. If you find that the patient is taking another ototoxic drug, inform the prescriber.

If the drug is to be given intravenously, always check the IV site for patency and signs of inflammation or infection.

⭐ *Priority actions to take* **after** *giving loop diuretics.* In addition to the general priority actions to take after giving diuretic therapy (p. 211), monitor serum potassium levels and report low values (less than 3.5 mEq/L or 3.5 mmol/L) to the prescriber. Give prescribed potassium supplements as ordered. Continue to monitor patients for any signs of hearing loss.

Be sure that urinary collection devices are within easy reach of patients and instruct them to call for help getting up to urinate. Frequently check and record urine output. Regularly empty urine collection devices. Check IV sites for patency at least every 8 hours and monitor for signs of phlebitis or infection (e.g., irritation, redness, swelling, warmth).

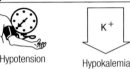

Common Side Effects

Loop Diuretics

Hypotension	Hypokalemia
Hyponatremia	Photosensitivity

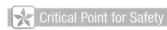

Critical Point for Safety

Give IV doses of furosemide (Lasix) slowly at a rate of 20 mg/min to avoid ototoxicity.

QSEN: Safety

⭐ *Teaching priorities for patients taking loop diuretics.* In addition to the general teaching priorities related to diuretic therapy (p. 211), include these teaching points and precautions:

- Remember that urine output can increase dramatically within an hour of taking a loop diuretic, which increases your risk for unexpected or uncontrolled urination.
- Limit alcohol intake because it increases your risk for dizziness, light-headedness, and fainting.
- Report any decrease in your hearing or the sensation of "ringing" in your ears to your prescriber because this may indicate the drug is damaging your ears.
- Stay out of direct sunlight and wear protective clothing and/or sunscreen when outdoors to reduce your risk for severe sunburn.
- Avoid using sunlamps and tanning beds because your skin's sensitivity to the sun is increased.
- Remember to eat foods that contain potassium, such as bananas, citrus foods, avocados, asparagus, broccoli, sweet potatoes, and meat to help prevent excessive loss of potassium.
- Take any prescribed potassium supplement with food or liquids to prevent stomach irritation.

Life span considerations for loop diuretics

Considerations for pregnancy and lactation. Loop diuretics have a moderate level of increased risk for birth defects or fetal damage, and they should not be given to women who are pregnant or breastfeeding. Animal studies have shown these drugs to cause fetal harm (are teratogenic). Furosemide passes into breast milk and should not be used while breastfeeding.

Considerations for older adults. Older adults are more sensitive to the effects of loop diuretics and are more likely to develop dizziness and light-headedness, which increases their risk for falls. They are also more likely to develop blood clots and signs of low blood potassium. Teach them to report new-onset muscle weakness to the prescriber. Older adults are more likely to have tinnitus and hearing loss with these drugs. Teach them to note whether they are having more difficulty hearing what is said and whether they need to set the volume higher on the radio or television.

Potassium-Sparing Diuretics

How potassium-sparing diuretics work. Potassium-sparing diuretics slow the sodium pumps so more sodium and water are excreted in the urine, but these drugs do **not** increase the loss of potassium. They prevent potassium loss in the urine and cause more potassium to be returned to the blood. These drugs work in a place in the nephron tubes that is different from other diuretics (see Figure. 12.1).

Commonly prescribed potassium-sparing diuretics are listed in the following table. Be sure to consult a reliable source for more information on a specific potassium-sparing diuretic.

 Critical Point for Safety

Teach patients taking loop diuretics about foods that contain potassium, such as bananas and oranges, or to drink citrus fruit juices.

QSEN: Safety

 Critical Point for Safety

Instruct older adults to report indicators of difficulty with hearing, including the need to increase the volume setting on the radio or television.

QSEN: Safety

Adult Dosages for Commonly Prescribed Natriuretic Potassium-Sparing Diuretic Drugs[a]

Drug Category	Drug Name	Usual Maintenance Dose
Natriuretics: Potassium-Sparing	spironolactone (Aldactone, CaroSpir)	25–100 mg orally daily in single or divided doses
	triamterene (Dyrenium)	100 mg orally twice daily. Max: 500 mg/day
	amiloride (Midamor)	5–10 mg orally daily. Max: 20 mg/day

[a]Some potassium-sparing diuretics are combined with a thiazide diuretic used to treat hypertension and to reduce edema due to salt and water retention in disorders of the heart, kidneys, liver, and lungs (e.g., Dyazide [hydrochlorothiazide/triamterene], Aldactazide [hydrochlorothiazide/spironolactone])

Intended responses of potassium-sparing diuretics
- Urine output is increased.
- Urine is lighter in color.
- Blood pressure is lower.
- Serum potassium levels stay within the normal range (3.5 to 5 mEq/L).

Common side effects of potassium-sparing diuretics. Blood pressure drops faster when the patient who is taking potassium-sparing diuretics moves from a sitting or lying position to a standing position, causing some dizziness or light-headedness (orthostatic, also called postural hypotension). Patient falls are more likely.

Blood levels of sodium decrease (hyponatremia). Symptoms of low sodium levels include drowsiness, dry mouth, increased thirst, lack of energy, and muscle weakness.

Other common side effects of potassium-sparing diuretics include nausea, vomiting, stomach cramps, and diarrhea.

Women may develop *hirsutism* (facial hair), irregular menstrual cycles, and deepening of the voice. Men may have trouble getting or keeping an erection. Both men and women may develop breast enlargement (*gynecomastia* in men).

Triamterene may cause the skin to become more sensitive to sunlight (*photosensitivity*), possibly with skin rash, itching, redness, or severe sunburn.

Possible adverse effects of potassium-sparing diuretics. Fainting or falling when changing positions may occur because of the decrease in blood volume and blood pressure.

Because these drugs "spare" potassium, the patient is at risk for increased potassium levels (hyperkalemia). A life-threatening side effect of high potassium level is the development of an irregular heartbeat (*dysrhythmia*). Symptoms of a high potassium level include confusion, irregular heartbeat, nervousness, numbness or tingling (in the hands, feet, or lips), shortness of breath or difficulty breathing, unusual fatigue or weakness, and weakness or a heavy feeling in the legs.

⭐ ***Priority actions to take** before **giving potassium-sparing diuretics.*** In addition to the general priority actions to take before giving diuretic therapy (p. 210), check the most recent serum electrolyte levels. If the potassium level is greater than 5 mEq/L or 5 mmol/L or the sodium level is less than 135 mEq/L or 135 mmol/L, inform the prescriber.

⭐ ***Priority actions to take** after **giving potassium-sparing diuretics.*** In addition to the general priority actions to take after giving diuretic therapy (p. 211), monitor the patient for signs and symptoms of high potassium. These include dry mouth, increased thirst, irregular heartbeat, mood changes, muscle cramps, nausea, vomiting, fatigue or weakness, and weak pulses. Also monitor for signs and symptoms of low sodium levels, including confusion, convulsions, decreased mental activity, irritability, muscle cramps, and unusual fatigue or weakness.

⭐ ***Teaching priorities for patients taking potassium-sparing diuretics.*** In addition to the general teaching priorities related to diuretic therapy (p. 211), include these teaching points and precautions:
- Avoid eating excessive amounts of high-potassium-containing foods, such as meats, dairy products, dried fruits, bananas, cantaloupe, kiwis, oranges, avocados, broccoli, dried beans or peas, lima beans, soybeans, and spinach.
- Do not use salt substitutes because these products contain potassium instead of sodium.

Life span considerations for potassium-sparing diuretics
Considerations for pregnancy and lactation. Spironolactone has a high likelihood of increasing the risk of birth defects or fetal damage and should be avoided during

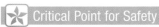

Common Side Effects
Potassium-Sparing Diuretics

Hyponatremia   Hyperkalemia

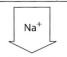

Nausea   Breast enlargement

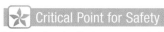

Critical Point for Safety

Do not give potassium supplements, salt substitutes, or angiotensin-converting enzyme inhibitors to patients taking potassium-sparing diuretics because these drugs can increase the risk of developing high to extremely high blood potassium levels.

QSEN: Safety

Critical Point for Safety

Most salt substitutes are made by replacing sodium with potassium. Therefore, salt substitutes should be avoided while taking a potassium-sparing diuretic.

QSEN: Safety

pregnancy. Triamterene and amiloride have a low likelihood of increasing the risk for birth defects or fetal damage.

REVIEW OF RELATED PHYSIOLOGY AND PATHOPHYSIOLOGY FOR OVERACTIVE BLADDER

Normally, the bladder's detrusor muscle contracts and relaxes appropriately in response to the amount of urine in the bladder and controls the initiation of urination. **Overactive bladder** (OAB) results when the layered detrusor contracts spastically, sometimes without a known cause. This results in continuous high bladder pressure and the urgent need to urinate—also known as *urgency* (Figure 12.2).

People with OAB often have a sudden, unstoppable need to urinate at inconvenient and unpredictable times and sometimes lose control before reaching a toilet *(incontinence)*. Thus, OAB interferes with work, daily routine, intimacy, and sexual function; causes embarrassment; and can diminish self-esteem and quality of life. OAB is fairly common in older adults. Drugs for OAB are used to treat the symptoms of the disorder but do not cure the cause of the problem.

TYPES OF DRUGS FOR OVERACTIVE BLADDER

Urinary Antispasmodics

How urinary antispasmodics work. Drugs for OAB (urinary **antispasmodics**) are prescribed to treat and improve symptoms, including frequent urination, urgency of urination, and urinary incontinence. These drugs decrease the spasms of the detrusor muscle.

Commonly prescribed drugs for OAB are listed in the following table. Be sure to consult a valid drug resource for more information about a specific drug for OAB.

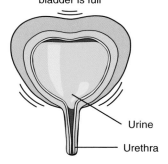

Normal Bladder
Detrusor muscle contracts when bladder is full

Urine

Urethra

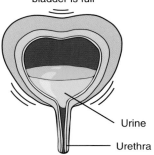

Overactive Bladder
Detrusor muscle contracts before bladder is full

Urine

Urethra

FIG. 12.2 Pathophysiology of overactive bladder.

Adult Dosages for Commonly Prescribed Urinary Antispasmodic Drugs

Drug Category	Drug Name	Usual Maintenance Dose
Urinary Antispasmodics	oxybutynin (Ditropan, Ditropan XL, Oxytrol)	5 mg orally 2–3 times per day. Max: 5 mg 4 times/day Extended-release 5–10 mg orally once daily. Max: 30 mg/day
	oxybutynin transdermal system patch (Oxytrol; Gelnique)	Apply 1 patch (delivering 3.9 mg/day of oxybutynin) topically twice weekly (every 3–4 days) to the a bdomen, hip, or buttock *Special Considerations:* **Rotate patch site at each application**
	tolterodine (Detrol, Detrol LA)	2 mg orally twice daily Extended-release 4 mg orally once daily
	solifenacin (VESIcare, Vesicare LA)	5–10 mg orally once daily
	darifenacin (Enablex)	7.5–15 mg orally once daily
	trospium chloride (Sanctura, Sanctura XR)	20 mg orally twice daily Extended-release: 60 mg orally once daily in the morning 1 hr before breakfast *Special Considerations:* **Give 1 hr before meals or on an empty stomach**

Intended responses of urinary antispasmodics
- Urinary frequency is decreased.
- Urinary urgency is decreased.
- Urinary incontinence is decreased.

Common Side Effects
Urinary Antispasmodics

Dizziness

Constipation

Dry mouth

Dry eyes

Common side effects of urinary antispasmodics. Frequent side effects of drugs for OAB include dry mouth, dry eyes, headache, dizziness, and constipation.

Possible adverse effects of urinary antispasmodics. Adverse effects of these drugs include chest pain, fast or irregular heart rate, shortness of breath, swelling (edema) and rapid weight gain, confusion, and hallucinations. In addition, these drugs may cause decreased urination or no urine output, and painful or difficult urination.

Signs of an allergic reaction include rash (hives), difficulty breathing, and swelling of the face, lips, tongue, or throat.

Patients may be at increased risk for heatstroke during exercise or hot weather because these drugs decrease perspiration (sweating).

⭐ *Teaching priorities for patients taking urinary antispasmodics.* Because most of these drugs are prescribed for outpatients, emphasize the following teaching points and precautions:

- Take these drugs on an empty stomach with water. If you experience stomach upset, the drugs may be taken with milk or food.
- Do not crush, chew, break, or open extended-release or long-acting capsules. Instead, swallow the capsule whole because these drugs are made to release the medication slowly into the body. When the capsules are opened in any way, the drug is released all at once and can cause an overdose with more side effects. Also, the drug will not be effective throughout the day.
- If you miss a dose, take it as soon as possible. If it is almost time for the next dose, skip the missed dose and take the drug at the next scheduled time.
- Do not take extra pills to make up for the missed dose.
- Avoid becoming overheated or dehydrated during exercise or hot weather because these drugs may decrease sweating and increase the risk for heatstroke.
- Weigh yourself daily at the same time of day, on the same scale, and wearing the same amount of clothing, and keep a record of your weights.
- If you gain more than 2 lb in 1 day or 3 lb in a week, notify your prescriber.
- If you take your blood pressure daily, notify your prescriber if it is lower than 90/60, or if you are frequently light-headed.
- Notify your prescriber if your heartbeat becomes irregular, consistently lower than 60 beats per minute, or higher than 100 beats per minute.
- Report urinary urgency, frequency, difficulty urinating, or incontinence to your prescriber.
- Keep track of your fluid intake and output. If urinary symptoms do not improve, or if they become worse while taking these drugs, immediately contact your prescriber.
- Because these drugs may blur your vision or cause drowsiness, avoid driving, or any other activities that require clear vision and mental alertness, until you know how the drugs will affect you.
- Do not drink alcohol within 2 hours of these drugs because side effects such as drowsiness are increased. Drink alcohol only when you do not plan to drive or operate dangerous equipment.
- If you use the transdermal patch system, apply a new patch to your skin every 3 to 4 days (as prescribed), and rotate the application sites.
- Apply the fresh patch to a different clean, dry, and smooth area, and press it firmly to ensure that it stays in place. Be sure to remove the old patch.
- Report any skin redness, itchiness, or irritation to your prescriber.

Life span considerations for urinary antispasmodics
Considerations for pregnancy and lactation. Oxybutynin has a low likelihood of increasing the risk for birth defects or fetal damage. Other OAB drugs have a moderate likelihood of increasing the risk for birth defects or fetal damage. They are not recommended for use with pregnant or breastfeeding women.

⭐ **Critical Point for Safety**

Patients taking drugs for OAB are at risk for heatstroke during exercise or in hot weather.

QSEN: Safety

⭐ **Critical Point for Safety**

Teach patients using the transdermal patch system to remove the old patch before applying a new one to avoid excessive dosage.

QSEN: Safety

Get Ready for the NCLEX® Examination!

Key Points

- Most commonly prescribed diuretics work on the nephrons in the kidneys to increase urine output.
- Diuretics are prescribed to treat hypertension, heart failure, kidney disease, and liver disease.
- The five classes of diuretics include thiazides and thiazide-like diuretics, loop diuretics, carbonic anhydrase inhibitors, potassium-sparing diuretics, and osmotic diuretics.
- The three most commonly prescribed diuretics are called natriuretic diuretics (thiazide, loop, potassium-sparing).
- The most common side effects of diuretics are dizziness and light-headedness related to hypotension.
- After giving any diuretic drug, monitor blood pressure at least once every 8 hours. Rapid water loss decreases blood volume and lowers blood pressure.
- Check the apical pulse of patients receiving a thiazide diuretic for a full minute to determine whether the rhythm is regular.
- If a patient forgets to take a diuretic, a double dose should **not** be taken the next day.
- Thiazide diuretics should **not** be given during pregnancy or to breastfeeding mothers because they cause side effects, pass into breast milk, and may cause a decrease in the flow of breast milk.
- Give IV doses of furosemide (Lasix) slowly at a rate of 20 mg per minute to avoid ototoxicity.
- Teach patients that diuresis (increased urine output) can occur rapidly after IV administration of a loop diuretic and may lead to incontinence.
- Teach patients taking loop diuretics about foods that contain potassium, such as bananas and oranges, or to drink citrus fruit juices.
- Instruct older adults to report indicators of difficulty with hearing, including the need to increase the volume setting on the radio or television.

- Teach patients taking potassium-sparing diuretics to avoid the use of salt substitutes because these substitutes are made with potassium instead of sodium.
- Do not give potassium supplements, salt substitutes, or angiotensin-converting enzyme inhibitors to patients taking potassium-sparing diuretics because these drugs can increase the risk of developing high to extremely high blood potassium levels (hyperkalemia).
- Unless a patient is on a fluid restriction, be sure that fluid intake closely matches the urine output in a patient taking diuretics.
- Monitor patients taking diuretics for signs and symptoms of dehydration.
- Monitor electrolytes carefully when a patient is taking a diuretic.
- Check the blood pressure of a patient who is taking diuretics at least once per shift, even if it is not ordered.
- Drugs for OAB decrease detrusor muscle spasms and relieve symptoms.
- Patients taking OAB drugs are at risk for heatstroke.
- Teach patients using the transdermal patch system to remove the old patch before applying a new one.

Additional Learning Resources

🌐 Be sure to visit your Evolve website (http://evolve.elsevier.com/Workman/pharmacology/) for additional online resources.

SG Go to your Study Guide for additional learning activities to help you master this chapter's content

Review Questions

See *Answers to In-Text Review Questions* in the back of the book for answers to these questions.

1. **For which complication does the nurse remain alert when a patient is taking any type of diuretic?**

   A. Loss of appetite
   B. Bladder spasms
   C. Hypertension
   D. Dehydration

2. **A patient who has been prescribed a diuretic for the past 2 weeks is now experiencing all the following changes. Which change indicates to the nurse that the diuretic is effective?**

   A. Weight loss of 7 lb.
   B. Heart rate increased from 72 to 80 beats per minute
   C. Respiratory rate decreased from 20 to 16 breaths per minute
   D. Morning blood glucose decreased from 142 mg/dL to 110 mg/dL

3. **A patient prescribed a once-daily diuretic calls the office to report that yesterday's drug dose was missed. What is the nurse's best advice?**

   A. "Take today's dose now and restrict today's fluid intake to 1 L."
   B. "Take yesterday's dose now and take today's dose after another 6 hours."
   C. "Take today's dose now and maintain your normal intake of food and fluids."
   D. "Skip today's doses of all your medications, and then begin everything fresh tomorrow."

4. **The nurse is teaching a patient about diuretic therapy. Which statement made by the patient indicates that more teaching is needed?**

   A. "I am so thankful that my high blood pressure has been cured by this drug."
   B. "I always try to drink just about the same amount of fluid that I urinate each day."

C. "I will call my health care provider if my heart rate is less than 60 beats per minute."

D. "I have been taking this drug early in the day so that I don't have to get up during the night."

5. A patient taking a thiazide diuretic has the following blood laboratory values for kidney function. Which value does the nurse report to the prescriber **immediately to prevent harm**?

A. Sodium 136 mEq/L
B. Potassium 2.6 mEq/L
C. Creatinine 0.9 mg/dL
D. Blood urea nitrogen 6 mg/dL

6. The nurse administers 20 mg of furosemide (Lasix) to a patient by the intravenous (IV) route. Which action is **most important** for the nurse to take **to prevent harm**?

A. Give the drug slowly over at least 2 minutes.
B. Check the patient carefully for symptoms of low blood glucose levels.
C. Mix the drug with potassium chloride to prevent a rapid drop in serum potassium levels.
D. Monitor the IV site after giving the drug because furosemide causes severe tissue damage if infiltration occurs.

7. A patient who is prescribed spironolactone asks why he or she must avoid salt substitutes. What is the nurse's **best** response?

A. They may increase your risk for a high potassium level.
B. Your hypertension will be worse while taking salt substitutes.
C. These condiments may lead to hypokalemia.
D. Water retention is more likely to occur.

8. A patient is prescribed an extended-release drug for overactive bladder. Which precaution is **most important** for the nurse to teach the patient **to prevent harm**?

A. "Avoid taking this drug at bedtime."
B. "Drink at least 3 L of fluid daily."
C. "Swallow the tablet or capsule whole."
D. "Perform a home pregnancy test monthly."

9. A patient with overactive bladder has been prescribed tolterodine. While assessing the patient, the nurse discovers the presence of the following health problems. Which problem causes the nurse to contact the prescriber and question the drug order?

A. Asthma
B. Glaucoma
C. Hypotension
D. Diabetes mellitus

Clinical Judgment

1. Which priority teaching will the nurse be sure to include when instructing a patient about the patch form of oxybutynin to treat overactive bladder? **Select all that apply.**

A. Removing the old patch before applying the new patch
B. Examining the skin under the old patch for redness or irritation
C. Changing the patch every day in the morning
D. Removing the adhesive backing on the patch before applying
E. Reminding the patient that increased tearing and saliva are side effects
F. Placing the new patch in the same area as the old patch
G. Expecting an increase in frequency and urgency of urination
H. Pressing the new patch firmly, and holding it in place for 15 seconds
I. Reporting any itchiness under the patch
J. Carefully cleaning and drying the site before applying the new patch

2. A 68-year-old patient with hypertension is prescribed hydrochlorothiazide for blood pressure control. The nurse is teaching the patient about this drug. Which statements by the patient indicate that the patient understands the teaching or requires further teaching? **Use an X to indicate which patient statement about issues related to this therapy is either Understood or Requires Further Teaching.**

PATIENT STATEMENT	UNDERSTOOD TEACHING	REQUIRES FURTHER TEACHING
"While I'm taking this drug, my urine will be lighter in color, and the amount will increase."		
"I will avoid foods like bananas and broccoli."		
"I will sit on the side of the bed for 1 to 2 minutes before standing up."		
"If my blood pressure is 120/70 mm Hg., I will report it to my doctor immediately."		
"I will check my heart rate and report any irregular rhythms."		
"If I miss taking my morning dose, I will take 2 pills the next day."		
"I will get my blood potassium tested as ordered by my doctor."		

Drug Therapy for Hypertension

Learning Objectives

The content presented in this chapter should help you to:

1. Explain how antihypertensive drugs lower blood pressure.
2. Describe the common names, actions, usual adult dosages, possible side effects, and adverse effects of angiotensin-converting enzyme (ACE) inhibitors and angiotensin II receptor blockers (ARBs).
3. Discuss the priority actions to take before and after giving ACE inhibitors and angiotensin II receptor blockers.
4. Prioritize essential information to teach patients about ACE inhibitors and angiotensin II receptor blockers to manage hypertension.
5. Describe the common names, actions, usual adult dosages, possible side effects, and adverse effects for calcium

channel blockers, beta blockers, alpha blockers, alpha-beta blockers, central-acting adrenergic drugs, and direct vasodilators.

6. Discuss the priority actions to take before and after giving calcium channel blockers, beta blockers, alpha blockers, alpha-beta blockers, central-acting adrenergic drugs, and direct vasodilators.
7. Prioritize essential information to teach patients about calcium channel blockers, beta blockers, alpha blockers, alpha-beta blockers, central-acting adrenergic drugs, and direct vasodilators to manage hypertension.
8. Explain appropriate life span considerations for drugs used to treat hypertension.

Key Terms

ACE inhibitor (ĀS ĭn-HĪB-ĭ-tŭr) (p. 225) A drug that lowers blood pressure; ACE stands for angiotensin-converting enzyme.

alpha blocker (ĂL-fĕ BLŎ-kŭr) (p. 233) A drug that opposes the excitatory effects of norepinephrine released from sympathetic nerve endings at alpha receptors and causes vasodilation and a decrease in blood pressure. It is also referred to as an alpha-adrenergic blocking agent.

alpha-beta blocker (ĂL-fĕ BĀ-tĕ BLŎ-kŭr) (p. 234) Drugs that combine the effects of alpha blockers and beta blockers.

angiotensin II receptor blocker (ăn-jē-ō-TĔN-sĭn TŪ rĕ-SĔP-tŭr BLŎ-kŭr) (p. 228) Angiotensin II receptor blockers (ARBs), also called angiotensin II receptor antagonists, are a group of drugs that modulate the renin-angiotensin-aldosterone system and lower blood pressure.

antihypertensive (ăn-tē-hī-pŭr-TĔN-sĭv) (p. 224) A substance or drug that lowers blood pressure.

beta blocker (beta adrenergic blocker) (BĀ-tĕ BLŎ-kŭr [BĀ-tĕ ăd-rĕn-ŬR-jĭk BLŎ-kŭr]) (p. 231) A drug that limits the

activity of epinephrine (a hormone that increases blood pressure); beta blockers reduce the heart rate and the force of muscle contraction, thereby reducing the oxygen demand of the heart muscle.

calcium channel blocker (KĂL-sē-ŭm CHĂ-nĕl BLŎ-kŭr) (p. 230) A drug that slows the movement of calcium into the cells of the heart and blood vessels, relaxing blood vessels and reducing the workload of the heart.

central-acting adrenergic agents (SĔN-trŭl ĂK-tĭng ăd-rĕn-ŬR-jĭk Ā-jĕnts) (p. 236) Drugs that lower blood pressure by stimulating alpha receptors in the brain, which open peripheral arteries and ease blood flow.

direct vasodilators (dī-RĔKT văz-ō-DĪ-lā-tŭrz) (p. 237) Drugs that act directly on the smooth muscle of small arteries, causing these arteries to expand (dilate).

diuretics (dī-ŭr-ĔT-ĭk) Drugs that help rid the body of excess water and salt (sodium). (p. 225) See Chapter 12.

REVIEW OF RELATED PHYSIOLOGY AND PATHOPHYSIOLOGY

Blood pressure goes up when a person is active and down when resting or sleeping (Animation 13.1). Everyone's blood pressure goes up and down during a 24-hour period. Low blood pressure is called *hypotension*. When blood pressure remains abnormally high, it is called *hypertension*, which can cause many serious health problems. Often people are unaware of having high blood pressure because there are no specific symptoms. Sudden, dangerously high, and life-threatening blood pressure is called a *hypertensive crisis*.

Table **13.1**	American Heart Association Blood Pressure Categories			
BLOOD PRESSURE CATEGORY[a]	**SYSTOLIC (mm Hg) (UPPER NUMBER)**		**DIASTOLIC (mm Hg) (LOWER NUMBER)**	
Normal	Less than 120 mm Hg	and	Less than 80 mm Hg	
Elevated	120–129 mm Hg	and	Less than 80 mm Hg	
High Blood Pressure (Hypertension) Stage 1	130–139 mm Hg	or	80–89 mm Hg	
High Blood Pressure (Hypertension) Stage 2	140 mm/Hg or higher	or	90 mm Hg or higher	
Hypertensive Crisis **Consult your doctor immediately**	Higher than 180 mm Hg	and/or	Higher than 120 mm Hg	

[a]Blood Pressure Categories defined by the American Heart Association, May 2021. http://www.heart.org/HEARTORG/Conditions/HighBloodPressure/AboutHighBloodPressure/Understanding-Blood-Pressure-Readings_UCM_301764_Article.jsp. (Reprinted with permission © American Heart Association, Inc.)

Box **13.1**	Lifestyle Changes for Treating Hypertension

- Decrease salt (sodium) intake
- Decrease fat intake
- Lose weight
- Exercise regularly
- Quit smoking
- Decrease alcohol intake (not more than two alcohol drinks per day)
- Decrease and manage stress

Memory Jogger

High blood pressure stage 1 is a systolic blood pressure of 130–139 mm Hg and/or a diastolic blood pressure of 80–89 mm Hg according to the American Heart Association (see Table 13.1).

Critical Point for Safety

When hypertension is not treated, the following health problems may result:
- Arteriosclerosis (atherosclerosis)
- Heart attack (myocardial infarction)
- Stroke (cerebrovascular accident, brain attack)
- Enlarged heart (cardiomyopathy)
- Kidney damage (may lead to end-stage kidney disease)
- Blindness

QSEN: Safety

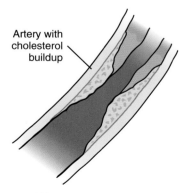

Artery with cholesterol buildup

FIG. 13.1 Atherosclerosis.

A sphygmomanometer and stethoscope are used to measure blood pressure. In some settings, automatic blood pressure monitoring machines are used. Blood pressure measurements include two numbers. The higher number is called the *systolic blood pressure (SBP)*. It represents pressure of blood against the artery walls when the heart contracts. The lower number is called the *diastolic blood pressure (DBP)*. It represents pressure of blood against the artery walls when the heart relaxes.

As people age, they are more likely to develop hypertension. *Hypertension* is defined by the American Heart Association (2021) as a SBP of greater than or equal to 140 mm Hg and/or a DBP of greater than or equal to 90 mm Hg. The new blood pressure classifications are: normal, elevated, high blood pressure stage 1, high blood pressure stage 2, and hypertensive crisis (Table 13.1). According to the Centers for Disease Control and Prevention (CDC, 2021), in the United States alone, nearly half of adults (108 million, or 45%) have hypertension. Only about one in four adults (24%) with hypertension have their condition under control.

Several risk factors have been associated with developing high blood pressure. Some, such as smoking, being overweight, and being physically inactive can be changed (are modifiable). Others, such as age, gender, family history, and race cannot be changed (are not modifiable). Yet, other risk factors (e.g., diabetes and hyperlipidemia) can be controlled with drugs. The use of oral contraceptives (birth control pills) increases the risk of hypertension in younger women, while being postmenopausal increases the risk for older women. Treatment of hypertension includes lifestyle changes (Box 13.1) and drugs that lower blood pressure (*antihypertensives*).

ARTERIOSCLEROSIS AND ATHEROSCLEROSIS

Arteriosclerosis is the thickening and stiffening of the arterial walls. High blood pressure causes arterial walls to thicken and stiffen and is also caused by these arterial wall changes. With *atherosclerosis*, plaques are formed inside the walls of arteries (Figure 13.1). As arterial walls stiffen and thicken, the arteries become narrow. Narrowed arteries decrease blood flow, and the body's organs and tissues may not receive enough blood. Narrowed arteries can also result in the formation of clots that block the flow of blood. Reduced or blocked blood flow to the heart can cause a heart attack, and reduced or blocked blood flow to the brain can cause a stroke.

High blood pressure also makes the heart work much harder to pump blood to the lungs and body. Over time, the extra work can cause the heart muscle to thicken and stretch. This can lead to an enlarged heart (*cardiomyopathy*) and heart failure.

High blood pressure can affect the ability of the kidneys to remove body wastes from the blood by hardening, thickening, and narrowing the arteries to the kidneys. This causes less blood flow to the kidneys and less filtering of waste products, which then build up in the blood. As kidney function becomes worse, kidney failure, including end-stage kidney disease (ESKD), can occur. When the kidneys fail, a patient needs either dialysis or a kidney transplant. About 25% of patients who are on kidney dialysis have kidney failure that was caused by hypertension.

HYPERTENSION

The two main types of hypertension include primary (essential) hypertension and secondary hypertension. Primary hypertension has no known cause. Secondary hypertension is caused by other diseases and drugs that raise blood pressure.

Primary hypertension is the most common form of high blood pressure, accounting for 85% to 90% of cases. Although it has no known cause, it is associated with certain risk factors (Table 13.2). A contributing factor may be the changes that occur in the arteries as people age. With increasing age blood pressure rises, large arteries become stiffer, and smaller arteries may become partly blocked. Examples of other factors that play a part in developing high blood pressure include smoking, an unhealthy diet (too much fat, salt, and alcohol), stress, obesity, and changes in the kidneys.

Secondary hypertension, the less common form of high blood pressure, is the result of other health problems or drugs. Examples of disorders that can cause this type of hypertension include partial blockages of the arteries to the kidneys (atherosclerosis) and diseases that damage the kidneys, such as infections and diabetes. Tumors of the adrenal glands, which sit on top of the kidneys, and sleep apnea may cause secondary hypertension (see Table 13.2).

Drugs that cause secondary hypertension include nonsteroidal antiinflammatory drugs (NSAIDs) and corticosteroids. Other drugs that may result in high blood

 Memory Jogger

The two main types of hypertension are primary (essential) and secondary.

Table **13.2**	Causes of Hypertension	
TYPE OF HYPERTENSION	**CAUSES**	
Primary (essential) hypertension	Cause is unknown Associated risk factors: Family history High sodium intake High calorie intake Physical inactivity Excessive alcohol intake Low potassium intake	
Secondary hypertension	Specific diseases: Renal vascular disease Primary aldosteronism Pheochromocytoma Cushing's disease Coarctation of the aorta Brain tumors Encephalitis Psychiatric disturbances Pregnancy Sleep apnea	Medications: Estrogen (oral contraceptives) Glucocorticoids Mineralocorticoids Sympathomimetics

From Ignatavicius, D., & Workman L. (2013). *Medical-surgical nursing: Patient-centered collaborative care* (7th ed.). St. Louis: Elsevier.

Critical Point for Safety

A patient with high blood pressure should not take over-the-counter allergy and cold drugs that contain phenylephrine because these drugs can worsen the hypertension.

QSEN: Safety

pressure include over-the-counter allergy and cold drugs that contain phenylephrine. Drugs that contain pseudoephedrine also cause elevated blood pressure.

GENERAL ISSUES FOR ANTIHYPERTENSIVE THERAPY

Antihypertensive drugs are prescribed to control and manage high blood pressure. Awareness and treatment of hypertension are extremely important because, when left untreated, it can cause diseases that damage the heart and arteries, kidneys, and brain. Untreated hypertension also decreases life expectancy in adults. Treating the cause of secondary hypertension can cure the problem. Managing primary hypertension is a lifelong process and usually requires that patients continue with lifestyle changes and antihypertensive drugs for the rest of their lives.

In addition to the priority practices listed for drug administration in Chapter 2, general priority actions to take for safe administration of antihypertensive drugs are listed in the following paragraphs. Specific actions are discussed with each individual class of drugs.

PRIORITY ACTIONS TO TAKE *BEFORE* GIVING ANY ANTIHYPERTENSIVES

Always get a complete list of drugs that the patient is currently using, including herbal and over-the-counter drugs.

Obtain a baseline set of vital signs. If the patient's blood pressure is low (less than 90/60 mm Hg) or the heart rate is low (less than 60 beats/min), notify the prescriber and ask if the patient should receive the drug. Ask the patient about signs and symptoms such as dizziness, light-headedness, or headaches.

Ask women of childbearing years if they are pregnant, planning to become pregnant, or breastfeeding because many antihypertensive drugs can harm the fetus directly or reduce blood pressure in the fetus.

PRIORITY ACTIONS TO TAKE *AFTER* GIVING ANY ANTIHYPERTENSIVES

Recheck and continue to monitor the patient's vital signs every 4 to 8 hours. Ask the patient about dizziness or light-headedness as these are signs of hypotension. If these symptoms occur, check the patient's blood pressure and heart rate while the patient is lying down, sitting, and standing (orthostatic vital signs). Notify the prescriber of positive orthostatic vital signs. *Orthostatic hypotension* is said to occur if, within 3 minutes of standing, systolic pressure drops by at least 20 mm Hg, diastolic pressure drops by at least 10 mm Hg, or heart rate increases more than 20 beats/min. Instruct the patient to call for help when getting out of bed and make sure the call light is within easy reach. Help the patient change positions slowly.

 Memory Jogger

Orthostatic hypotension criteria:
• Decreased SBP of 20 mm Hg or more
• Decreased DBP of 10 mm Hg or more
• Increased heart rate of 20 beats/min or more

TEACHING PRIORITIES FOR PATIENTS TAKING ANY ANTIHYPERTENSIVES

Antihypertension drugs are commonly prescribed and can be very effective when used correctly. The following points are essential for patient and family education when antihypertensives are prescribed:
• Check and keep a daily record of blood pressure and heart rate measurements using the techniques you have been taught.
• Change positions slowly to avoid the symptoms of low blood pressure, which are light-headedness and dizziness.
• Do not drive, operate machines, or do anything that is dangerous until you know how the antihypertensive drug will affect you. Also avoid these activities whenever you have symptoms of low blood pressure.
• Keep all follow-up appointments with your prescriber to monitor blood pressure and side effects of antihypertensive drugs.
• Take all prescribed doses as directed. If you miss a dose and the next dose is not due for more than 4 hours, take the dose as soon as possible. If the next dose is due in less than 4 hours, skip the missed dose and return to the regular dosing schedule.
• Never take double doses of antihypertensive drugs.

 Critical Point for Safety

Teach patients to take missed doses as soon as possible. If it is almost time for the next dose, the patient may skip the missed dose and return to the regular dosing schedule.

QSEN: Safety

- Notify their prescriber for any signs of low blood pressure or chest pain.
- Consult with their prescriber before taking over-the-counter drugs.
- Remember that lifestyle changes will help manage and reduce hypertension. These include weight loss, exercise, stress reduction, smoking cessation, and a low-salt–low-fat diet.
- These drugs will help to control, but *not* cure, high blood pressure and you may need to take these drugs for the rest of your life.
- Remember that controlling high blood pressure is important to prevent other serious health problems such as heart failure, kidney disease, and stroke.
- Obtain and wear a medical alert bracelet that states the drug and dose you are taking, along with your diagnosis.

TYPES OF ANTIHYPERTENSIVE DRUGS

Several types of drugs are used to control hypertension. They may be used alone or in combination with other drugs. Antihypertensive drugs have several classes:
- **Diuretics**—drugs that eliminate excess water and salt from the body (see Chapter 12).
- **Angiotensin-converting enzyme (ACE) inhibitors**—drugs that lower blood pressure. For people with diabetes, especially those with protein (albumin) in their urine, ACE inhibitors also help slow kidney damage.
- **Angiotensin II receptor blockers (ARBs)**—drugs that change the action of the renin-angiotensin-aldosterone system. These drugs block the activation of angiotensin II type 1 receptors. ARBs are mainly used in the treatment of hypertension when the patient is intolerant of ACE inhibitor therapy. These drugs are also called *angiotensin receptor antagonists.*
- **Calcium channel blockers**—drugs that slow the movement of calcium into the cells of the heart and blood vessels. This in turn relaxes the blood vessels, increases the supply of oxygen-rich blood to the heart, and reduces the workload of the heart.
- **Beta blockers (beta-adrenergic blockers)**—drugs that limit the activity of epinephrine (a hormone that increases blood pressure). Beta blockers reduce the heart rate and force of contraction, leading to decreased oxygen demand by the heart muscle.
- **Alpha blockers**—drugs that oppose the excitatory effects of norepinephrine released from sympathetic nerve endings at alpha receptors and cause blood vessel relaxation and vasodilation, leading to a decrease in blood pressure. These drugs are also called alpha-adrenergic blocking agents.
- **Alpha-beta blockers**—drugs that combine the effects of alpha and beta blockers.
- **Central-acting adrenergic agents**—drugs that lower blood pressure by stimulating alpha receptors in the brain, which widen (dilate) peripheral arteries and ease blood flow. Central-acting adrenergic agents such as clonidine are usually prescribed when all other antihypertensive medications have failed. For treating hypertension, these drugs are usually administered in combination with a diuretic.
- **Direct vasodilators**—drugs that act directly on the smooth muscle of small arteries, causing these arteries to expand (dilate).

DIURETICS

Diuretics are drugs that help rid the body of excess water and salt (sodium) to control blood pressure. Those most commonly used to treat hypertension include thiazide, loop, and potassium-sparing diuretics. See Chapter 12 for additional information on diuretic drugs.

ANGIOTENSIN-CONVERTING ENZYME INHIBITORS

How Angiotensin-Converting Enzyme Inhibitors Work

ACE inhibitors block the production of substances that constrict (narrow) blood vessels. They also help decrease the buildup of water and salt in the blood and body tissues. ACE inhibitors block an enzyme in the body that is necessary for production of angiotensin II (a substance that causes blood vessels to tighten or constrict). The result is that blood vessels relax and blood pressure is decreased. This also decreases

 Critical Point for Safety

Patients with hypertension should not take over-the-counter drugs (such as drugs for appetite control, asthma, colds, and hay fever) without consulting with their prescriber.

QSEN: Safety

 Critical Point for Safety

Antihypertensive drugs will help control but will **not** cure hypertension. To be effective these drugs need to be taken daily as prescribed to lower blood pressure. Many patients may need to take these drugs for the rest of their lives.

QSEN: Safety

the heart's workload and increases the blood flow and oxygen to the heart and other organs. In the kidneys, reduction of angiotensin II improves urine output and sodium excretion, which also helps lower blood pressure.

These drugs are often given to patients with health problems such as heart failure, kidney disease, and diabetes. ACE inhibitors are often prescribed *along with* diuretics to control hypertension, and combined ACE inhibitor/diuretic drug forms are available. For example, lisinopril/hydrochlorothiazide (Prinzide, Zestoretic) is often prescribed for the management of hypertension; lisinopril is an ACE inhibitor, and hydrochlorothiazide is a thiazide diuretic.

Usually, the first doses of an ACE inhibitor are lower when the patient is also taking a diuretic or has renal (kidney) impairment. Be sure to consult a reliable drug resource for information on any specific ACE inhibitor.

Usual Adult Dosages for Commonly Prescribed ACE Inhibitors

Drug Category	Drug Name	Usual Maintenance Dose
ACE Inhibitors	benazepril (Lotensin)	10–40 mg/day orally in one to two divided doses. Max: 80 mg/day
	captopril (Capoten)	12.5–25 mg orally two to three times daily
	enalapril (Epaned, Vasotec)	5–40 mg orally once daily or in two divided doses. Max: 450 mg/day 1.25 mg IV every 6 hr. Max: 20 mg/day
	fosinopril (Monopril)	20–40 mg orally once daily once daily or in two divided doses. Max: 80 mg/day
	lisinopril (Prinivil, Zestril)	20–40 mg orally once daily. Max: 80 mg/day
	moexipril (Univasc)	7.5–30 mg/day orally given once daily or in two divided doses. Max: 30 mg/day
	perindopril (Aceon)	4–8 mg orally once daily or in two divided doses. Max: 16 mg/day
	quinapril (Accupril)	20–80 mg orally daily as single dose or two divided doses. Max: 80 mg/day
	ramipril (Altace)	2.5-20 mg/day orally, given in one to two divided doses. Max 20 mg/day
	trandolapril (Mavik)	1–4 mg orally once daily. Max: 8 mg/day *Special Considerations:* **For Black patients, begin with 2 mg orally daily**

Intended Responses of Angiotensin-Converting Enzyme (ACE) Inhibitors
- Production of angiotensin II is decreased.
- Vasodilation of blood vessels is increased.
- Excess tissue water and salt are decreased.
- Blood pressure is lowered.
- Workload on the heart is decreased.

Common Side Effects of Angiotensin-Converting Enzyme (ACE) Inhibitors
The most common side effects of ACE inhibitors include hypotension; protein in the urine; taste disturbances; increased blood potassium level (*hyperkalemia*); headache; and a persistent, dry cough. If one ACE inhibitor causes a cough, it is likely that others will as well, and the patient may need to be prescribed another type of antihypertensive drug if the cough is severe or bothers him or her.

Possible Adverse Effects of Angiotensin-Converting Enzyme (ACE) Inhibitors
Adverse effects include fever and chills; hoarseness; swelling in the face, hands, or feet; trouble swallowing or breathing; stomach pain; chest pain; rashes and itching skin; and yellow eyes or skin. Some patients also develop dizziness, light-headedness, or fainting.

 Memory Jogger

The generic names for ACE inhibitors end in "-pril" (e.g., enalapril, captopril, lisinopril).

 Do Not Confuse

Accupril *with* **Aciphex**

An order for Accupril may be confused with Aciphex. Accupril is an ACE inhibitor, whereas Aciphex is a proton pump inhibitor used for healing gastrointestinal ulcers.

QSEN: Safety

 Do Not Confuse

Zestril *with* **Zetia**

An order for Zestril may be confused with Zetia. Zestril is an ACE inhibitor, whereas Zetia is a cholesterol-lowering drug.

QSEN: Safety

 Do Not Confuse

benazepril *with* **Benadryl**

An order for benazepril may be confused with Benadryl. Benazepril is an ACE inhibitor, whereas Benadryl is an antihistamine.

QSEN: Safety

Common Side Effects

ACE Inhibitors

Hypotension

Taste changes

Na⁺ Na⁺
Na⁺ Na⁺
Na⁺ Na⁺
Hyperkalemia

Headache

Critical Point for Safety

If a patient taking an ACE inhibitor develops a severe, persistent, dry cough, the prescriber is notified, and the drug may be discontinued, requiring the prescribing of a different type of antihypertensive drug.

QSEN: Safety

Allergic reactions and kidney failure are serious but rare adverse effects of ACE inhibitors.

Angioedema is a diffuse swelling of the eyes, lips, and tongue (see Figure 1.6). It may occur with allergic reactions to these drugs and may be life threatening. Swelling of the trachea (windpipe/airway) can interfere with breathing, which is a life-threatening event. Angioedema can occur months or even years after ACE inhibitor therapy is started.

Neutropenia (decreased leukocytes in the blood) may occur, increasing the risk of infections. Infections may develop in the throat, intestinal tract, other mucous membranes, or the skin. Symptoms of neutropenia include any signs of infection such as chills, fever, or sore throat.

Some ACE inhibitors (for example, enalapril, quinapril, and ramipril) cause increased sun sensitivity (photosensitivity).

Priority Actions to Take *Before* Giving Angiotensin-Converting Enzyme (ACE) Inhibitors

In addition to the general priority actions to take before giving any antihypertensive drug therapy (p. 224), ask about any allergies to drugs, foods, preservatives, or dyes because more people develop allergies with ACE inhibitors than with any other type of blood pressure drugs. Ask patients if they are also taking diuretics to control blood pressure, because ACE inhibitors enhance the blood pressure–lowering effects of diuretics.

Priority Actions to Take *After* Giving Angiotensin-Converting Enzyme (ACE) Inhibitors

In addition to the general priority actions to take after giving any antihypertensive drug therapy (p. 224), check patients' blood potassium levels because these drugs reduce the excretion of potassium. This is even more important if the patient is also prescribed a potassium-sparing diuretic. Keep track of urine output and weight because kidney failure is a rare but serious adverse effect of these drugs.

Check for any signs or symptoms of allergic reactions or infections.

Teaching Priorities for Patients Taking Angiotensin-Converting Enzyme (ACE) Inhibitors

In addition to the general priority teaching for patients taking any antihypertensive drug therapy (p. 224), include these teaching points and precautions:
- Take the drug at the same time every day.
- Take captopril (Capoten) 1 hour before eating or on an empty stomach.
- Do not drink alcohol until you talk with your prescriber because ACE inhibitors can increase the low blood pressure effect and the risk of dizziness or fainting.
- Avoid salt substitutes because they contain potassium, and a side effect of ACE inhibitors is increased blood potassium levels (hyperkalemia).
- Report any side effects of ACE inhibitors to your prescriber.
- Go to the emergency room immediately if any facial swelling occurs, because this is a sign of angioedema, a life-threatening adverse reaction.
- Remember that angioedema can occur even months to years after these drugs have been taken.
- If you are taking enalapril (Vasotec), quinapril (Accupril), or ramipril (Altace), remember to limit exposure to direct sunlight, wear protective clothing, and use sunscreens, because sun sensitivity (photosensitivity) is a side effect of taking these drugs.

Life Span Considerations for Angiotensin-Converting Enzyme (ACE) Inhibitors
Pediatric considerations. Children are at higher risk of severe side effects from taking these drugs. Parents should discuss the benefits and risks with their pediatric cardiologist before ACE inhibitors are prescribed.

Considerations for pregnancy and lactation. ACE inhibitors have a high likelihood of increasing the risk of birth defects or fetal damage. They are not prescribed for women who are pregnant or are thinking about becoming pregnant. Lisinopril has a moderate likelihood of increasing the risk of birth defects or fetal damage during the first trimester and a high likelihood of increasing the risk of birth defects or fetal

Critical Point for Safety

Monitor patients for swelling of the eyes, lips, and tongue, which indicates angioedema, a serious and life-threatening adverse effect of ACE inhibitors.

QSEN: Safety

Critical Point for Safety

ACE inhibitors may increase the effect of decreased blood pressure in patients who are also taking diuretics. ACE inhibitors and potassium-sparing diuretics cause much higher increases in blood potassium levels.

QSEN: Safety

Critical Point for Safety

Tell patients who are taking ACE inhibitors that drinking alcohol can increase the low blood pressure effect and the risk of dizziness or fainting.

QSEN: Safety

damage during the second and third trimesters. These drugs pass into breast milk and should not be used while breastfeeding because they can lower blood pressure and lead to kidney damage in the infant.

Considerations for older adults. Older adults are at greater risk of postural hypotension when taking ACE inhibitors due to the cardiovascular changes associated with aging. Remind patients to stand or sit up slowly, as rising too quickly may lower blood pressure rapidly, causing dizziness and an increased risk of falling. Also, instruct them to hold on to railings when going up or down steps.

ANGIOTENSIN II RECEPTOR BLOCKERS (ARBS)

How Angiotensin II Receptor Blockers (ARBs) Work

Angiotensin II receptor blockers (ARBs) block the effects of angiotensin II (vasoconstriction, sodium, and water retention) by directly blocking the binding of angiotensin II to angiotensin II type 1 receptors.

These drugs are prescribed alone or in combination with diuretics. Losartan combined with the thiazide diuretic hydrochlorothiazide (Hyzaar) is often prescribed to control high blood pressure. Lower doses of ARBs are used when a patient is taking a diuretic or has renal (kidney) or hepatic (liver) impairment. These drugs are inactivated by the liver and excreted from the body by the kidneys. Patients who have an impairment of either of these organs may have higher blood levels of the prescribed ARBs and are at greater risk of side effects or adverse effects. Be sure to consult a reliable resource for additional information regarding any angiotensin II receptor blocker.

Usual Adult Dosages for Commonly Prescribed Angiotensin-II Receptor Blockers (ARBs)

Drug Category	Drug Name	Usual Maintenance Dose
Angiotensin-II Receptor Blockers (ARBs)	candesartan (Atacand)	8–32 mg/day orally, given in one to two divided doses ***Special Considerations:* For volume-depleted patients, start with 8 mg orally once daily**
	eprosartan (Teveten)	400–800 mg/day orally, given in one to two divided doses
	irbesartan (Avapro)	150 mg orally once daily. 300 mg orally if more control is needed ***Special Considerations:* For volume-depleted patients, the starting dosage is 75 mg orally once daily**
	losartan (Cozaar)	50–100 mg/day orally, given in one to two divided doses
	olmesartan (Benicar)	20–40 mg orally once daily
	telmisartan (Micardis)	20–80 mg orally once daily
	valsartan (Diovan)	80–320 mg orally once daily

Intended Responses of Angiotensin-II Receptor Blockers (ARBs)
- Vasodilation of blood vessels is increased.
- Excess body water and salt are decreased.
- Blood pressure is lowered.
- Workload on the heart is decreased.

Common Side Effects of Angiotensin-II Receptor Blockers (ARBs)
There are few known side effects caused from ARBs. The documented side effects include dizziness, fatigue, headache, hypotension, diarrhea, and high blood potassium levels (hyperkalemia).

Possible Adverse Effects of Angiotensin-II Receptor Blockers (ARBs)

Adverse effects are rare but include kidney failure and life-threatening angioedema (swelling of the face, eyes, lips, tongue, and trachea, which can interfere with breathing) (see Figure 1.6 in Chapter 1).

An additional rare adverse effect is liver toxicity or drug-induced hepatitis. These drugs should not be given to patients who have known liver problems.

 Priority Actions to Take *Before* Giving Angiotensin-II Receptor Blockers (ARBs)

In addition to the general priority actions related to antihypertensive therapy (p. 224), check kidney function tests including blood urea nitrogen (BUN) and creatinine levels for preexisting kidney disease, because these drugs are excreted by the kidneys. Ask whether the patient has any kidney or liver problems because these drugs can worsen liver disease.

 Priority Actions to Take *After* Giving Angiotensin-II Receptor Blockers (ARBs)

In addition to the general priority actions related to antihypertensive therapy (p. 224), monitor for any swelling of the face, including the eyes, lips, or tongue (signs of angioedema). Report these to the prescriber immediately. Do not administer the ARB drug to the patient again because this is a life-threatening adverse reaction. Check the urine output and weight. Report decreased urine output or weight gain to the prescriber.

Check laboratory values for any changes in the blood potassium level because ARBs reduce potassium excretion by the kidneys. If the potassium level is higher than 5.5 mEq/L, notify the prescriber. Assess heart rate and rhythm, especially for a slow rate. If the patient has a heart monitor, assess for an increasing height of T waves, which is a sign of high potassium level. Check bowel sounds every shift. Increased bowel sounds and diarrhea are associated with high potassium levels.

 Teaching Priorities for Patients Taking Angiotensin-II Receptor Blockers (ARBs)

In addition to the general teaching priorities related to antihypertensive therapy (p. 224), include these teaching points and precautions:

- Remind patients to get up slowly to prevent dizziness and falls.
- Teach patients that alcohol use, standing for long periods, exercise, and hot weather may contribute to hypotension.
- Instruct female patients to consult with their prescriber if they are taking an angiotensin II receptor blocker and plan to become pregnant. These drugs can cause harm to the fetus.
- Tell patients to go to the emergency department immediately to report any facial swelling, because this is a sign of angioedema, a life-threatening adverse reaction.
- Remind patients that angioedema can occur months to years after these drugs have been taken. Teach them that if this happens, they should never take ARB drugs again.

Life Span Considerations for Angiotensin-II Receptor Blockers (ARBs)

Considerations for pregnancy and lactation. Angiotensin-II receptor blockers have a moderate likelihood of increasing the risk of birth defects or fetal damage during the first trimester and a high likelihood during the second and third trimesters. They should not be taken during the second or third trimesters of pregnancy. Valsartan (Diovan) has a high likelihood of increasing the risk of birth defects or fetal damage during all trimesters. These drugs can interfere with fetal blood pressure control and kidney function. They have been associated with problems in fetal kidney and skull development. It is not known if they pass into breast milk; however, a woman who plans to breastfeed should not use these drugs because there is not enough evidence that infants will be safe when a mother is breastfeeding while taking ARBs.

Common Side Effects
Angiotensin II Receptor Blockers

Fatigue

Headache

Hypotension

Diarrhea

Na⁺ Na⁺
Na⁺ Na⁺
Na⁺ Na⁺

Hyperkalemia

 Critical Point for Safety

When a patient has been given an ARB and experiences any swelling of the face, eyes, lips, or tongue, report this to the prescriber immediately. These are signs of the life-threatening adverse reaction, angioedema, and the patient should not receive these drugs again.

QSEN: Safety

CALCIUM CHANNEL BLOCKERS

How Calcium Channel Blockers Work

Calcium channel blockers block calcium from entering the muscle cells of the heart and arteries. Blocking calcium causes a decrease in the contraction of the heart and also dilates the arteries. Dilating the arteries lowers peripheral vascular resistance to decrease blood pressure and reduce the workload of the heart.

When these drugs are prescribed for older patients or patients with hepatic (liver) or renal (kidney) impairment, initial lower doses are used. Amlodipine (Norvasc) may be combined with atorvastatin (Caduet), with an ACE inhibitor (Lotrel), or with an ARB (Exforge). Be sure to consult a reliable drug resource for information on any calcium channel blocker drug.

Usual Adult Dosages for Commonly Prescribed Calcium Channel Blockers

Drug Category	Drug Name	Usual Maintenance Dose
Calcium Channel Blockers	amlodipine (Norvasc, Katerzia)	5–10 mg per orally once daily

	diltiazem (Cardizem, Cardizem CD, Cardizem LA, Cardizem SR, Cartia XT)	180–240 mg orally once daily
		Sustained release capsules:
		    120–360 mg orally once daily.
		    Max: 540 mg/day

	felodipine (Plendil)	2.5–10 mg orally once daily
	nicardipine (Cardene)	20–40 mg orally three times daily

	nifedipine (Adalat, Procardia, Procardia XL)	30–90 mg orally once daily.
		    Max: 120 mg/day
		Procardia XL is 120 mg orally
		    once daily

	verapamil (Calan, Calan SR, Isoptin)	80 mg orally three times daily
		Calan SR caplets or Isoptin SR
		    180 mg orally once daily in the
		    morning

Intended Responses of Calcium Channel Blockers

- Heart contraction is decreased.
- Artery dilation is increased.
- Heart workload is decreased.
- Blood pressure is lowered.
- Blood flow and oxygen to the heart are increased.
- Decreased episodes of supraventricular tachycardia.

Common Side Effects of Calcium Channel Blockers

The most common side effects of these drugs are constipation, nausea, headache, flushing, rash, edema (legs), hypotension, drowsiness, and dizziness.

Possible Adverse Effects of Calcium Channel Blockers

Dysrhythmias may occur with calcium channel blockers, including irregular, rapid, pounding, or excessively slow heart rhythms (less than 50 beats/min).

Patients with heart failure symptoms may worsen with verapamil and diltiazem because of the increased abilities of the drugs to reduce the strength and rate of heart contraction.

Stevens-Johnson syndrome (erythema multiforme) is a potentially lethal skin disorder resulting from an allergic reaction to drugs, infections, or illness. It causes damage to blood vessels of the skin. Symptoms include many different types of skin lesions (see Figure 1.5 in Chapter 1), itching, fever, joint aching, and generally feeling ill.

Rare but serious adverse effects include difficulty breathing; irregular, rapid, or pounding heart rhythm; slow heart rate (less than 50 beats/min); bleeding; chest pain; and vision problems (difficulty seeing).

⇄ Do Not Confuse

niCARdipine *with* **NIFEdipine**

An order for niCARdipine may be confused with NIFEdipine. Both are calcium channel blockers.

QSEN: Safety

⇄ Do Not Confuse

Norvasc *with* **Navane**

An order for Norvasc may be confused with Navane. Norvasc is a calcium channel blocker, whereas Navane is an antipsychotic drug used for schizophrenia and other psychotic disorders.

QSEN: Safety

Common Side Effects

Calcium Channel Blockers

Dizziness

Headache

Constipation, Nausea

Rash

✦ Critical Point for Safety

Calcium channel blockers can cause a severe skin disorder called Stevens-Johnson syndrome. Always check the patient for skin lesions, itching, fever, and achy joints.

QSEN: Safety

⊛ Priority Actions to Take *Before* Giving Calcium Channel Blockers

In addition to the general priority actions to take before giving any antihypertensive therapy (p. 224), find out if the patient has health problems that may be affected by taking these drugs, such as heart failure, blood vessel disease, and liver or kidney disease.

⊛ Priority Actions to Take *After* Giving Calcium Channel Blockers

In addition to the priority actions to take after giving any antihypertensive therapy (p. 224), report irregular heart rhythms to the prescriber. Watch for side effects or adverse effects of these drugs. If a patient develops skin lesions, itching, fever, and achy joints, report this to the prescriber at once because these are signs of Stevens-Johnson syndrome and an allergic reaction to the drug.

⊛ Teaching Priorities for Patients Taking Calcium Channel Blockers

In addition to the general teaching priorities related to antihypertensive therapy (p. 224), include these teaching points and precautions:

- Get up and change positions slowly to decrease dizziness.
- Avoid exercising in hot weather because that can cause dizziness and low blood pressure.
- Do not suddenly stop taking these drugs after taking them for several weeks because hypertension may return. Your prescriber can advise you on how to gradually stop taking the drug.

Life Span Considerations for Calcium Channel Blockers

Considerations for pregnancy and lactation. Calcium channel blockers have a moderate likelihood of increasing the risk of birth defects or fetal damage. While their effects have not been tested in human pregnancy, birth defects and stillbirths have occurred in studies of laboratory animals. Women should consult with their prescriber and pediatrician before using these drugs during pregnancy. Some calcium channel blockers pass into breast milk. Women who wish to take these drugs while breastfeeding should discuss this with their prescriber because they will have the same effects on the infant.

BETA BLOCKERS

How Beta Blockers Work

Beta blockers (beta adrenergic blockers) block the effects of epinephrine (adrenaline) on the heart. They decrease the heart rate and force of heart contractions, which leads to decreased blood pressure. As a result, the heart does not work as hard and requires less oxygen.

Beta blockers are classified as cardioselective and noncardioselective drugs. *Cardioselective* drugs work only on the cardiovascular system. *Noncardioselective* drugs have effects on all of the organs and systems of the body (systemic effects).

When beta blockers are prescribed for a patient with kidney damage, a lower dose of the drug is prescribed, or the time between doses is increased. An older adult may also be started on a lower drug dose. Be sure to consult a reliable drug resource for information about a specific beta blocker.

> 🧠 **Memory Jogger**
>
> The generic names of beta blockers end with "-olol" (for example, metoprolol, atenolol, labetolol).

Usual Adult Dosages for Commonly Prescribed Beta Blockers

Drug Category	Drug Name	Usual Maintenance Dose
Selective Beta Blockers	acebutolol ❶ (Sectral) selective	400–800 mg orally once daily
	atenolol ❶ (Tenormin) selective	25–100 mg orally in one or two divided doses
	betaxolol ❶ (Kerlone) selective	10–20 mg orally once daily
	bisoprolol ❶ (Zebeta) selective	5 mg orally once daily. Max: 20 mg/day

Continued

Do Not Confuse

Inderal *with* Adderall

An order for Inderal may be confused with Adderall. Inderal is a noncardioselective beta blocker, whereas Adderall is a stimulant used for narcolepsy and attention-deficit/hyperactivity disorder in children.

QSEN: Safety

Do Not Confuse

Toprol XL *with* Topamax

An order for Toprol XL may be confused with Topamax. Toprol XL is an extended-release form of metoprolol, a cardioselective beta blocker. Topamax is a central nervous system anticonvulsant.

QSEN: Safety

Common Side Effects

Beta Blockers

Impotence

Depression

Drowsiness, Lethargy, Fatigue

Insomnia

Critical Point for Safety

Beta blockers can decrease or increase blood glucose levels. Be sure to check blood glucose regularly in a patient with diabetes.

QSEN: Safety

Usual Adult Dosages for Commonly Prescribed Beta Blockers—cont'd

Drug Category	Drug Name	Usual Maintenance Dose
	metoprolol ❶ (Lopresor, Toprol XL) selective	100–200 mg orally per day in two divided doses. Max: 450 mg/day Extended-release capsules: 50–200 mg orally once daily. Max: 400 mg/day
Nonselective Beta Blockers	labetalol ❶ (Normodyne, Trandate) nonselective	200–400 mg orally twice daily. Max: 2,400 mg/day
	nadolol ❶ (Corgard) nonselective	40–80 mg orally once daily
	propranolol ❶ (Inderal, Inderal LA) nonselective	160–480 mg orally given in two to three divided doses Extended-release capsules: 80–160 mg orally once daily
	timolol ❶ (Blocadren, Istalol) nonselective	10–20 mg orally twice daily

❶ High-alert drug.

Intended Responses of Beta Blockers

- Heart rate is decreased.
- Force of heart contraction is decreased.
- Heart workload is decreased.
- Blood pressure is lowered.

Common Side Effects of Beta Blockers

Fairly common side effects of beta blockers include decreased sexual ability, dizziness or light-headedness, drowsiness, trouble sleeping *(insomnia)*, and fatigue or weakness.

Less common side effects that must be reported to the prescriber include difficulty breathing or wheezing; cold hands or feet; mental depression; shortness of breath; slow heart rate (less than 50 beats/min); and swelling in the ankles, feet, or lower legs.

Depression is another side effect that has been associated with taking beta blockers. A patient with a history of depression may notice that it becomes worse while taking these drugs. Beta blockers may also cause depression for the first time.

Possible Adverse Effects of Beta Blockers

Signs of drug overdose include a very slow heart rate, chest pain, severe dizziness or fainting, fast or irregular heart rate, difficulty breathing, bluish-colored fingernails and palms, and seizures. Report these signs and symptoms to the prescriber at once.

Adverse effects may also include "passing out" or falling when changing positions related to orthostatic (postural) hypotension.

Other adverse effects include back or joint pain, dark urine, dizziness or fainting when getting up, fever or sore throat, hallucinations, irregular heart rate, skin rash, unusual bleeding or bruising, and yellow eyes or skin. These drugs can affect the blood glucose level of a patient with diabetes and may cause hypoglycemia or hyperglycemia.

⭐ Priority Actions to Take *Before* Giving Beta Blockers

In addition to the general priority actions to take before giving any antihypertensive therapy (p. 224), check blood glucose levels regularly for patients with diabetes. Beta blockers can mask signs of hypoglycemia such as rapid heart rate, making it difficult to recognize and treat. Ask patients about a history of depression.

⭐ Priority Actions to Take *After* Giving Beta Blockers

In addition to the general priority actions to take after giving any antihypertensive therapy (p. 224), assess the heart rate and notify the prescriber if it is less than 60 beats/min. Continue to monitor blood glucose in patients with diabetes, because these drugs can mask the signs of hypoglycemia. Watch for signs and symptoms of depression.

✪ Teaching Priorities for Patients Taking Beta Blockers

In addition to the general teaching priorities related to antihypertensive therapy (p. 224), include these teaching points and precautions:

- Stand up or sit up slowly because these actions may lower blood pressure rapidly, causing dizziness and an increased risk for falls.
- Hold on to railings when going up or down steps to prevent falling.
- Check with your prescriber before stopping a beta blocker. It may be necessary to gradually decrease (wean) the daily dose of the drug because suddenly stopping beta blockers can increase your risk of a heart attack.
- Notify your prescriber for any weight gain or increase in shortness of breath because these are signs of worsening heart failure.
- Always inform health care providers that you are taking a beta blocker before any form of surgical or emergency treatment.
- Be sure to inform your health care providers about beta blocker use before medical tests and allergy shots, because these drugs can affect the results of medical tests and can cause serious reactions with allergy shots.
- Report any chest pain you experience during activity to your prescriber so safe levels of activity may be discussed.
- Stay out of direct sunlight, use a sun block skin protector, and wear protective clothing because beta blockers can cause increased sensitivity to sunlight and cold.
- Keep in mind the need to dress warmly during cold weather because decreased blood flow to the hands increases the risk of frostbite.
- Remember that these beta blockers can cause new-onset depression or worsen existing depression.

Life Span Considerations for Beta Blockers

Considerations for pregnancy and lactation. Most beta blockers have a moderate likelihood of increasing the risk of birth defects or fetal damage and should not be used during pregnancy unless absolutely necessary. Atenolol has a high likelihood of increasing risk and acebutolol has a low likelihood of increasing risk. These drugs are excreted in breast milk. No adverse effects on infants have been documented, but the possibility of a slowed heart rate and lowered blood pressure exists. Women who are breastfeeding should consult with their prescriber about the continued use of these drugs.

Considerations for older adults. Mental confusion is a side effect of beta blockers that is more likely to occur in older adults. Teach family members to watch for changes in mental status and report it to the prescriber. These drugs may also decrease a patient's ability to tolerate cool temperatures. Teach patients to dress warmly in cool weather and to wear hats and gloves when outdoors.

ALPHA BLOCKERS

How Alpha Blockers Work

Alpha blockers, also called alpha-adrenergic blockers, block receptors in arteries and smooth muscle. This relaxes the blood vessels and leads to an increase in blood flow and lower blood pressure. Be sure to consult a reliable drug resource for information about any specific alpha blocker.

 Critical Point for Safety

Patients should never suddenly stop taking beta blockers. This may cause unpleasant and harmful effects such as increased risk of heart attack.

QSEN: Safety

 Critical Point for Safety

Beta blockers can affect the results of medical tests, such as tests that raise heart rate and blood pressure.

QSEN: Safety

 Critical Point for Safety

Teach patients that beta blockers can cause new-onset depression or worsen existing depression.

QSEN: Safety

 Critical Point for Safety

Monitor older adults who have been prescribed beta blockers for mental confusion or changes in level of consciousness.

QSEN: Safety

Usual Adult Dosages for Commonly Prescribed Alpha Blockers

Drug Category	Drug Name	Usual Maintenance Dose
Alpha Blockers	doxazosin (Cardura, Cardura XL)	1 mg orally once daily. Max: 16 mg/day Extended release: 4–8 mg orally once daily
	prazosin (Minipress)	2–20 mg/day orally, given in divided doses two to three times a day. Max: 40 mg/day ***Special Considerations:*** **Give the first dose at bedtime for patients with hepatic impairment**

Continued

Common Side Effects

Alpha Blockers

Drowsiness

Headache

Hypotension

Runny nose

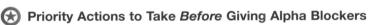
Muscle pain
in arms
and legs

 Critical Point for Safety

Teach men that they should not be prescribed phosphodiesterase type 5 inhibitors (erectile dysfunction drugs) if they are also taking alpha blocker therapy because of the risk of severe hypotension.

QSEN: Safety

 Critical Point for Safety

Give the first dose of prazosin and terazosin at bedtime and caution the patient not to get up without assistance. Orthostatic hypotension is a common side effect after the first doses of these drugs.

QSEN: Safety

Critical Point for Safety

Teach patients that weight gain and ankle swelling are signs that the body is holding extra fluid and should be reported immediately to the prescriber.

QSEN: Safety

 Critical Point for Safety

Alpha blockers pass into breast milk. Teach women who are breastfeeding or planning to breastfeed that it may be necessary to stop breastfeeding while on alpha blockers.

QSEN: Safety

Usual Adult Dosages for Commonly Prescribed Alpha Blockers—cont'd

Drug Category	Drug Name	Usual Maintenance Dose
	terazosin (Hytrin)	1–20 mg orally in one or two divided doses *Special Considerations:* **Give the first dose at bedtime**

Intended Responses of Alpha Blockers
- Artery relaxation and dilation are increased.
- Blood flow is increased.
- Blood pressure is lowered.

Common Side Effects of Alpha Blockers
The most common side effects of alpha blockers are dizziness, drowsiness, fatigue, headache, nervousness, irritability, stuffy or runny nose, nausea, pain in the arms and legs, hypotension, and weakness.

A side effect of prazosin and terazosin is first-dose orthostatic hypotension because initially the patient is more sensitive to the blood pressure lowering effects. As patients continue to take these drugs, they become less sensitive and have fewer problems with hypotension.

Possible Adverse Effects of Alpha Blockers
Alpha blockers can lower blood pressure more than is desired and cause side effects. Life-threatening effects are rare. Adverse effects to report to the prescriber include fainting; shortness of breath or difficulty breathing; fast, pounding, or irregular heart rhythm; chest pain; and swollen feet, ankles, or wrists.

⭐ Priority Actions to Take *Before* Giving Alpha Blockers
In addition to the general priority actions to take before giving any antihypertensive therapy (p. 224), ask male patients if they are taking any phosphodiesterase type 5 inhibitor erectile dysfunction drugs (e.g., sildenafil [Viagra], tadalafil [Cialis], or vardenafil [Levitra]).

⭐ Priority Actions to Take *After* Giving Alpha Blockers
Be sure to review and use the general priority actions to take after giving any antihypertensive drug (p. 224).

⭐ Teaching Priorities for Patients Taking Alpha Blockers
In addition to the general teaching priorities related to giving any antihypertensive therapy (p. 224), include these teaching points and precautions:
- Do not to drive or use dangerous machines for at least 24 hours after taking your first dose of an alpha blocker because a sudden drop in blood pressure can cause dizziness or confusion.
- Get up slowly, especially during the middle of the night.
- Weigh yourself twice a week and check your ankles for swelling. Weight gain and ankle swelling are signs that the body is holding on to extra fluid and should be reported to your prescriber.

Life Span Considerations for Alpha Blockers
Considerations for pregnancy and lactation. Alpha blockers have a moderate likelihood of increasing the risk of birth defects or fetal harm. Women who are pregnant or planning to become pregnant should inform their prescriber. Alpha blockers pass into breast milk; mothers who wish to breastfeed should discuss this with their prescriber and pediatrician. It may be necessary to avoid breastfeeding while taking these drugs.

ALPHA-BETA BLOCKERS

How Alpha-Beta Blockers Work
Alpha-beta blockers combine the effects of alpha blockers and beta blockers. They relax blood vessels like alpha blockers, and they slow the heart rate and decrease the

force of heart contractions like beta blockers. These actions result in lower blood pressure. Be sure to consult a reliable drug resource for information on any specific alpha-beta blocker drug.

Usual Adult Dosages for Commonly Prescribed Alpha-Beta Blockers

Drug Category	Drug Name	Usual Maintenance Dose
Alpha-Beta Blockers	carvedilol ❶ (Coreg, Coreg CR)	6.25–25 mg orally twice daily Extended release: 20–80 mg orally once daily in the morning ***Special Considerations:* Give with food**
	labetalol HCL ❶ (Normodyne, Trandate)	200–400 mg orally twice daily 10–20 mg IV, then 20–80 mg IV every 10–30 min until goal blood pressure is attained

❶ High-alert drug.

Intended Responses of Alpha-Beta Blockers
- Artery relaxation and dilation (widening) are increased.
- Heart rate is decreased.
- Force of heart contraction is decreased.
- Heart workload is decreased.
- Blood pressure is lowered.
- Blood flow and oxygen to the heart are increased.

Common Side Effects of Alpha-Beta Blockers
Common side effects of alpha-beta blockers include dizziness, fatigue, muscle weakness, orthostatic hypotension, diarrhea, impotence, and increased blood glucose levels (hyperglycemia).

Possible Adverse Effects of Alpha-Beta Blockers
Suddenly stopping alpha-beta blockers can cause life-threatening heart dysrhythmias, hypertension, or chest pain. Bradycardia, heart failure, and pulmonary edema can also occur.

Other adverse effects of these drugs may include yellow skin or eyes, swelling in the feet or ankles, weight gain, wheezing or trouble breathing, cold hands or feet, and difficulty sleeping.

⊛ Priority Actions to Take *Before* Giving Alpha-Beta Blockers
In addition to the general priority actions to take before giving any antihypertensive therapy (p. 224), obtain a baseline weight. Use this information to compare for changes after therapy is started and to determine whether an adverse reaction is occurring. Check the patient for swelling in the feet or ankles. If the patient has diabetes, check the blood glucose level regularly.

⊛ Priority Actions to Take *After* Giving Alpha-Beta Blockers
In addition to the general priority actions to take after giving any antihypertensive therapy (p. 224), check blood glucose levels frequently for patients with diabetes, because these drugs may cause an increase in glucose levels.

Check intake and output and daily weights. Look for any signs of fluid overload (e.g., swelling, difficulty breathing, crackles, and weight gain).

⊛ Teaching Priorities for Patients Taking Alpha-Beta Blockers
In addition to the general teaching priorities related to antihypertensive therapy (p. 224), include these teaching points and precautions:
- Suddenly ceasing to take these drugs can lead to life-threatening problems.
- Contact your prescriber if you develop an irregular heart rate, a heart rate less than 50 beats/min, or changes in blood pressure.

Common Side Effects
Alpha-Beta Blockers

Muscle weakness

Hypotension

Diarrhea

Hyperglycemia

Impotence

⊛ **Critical Point for Safety**

Because alpha-beta blockers can cause elevated blood glucose, be sure to monitor blood glucose levels regularly in patients with diabetes.

QSEN: Safety

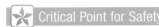
- Do not to drive or operate dangerous machines until you know how the drug affects you, because it may cause dizziness or drowsiness.
- Change positions slowly to prevent falls.
- If you take labetalol (Normodyne), you may become more sensitive to cold and may need to dress warmly.
- If you have diabetes, carefully watch for signs of changes in blood sugar. These drugs may interfere with or mask some of the signs of low blood sugar. You may need to check your glucose levels more frequently and adjust the timing of your meals.

Life Span Considerations for Alpha-Beta Blockers
Considerations for pregnancy and lactation. Alpha-beta blockers have a moderate likelihood of increasing the risk of birth defects or fetal damage. These drugs cross the placenta and are present in breast milk. They may cause slowed heart rate, hypotension, hypoglycemia, and respiratory depression in the newborn.

CENTRAL-ACTING ADRENERGIC AGENTS

How Central-Acting Adrenergic Agents Work
Central-acting adrenergic agents stimulate central nervous system receptors to decrease constriction of blood vessels, which leads to dilation of arteries, and lower blood pressure. Be sure to consult a reliable drug resource for information about any specific central-acting adrenergic agent.

Usual Adult Dosages for Commonly Prescribed Central-Acting Adrenergic Agents

Drug Category	Drug Name	Usual Maintenance Dose
Central-Acting Adrenergic Agents	clonidine (Catapres, Catapres TTS)	0.1–0.8 mg orally in 2 divided doses. Max: 2.4 mg/day Transdermal patch: 0.1–0.3 mg patch every 7 days
	methyldopa (Aldomet)	250 to 2000 mg/day in 2 to 4 divided doses. Max: 3000 mg/day

Common Side Effects

Central-Acting Adrenergic Agents

Dry mouth   Nasal congestion   Drowsiness

Intended Responses of Central-Acting Adrenergic Agents
- Vasodilation of arteries is increased.
- Blood pressure is lowered.
- Heart workload is decreased.

Common Side Effects of Central-Acting Adrenergic Agents
Central-acting adrenergic agents have a higher incidence of side effects than other blood pressure–lowering drugs. Common side effects include drowsiness, lethargy, dry mouth, and nasal congestion

Possible Adverse Effects of Central-Acting Adrenergic Agents
Myocarditis associated with allergic type reactions to methyldopa are rare but have been known to cause death.

⊛ Priority Actions to Take *Before* Giving Central-Acting Adrenergic Agents
In addition to the general priority actions to take before giving any antihypertensive therapy (p. 224), obtain a baseline weight on the patient.

When administering a clonidine patch, be aware that it is packaged with two patches. The smaller patch contains the drug, and the larger patch is used to cover the drug patch. If the patch falls off, a new patch should be placed on the patient. Be sure to record the date and time and initial the patch before placing it on the patient.

⭐ **Priority Actions to Take *After* Giving Central-Acting Adrenergic Agents**

In addition to the general priority actions to take after giving any antihypertensive therapy (p. 224), keep track of the patient's intake and output: check feet and ankles for swelling; listen to the patient's lungs for crackles; watch for signs of mental status changes suggesting that blood pressure may be too low; and look for behavioral signs of depression such as difficulty concentrating, sleep changes, or a loss of interest in daily activities. Be sure to remove the old clonidine patch when a new patch is applied.

⭐ **Teaching Priorities for Patients Taking Central-Acting Adrenergic Agents**

In addition to the general teaching priorities related to antihypertensive therapy (p. 224), include these teaching points and precautions:

- When prescribed to do so, ceasing to take these drugs should be done gradually. If they are stopped suddenly, blood pressure could become dangerously high.
- To ease dry mouth symptoms, perform frequent mouth care with rinses, tooth brushing, and the use of sugarless gum.
- If you use transdermal clonidine, the patch can stay on during bathing or swimming.
- Remember that the transdermal form of this drug is packaged with two patches. The smaller patch contains the actual drug; and the larger patch, which does not contain medication, is used to cover the drug patch. If the patch falls off, apply a new one.

Life Span Considerations for Central-Acting Adrenergic Agents

Considerations for pregnancy and lactation. Clonidine has a moderate likelihood of increasing the risk of birth defects or fetal damage and should be avoided during pregnancy and breastfeeding. Methyldopa (Aldomet) has a low likelihood of increasing the risk of birth defects or fetal damage when prescribed by mouth and a moderate likelihood when prescribed intravenously. Oral methyldopa has been used safely during both pregnancy and breastfeeding. This drug is also safely used to treat pregnancy-induced hypertension.

Considerations for older adults. Older adults are very sensitive to the actions of central-acting adrenergic agents and tend to have an increased risk of orthostatic hypotension, dizziness, and falls. Teach older adults to change positions slowly and to ask for help getting up.

DIRECT VASODILATORS

How Direct Vasodilators Work

A *vasodilator* is any drug that relaxes blood vessel walls. **Direct vasodilators** act directly on the peripheral arteries, causing them to dilate, which leads to lower blood pressure. Be sure to consult a reliable drug resource for information on any specific direct vasodilator.

Usual Adult Dosages for Commonly Prescribed Direct Vasodilators

Drug Category	Drug Name	Usual Maintenance Dose
Direct Vasodilators	hydralazine (Apresoline)	10–25 mg orally four times daily. Max: 300 mg/day 10–20 mg IV bolus every 4–6 hr as needed
	minoxidil (Loniten)	5–100 mg orally daily in 1 to 3 divided doses

Intended Responses of Direct Vasodilators

- Vasodilation (widening) of arteries is increased.
- Blood pressure is lowered.
- Heart workload is decreased.

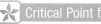

Critical Point for Safety

Frequent mouth rinses, oral care, and chewing sugarless gum can relieve the dry-mouth side effect of central-acting adrenergic agents.

QSEN: Safety

Critical Point for Safety

Clonidine should be avoided during pregnancy because it has a moderate likelihood of increased risk of birth defects and fetal damage.

QSEN: Safety

Common Side Effects of Direct Vasodilators

Direct vasodilators, along with central-acting adrenergic agents, have a higher incidence of side effects. Common side effects include tachycardia and salt (sodium) retention (hypernatremia).

Possible Adverse Effects of Direct Vasodilators

Stevens-Johnson syndrome may occur with minoxidil. This is a severe inflammatory eruption of the skin and mucous membranes (see Figure 1.5 in Chapter 1).

⭐ Priority Actions to Take *Before* Giving Direct Vasodilators

In addition to the general priority actions to take before giving any antihypertensive therapy (p. 224), be sure to get a baseline weight for the patient.

⭐ Priority Actions to Take *After* Giving Direct Vasodilators

In addition to the general priority actions to take after giving any antihypertensive therapy (p. 224), keep track of intake and output. Check the patient's feet and ankles for swelling. Listen to the patient's lungs for crackles. These drugs increase the risk of fluid retention and edema formation.

⭐ Teaching Priorities for Patients Taking Direct Vasodilators

In addition to general teaching priorities related to antihypertensive therapy (p. 224), include these teaching points and precautions:

* Contact your prescriber if you miss more than two doses. Remember that these drugs should be stopped gradually because blood pressure can become dangerously high if they are stopped suddenly.
* Report any persistent heart rate increase of more than 20 beats/min to your prescriber. This may be a sign of heart failure.
* Weigh yourselves and check your feet and ankles for swelling twice a week.
* Report weight gain of more than 3 pounds in 1 week to your prescriber because this may indicate heart failure.

Life Span Considerations for Direct Vasodilators

Considerations for pregnancy and lactation. Hydralazine (Apresoline) has a low likelihood of increasing the risk of birth defects or fetal damage and has been used safely during both pregnancy and breastfeeding to decrease high blood pressure in women. Small amounts of this drug pass into breast milk, putting infants at minimal risk of side effects. A woman who plans to breastfeed should discuss this with the prescriber.

⭐ Critical Point for Safety

With vasodilator drugs, report a sustained increase in heart rate of more than 20 beats/min to the prescriber immediately because this may indicate heart failure.

QSEN: Safety

Get Ready for the NCLEX® Examination!

Key Points

* Hypertension is defined as a systolic blood pressure (SBP) of greater than or equal to 140 mm Hg and/or a diastolic blood pressure (DBP) of greater than or equal to 90 mm Hg.
* Untreated hypertension can lead to many health problems, including heart attack, stroke, and kidney disease.
* A patient with high blood pressure should not take over-the-counter allergy and cold drugs that contain phenylephrine because these drugs can worsen the hypertension.
* Orthostatic hypotension criteria include decreased SBP of 20 mm Hg or more, decreased DBP of 10 mm Hg or more, and increased heart rate of 20 beats/min or more.
* Teach patients who are prescribed drugs to lower blood pressure to sit up and stand slowly, because dizziness and hypotension are common side effects of these drugs.

* Teach patients to take missed doses as soon as possible. If it is almost time for the next dose, they should skip the missed dose and return to the regular dosing schedule.
* Antihypertensive drugs will help control but will not cure hypertension. Teach patients that they may need to take these drugs for the rest of their lives.
* Patients with hypertension should not take over-the-counter drugs (such as drugs for appetite control, asthma, colds, and hay fever) without asking their prescriber.
* If you are taking an ACE inhibitor and develop a severe or bothersome and persistent dry cough, notify your prescriber because the drug may need to be discontinued.
* Monitor patients for swelling of the eyes, lips, and tongue, which indicates angioedema, a serious and life-threatening adverse effect of ACE inhibitors.

- ACE inhibitors may increase the effect of decreased blood pressure in patients who are also taking diuretics.
- ACE inhibitors and potassium-sparing diuretics cause much higher increases in blood potassium levels.
- Tell patients who are taking ACE inhibitors that drinking alcohol can increase the low blood pressure effect and the risk of dizziness or fainting.
- ACE inhibitors should not be prescribed for women who are pregnant. They can cause low blood pressure, severe kidney failure, increased potassium, and even death in a newborn when used after the first trimester of pregnancy.
- Angiotensin II receptor blockers (ARBs) block the action of angiotensin II, leading to increased vasodilation (widening) of arteries.
- Angioedema (swelling of the face, eyes, lips, and tongue) is a life-threatening adverse effect of angiotensin II receptor blockers and ACE inhibitors.
- Report any swelling of the face, eyes, lips, or tongue to the prescriber immediately when a patient is given an ARB. These are signs of the life-threatening adverse reaction, angioedema, and the patient should not receive these drugs again.
- Calcium channel blockers can cause a severe skin disorder called Stevens-Johnson syndrome. Always check the patient for skin lesions, itching, fever, and achy joints.
- Beta blockers can decrease or increase blood glucose levels. Be sure to check blood glucose regularly in a patient with diabetes.
- Patients should never suddenly stop taking beta blockers. This may cause unpleasant and harmful effects such as increased risk of heart attack.
- Beta blockers can affect the results of medical tests such as tests that raise heart rate and blood pressure.
- Teach patients that beta blockers can cause new-onset depression or worsen existing depression.
- Monitor older adults who have been prescribed beta blockers for mental confusion or changes in level of consciousness.
- Teach men that they should not be prescribed phosphodiesterase type 5 inhibitors (erectile dysfunction drugs) if they are also taking alpha blocker therapy because of the risk of severe hypotension.
- Give the first dose of prazosin and terazosin at bedtime and caution the patient not to get up without assistance. Orthostatic hypotension is a common side effect of the first doses.
- Teach patients that weight gain and ankle swelling are signs that the body is holding extra fluid and should be reported immediately to the prescriber.
- Alpha blockers pass into breast milk. Teach women who are breastfeeding or planning to breastfeed that it may be necessary to stop breastfeeding while on alpha blockers.
- Monitor patients with diabetes carefully when taking alpha-beta blockers because these drugs cause hyperglycemia (high blood sugar).
- Many blood pressure–lowering drugs can cause drowsiness or dizziness. Teach patients taking these drugs not to drive or operate machines.
- Methyldopa (Aldomet), a central-acting adrenergic drug, is the drug of choice for controlling high blood pressure during pregnancy.
- Frequent mouth rinses, oral care, and chewing sugarless gum can relieve the dry-mouth side effect of central-acting adrenergic agents.
- A sustained heart rate increase of more than 20 beats/min should be reported to the prescriber when a patient is taking a direct vasodilator drug.
- Always check blood pressure, heart rate, and weight and look for swelling of the ankles or feet before and after giving antihypertensive drugs.
- Encourage patients to adopt lifestyle changes, such as weight loss, regular exercise, and low-salt diets, which will help to control high blood pressure.
- Be sure that patients know how to check their heart rate and blood pressure and understand the importance of follow-up checks.

Additional Learning Resources

🌐 Be sure to visit your Evolve website (http://evolve.elsevier.com/Workman/pharmacology/) for additional online resources.

SG Go to your Study Guide for additional learning activities to help you master this chapter.

Review Questions

See *Answers to In-Text Review Questions* in the back of the book for answers to these questions.

1. The nurse is reviewing a patient's blood pressure, which has been consistently around 138/88 mm Hg. What does this reading represent to the nurse?

   A. Normal blood pressure
   B. Elevated blood pressure
   C. Stage 1 high blood pressure
   D. Stage 2 high blood pressure

2. The nurse is caring for a patient with newly diagnosed untreated hypertension. Which health problems is the patient at increased risk of developing? Select all that apply.

   A. Kidney damage
   B. Stroke
   C. Diabetes mellitus
   D. Seizures
   E. Cardiomyopathy
   F. Blindness

3. The nurse is teaching a patient about antihypertensive therapy. Which statement made by the patient indicates a need for further teaching?

   A. "Now that my blood pressure is normal, I won't need to take my medication anymore."
   B. "When I take my blood pressure at home, I always try to take it at just about the same time every day."
   C. "I check the labels on cans and other food packages to be sure they do not have too much sodium."
   D. "I hope that by continuing to lose weight, I might not have to take medications to manage my high blood pressure."

4. Which action or precaution is **most important** for the nurse to perform before giving any type of drug for hypertension to a patient?

   A. Ensuring that the patient is in a sitting position
   B. Checking the patient's blood pressure
   C. Having the patient drink a full glass of water
   D. Checking the patient's pulse for regularity

5. The nurse has checked a patient's blood pressure before administering an oral dose of enalopril, 10 mg. What is the nurse's **best** action when the reading is 88/52 mm Hg?

   A. Give the patient a cup of coffee and retake the blood pressure in 30 minutes.
   B. Document the finding as the only action and administer the drug as usual.
   C. Raise the side rails and apply oxygen by mask or nasal cannula.
   D. Hold the dose and notify the prescriber.

6. When the nurse gives the first dose of any antihypertensive drug to a patient, which **priority** instruction does the nurse give to the patient?

   A. "Stay in bed and call for help if you need to get up for any reason."
   B. "Urinate in a container so that we can keep track of your urine output."
   C. "If you develop a headache, we can give you some acetaminophen."
   D. "Avoid selecting salty foods from your menu."

7. A patient asks the nurse how atenolol will help reduce his high blood pressure. What is the nurse's **best** response?

   A. "It will help your body rid itself of excess fluids and decrease the work your heart must do to pump blood."

   B. "It will help decrease built-up water and salt in your blood and tissues."
   C. "It will block vasoconstriction as well as salt and water retention."
   D. "It will decrease your heart rate and how hard your heart pumps."

8. What is the nurse's **best** action when a patient who has been taking lisinopril develops swollen lips and reports that his or her tongue feels thick?

   A. Documenting the report and reassuring the patient that this is a common drug side effect
   B. Checking the patient's pulse for rhythm and taking the patient's blood pressure
   C. Holding the lisinopril dose and notifying the prescriber immediately
   D. Asking the patient whether this has ever happened before

9. A female patient has been prescribed losartan. Which substance is **most important** for the nurse teach the patient to avoid?

   A. Oral contraceptives
   B. Salt substitutes
   C. Caffeine
   D. Alcohol

10. A patient with hypertension and type 2 diabetes is taking carvedilol. What **priority** precaution does the nurse take when giving this drug?

    A. Assessing blood pressure in both arms
    B. Monitoring strict intake and output
    C. Checking blood sugar levels regularly
    D. Watching for sacral swelling

Clinical Judgment

1. Which **priority** precautions or actions will the nurse be sure to include when instructing a 25-year-old hospitalized female patient about the taking the first dose of prazosin for hypertension? **Select all that apply.**

   A. Do not drive for at least 24 hours.
   B. Examine your skin for bruising, redness, or irritation.
   C. Get up slowly from bed or a chair.
   D. Weigh yourself every day.
   E. Avoid the use of hair dyes while taking this drug.
   F. Your first dose of this drug will be given at bedtime.
   G. Discuss the use of this drug with your prescriber if you plan to become pregnant.
   H. Check your ankles for any swelling.
   I. Report any weight loss to your prescriber.
   J. Be sure to call for help when getting out of bed.

2. An older adult patient with difficult-to-control hypertension is prescribed a thiazide diuretic, an angiotensin II receptor blocker (ARB), a beta blocker and a direct vasodilator for blood pressure control. The nurse is teaching the patient about these drugs. Which statements made by the patient indicate that the patient understands the teaching or requires further teaching? **Use an X to indicate which patient statement about issues related to this therapy is either Understood or Requires Further Teaching.**

PATIENT STATEMENT	UNDERSTOOD TEACHING	REQUIRES FURTHER TEACHING
"While I'm taking this drug my urine will be darker and the amount will decrease."		
"I will check and keep a record of my blood pressure every day."		
"I will get up slowly from bed or from the chair."		
"If my blood pressure is 120/70 mm Hg, I will report it to my doctor immediately."		
"I will get to the emergency department if I notice any swelling in my face or throat."		
"When I'm working outside, I will be sure to wear protective clothing."		
"If my heart rate is 90 beats a minute, I will increase the dosage of my beta blocker."		
"I will be sure to let my prescriber know if I notice any weight gain or ankle swelling."		

14

Drug Therapy for Heart Failure

http://evolve.elsevier.com/Workman/pharmacology/

Learning Objectives

The content presented in this chapter should help you to:

1. Describe the common names, actions, usual adult dosages, possible side effects, and adverse effects of vasodilators and cardiac glycosides (digoxin).
2. Discuss the priority actions to take before and after giving vasodilators and cardiac glycosides.
3. Prioritize essential information to teach patients taking vasodilators and cardiac glycosides.
4. Describe the common names, actions, usual adult dosages, possible side effects, and adverse effects of human B-type

natriuretic peptides, positive inotropes, potassium, and magnesium.

5. Discuss the priority actions to take before and after giving human B-type natriuretic peptides, positive inotropes, potassium, and magnesium.
6. Prioritize essential information to teach patients taking human B-type natriuretic peptides, positive inotropes, potassium, and magnesium.
7. Explain life span considerations for drugs used to treat heart failure.

Key Terms

cardiac glycoside (CAR-dē-ak GLĬ-kō-sīd) (p. 252) A class of drugs that improve heart failure by slowing down a heart rate that is too fast, allowing more time for the left ventricle to fill.

human B-type natriuretic peptide (HŪ-măn B TĬP NĀ-trē-yū-RĚT-ik PĚP-tīd) (p. 254) A hormone that is produced by the heart ventricles and a synthetic drug with actions that include increased water elimination and blood vessel dilation.

magnesium (măg-NĒ-zē-ŭm) (p. 257) A major mineral that is the fourth most abundant in the human body. It helps the heart rhythm remain steady and keeps the bones strong.

positive inotrope (PŎS-ĭh-tĭv ĬN-ō-trōp) (p. 256) Heart pump drugs that make the heart muscle contract more forcefully. They also relax blood vessels so blood can flow better.

potassium (pō-TĂS-ē-ŭm) (p. 257) A very important electrolyte that is essential for a healthy nervous system and a regular heart rhythm.

vasodilator (VĀ-sō-dī-LĀ-tŏr) (p. 249) A class of drugs that act directly on the peripheral arteries to cause them to dilate.

REVIEW OF RELATED PHYSIOLOGY AND PATHOPHYSIOLOGY

Heart failure can occur at any age; however, it is much more common in older people because they often have disorders that damage the heart muscle (e.g., high blood pressure or heart attack), and age-related changes in the heart can make it pump less efficiently. As the world population ages, the number of people diagnosed with heart failure continues to increase. Around the world, an estimated 64.3 million people are living with *heart failure*. About 6.2 million people live with heart failure in the United States alone, and as many as 550,000 new cases occur each year.

Heart failure occurs when the heart cannot pump enough blood to meet the needs of the body. Most heart failure is caused by hypertension. Many of the drugs used to treat hypertension are also used to treat heart failure. Other causes of heart failure include myocardial infarction, coronary artery disease, cardiomyopathy, substance abuse (e.g., alcohol and illicit or prescribed drugs), heart valve disease, congenital defects, cardiac infections and inflammations, and conditions that increase cardiac output and energy demands such as sepsis.

The heart is a muscular organ that is hollow and divided into four chambers: right atrium, right ventricle, left atrium, and left ventricle (Animations 14.1 and 14.2). The

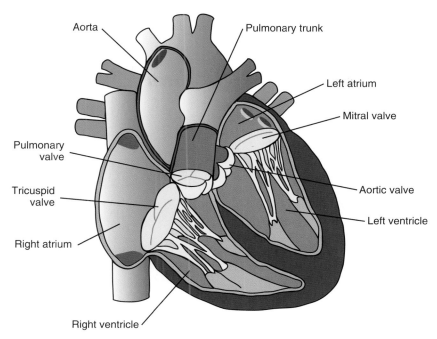

FIG. 14.1 Heart chambers and valves.

atrial and ventricular chambers are separated by one-way valves that open when the pressure in the first chamber is higher than that in the second chamber (Figure 14.1).

Blood enters the heart from the vena cava into the right atrium. This blood comes from the rest of the body; most of the oxygen has been used. From the right atrium, the blood moves through the tricuspid valve into the right ventricle. The muscle of the right ventricle contracts to make the pressure in this chamber higher than the pressure in the pulmonary artery. When right ventricular pressure is high enough, the pulmonary valve opens and allows blood to move from the right ventricle into the pulmonary artery. From there, blood moves into the lungs, where it picks up oxygen. The oxygenated blood then moves into the left atrium. When the pressure in the left atrium is high enough, the blood moves through the mitral valve (also called the bicuspid valve) into the left ventricle. The muscles of the left ventricle are the strongest ones in the heart. They must contract and increase the pressure in the left ventricle to force the blood to leave the left ventricle through the aortic valve and into the aorta. Once oxygenated blood enters the aorta, it circulates throughout the entire body to deliver oxygen to every tissue and organ. So, it is important that the muscles of the left ventricle have the best contraction to force blood into the aorta.

The muscles of the left ventricle are similar to other body muscles in that they contract best and are strongest after a stretch. Think of a baseball pitcher winding up to throw a fastball. He or she first moves the arm back as far as possible to stretch the throwing muscles. This stretching before throwing allows the muscles to contract harder and faster, resulting in a better throw. When the muscles of the left ventricle are stretched to the best level, the result is a stronger contraction that moves more blood from the left ventricle into the aorta. Usually, this stretch occurs naturally when the right amount of blood fills the ventricle *(preload)*. If the muscle is not stretched enough, the resulting contraction is weak and moves only a small amount of blood into the aorta (just as a small windup before a pitch results in a weak and short throw).

One problem that can occur with the muscle of the left ventricle is that it can become *overstretched*. When any muscle is overstretched, its contraction is weaker. Think about a person with a rubber band. Not stretching the rubber band, or stretching it only a little, results in a weak snap. Stretching it more increases the snap. However, if the rubber band is overstretched, it becomes so flabby that it cannot "snap" back. When the muscles of the left ventricle are overstretched or flabby and

 Memory Jogger

When the left ventricular muscle is stretched, a stronger heart contraction moves more blood from the left ventricle into the aorta and out to the body.

 Memory Jogger

Preload is the "stretching" of the muscle caused by blood filling the left ventricle.

Normal   **Heart Failure**

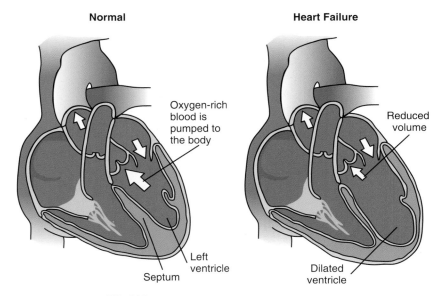

FIG. 14.2 Normal heart and heart with heart failure.

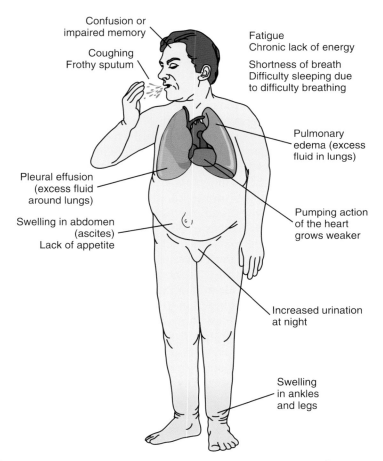

FIG. 14.3 Signs and symptoms of heart failure and peripheral and pulmonary congestion.

the contraction is weak, too much blood remains in the left ventricle, and more blood arriving from the left atrium is added to it. This overstretches the muscle more and continues to weaken contractions, leading to heart failure (Figure 14.2). Blood then backs up into other heart chambers, leading to congestion in the lungs and the peripheral veins (Figure 14.3).

Some of the drugs used to treat heart failure work by actually making the muscles contract better. Others work by reducing the amount of blood in the left ventricle (preventing overstretching). Still, others work by lowering the pressure in the aorta *(afterload)*, so muscles of the left ventricle do not have to contract as hard or as strong to move blood out of the ventricle and into the aorta.

Heart function and blood pressure work together for good blood circulation and blood flow to ensure that oxygen is delivered to all body tissues and organs. Heart contractions must be strong enough to move blood into the arteries. Then arterial pressure must be high enough to move blood through the arteries and into the tissues and organs. *Mean arterial pressure (MAP)* is the average systolic blood pressure in the large arteries, including the aorta. For the average healthy adult, the normal MAP range is between 70 and 100 mm Hg, which ensures good blood circulation to tissues. If the MAP is too low (<60 mm Hg), tissues and organs will not receive enough blood to ensure oxygenation. MAP also is the pressure that the left ventricle must overcome to move blood from the left ventricle into the aorta during contraction (afterload). If MAP is higher than normal (>110 mm Hg), the heart, especially the left ventricle, has to work harder to move blood into the aorta. Heart attacks (myocardial infarction) and heart failure can occur when the heart has to work too hard for too long.

LEFT HEART FAILURE

When blood collects in the left side of the heart, it starts to backflow into the pulmonary system and results in congestion in the lungs, decreased lung function, and difficulty breathing. Because the left ventricle pumps blood to the body, symptoms include signs of decreased cardiac output (such as fatigue and weakness) and signs of pulmonary congestion (such as crackles and wheezes detected with a stethoscope). Box 14.1 lists the key signs and symptoms associated with left ventricular heart failure.

Left heart failure can be either systolic or diastolic. *Systolic left heart failure* is more common. It happens when the heart contractions are too weak to circulate enough blood to meet the needs of the body. The decrease in contractility causes a decrease in the amount of blood pumped out with each contraction, leaving more blood in the ventricle and causing an increase in preload. Afterload increases because of increased peripheral resistance usually as a result of high blood pressure. These two changes cause a decrease in *ejection fraction* (percentage of blood pumped with each cardiac contraction) from a normal of 50% to 70% to less than 40%. The lower ejection fraction leads to less blood (cardiac output) for tissue perfusion. Blood collects in the pulmonary blood vessels, causing signs of lung congestion.

Diastolic left heart failure occurs when the left ventricle is not able to relax enough during diastole and causes a decrease in filling of the ventricles (preload) before contraction. A decrease in cardiac output results and not enough blood is pumped to

 Memory Jogger

Afterload is the pressure in the aorta that the left ventricle must overcome before blood can move from it into the aorta.

 Memory Jogger

Mean arterial pressure (MAP) is the average systolic blood pressure in the large arteries, including the aorta. The normal MAP range for a healthy adult is between 70 and 100 mm Hg

 Memory Jogger

Heart failure most commonly occurs in the left ventricle.

Memory Jogger

The normal ejection fraction is 50%–70%. With systolic heart failure, the ejection fraction is less than 40%.

| Box **14.1** | Signs and Symptoms of Left Heart Failure |

DECREASED CARDIAC OUTPUT
- Fatigue
- Weakness
- Oliguria (decreased urine output) during the day
- Angina
- Confusion, restlessness
- Dizziness
- Tachycardia, palpitations
- Paleness (pallor)

- Weak peripheral pulses
- Cool extremities

PULMONARY CONGESTION
- Hacking cough, worse at night
- Dyspnea/breathlessness
- Crackles or wheezes in lungs
- Frothy, pink-tinged sputum
- Tachypnea
- S₃/S₄ summation gallop (abnormal heart sounds)

Modified from Ignatavicius, D., Workman, M. L., Rebar, C., & Heimgartner, N. (2021). *Medical-surgical nursing: Concepts for interprofessional collaborative care* (10th ed., p. 671). Philadelphia: Elsevier.

meet the needs of the body. With diastolic failure the patient's ejection fraction may be very close to normal; however, the actual volume ejected is less.

RIGHT HEART FAILURE

With right heart failure, the right ventricle does not empty. This causes increased volume and pressure in the right side of the heart. When the right ventricle contracts poorly, signs and symptoms of peripheral congestion occur (Box 14.2) such as weight gain, swelling in the legs, *jugular vein distention* (Figure 14.4), and increased blood pressure. The pathophysiology of heart failure is summarized in Figure 14.5.

COMPENSATORY MECHANISMS FOR HEART FAILURE

The body has several ways to compensate for heart failure. In response to tissue hypoxia (not enough oxygen), the sympathetic nervous system is stimulated, and the catecholamine hormones, epinephrine and norepinephrine, are released. These

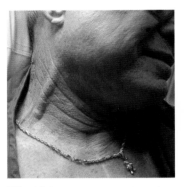

FIG. 14.4 Jugular vein distention. (From Goldman, L., & Ausiello, D. [2007]. *Cecil medicine* [23rd ed.]. Philadelphia: Saunders.)

Box 14.2	Signs and Symptoms of Right Heart Failure
SYSTEMIC CONGESTION <ul><li>Jugular (neck vein) distention</li><li>Enlarged liver and spleen</li><li>Anorexia and nausea</li><li>Dependent edema (legs and sacrum)</li><li>Distended abdomen</li></ul>	<ul><li>Swollen hands and fingers</li><li>Increased urine output (polyuria) at night</li><li>Weight gain</li><li>Increased blood pressure (from excess volume) or decreased blood pressure (from heart failure)</li></ul>

Modified from Ignatavicius, D., Workman, M. L., Rebar, C., & Heimgartner, N. (2021). *Medical-surgical nursing: Concepts for interprofessional collaborative care* (10th ed., p. 671). Philadelphia: Elsevier.

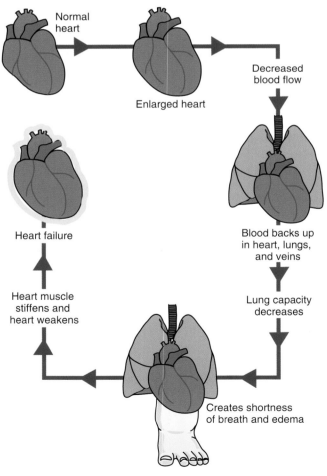

FIG. 14.5 Pathophysiology of heart failure.

hormones act on the heart in two ways. First, they increase the heart rate. Second, they increase the power of the heart muscle fibers to contract or shorten so the heart pumps more forcefully. The ability of the heart fibers to shorten is called *contractility*. These actions increase the amount of blood pumped by the heart in 1 minute, known as the *cardiac output*.

Sympathetic nervous system stimulation also causes arterial vasoconstriction (narrowing of the arteries). This helps the body to maintain blood pressure and improve blood flow to the tissues. The downside to this compensation is that narrowing of the arteries leads to increased afterload, more work for the heart, and increased oxygen needs. *Increased afterload can lead to worsening heart failure.*

When heart failure causes decreased blood flow to the kidneys, another compensation process called the *renin-angiotensin system (RAS)* is activated. This pathway causes the release of two body chemicals: angiotensin II and aldosterone. *Angiotensin II* causes blood vessel constriction (increased afterload), whereas *aldosterone* leads to sodium and water retention (increased preload). Activation of the RAS leads to increased blood pressure.

A third way that the body can compensate for heart failure is by *myocardial hypertrophy* (enlargement) of the heart muscle. An increase in the heart muscle size can lead to more forceful contractions and increased cardiac output. But when the heart muscle becomes too big, it outgrows its blood supply. The thickened muscle also becomes "stiff," resulting in less effective contractions and diastolic heart failure.

TREATMENT FOR HEART FAILURE

Continuous heart function is needed for life. Unmanaged heart failure leads to death. Heart failure is usually a chronic disorder and can be "cured" only with a heart transplant. Goals for treatment and management include (1) making physical activity more comfortable, (2) improving quality of life, and (3) prolonging life. Interventions focus on:
- Treating the cause of heart failure.
- Controlling factors that can cause it to worsen.
- Treating its symptoms.

Lifestyle changes are an important part of a treatment plan. Suggested changes include weight loss, smoking cessation, and a low-salt and low-fat diet. Drug therapy only improves heart function; drugs do *not* cure heart failure. Because the damage to the heart muscle is not reversible, the only real cure for heart failure is a heart transplant.

GENERAL ISSUES IN HEART FAILURE THERAPY

There are several classes of drugs for heart failure that have both common and different actions and effects. Priority actions for these common actions and effects are listed in the following discussion. Specific responsibilities are listed with each class of heart failure drugs.

⭐ PRIORITY ACTIONS TO TAKE *BEFORE* GIVING ANY HEART FAILURE DRUG

Always obtain a complete list of drugs that the patient is currently taking, including over-the-counter and herbal drugs, some of which could cause heart failure or make it worse. Check the patient's blood pressure and heart rate. If the blood pressure is low (less than 90/60 mm Hg) or the heart rate is low (less than 60 beats/min), check with the prescriber about whether the patient should receive the drug because many of these drugs can lower heart rate even further. Assess the apical pulse for a full minute because a patient with heart failure may have extra heart sounds and dysrhythmias causing irregular heartbeats. Check the drug order because some prescribers provide guidelines for when to administer and when to hold these drugs. Obtain a baseline weight for each patient because weight gain is a sign of worsening heart failure. Assess for and document symptoms of heart failure. Ask female patients of

Memory Jogger

Cardiac output (CO) is the product of heart rate (HR) and stroke volume (SV). The formula for this is $CO = HR \times SV$. An increase in heart rate and/or stroke volume results in an increase in cardiac output.

Memory Jogger

The renin-angiotensin system causes vasoconstriction and body retention of sodium and water to increase blood pressure.

Memory Jogger

The only real cure for heart failure is a *heart transplant* because the damage to the heart muscle is irreversible.

Memory Jogger

Remember that the apical pulse is displaced lateral to the midclavicular line with left heart failure.

childbearing years if they are pregnant, breastfeeding, or planning to become pregnant because many drugs for heart failure should be avoided during pregnancy.

⭐ PRIORITY ACTIONS TO TAKE *AFTER* GIVING ANY HEART FAILURE DRUG

Reassess and continue to monitor the patient's blood pressure and apical heart rate. Notify the prescriber if either measure is low. Ensure that the call light is within easy reach and tell the patient to call for assistance when getting out of bed because of the increased risk for dizziness, light-headedness, and hypotension with these drugs. Reassess for symptoms of heart failure and document your findings. Check for any signs or symptoms of allergic reactions or infections.

⭐ TEACHING PRIORITIES FOR PATIENTS TAKING ANY HEART FAILURE DRUG

Teaching priorities for patients taking any drug for heart failure include:
* Change positions slowly to prevent dizziness and falls. When you get up, go from a lying position to sitting before standing.
* Remember that these drugs will help to control but will **not** cure heart failure; heart failure drugs may be prescribed for life.
* Check and keep a daily record of your blood pressure and heart rate measurements using the techniques taught to you.
* Keep regular follow-up visits with your prescriber to check and maintain control of your heart failure.
* Consult with your prescriber before taking any over-the-counter drugs, including cough or allergy remedies or herbal preparations.
* Notify your prescriber of any weight gain or increase in shortness of breath because these are signs of worsening heart failure.
* If you experience dizziness, drowsiness, or light-headedness do not drive, use heavy or dangerous equipment, or do anything that could be dangerous or require increased alertness until you know how the drug affects you.
* Get a medical alert bracelet identifying your diagnosis and the heart failure drugs you are prescribed.

? Did You Know?

Most over-the-counter cold and allergy medications constrict blood vessels and raise blood pressure.

TYPES OF DRUGS USED TO TREAT HEART FAILURE

Heart failure is a complex problem in which more than one normal action is disrupted. For this reason, usually, a combination of drugs is prescribed to manage symptoms and improve heart-pumping function. Some of these drugs have other uses. For example, antihypertensive drugs are commonly used in heart failure therapy for several reasons. First, hypertension is a common cause of heart failure. In addition, by lowering blood pressure these drugs allow the heart to pump more easily. Therefore, drugs such as angiotensin-converting enzyme (ACE) inhibitors, angiotensin II receptor blockers (ARBs), and most beta-adrenergic blockers are part of drug therapy for heart failure. Diuretics help in the treatment of heart failure by reducing blood volume, relaxing arteries, and improving heart muscle pumping. Diuretic drugs are discussed in detail in Chapter 12. Chapter 13 discusses antihypertensive drugs. Other drugs used in the treatment of heart failure include anticoagulants (Chapter 17), which may be used to prevent clots from forming in the heart chambers; and antidysrhythmic drugs (Chapter 15), which may be prescribed for abnormal heart rhythms. This chapter focuses on the drugs with intended actions that are specific to the heart.

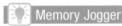

Memory Jogger

The major classes of drugs to treat heart failure are:
* ACE inhibitors
* Beta blockers
* Vasodilators
* Cardiac glycosides
* Diuretics
* Human B-type natriuretic peptides
* Positive inotropes

ANGIOTENSIN CONVERTING ENZYME (ACE) INHIBITORS

ACE inhibitors are often among the first drugs prescribed to treat heart failure. Dosages for these drugs are different when used to treat heart failure rather than high blood pressure. The most common ACE inhibitors used to treat heart failure are listed in the following table. Be sure to consult a reliable drug resource for information about any specific ACE inhibitor. Refer to Chapter 13 for more general information about ACE inhibitors.

Usual Adult Dosages for Commonly Prescribed ACE Inhibitors

Drug Category	Drug Name	Usual Maintenance Dose
ACE Inhibitors	benazepril (Lotensin)	10–40 mg orally once daily as a single dose or in two divided doses
	captopril (Capoten)	50–100 mg orally three times daily. Max: 450 mg/day
	enalapril (Epaned, Vasotec)	10–20 mg orally twice daily
	fosinopril (Monopril)	5–40 mg orally once daily as a single dose or in two divided doses
	lisinopril (Prinivil, Zestril)	Initially 2.5–5 mg orally once daily; may increase to 20–40 mg orally once daily
	moexipril (Univasc)	7.5–30 mg/day orally given once daily or in two divided doses every 12 hr *Special Considerations:* **Give doses at least 1 hr before meals**
	perindopril (Aceon)	2–16 mg orally once daily
	quinapril (Accupril)	5–20 mg orally twice a day
	ramipril (Altace)	2.5–20 mg/day orally, given in one to two divided doses. Max: 10 mg/day
	trandolapril (Mavik)	1–4 mg orally once daily

BETA BLOCKERS

How Beta Blockers Work

Beta blockers block the effects of epinephrine (adrenaline) on the heart. They decrease the heart rate and the force of heart contractions, which results in a decrease in blood pressure. As a result, the heart does not work as hard and requires less oxygen.

These drugs are often used with ACE inhibitors to treat heart failure. They may temporarily worsen heart failure symptoms but, when taken over a long period, they improve heart function.

Most dosages are the same as when used for high blood pressure. See Chapter 13 for the usual dosages and ranges. Those drugs with specific limits, when used for heart failure, are listed in the following table. Only the sustained-release form of metoprolol is used to treat heart failure. Be sure to consult a reliable drug reference for specific information about any specific beta blocker. Refer to Chapter 13 for more general information about beta blockers.

Adult Dosages for Commonly Prescribed Beta Blockers

Drug Category	Drug Name	Usual Maintenance Dose
Beta Blockers	carvedilol ❶ (Coreg, Coreg CR)	3.125–25 mg orally twice daily CR (controlled release) 10–80 mg daily *Special Considerations:* **With CR, reduce dose for bradycardia**
	metoprolol ❶ (Toprol XL)	*Adults:* 25–200 mg orally once daily

❶ High-alert drug.

VASODILATORS

How Vasodilators Work

Vasodilators are a class of drugs that act directly on the peripheral arteries to cause them to dilate. This leads to the lowering of blood pressure and decreasing the workload of the heart. Vasodilators are often given to patients who cannot take ACE inhibitors or angiotensin II receptor blockers (ARBs). The vasodilator that is most commonly prescribed for heart failure is hydralazine (Apresoline).

Other vasodilators used for treating chronic heart failure include isosorbide dinitrate (Isordil) and nitroglycerin. Isosorbide dinitrate and nitroglycerin (NTG) produce greater venous vasodilation than arterial vasodilation. Nitroglycerin also increases coronary blood flow by dilating the coronary arteries. With vasodilation, the heart is better able to pump blood out to meet the needs of the body. Be sure to consult a reliable drug resource for information about any specific vasodilator.

Do Not Confuse

Apresoline *with* **Priscoline**

An order for Apresoline may be confused with Priscoline. Apresoline is a vasodilator, whereas Priscoline is an alpha-adrenergic antagonist often used for persistent pulmonary hypertension in newborns.

QSEN: Safety

Do Not Confuse

Isordil *with* **Plendil**

An order for Isordil may be confused with Plendil. Isordil is a vasodilator, whereas Plendil is a calcium channel blocker.

QSEN: Safety

Common Side Effects
Vasodilators

Hypernatremia   Headache   Dizziness

Hypotension   Tachycardia

Critical Point for Safety

Wear gloves to administer nitroglycerin ointment to prevent absorbing the drug through your skin, which can cause headache or hypotension.

QSEN: Safety

Adult Dosages for Commonly Prescribed Vasodilators

Drug Category	Drug Name	Usual Maintenance Dose
Vasodilators	hydralazine (Apresoline)	25–100 mg orally three times daily
	isosorbide dinitrate (Dilatrate SR, Isochron, IsoDitrate, Isordil Titradose)	20–40 mg orally three times daily
	nitroglycerin (many brand names)	Sublingual or buccal tablets: 0.3–0.6 mg; may repeat every 5 min three times Sublingual or lingual spray: one to two sprays; may repeat every 5 min three times Oral (sustained-release capsules): 2.5–9 mg every 6–8 hr IV: 5–20 mcg/min Transdermal ointment: 1–2 inches every 6–8 hr Transdermal patch: 0.1–0.8 mg/hr up to 0.8 mg/hr; patch is worn 12–14 hr/day *Special Considerations:* **For transdermal ointment and patch, remove during the longest sleeping period**

Intended Responses of Vasodilators
- Vasodilation of arteries (hydralazine) is increased.
- Venous vasodilation (nitroglycerin, isosorbide) is increased.
- Blood flow to coronary arteries (nitroglycerin) is increased.
- Blood pressure is lowered.
- Heart workload is decreased.

Common Side Effects of Vasodilators
Common side effects of hydralazine include tachycardia and salt retention (hypernatremia). Common side effects of nitroglycerin and isosorbide include hypotension, headache, dizziness, and tachycardia. Allergic reactions include skin rash, especially on the face.

Possible Adverse Effects of Vasodilators
Adverse effects are very rare with hydralazine. They include neutropenia and shock with overdose. Neutropenia is an acute disease marked by high fever and a sharp drop in circulating white blood cells. Decreased white blood cells can lead to life-threatening infections. Adverse effects of nitroglycerin and isosorbide are also very rare. Circulatory collapse and shock may occur with nitroglycerin overdose.

Priority Actions to Take *Before* Giving Vasodilators
In addition to the general priority actions to take before giving any drug for heart failure (p. 247), wear gloves when administering nitroglycerin ointment. This drug can cause headaches if it is absorbed through the skin. Squeeze the ointment onto the special-ruled paper. Choose an unused site on a hairless area of the patient's chest, back, or upper arm. Place the application paper on the skin drug side down. Gently press on the paper to evenly disperse the drug. Be careful not to spread ointment outside the borders of the paper. Put tape over the paper to keep it in place (Figure 14.6).

Priority Actions to Take *After* Giving Vasodilators
In addition to the general priority actions to take after giving any drug for heart failure (p. 248), for safe skin-care, be sure to apply nitroglycerin drug patches or

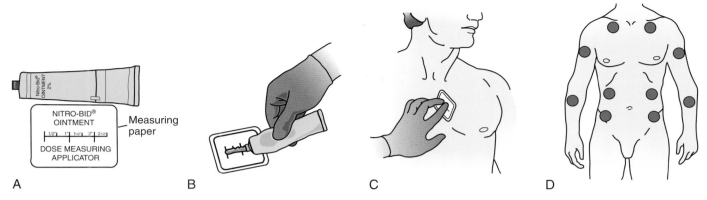

FIG. 14.6 Application of nitroglycerin ointment. (A) Check ointment dose and paper. (B) Apply dose to the paper. (C) Apply paper with the drug to the patient. (D) Appropriate sites for drug application.

ointments to a different site with each dose. Remove the previous dose and use a tissue to clean off any ointment left on the patient's skin before applying the next dose. Avoid rubbing the skin too much because this can cause more ointment to be absorbed or could tear the skin. Note that leaving the ointment from the previous dose on a patient's skin is like giving a double dose of the drug.

Nitroglycerin (ointment or patch) loses its effectiveness when used continuously. This is why it is good to have some "drug-free" time during a 24-hour period. Be sure to remove the patches at night or whenever the patient has his or her longest sleeping period because the heart is less stressed during that time.

Monitor intake and output. Check the patient's feet and ankles for swelling. Listen with a stethoscope for crackles in the lungs. Ask the patient about headaches or dizziness. A mild headache pain reliever such as acetaminophen (Tylenol) may be required for headaches related to nitroglycerin.

⊛ Teaching Priorities for Patients Taking Vasodilators

In addition to general teaching priorities related to any drugs for heart failure (p. 248), include these teaching points and precautions:

- Contact the prescriber if more than two doses are missed because these drugs should be discontinued gradually. Do not stop the drug suddenly, because blood vessels constrict too much (known as a rebound response), causing decreased blood flow to the heart and a rapid rise in blood pressure.
- Report any heart rate increase of more than 20 beats/min to your prescriber.
- Remember to report any increase in headaches, dizziness, or light-headedness to your prescriber.
- Keep sublingual and buccal nitroglycerin in place until completely dissolved. Nitroglycerin should cause a tingling sensation, which indicates that the drug is potent. Do not eat or drink until the tablet is dissolved. Note that if one tablet does not relieve chest pain, you should notify the prescriber.
- Be sure to store nitroglycerin tablets in the drug container distributed by the pharmacy. Remember that the drug degrades (loses its strength or potency) quickly, especially when exposed to light or moisture. *A nitroglycerin tablet that has lost its potency will not have any helpful effect.*
- Be certain the drug container is labeled so that if another person is helping you during an attack of chest pain, the right drug will be given.
- Use the proper techniques for applying nitroglycerin ointment or patches. Remove the ointment or patch at night or during the period of your longest rest or sleep (e.g., if you work at night, the drug is removed before you go to sleep during the day).
- Although acetaminophen may be needed at first to relieve headaches, you will likely develop a tolerance for nitroglycerin and isosorbide, and the headaches will decrease or disappear.

⬥ **Critical Point for Safety**

Remove a patient's nitroglycerin ointment or patch during the time when he or she has his or her longest sleep period, usually at night before bedtime to avoid loss of drug effectiveness.

QSEN: Safety

⬥ **Critical Point for Safety**

Teach patients that a tingling sensation indicates a potent nitroglycerin tablet.

QSEN: Safety

⬥ **Critical Point for Safety**

Sublingual and buccal nitroglycerin should not be swallowed. When swallowed, the liver destroys most of the drug, so it is not effective.

QSEN: Safety

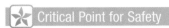

Critical Point for Safety

Intravenous (IV) hydralazine can also be used to treat high blood pressure associated with eclampsia (a serious condition that leads to seizures caused by high blood pressure) during pregnancy.

QSEN: Safety

- Weigh yourself and check your feet and ankles for swelling at least twice a week.
- Report a weight gain of more than 3 pounds in 1 week because it usually is a result of water retention, which is an indicator of worsening heart failure. Also report increased swelling to your prescriber.

Life Span Considerations for Vasodilators

Considerations for pregnancy and lactation. Isosorbide and nitroglycerin have a low to moderate likelihood of increasing the risk for birth defects or fetal damage. They may affect fetal circulation and should be used with caution during pregnancy. Hydralazine has been used safely for blood pressure control during pregnancy.

Considerations for older adults. Older adults may be more sensitive to the hypotensive effects of vasodilators and may need to be started on lower doses. Older adults are more likely to develop orthostatic hypotension while taking vasodilators, and their risk of falls is increased. Stress the need to change positions slowly and use handrails when going up or down steps. Also, warn older adults not to drive or operate dangerous or heavy equipment until they know how vasodilators affect them.

CARDIAC GLYCOSIDES (DIGOXIN)

How Cardiac Glycosides Work

Cardiac glycosides are a class of drugs that improve heart failure by slowing down a heart rate that is too fast and allowing more time for the left ventricle to fill. They also work on the muscle fibers in the heart and increase the force of each heartbeat (contractility). Both of these actions improve cardiac output. For many years, these drugs were the mainstay of heart failure therapy. Often now, newer drugs are prescribed although some patients are still prescribed a cardiac glycoside. Digoxin is used for maintenance therapy with heart failure. It comes in oral (tablet, capsules, elixir) and intravenous (IV) forms. Prescribed doses are age and weight dependent. Digoxin doses also vary according to whether the dose is a loading or a maintenance dose. Be sure to consult a reliable drug reference for information about any specific cardiac glycoside.

Adult Dosages for Commonly Prescribed Cardiac Glycosides

Drug Category	Drug Name	Usual Maintenance Dose
Cardiac Glycosides	digoxin ❶ (Digitek, Lanoxicaps, Lanoxin, Nativelle)	Tablets: Loading dose 10–15 mcg/kg orally given in three divided doses. Administer one-half (50%) the total loading dose initially, then one-fourth (25%) the loading dose every 6 to 8 hr for 2 doses Maintenance dose 3.4–5.1 mcg/kg/day orally once daily Liquid: Loading dose same as tablets Maintenance dose 3–4.5 mcg/kg/day orally once daily IV/IM: Loading dose 8 to 12 mcg/kg/total loading dose IV or IM divided into three doses, with the first dose equaling one-half the total. Administer the remaining half in two equally divided doses at 6- to 8-hr intervals Maintence dose 2.4–3.6 mcg/kg/day IM or IV once daily

❶ High-alert drug.

Intended Responses of Cardiac Glycosides
- Contractility is increased.
- Cardiac output is increased.
- Heart rate is decreased.

Common Side Effects of Cardiac Glycosides

The most common side effects of digoxin (Lanoxin) are heart rhythm disturbances that are related to digoxin toxicity. Other common side effects to watch for include fatigue, bradycardia (slow heart rate less than 60 beats/min), anorexia (loss of appetite), nausea, and vomiting.

Possible Adverse Effects of Cardiac Glycosides

Signs and symptoms of overdose include early signs such as loss of appetite, nausea, vomiting, diarrhea, or vision problems. Other signs and symptoms include changes in heart rate or rhythm (irregular or slow), palpitations, or fainting. In infants and small children, the earliest signs of overdose are changes in heart rate and rhythm. Children may not have the same symptoms as adults.

Dysrhythmias (abnormal and irregular heart rhythms) caused by digoxin can be life-threatening.

⭐ Priority Actions to Take *Before* Giving Cardiac Glycosides

In addition to the general priority actions to take before giving any heart failure drug (p. 247), check the apical heart rate with a stethoscope for a full minute because these drugs can decrease heart rate and cause dysrhythmias. Note whether the heart rate is regular or irregular. If it is less than 60 beats/min, greater than 100 beats/min, or irregular, notify the prescriber. For a heart rate lower than 60 beats/min, hold the dose, notify the prescriber, and ask whether the patient should receive this drug.

If the prescriber has ordered a cardiac monitor for the patient, make sure that the monitor is in place and ask the monitor watcher about the patient's baseline rhythm.

Ask female patients of childbearing years if they are pregnant, breastfeeding, or planning to become pregnant because digoxin passes from the mother to the fetus and also passes into breast milk.

Ask patients if they have a history of electrolyte disorders, heart rhythm problems, kidney or liver disease, or thyroid disease. Check the patient's serum potassium level and notify the prescriber if it is low (a low potassium level increases the risk for digoxin toxicity).

⭐ Priority Actions to Take *After* Giving Cardiac Glycosides

In addition to the general priority actions to take after giving any heart failure drug (p. 248), check the apical heart rate for a full minute after giving each dose of this drug. After giving the drug, if the heart rate is less than 60 beats/min or irregular, notify the prescriber.

If the patient is on a heart monitor, ask the monitor watcher whether the patient's heart rate and rhythm have changed after each dose. Check the patient's current potassium, magnesium, and calcium laboratory values. Abnormal values may affect how this drug works. Monitor the patient for signs and symptoms of digoxin overdose such as loss of appetite, nausea, vomiting, bradycardia, and vision problems.

⭐ Teaching Priorities for Patients Taking Cardiac Glycosides

In addition to the general teaching priorities related to drugs for heart failure (p. 248), include these teaching points and precautions:
- Check and record your heart rate every day before taking digoxin.
- Notify your prescriber if your heart rate drops below 60 beats/min, is greater than 100 beats/min, or becomes irregular.
- Report any signs or symptoms of digoxin overdose (e.g., confusion, irregular pulse, loss of appetite, nausea, vomiting, diarrhea, fast heart rate, or vision changes) to your prescriber.
- Weigh yourself every day and report a weight gain of greater than 2 pounds per day to your prescriber.

Common Side Effects

Vasodilators

Fatigue   Anorexia,   Dizziness
            Nausea/
            Vomiting

Hypotension   Bradycardia   Dysrhythmias

⭐ **Critical Point for Safety**

Report common side effects of digoxin to the prescriber immediately because they are probably signs of digoxin toxicity, which can be life-threatening.

QSEN: Safety

⭐ **Critical Point for Safety**

Digoxin has a very narrow therapeutic range (0.8–2 ng/mL), and levels above 2 ng/mL are considered toxic. When a patient shows any signs of overdose (digoxin toxicity), a blood level for digoxin is drawn, and the dose is held.

QSEN: Safety

⭐ **Critical Point for Safety**

Always check the apical heart rate for a full minute before giving a cardiac glycoside.

QSEN: Safety

⭐ **Critical Point for Safety**

Always check a patient's serum potassium level before giving a dose of digoxin. Prescribed diuretics can lead to low potassium (hypokalemia), which increases the risk of digoxin toxicity.

QSEN: Safety

⭐ **Critical Point for Safety**

Teach patients taking digoxin to check their pulse before taking the drug. Tell them to notify the prescriber if their heart rate is slower than 60 beats/min, faster than 100 beats/min, or irregular.

QSEN: Safety

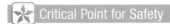

- Take your digoxin exactly as ordered by your prescriber. Digoxin should be taken every day at the same time, and a dose should *never* be skipped. A missed dose may be taken within 12 hours of its scheduled time. After that time, it should be skipped because a double dose can lead to toxicity.
- Avoid taking antacids within 2 hours of digoxin because antacids can affect the absorption of this drug.

Life Span Considerations for Cardiac Glycosides

Pediatric considerations. Doses of digoxin are specific and age-related. This drug has been used in newborns and children of all ages.

Considerations for pregnancy and lactation. Digoxin has a low to moderate likelihood of increasing the risk for birth defects or fetal damage. It passes from the mother to the fetus during pregnancy. It also passes to the baby through breast milk. Therefore, breastfeeding is not recommended during digoxin therapy.

Considerations for older adults. Older adults are more sensitive to the effects of this drug and more likely to develop side effects, including digitalis toxicity. In addition, older adults may be taking diuretics that alter blood potassium levels, increasing the risk for changes in the activity of cardiac glycosides. Teach older adults to take their medication exactly as prescribed and to keep all appointments for laboratory work to measure potassium and drug levels.

DIURETICS

Spironolactone (Aldactone), a potassium-sparing diuretic, is used to treat heart failure when systolic dysfunction is present. When prescribed in low doses, this drug blocks the action of aldosterone, which causes the body to hold on to salt and water. When spironolactone is prescribed, another diuretic usually will also be prescribed at its regular dose to decrease the volume of fluid in the blood vessels and reduce the workload of the heart. Used together, these drugs help the body maintain a more normal blood potassium level.

For more information on diuretics and the usual doses of thiazide and loop diuretics, see Chapter 12. The doses of potassium-sparing diuretics when they are used to treat heart failure are listed in the following table. Be sure to consult a reliable drug resource for information about any specific diuretic.

Adult Dosages for Commonly Prescribed Potassium-Sparing Diuretics

Drug Category	Drug Name	Usual Maintenance Dose
Potassium-Sparing Diuretics	amiloride (Midamor)	5–10 mg orally once daily. Max: 20 mg/day
	spironolactone (Aldactone, Carospir)	25–200 mg orally once daily ***Special Considerations:*** **Usually given with another diuretic for adequate diuretic response**
	triamterene (Dyrenium)	100 mg orally twice daily. Max: 300 mg/day

HUMAN B-TYPE NATRIURETIC PEPTIDES

How Natriuretic Peptides Work

Nesiritide (Natrecor) is a **human B-type natriuretic peptide**, which is a hormone that is produced by the heart ventricles and also is a synthetic drug. The actions of this drug include increased water elimination and blood vessel dilation. Both are helpful when treating a patient with heart failure. This drug is given by the IV route and helps the body get rid of extra sodium and water, thus lowering blood pressure. As a result, the patient is less short of breath and has less edema. Be sure to consult a reliable drug resource for more information about nesiritide.

Adult Dosages for Commonly Prescribed Natriuretic Peptides

Drug Category	Drug Name	Usual Maintenance Dose
Natriuretic Peptides	nesiritide (Natrecor ❶)	2 mcg/kg IV bolus followed by 0.01 mcg/kg/min continuous infusion

❶ High-alert drug.

Intended Responses of Natriuretic Peptides
- Excess sodium and water in the body are decreased.
- Urine output is increased.
- Vasodilation is increased.
- Blood pressure is lowered
- Shortness of breath and swelling are decreased.

Common Side Effects of Natriuretic Peptides
Side effects of natriuretic peptides include hypotension, dizziness, light-headedness, frequent urination, nausea, vomiting, nervousness, confusion, and palpitations.

Possible Adverse Effects of Natriuretic Peptides
Apnea (absence of breathing) is a life-threatening adverse effect of nesiritide.

⭐ Priority Actions to Take *Before* Giving Nesiritide
In addition to the general priority actions to take before giving any heart failure drug (p. 247), monitor for normal heart rate (60 to 100 beats/min), blood pressure, and respiratory rate (12 to 20 breaths/min). Remember that apnea is a life-threatening adverse effect of this drug.

Check the IV site for patency. Look for any signs of infection. This drug is given as an IV bolus followed by a continuous infusion. Double check the prescribed IV rate with another professional RN to be sure that it is accurate. Place the IV bolus and continuous IV infusions on an infusion pump to control the infusion rate. Document these actions.

⭐ Priority Actions to Take *After* Giving Nesiritide
In addition to the general priority actions to take after any heart failure drug (p. 248), continue to monitor blood pressure, heart rate, and respiratory rate during nesiritide infusion. Continue to check the IV line for patency and signs of infection. Tell the patient to report any pain or discomfort at the IV site. Continue to monitor and document the IV pump rate to make sure the infusion is at the correct prescribed rate.

⭐ Teaching Priorities for Patients Taking Nesiritide
In addition to the general teaching priorities related to giving any drugs for heart failure (p. 248), include these teaching points and precautions:
- Remember why this drug has been prescribed and how it will help your heart failure.
- Frequent blood pressure checks are necessary to screen for hypotension and you will be measuring urine output.

Life Span Considerations for Nesiritide
Considerations for pregnancy and lactation. Nesiritide appears to have a low to moderate likelihood of increasing the risk for birth defects or fetal harm.

Considerations for older adults. Older adults are at greater risk for confusion. Teach family members to assess the level of alertness and thought processes of an older

Common Side Effects
Natriuretic Peptides

Dizziness

Frequent urination

Nausea

Confusion

Palpitations

Hypotension

⭐ **Critical Point for Safety**

Nesiritide is incompatible with injectable forms of heparin, insulin, ethacrynic acid, bumetanide, enalapril; enalaprilat, hydralazine, and furosemide. These drugs should not be administered through the same IV catheter as nesiritide.

QSEN: Safety

adult who has recently started receiving prescribed IV nesiritide, especially during the first week of drug therapy.

POSITIVE INOTROPES (HEART PUMP DRUGS)

How Positive Inotropes Work

Positive inotropes are heart pump drugs that make the heart muscle contract more forcefully. They also relax blood vessels so the blood flow is increased. These drugs are used for people with severe heart failure symptoms. They are given intravenously to stimulate stronger heart contractions and keep blood circulating. Although some patients with heart failure receive these drugs while in the hospital, many also receive them at home using an infusion pump. Be sure to consult a reliable drug resource for more information about positive inotropes.

Adult Dosages for Commonly Prescribed Positive Inotropes

Drug Category	Drug Name	Usual Maintenance Dose
Positive Inotropes	dobutamine ❶ (Dobutrex)	0.5–1 mcg/kg/min continuous IV infusion; titrate up as needed (usual range is 2–20 mcg/kg/min) *Special Considerations:* **On rare occasions, 40 mcg/kg/minute IV have been required to obtain the desired clinical response**
	dopamine ❶ (Intropin)	2–5 mcg/kg/min continuous IV infusion, initially. Titrate by 5–10 mcg/kg/min until goal hemodynamic and/or renal response is attained (usual range is 5–15 mcg/kg/min) *Special Considerations:* **Infusion rates more than 20 mcg/kg/minute may result in vasoconstriction or arrhythmias**
	inamrinone ❶ (Inocor)	0.75 mg/kg loading dose over 10–15 minutes followed by 5–10 mcg/kg/min continuous infusion *Special Considerations:* **An additional loading dose of 0.75 mg/kg IV may be given 30 minutes after the initial dose. Maximum total dosage, including loading doses, is 10 mg/kg/day IV. Following cardiopulmonary resuscitation to stabilize or maintain cardiac output, the maximum maintenance infusion rate suggested is 15 mcg/kg/minute IV**
	milrinone ❶ (Primacor)	Loading dose 50 mcg/kg IV, then 0.125–0.75 mcg/kg/min continuous IV infusion

❶ High-alert drug.

Intended Responses of Positive Inotropes
- Contractility is increased.
- Cardiac output is increased.
- Blood vessel dilation is increased.
- Preload and afterload are decreased.
- Heart function and contractility are improved.
- Blood pressure is lowered.
- Circulation is improved.

Common Side Effects of Positive Inotropes

Common side effects of positive inotrope drugs include hypertension, increased heart rate, premature ventricular contractions, and other dysrhythmias.

Inamrinone and milrinone can cause hypotension.

Do Not Confuse

DOPamine *with* **DOBUTamine**

An order for DOPamine can be confused with DOBUTamine. Both drugs are positive inotropes that increase the force of heart contractions.

QSEN: Safety

Critical Point for Safety

The effects of dopamine are dose-related. Low-dose dopamine (0.5–3 mcg/kg/min) causes renal vasodilation and increased urine output. Moderate-dose dopamine (2–20 mcg/kg/min) causes the increased force of heart contraction. High-dose dopamine (more than 10 mcg/kg/min) causes peripheral vasoconstriction to increase blood pressure.

QSEN: Safety

Common Side Effects

Positive Inotropes

Hypertension

Tachycardia, Dysrhythmias

Possible Adverse Effects of Positive Inotropes

Ventricular dysrhythmias may occur with milrinone and may be life-threatening. Rarely, a patient may have allergic reactions to these drugs, including rash, fever, bronchospasm, and chest pain.

Priority Actions to Take *Before* Giving Positive Inotropes

In addition to the general priority actions to take before giving any heart failure drug (p. 247), during infusion of a heart-pump drug, frequently monitor the patient's heart rate and blood pressure (at least every 1 to 2 hours). Make sure that the patient's IV line is patent. Double-check the prescribed correct IV rate by asking another professional nurse to check the calculation. Place the IV bolus and continuous IV infusions on an infusion pump to control the infusion rate. Document these actions. These drugs cause vasoconstriction, so if infiltration occurs, reduced blood flow to the tissues can result in severe tissue damage and even tissue necrosis.

Ask whether the patient has a history of high blood pressure or heart dysrhythmias.

Priority Actions to Take *After* Giving Positive Inotropes

In addition to the general priority actions to take after giving any heart failure drug (p. 248), watch the IV site for patency and any signs of infection such as pain, redness, swelling, and warmth. Remind the patient to immediately report any pain or discomfort at the IV site. Continue to monitor and document the IV pump rate to make sure the infusion is at the correct prescribed rate. Continue to check blood pressure and heart rate while a patient is receiving these drugs.

Teaching Priorities for Patients Taking Positive Inotropes

In addition to the general teaching priorities related to giving any drugs for heart failure (p. 248), include these teaching points and precautions:

* Immediately report any signs and symptoms of IV lines that are no longer patent or that have developed an infection (e.g., burning or pain, redness, swelling, warmth) to your nurse or prescriber.
* If you are receiving these drugs at home, use the infusion techniques you have been taught. Report any problems with the IV pump immediately to the home care nurse.
* Remember why this drug has been ordered and do not stop the drug unless told to do so by your prescriber.
* Report any chest pain, dyspnea, numbness, or tingling or burning in the extremities to your provider immediately.

Life Span Considerations for Positive Inotropes

Considerations for pregnancy and lactation. Positive inotrope drugs have a low to moderate likelihood of increasing the risk for birth defects or fetal harm.

Considerations for older adults. Older adults are more likely to experience adverse effects of these drugs, especially chest pain and hypertension. Monitor the older adult receiving any positive inotropic drug at least every 2 hours for changes in blood pressure, heart rate, and heart rhythm.

POTASSIUM AND MAGNESIUM

How Potassium and Magnesium Work

Potassium is an important electrolyte that is essential for a healthy nervous system and a regular heart rhythm. **Magnesium** is a major mineral and is the fourth most abundant mineral in the human body. It helps the heart rhythm to remain steady.

Patients taking diuretic drugs for heart failure can lose potassium and magnesium in their urine. To keep blood levels of potassium and magnesium within normal ranges, supplements are often prescribed. Be sure to consult a reliable drug resource for more information about potassium and magnesium.

 Critical Point for Safety

Positive inotropic (heart-pump) drugs are given intravenously. Be sure that the IV line is patent so that the drug does not go into the patient's tissues and cause damage.

QSEN: Safety

 Critical Point for Safety

Positive inotropes are often given in the home setting because heart failure is a chronic disease. It is important to teach patients and caregivers how to monitor the IV site, how to use the infusion pump, and what to report to the prescriber of home health nurse.

QSEN: Safety

Adult Dosages for Commonly Prescribed Potassium and Magnesium Supplements

Drug Category	Drug Name	Usual Maintenance Dose
Potassium Supplements	potassium ❶ (K-Dur, K-Lor, Kaon CL, K-Lyte, Slow-K, Klotrix, Kaochlor 10%)	20 mEq orally once daily to prevent potassium deficit with or after a meal 40–100 mEq orally in 2–5 daily doses to treat potassium deficit with or after meals Max: 200 mEq/day IV: Up to 200–400 mEq IV drip daily ***Special Considerations:* Do *not* exceed 10 mEq/hr by IV**
Magnesium Supplements	magnesium ❶ (Max-Oxide, Uro-Mag)	270–400 mg orally daily

❶ High alert drug.

Common Side Effects

Potassium and Magnesium

IV site irritation   Nausea, Vomiting, Diarrhea, Gas, Abdominal discomfort

Intended Responses of Potassium and Magnesium

- Blood values for potassium and magnesium are normal (see Table 1.4 in Chapter 1).
- Low potassium and magnesium levels are prevented or corrected.
- Some abnormal heart rhythms are prevented.
- Heart muscle excitability is decreased.

Common Side Effects of Potassium and Magnesium

Common side effects of potassium and magnesium include nausea, vomiting, diarrhea, gas, and abdominal discomfort. When potassium is given intravenously, it can cause burning or irritation at the IV site.

Possible Adverse Effects of Potassium and Magnesium

High potassium or magnesium levels can cause life-threatening electrocardiogram (ECG) changes and abnormal heart rhythms. Potassium should **never** be given via IV push.

Black, tarry, or bloody stools are signs of stomach bleeding and should be reported to the prescriber immediately.

Adverse effects with magnesium sulfate are rare and include complete heart block and respiratory arrest. With higher doses, muscle weakness and a loss of deep tendon reflexes can occur.

⭐ Priority Actions to Take *Before* Giving Potassium or Magnesium

In addition to the general priority actions to take before giving any heart failure drug (p. 247), check and recheck the dosage of potassium prescribed and the concentration of the drug in the vial. Concentrations vary considerably. An overdose of intravenous potassium can be lethal.

If the patient is on a heart monitor, check the heart rhythm or ask the monitor watcher about it. Check the patient's current laboratory values for potassium and magnesium. If these values are outside of the normal range, notify the prescriber (see Table 1.4 in Chapter 1 for a listing of normal ranges). If the potassium level is low (less than 3.5 mEq/L), assess handgrip strength and bowel sounds at least every shift. Also, assess respiratory rate and effort, and oxygen saturation. Notify the prescriber if oxygen saturation drops below 90%. If the magnesium level is low (less than 1.3 mEq/L), assess the patient for nausea and/or vomiting, weakness and sleepiness, personality changes, muscle spasms or tremors, and loss of appetite.

⭐ Priority Actions to Take *After* Giving Potassium or Magnesium

In addition to the general priority actions to take after giving any heart failure drug (p. 248), make sure that any follow-up laboratory values are drawn and sent to the laboratory.

If the patient has an IV site, recheck it for signs of irritation every 2 to 4 hours. Instruct the patient to report any pain or discomfort in the IV site immediately.

Watch for signs of potassium overdose *(hyperkalemia)*, including slow and irregular heart rhythm, fatigue, muscle weakness, *paresthesia* (numbness and tingling), confusion, difficulty breathing, and ECG changes.

Also, watch for signs of increased magnesium level (hypermagnesemia) such as muscle and generalized weakness, decreased reflexes (neuromuscular depression), hypotension, abnormal cardiac rhythm, drowsiness, decreased alertness and concentration, decreased rate of breathing/respiratory paralysis, central nervous system (CNS) depression, and coma.

Cardiac changes with high levels of magnesium include bradycardia, peripheral vasodilation, and hypotension. ECG changes show a prolonged PR interval and a widened QRS complex. Bradycardia can be severe and cardiac arrest is possible. Hypotension is also severe with a diastolic pressure lower than normal. *Patients with severe hypermagnesemia are in grave danger of cardiac arrest.*

⊛ Teaching Priorities for Patients Taking Potassium and Magnesium

In addition to the general teaching priorities related to any drugs for heart failure (p. 248), include these teaching points and precautions:

- Remember why a potassium or magnesium supplement has been ordered.
- If you miss a dose, take it within 2 hours. Do **not** take a double dose of either potassium or magnesium.
- Take oral potassium and magnesium supplements with food or right after meals with a full glass of water or fruit juice. Taking potassium on an empty stomach can cause nausea and vomiting.
- Avoid using salt substitutes that contain potassium. Consult a list of dietary sources of potassium (Box 14.3) and magnesium (Box 14.4).
- Report any signs of too much potassium (e.g., palpitations, skipped heartbeats, muscle twitching or weakness, or numbness and tingling) to your prescriber immediately.
- Be sure to have any prescribed laboratory values drawn to monitor responses to these supplements as instructed by your prescriber.

Life Span Considerations for Potassium and Magnesium

Considerations for pregnancy and lactation. Potassium has a low to moderate likelihood of increasing the risk for birth defects or fetal harm. Magnesium sulfate is safe

 Memory Jogger

Signs of increased blood potassium level include slow and irregular heart rhythm, fatigue, muscle weakness, paresthesia (numbness and tingling), confusion, difficulty breathing, and ECG changes.

Memory Jogger

Signs of increased blood magnesium level include muscle and generalized weakness, decreased reflexes (neuromuscular depression), hypotension, abnormal cardiac rhythm, drowsiness, decreased alertness and concentration, decreased rate of breathing/respiratory paralysis, CNS depression, and coma.

Box 14.3   Dietary Sources of Potassium

- Baked potato
- Bananas
- Beet greens
- Clams
- Halibut, tuna, cod fish
- Molasses
- Prune, carrot, tomato juice
- Soybeans
- Spinach
- Sweet potato
- Tomato paste, sauce, puree
- White, lima beans
- Winter squash
- Yogurt

Box 14.4   Dietary Sources of Magnesium

- Almonds
- Black beans
- Bran cereal
- Brazil nuts
- Buckwheat flour
- Cashews
- Halibut
- Mixed nuts
- Pumpkin and squash seed kernels
- Sesame seeds
- Soybeans
- Spinach
- Walnuts
- White beans
- Whole grain rice

to give during pregnancy. It is used during labor to lower the risk of seizures for patients with eclampsia. The infant may have decreased reflexes for the first 24 hours after birth when magnesium is used during labor.

ENTRESTO

How Entresto Works

Entresto is a combination drug containing sacubitril (a neprilysin inhibitor) and valsartan (an angiotensin II receptor blocker [ARB]). Sacubitril increases the levels of certain proteins in the body that dilate blood vessels to lower blood pressure. Valsartan is an ARB which keeps blood vessels from narrowing to decrease blood pressure and increase blood flow. Entresto is used to treat heart failure in adults and children who are at least a year old. The use of Entresto with patients who have chronic heart failure helps decrease the risk of hospitalization when symptoms worsen and decreases the risk of death due to heart failure. It is usually given with other heart failure medications. Be sure to consult a reliable drug resource for more information about Entresto.

Adult Dosages for Entresto

Drug Category	Drug Name	Usual Maintenance Dose
Combination Drugs	sacubitril (a neprilysin inhibitor) and valsartan (an ARB) (Entresto)	Initial dose: sacubitril 49 mg and valsartan 51 mg orally twice a day Maintenance dose: sacubitril 97 mg and valsartan 103 mg orally twice a day *Special Considerations:* **The drug comes in an oral suspension if a patient has difficulty swallowing tablets**

Intended Responses of Entresto
- Vasodilation of blood vessels is increased.
- Excess body sodium is decreased.
- Blood pressure is lowered.
- Workload on the heart is decreased.
- Blood flow is improved.

Common Side Effects of Entresto

Common side effects of Entresto include reduced kidney function, increased potassium level (hyperkalemia), dizziness, lightheadedness, and cough.

Possible Adverse Effects of Entresto

Adverse effects of Entresto include signs of an allergic reaction such as hives; difficulty breathing; and swelling of the face, lips, tongue, or throat (angioedema).

With hyperkalemia, the patient may have a slow heart rate, weak pulse, muscle weakness, or tingling.

Kidney problems can include little or no urination, difficult or painful urination, swelling of the ankles and feet, and feeling very tired and short of breath.

⭐ Priority Actions to Take *Before* Giving Entresto

In addition to the general priority actions to take before giving any heart failure drug, (p. 247), be sure to ask the patient about health problems including liver disease, kidney disease, diabetes, hereditary problems, and angioedema. Ask if the patient is prescribed a low salt diet or is dehydrated. Ask any female patient of childbearing age if she is pregnant or planning to become pregnant. Check the patient's laboratory values for current liver and kidney function values (see Tables 1.3 and 1.4 for normal values).

Ask the patient about allergies to any ARB drugs or angiotensin converting enzyme (ACE) inhibitors. Entresto should *not* be taken within 36 hours before or after any ACE inhibitor.

⭐ Priority Actions to Take *After* Giving Entresto

In addition to the general priority actions to take after giving any heart failure drug (p. 248), monitor for any swelling of the face, including the eyes, lips, or tongue

Common Side Effects

Entresto

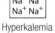

Hyperkalemia

Dizziness, Lightheadedness

Cough

Reduced kidney function

⭐ **Critical Point for Safety**

Entresto should **not** be given within 36 hours before or after any ACE inhibitor drug.

QSEN: Safety

(signs of angioedema). Report this immediately to the prescriber. Ask the patient about side effects such as dizziness and tiredness. Continue to monitor liver and kidney function laboratory values.

If the drug is given as an oral suspension, be sure to shake the liquid well before measuring the correct dosage. Use the dosing syringe to measure the dosage.

⭐ Teaching Priorities for Patients Taking Entresto
In addition to the general teaching priorities related to any heart failure drug (p. 248), include these teaching points and precautions:
- Check and record your blood pressure and heart rate every day. Report any abnormalities to the prescriber.
- Remember to store the drug at room temperature.
- Discard any oral suspension not used within 15 days.
- For the oral suspension, use the measuring device that comes with the drug. Do *not* use ordinary kitchen spoons.
- Report any increasing tiredness, dizziness or lightheadedness, changes in urine output or signs of angioedema to your prescriber immediately.
- Be sure to keep follow-up appointments with your prescriber and to have any lab tests done as ordered.
- Do not use potassium supplements unless instructed to do so by your prescriber.
- Avoid drinking alcohol because it can lower your blood pressure and cause increased side effects of Entresto.

Life Span Considerations for Entresto
Considerations for pregnancy and lactation. Entresto should not be used during pregnancy because it can cause injury or death to the fetus if taken during the second or third trimester.

OTHER DRUGS USED TO TREAT HEART FAILURE
Anticoagulants such as heparin and warfarin (Coumadin) prevent clots from forming or getting bigger and may be prescribed to treat heart failure. See Chapter 17 for more information on these drugs. The antidysrhythmic drug amiodarone (Cordarone) may be used to prevent or treat irregular heart rhythms that begin in the ventricles such as ventricular tachycardia. See Chapter 15 for more information on this drug. Irregular heart rhythms can be life-threatening.

> **⭐ Critical Point for Safety**
> Entresto should be stored at room temperature. Discard any oral suspension not used within 15 days after it was mixed. Do **not** keep the oral suspension refrigerated.
>
> QSEN: Safety

Get Ready for the NCLEX® Examination!

Key Points
- Most heart failure is caused by high blood pressure and begins in the left ventricle then progresses to right heart failure.
- Left heart failure causes symptoms in the lungs, and right heart failure causes peripheral symptoms.
- Drugs for heart failure are prescribed to make physical activity more comfortable, improve quality of life, and prolong life.
- The only cure for heart failure is a heart transplant because the damage to the heart muscle is not reversible.
- Angiotensin-converting enzyme (ACE) inhibitors, angiotensin II receptor blockers (ARBs), vasodilators, and human B-type natriuretic peptides may be prescribed to decrease afterload.
- Diuretics may be prescribed to decrease preload by reducing the circulating blood volume.
- Low-dose spironolactone (Aldactone) is used to block the action of aldosterone, a hormone that causes the body to hold on to salt and water.
- Wear gloves to administer nitroglycerin ointment to prevent absorbing the drug through your skin, which can cause headache or hypotension.
- Remove a patient's nitroglycerin ointment or patch during the time when he or she has his or her longest sleep period, usually at night before bedtime.
- Teach patients that a tingling sensation indicates a potent nitroglycerin tablet.
- Sublingual and buccal nitroglycerin should not be swallowed. When swallowed, the liver destroys most of the drug so it is not effective.
- The dosages for digoxin are very low compared with those for most drugs. Be sure to calculate the correct dose carefully.
- Report common side effects of digoxin to the prescriber immediately because they are probably signs of digoxin toxicity, which can be life-threatening.
- Digoxin has a very narrow therapeutic range (0.8 to 2 ng/mL), and levels above 2 ng/mL are considered toxic. When a pa-

tient shows any signs of overdose (digoxin toxicity), a blood level for digoxin is drawn, and the dose is held.

- Always check the apical heart rate for a full minute before giving digoxin.
- Always check a patient's serum potassium level before giving a dose of digoxin. Prescribed diuretics can lead to low potassium, which increases the risk of digoxin toxicity.
- Positive inotropic (heart-pump) drugs are given intravenously. Be sure that the IV line is patent so the drug does not go into the patient's tissues and cause damage.
- Check and recheck the concentration of potassium to be sure it matches the prescriber's order before administering the drug. **Never** give potassium via IV push.
- Potassium is a high-alert drug because it can lead to serious harm if given at too high a dose, given to a patient for whom it was not prescribed, or not given to a patient for whom it was prescribed.
- Instruct patients to report weight gain of more than 2 pounds in a day or 5 pounds in a week to the prescriber.
- Nesiritide is a human B-type natriuretic peptide that causes water elimination and blood vessel dilation.

- Dopamine is a positive inotropic drug that has effects that are dose-related. At low doses, it increases kidney perfusion; at moderate doses, it increases the contractility of the heart muscle; and at high doses, it causes constriction of the blood vessels.
- Rates of IV drugs for heart failure should always be controlled by an infusion controller device.
- Entresto should not be given within 36 hours before or after any ACE inhibitor drug.
- Entresto should be stored at room temperature. Discard any oral suspension not used within 15 days after it was mixed. Do not keep the oral suspension refrigerated.

Additional Learning Resources

Be sure to visit your Evolve website (http://evolve.elsevier.com/Workman/pharmacology/) for additional online resources.

SG Go to your Study Guide for additional learning activities to help you master this chapter content.

Review Questions

See *Answers to In-Text Review Questions* in the back of the book for answers to these questions.

1. **Which symptom will the nurse assess for in a patient who has left ventricular heart failure?**

   A. Weight gain
   B. Swelling in the legs
   C. Jugular vein distention
   D. Crackles in the lungs

2. **Which condition alerts the nurse to assess a patient for worsening heart failure?**

   A. Blood pressure of 106/40 mm Hg
   B. Pounding headache
   C. Ankle swelling
   D. Foul urine odor

3. **The nurse prepares to administer a drug for heart failure to a patient. Which assessment finding does the nurse report to the prescriber before administering the drug?**

   A. Increased systolic blood pressure from 128 to 136
   B. Urine output of 2100 mL in 24 hours
   C. Weight gain of 1 pound in 3 days
   D. Heart rate of 54 beats/min

4. **Which statement made by a patient with heart failure indicates to the nurse that additional teaching is needed about the prescribed drug therapy?**

   A. "I always try to take my heart failure drugs at the same time each day."
   B. "Now I am using a weekly pill dispenser to keep my drugs straight."
   C. "Now that my heart failure is cured, I can cut back on the drugs I take."
   D. "If I gain more than 3 pounds in a week, I will call my doctor."

5. **The nurse is creating a care plan for a patient with heart failure. Which lifestyle changes does the nurse include in the plan of care? Select all that apply.**

   A. Fluid restriction of 1000 mL/day
   B. Weight loss program
   C. Smoking cessation program
   D. Aerobic exercise program
   E. Low-salt, low-fat diet
   F. Limiting alcohol intake

6. **A patient with heart failure is prescribed oral captopril (Capoten) and carvedilol (Coreg). The heart rate after giving these drugs is decreased from 84 per minute to 68 per minute. What is the nurse's best action?**

   A. Holding the next dose
   B. Immediately notifying the prescriber
   C. Documenting the finding as the only action
   D. Scheduling the captopril and carvedilol to be given at different times

7. **A patient is prescribed nitroglycerin ointment. What technique does the nurse use for protection and to avoid experiencing side effects from this drug during drug administration?**

   A. Squeezing the ointment onto the special paper
   B. Cleansing the skin before applying the drug
   C. Rotating the drug application skin sites
   D. Wearing a pair of disposable gloves

8. **A patient is to receive nesiritide (Natrecor). Which patient assessments are most important for the nurse to perform before giving this drug? Select all that apply.**

   A. Measuring heart rate
   B. Assessing the swallowing reflex
   C. Checking the IV line for patency
   D. Calculating oral intake

E. Assessing respiratory rate factors
F. Taking blood pressure

9. Which action or precaution is **most important** for the nurse to teach a patient who has been prescribed an oral potassium supplement?

A. "If you miss a dose, double your next dose to keep your blood level of potassium normal."
B. "Take your potassium with food or a full glass of water to avoid nausea and vomiting."
C. "Be sure to use salt substitutes instead of salt so that your body will not retain water."
D. "Eat lots of foods that are high in potassium such as bananas, spinach, broccoli, and sweet potatoes."

10. What is the **most important** action for the nurse to perform before administering a patient's daily dose of digoxin?

A. Checking the patient's apical pulse for a full 60 seconds
B. Assessing the patient's dependent body areas for edema formation
C. Asking whether the patient has experienced any heart palpitations during the last 24 hours

D. Verifying that the time of administration today is within one-half hour of the time the drug was administered yesterday

11. Which benefits will the nurse discuss with a patient newly prescribed to take Entresto? **Select all that apply.**

A. Lowering the risk of hospitalization
B. Decreasing the risk of kidney failure
C. Lowering blood pressure by increasing sodium level
D. Decreasing the risk of death
E. Increasing the dilation of blood vessels
F. Improving blood flow

12. A patient prescribed digoxin 0.25 mg orally per day has all of the following laboratory blood values. Which value will the nurse report to the prescriber before administering the next dose of digoxin?

A. Sodium 133 mEq/L
B. Potassium 2.8 mEq/L
C. Blood urea nitrogen 9 mg/dL
D. White blood cell count 11,000 cells/mm^3

Clinical Judgment

1. The nurse is providing care for a 53-year-old patient on a cardiac monitor, who is prescribed digoxin 0.125 mg orally each day in the morning for heart failure. The patient's morning potassium level is 2.2 mEq/L. The prescriber orders 2 doses of IV potassium 10 mEq. **Use an X to indicate which actions are Relevant, which are Less Relevant, and which are Potentially Harmful.**

ACTION	RELEVANT	LESS RELEVANT	POTENTIALLY HARMFUL
Checking the patient's saline lock for patency and signs of infiltration or irritation			
Giving the potassium by the IV push route			
Using an IV pump when infusing each dose of potassium			
Diluting the potassium in 20 mL of normal saline			
Infusing each dose over a full hour			
Instructing the patient to report if the infusion is burning or painful			
Sending a blood sample for potassium after the first dose is given			
Checking the patient's heart monitor rhythm before and after giving each dose of potassium			

2. The nurse is providing care for a 62-year-old male patient with heart failure who is prescribed a continuous IV infusion of dobutamine. Which **intended** responses to this drug therapy will the nurse expect? Select all that apply.

A. Improved blood flow and circulation
B. Decreased heart muscle contractility
C. Decreased blood pressure
D. Irregular heart rate
E. Improved heart function
F. Decreased preload and afterload
G. Tachycardic heart rate
H. Discomfort at the IV site
I. Increased blood vessel dilation
J. Improved cardiac output

Learning Objectives

The content presented in this chapter should help you to:

1. Explain how different classes of drugs are used to treat abnormal heart rhythms.
2. Describe the common names, actions, usual adult dosages, possible side effects, and adverse effects of atropine, digoxin, adenosine, and magnesium sulfate.
3. Discuss the priority actions to take before and after giving atropine, digoxin, adenosine, and magnesium sulfate.
4. Prioritize essential information to teach patients taking atropine, digoxin, adenosine, and magnesium sulfate.
5. Describe the common names, actions, usual adult dosages, possible side effects, and adverse effects of class I, II, III,

and IV antidysrhythmic drugs used to treat rapid abnormal heart rhythms.
6. Discuss the priority actions to take before and after giving class I, II, III, and IV antidysrhythmic drugs used to treat rapid abnormal heart rhythms.
7. Prioritize essential information to teach patients taking class I, II, III, and IV antidysrhythmic drugs used to treat rapid abnormal heart rhythms.
8. Describe life span considerations for antidysrhythmic drugs used to treat abnormal heart rhythms.

Key Terms

adenosine (ă-DĔN-ō-sēn) (p. 280) A drug administered intravenously for supraventricular tachycardia (SVT); adenosine can help identify SVT. Certain SVTs can be successfully terminated with adenosine.

antidysrhythmic drugs (ăn-tī-dĭs-RĬTH-Mĭk DRŬGZ) (p. 269) Drugs used to treat abnormal heart rhythms.

atropine (Ă-trō-pēn) (p. 270) A competitive muscarinic acetylcholine receptor antagonist used as a temporary treatment for abnormally slow heart rates.

beta blockers (BĔ-tă BLŎK-ĕrz) (p. 277) (See Chapter 13.)

bradycardia (brā-dē-KĂR-dē-ă) (p. 267) Slow heart rate, usually considered to be less than 60 beats/min.

bradydysrhythmia (brā-dē-dĭs-RĬTH-mē-ă) (p. 270) An abnormally slow heart rhythm.

calcium channel blockers (KĂL-sē-ŭm CHĂN-ŭl BLŎK-ĕrz) (p. 280) (See Chapter 13.)

digoxin (dĭ-JŎK-sĭn) (p. 271) (See Chapter 14.)

dysrhythmia (dĭs-RĬTH-mē-ă) (p. 267) An abnormal heart rhythm.

magnesium sulfate (mă-NĔ-zē-ŭm SŬL-fāt) (p. 282) (See Chapter 14.)

potassium channel blockers (pō-TĂS-ē-ŭm BLŎK-ĕrz) (p. 278) A class of drugs that act by inhibiting potassium movement through cell membranes. Blocking potassium channels lengthens the duration of action potentials.

sodium channel blockers (SŌ-dē-ŭm CHĂN-ŭl BLŎK-ĕrz) (p. 272) A class of drugs that act by inhibiting sodium movement through cell membranes. Results include slowing of the heart rate, reducing heart muscle cell excitability, and reducing speed of conduction.

REVIEW OF RELATED PHYSIOLOGY AND PATHOPHYSIOLOGY

One of the heart's functions is to pump blood to the body and the lungs. The left side of the heart receives oxygen-rich blood from the lungs and pumps it out to the body. The right side of the heart receives oxygen-poor blood from the body and sends it to the lungs (Figure 15.1). The heart muscle must be strong and have its own well-oxygenated blood supply to perform well. The coronary arteries deliver the blood supply to the heart muscle.

PACEMAKERS AND THE CARDIAC CONDUCTION SYSTEM

The electrical conduction system controls heart rate and rhythm through the heart's own system of electrical impulses that travel through the heart muscle, causing the heart to contract and pump blood. The part of the system that sets the heart rate and

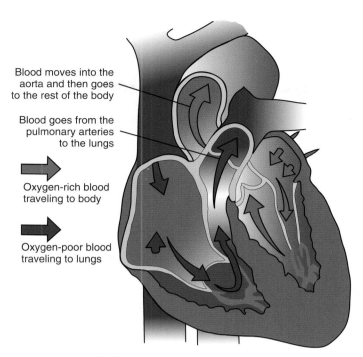

FIG. 15.1 Blood flow through the heart.

Blood moves into the aorta and then goes to the rest of the body

Blood goes from the pulmonary arteries to the lungs

Oxygen-rich blood traveling to body

Oxygen-poor blood traveling to lungs

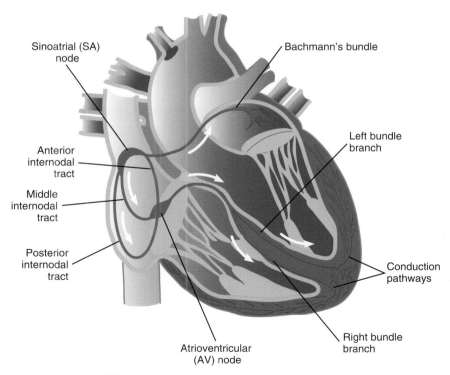

Sinoatrial (SA) node

Anterior internodal tract

Middle internodal tract

Posterior internodal tract

Atrioventricular (AV) node

Bachmann's bundle

Left bundle branch

Conduction pathways

Right bundle branch

FIG. 15.2 Electrical conduction system of the heart.

rhythm by generating impulses is called the *pacemaker.* Under normal circumstances, the *sinoatrial (SA) node,* composed of special muscle fibers capable of causing electrical impulses, is the pacemaker and controls the heart rate. The SA node initiates electrical impulses at a rate of 60 to 100 per minute. These impulses travel across pathways to the *atrioventricular (AV) node* and then down through the *His-Purkinje system* to cause the ventricles to contract and pump blood out of the heart (Figure 15.2).

 Memory Jogger

The normal pacemaker of the heart, the SA node, initiates 60–100 electrical impulses per minute.

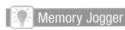
When the SA node does not function, the AV node takes over as the secondary pacemaker of the heart. This secondary pacemaker usually initiates 40 to 60 electrical impulses per minute, which results in a slower heart rate. If both the SA and the AV nodes are not working, the ventricular muscle cells become the third pacemaker of the heart, with a very slow rate of 20 to 40 impulses per minute. This slow rate of heart contractions is not enough to supply the body with the blood and oxygen it needs to function, and the patient may have symptoms such as confusion or a change in level of consciousness.

HEART RATE

Sometimes it is normal for the heart to beat faster or slower. Heart rate is related to a person's state of health and whether he or she is exercising or resting. For example, a young athlete may have a normal resting heart rate of 50 beats per minute with an exercising heart rate of 100, whereas an older adult may have a resting heart rate of 80 or 90 beats per minute and an exercising heart rate of 120 to 140. Normal heart rate ranges for adults and children are summarized in Table 15.1.

How fast the heart beats depends upon how much oxygen-rich blood the body needs. During activity, excitement, fever, or shock, the body needs more oxygen-rich blood, so the heart rate may increase to 100 beats per minute or more. When a person is resting or sleeping, the body needs less oxygen-rich blood, so the heart rate decreases, sometimes to less than 60 beats per minute.

NORMAL HEART RHYTHM

When the heart beats normally, each impulse that starts from the SA node causes the atria and ventricles to contract regularly and in sequence at a rate between 60 and 100 beats per minute (Animation 15.1). This normal rhythm of the heart is called *normal sinus rhythm* (Figure 15.3) (Animation 15.2). This means that the impulse begins in the SA node and travels normally to cause the atria to contract and then to

Table **15.1**	**Normal Heart Rates**
AGE-GROUP	**RANGE (BEATS/MIN)**
Adults	60–100
Children	70–120
Toddlers	90–150
Infants	120–160

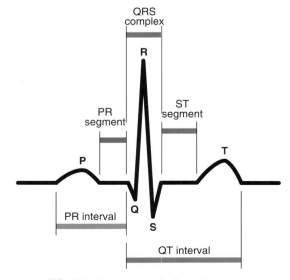

FIG. 15.3 Normal sinus rhythm of the heart.

the ventricles to contract. A slow heart rhythm started by the SA node is called sinus **bradycardia** (less than 60 beats per minute). A rapid heart rhythm started by the SA node is called sinus **tachycardia** (more than 100 beats per minute).

DYSRHYTHMIAS

Dysrhythmias are abnormal heart rhythms (Box 15.1). They often begin with an abnormal unexpected impulse somewhere in the heart muscle tissue (but *not* from the SA node). Abnormal rhythms are often caused by problems with the electrical conduction system of the heart. Dysrhythmias may also be caused by heart muscle contractions that are irregular or faster or slower than normal. Most dysrhythmias have a negative effect on how well the heart works as a pump, resulting in a decrease in *cardiac output* (the amount of blood the heart pumps in a minute).

Dysrhythmias can be named according to where they begin. *Atrial dysrhythmias* begin in the atria, whereas *supraventricular dysrhythmias* originate above the ventricles and *ventricular dysrhythmias* begin within the ventricles.

Heartbeats that occur earlier than expected are called *premature contractions.* They can begin in the atria (premature atrial contractions [PACs]), in the AV node region (premature junctional contractions [PJCs]), or ventricles (premature ventricular contractions [PVCs]). A patient may notice the feeling of a skipped beat. An occasional premature beat is usually not serious; however, premature beats may lead to other serious dysrhythmias. When premature beats are frequent, cardiac output is decreased.

Other dysrhythmias cause the chambers of the heart (atria and ventricles) to quiver (*fibrillate*) instead of contracting normally and effectively. This fibrillation results from totally disorganized electrical activity and produces ineffective contraction and pumping of blood. When the atria fibrillate, it is called *atrial fibrillation*. Atrial fibrillation decreases cardiac output because the atrial portion of cardiac output is lost when the atria do not contract. *Ventricular fibrillation* is the name for the condition in which the ventricles fibrillate. Ventricular fibrillation is life threatening and can lead to death in minutes because no blood is pumped from the heart (no cardiac output) when the ventricles quiver and do not contract.

Box 15-1   List of Common Dysrhythmias

ATRIAL
- Atrial fibrillation
- Atrial flutter
- Premature atrial contractions
- Sick sinus syndrome
- Supraventricular tachycardia

VENTRICULAR
- Asystole
- Premature ventricular contractions
- Pulseless electrical activity
- Ventricular fibrillation
- Ventricular tachycardia

JUNCTIONAL
- Junctional tachycardia
- Premature junctional contractions

HEART BLOCKS
- First-degree heart block
- Second-degree heart block
- Mobitz type I/Wenckebach
- Mobitz type II
- Third-degree heart block (complete heart block)

Dysrhythmia Symptoms

Dysrhythmias may or may not cause symptoms in patients (Box 15.2). Often abnormal rhythms cause symptoms such as a fluttery feeling in the chest, racing heartbeats, slow heartbeats, irregular heart beats (Animation 15.3), chest pain, shortness of breath, light-headedness, dizziness, and fainting *(syncope)*. Having symptoms does not always mean having a serious dysrhythmia. Some people with symptoms do not have a serious dysrhythmia, whereas others with no symptoms may have a life-threatening dysrhythmia.

 Memory Jogger

The electrical impulses that cause normal sinus rhythm begin in the SA node.

 Memory Jogger

A slow heart rate (less than 60 beats per minute) is bradycardia. A fast heart rate (more than 100 beats per minute) is tachycardia.

 Memory Jogger

Dysrhythmias decrease cardiac output, which leads to symptoms such as dizziness, light-headedness, fainting *(syncope)*, and decreased peripheral pulses.

 Critical Point for Safety

Without immediate intervention, ventricular fibrillation leads to death within minutes.

QSEN: Safety

 Critical Point for Safety

Some patients with symptoms do not have serious dysrhythmias, whereas others without symptoms may have life-threatening dysrhythmias.

QSEN: Safety

Box **15.2**   Common Symptoms of Dysrhythmias

- Chest pain
- Dizziness
- Fainting (syncope)
- Fluttering in the chest
- Light-headedness

- May have *no* symptoms
- Rapid heart rate
- Shortness of breath
- Slow heart rate

Box **15.3**   Risk Factors for Developing Dysrhythmias

- Age (older adults)
- Genetics (family history)
- Coronary artery disease
- Thyroid problems
- Hypothyroidism—bradycardia
- Hyperthyroidism—tachycardia
- Drugs and supplements
- Cough/cold remedies with pseudoephedrine
- High blood pressure
- Obesity
- Diabetes
- Low blood sugar (hypoglycemia)

- Obstructive sleep apnea
- Electrolyte imbalance
- Potassium
- Sodium
- Calcium
- Magnesium
- Alcohol abuse
- Stimulant use
- Caffeine
- Nicotine
- Illicit drugs
- Cocaine
- Amphetamines

Risk Factors for Dysrhythmias

Several factors increase the risk for a person developing a heart dysrhythmia (Box 15.3). Older adults with age-related heart changes are more likely to have dysrhythmias. Genetics and family history increase the risk for them. For example, some people are born with an extra electrical impulse pathway and may develop *Wolff-Parkinson-White syndrome*, a specific type of dysrhythmia. Some disease processes may lead to dysrhythmias. Diabetes increases the risk for developing high blood pressure and coronary artery disease. High blood pressure and obesity increase the risk for developing coronary artery disease, with narrow arteries and heart damage that may cause abnormal heart rhythms. Thyroid problems may cause rapid or slow heart rates. *Obstructive sleep apnea* (a sleep disorder with pauses in breathing during sleep) can cause bradycardia and episodes of atrial fibrillation. Electrolyte imbalances can cause the heart to initiate abnormal electrical impulses. When electrolyte levels (such as potassium, sodium, calcium, and magnesium) are too high or too low, dysrhythmias may occur.

Drugs may also affect heart rhythm. Over-the-counter cold and cough drugs containing pseudoephedrine (e.g., pseudoephedrine [Sudafed]) can cause tachycardia. Stimulants such as caffeine and nicotine can cause premature heartbeats and rapid (tachycardic) rhythms. Too much alcohol also can change the conduction of electrical impulses and increase the chance for atrial fibrillation. Illegal drugs such as cocaine and amphetamines can cause serious heart rhythm problems, including ventricular fibrillation, which can lead to sudden death.

Measuring the Heart Rate

The most accurate way to measure a patient's heart rate is to listen with a stethoscope over the apical region of the chest for a full minute. The apical heart rate is measured at the left fifth intercostal space in the midclavicular area (usually two fingers below the left nipple in a male) (Figure 15.4). Listen with a stethoscope for a full minute. Count the number of heartbeats. Note any irregular rhythms.

An important part of teaching for a patient with an abnormal heart rate is how to count the heart rate. Tell the patient to obtain a watch or clock that has a second hand. Instruct him or her to place the index and middle finger of the dominant hand

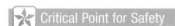

Critical Point for Safety

Over-the-counter cough and cold drugs that contain pseudoephedrine (Sudafed) can cause abnormal rapid heart rhythms.

QSEN: Safety

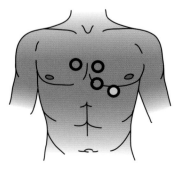

FIG. 15.4 Location of the apical pulse.

on the inner wrist of the opposite arm just below the base of the thumb (Figure 15.5). In this way the patient should feel the pulsing of the radial artery against the fingers. Have him or her count the number of pulse beats for a full minute. Also tell the patient to note whether the heart rhythm is regular or irregular when measuring the heart rate. A normal heart rhythm is regular.

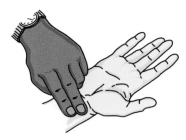

FIG. 15.5 Checking the radial pulse.

GENERAL ISSUES RELATED TO ANTIDYSRHYTHMIC THERAPY

Antidysrhythmic drugs are used to treat abnormal heart rhythms and may be prescribed to increase or decrease the heart rate. The actions of drugs prescribed to treat rapid heart rates may be to decrease spontaneous contraction of myocardial cells, including pacemaker cells *(automaticity)*, slow ability of heart muscle cells to transmit electrical impulses *(conductivity)*, or prolong the refractory period of heart cells. The *refractory period* is the period of time after an impulse generation during which normal stimulation will not cause another impulse. During the absolute refractory period, an impulse *cannot* be conducted. During the relative refractory period, an impulse must be stronger than normal to be conducted.

⭐ PRIORITY ACTIONS TO TAKE *BEFORE* GIVING ANY ANTIDYSRHYTHMIC DRUG

Before giving any antidysrhythmic drug, be sure to get a complete list of the drugs that the patient is using, including over-the-counter and herbal drugs. Check the patient's heart rate and blood pressure. Watch for decreased or increased heart rate (less than 60 beats per minute or more than 100 beats per minute) and decreased blood pressure (less than 90/60 mm Hg), which may indicate decreased blood flow to the tissues. *Be sure to check the heart rate by listening to the apical pulse for a full minute.* If a cardiac monitor is being used, ask the monitor watcher, charge nurse, or prescriber about the patient's rhythm. Get a baseline weight for each patient because the dosage of many of these drugs is based on weight.

 Critical Point for Safety

A patient with liver or kidney problems often needs *smaller* doses of most antidysrhythmic drugs to avoid drug overdose and drug toxicity.

QSEN: Safety

⭐ PRIORITY ACTIONS TO TAKE *AFTER* GIVING ANY ANTIDYSRHYTHMIC DRUG

After giving any antidysrhythmic drug, be sure to recheck the patient's heart rate and blood pressure in 30 minutes. Ask the monitor watcher about changes in the heart rhythm because all antidysrhythmic drugs can cause dysrhythmias. Ensure that the call light is within easy reach, and instruct the patient to call for help before getting out of bed, especially after the first dose of any antidysrhythmic drug, and until the patient's response to the drug is determined. Instruct patients to get up and change positions slowly because of the possibility of decreased blood pressure, which can cause dizziness or fainting.

 Critical Point for Safety

Monitor heart rate and rhythm after giving any antidysrhythmic drug because these drugs can also cause dysrhythmias.

QSEN: Safety

⭐ TEACHING PRIORITIES FOR PATIENTS TAKING ANY ANTIDYSRHYTHMIC DRUG

- Check and record your heart rate and blood pressure using the proper techniques taught by your nurses and prescriber.
- Take your prescribed drugs exactly as instructed by the prescriber. *Never take a double dose.*
- Consult with your prescriber before taking any over-the-counter drugs.
- Keep all follow-up appointments with the prescriber to monitor the progress of your dysrhythmia treatment.
- Wear a medical identification bracelet stating which antidysrhythmic drugs are being used and the reason for their use.
- Get up and change positions slowly because of the side effects of dizziness and drowsiness.
- Sit on the side of the bed for a few minutes before standing up.
- Avoid driving or operating dangerous machines that require alertness until you know how these drugs affect you.

 Critical Point for Safety

Teach patients who have been prescribed antidysrhythmic drugs to check and record their heart rate and blood pressure daily.

QSEN: Safety

TYPES OF DRUGS TO TREAT DYSRHYTHMIAS

Antidysrhythmic drugs are used to convert a dysrhythmia to a normal rhythm with normal impulse conduction, or to control and prevent more serious dysrhythmias. These drugs may not cure abnormal rhythms and may need to be taken for a lifetime.

ATROPINE FOR BRADYDYSRHYTHMIAS

How Atropine Works

Atropine is a competitive muscarinic acetylcholine receptor antagonist used to treat abnormally slow heart rhythms known as **bradydysrhythmias**. Atropine blocks the actions of the vagus nerve on the heart. The vagus nerve slows down the heart rate. By blocking the action of this nerve, atropine causes an increase in electrical impulse conduction and heart rate. This drug is used for a patient who has symptomatic bradycardia. Atropine may also be used in emergency situations when a patient's heart rhythm is in asystole. *Asystole* is the absence of electrical or contraction activity within the heart. It appears on the electrocardiogram (ECG) monitor as a straight line or "flatline." In emergency settings atropine may also be given through the endotracheal (ET) tube of a patient who has been intubated. Usually twice the normal dose is used, and it is mixed with 5 to 10 mL of normal saline.

Atropine may also be given by the intraosseous (into the bone) route. Specially trained emergency care providers give drugs by endotracheal tube and intraosseous routes. Other uses for atropine include as a preoperative drug to decrease production of gastrointestinal and respiratory secretions and prevention of laryngospasm, bradycardia, and hypotension during anesthesia. This drug is also used topically to dilate pupils before eye examinations. Be sure to consult a reliable drug resource for more specific information about atropine.

Adult Dosages for Commonly Prescribed Atropine

Drug Category	Drug Name	Usual Maintenance Dose
Muscarinic Acetylcholine Receptor Antagonists	atropine (atropine sulfate)	0.5–1 mg IV every 3–5 min as needed up to 3 mg ***Special Considerations:* Doses less than 0.5 mg IV have been associated with paradoxical bradycardia**

Intended Responses of Atropine
- Heart rate is increased.
- Cardiac output is increased.
- Symptoms such as dizziness and light-headedness are decreased.

Common Side Effects of Atropine
Common side effects of atropine include tachycardia, drowsiness, blurred vision, dry mouth, and urinary hesitancy or retention.

Possible Adverse Effects of Atropine
A rare but serious and life-threatening effect of atropine is the occurrence of ventricular fibrillation (a chaotic dysrhythmia that causes the ventricles to quiver and not pump blood to the body). Because atropine increases heart rate and workload, it can also worsen heart ischemia (decreased blood flow to the heart muscle, causing chest pain) and heart blocks. Atropine can also cause premature ventricular contractions (PVCs) or ventricular tachycardia.

Doses of atropine smaller than 0.5 mg may make bradycardia worse (paradoxical bradycardia).

 Critical Point for Safety

Give twice the normal dose when atropine is given by ET tube. Mix the dose with 5–10 mL normal saline.

QSEN: Safety

Memory Jogger

Use the acronym NAVEL to remember drugs that may be given by ET tube: Narcan (naloxone), atropine, Valium (diazepam), epinephrine, and lidocaine.

Critical Point for Safety

Do not give large doses of atropine to older adults because they are more sensitive to its effects and may experience confusion.

QSEN: Safety

Common Side Effects

Atropine

Blurred vision   Tachycardia   Dry mouth

Urinary retention   Drowsiness

Critical Point for Safety

Administering a dose of atropine less than 0.5 mg may make bradycardia worse (paradoxical bradycardia).

QSEN: Safety

⭐ Priority Actions to Take *Before* Giving Atropine

In addition to the general priority actions to take before giving any antidysrhythmic drug (p. 269), check the patient's heart rate and blood pressure. Look for decreased heart rate and blood pressure, which may indicate decreased blood flow to the tissues.

Bring the emergency cart to the patient's bedside because he or she may need to be given other emergency drugs or to have the heart paced using a transthoracic temporary pacemaker.

Assess the intravenous (IV) site for patency and signs of infection or infiltration such as redness, swelling, warmth, or decreased IV flow. Ask the patient if the IV site is causing any discomfort.

Ask patients about vision problems such as glaucoma, because atropine can make this problem worse.

⭐ Priority Actions to Take *After* Giving Atropine

In addition to the general priority actions to take after giving any antidysrhythmic drug (p. 269), recheck the patient's heart rate and blood pressure because these should improve after atropine is given. Continue to monitor the IV site for patency. Check the patient's pulse for regularity and strength.

Monitor urine output because urinary retention can be a side effect of atropine. Ask whether the patient is experiencing any problems with dry mouth, blurred vision, or drowsiness. Report serious side effects to the prescriber. Check for bowel sounds and abdominal tenderness because atropine can also cause constipation.

⭐ Teaching Priorities for Patients Taking Atropine

In addition to the general teaching priorities related to any antidysrhythmic drugs (p. 269), include these teaching points and precautions:
- Atropine is not prescribed for long-term use and is usually given in a patient care setting and should be administered exactly as ordered by the prescriber. It may cause drowsiness, so you should call for assistance when getting up.
- Remember that the action of atropine is to increase heart rate and blood pressure. Improved blood flow to the tissues usually leads to decreased symptoms such as dizziness.
- Atropine is used for short-term treatment for bradydysrhythmias (slow abnormal rhythms).
- You will likely need a more permanent solution such as a pacemaker.
- Using mouth rinses and frequent mouth hygiene will help relieve dry mouth and prevent tooth decay.
- Notify your prescriber or nurse if you experience any vision problems.
- Atropine can affect the ability of the body to regulate heat, so avoid strenuous activity in a hot setting.

Life Span Considerations for Atropine

Considerations for pregnancy and lactation. Atropine has a low to moderate likelihood of increasing the risk for birth defects or fetal harm. IV atropine may cause tachycardia in the fetus and should be used with caution in pregnant women. However, it may be necessary to use this drug when the mother's heart rate becomes so slow that the fetus may not receive enough oxygen and damage may occur.

Considerations for older adults. The risk for drug-induced myocardial infarction (heart attack) is greater in the older adult. Although all patients receiving atropine must be monitored, extra-close monitoring is needed when the drug is used for older adults.

DIGOXIN

How Digoxin Works

Digoxin (Lanoxin) is a cardiac glycoside that may be used in small doses to increase contractility and slow conduction through the AV node, causing slowing of the heart

 Critical Point for Safety

Teach patients to use mouth rinses and frequent oral hygiene to relieve dry mouth and prevent tooth decay.

QSEN: Safety

rate. It is used for atrial fibrillation because it helps to slow the ventricular rate by blocking the number of electrical impulses that pass through the AV node to the heart ventricles. Digoxin also helps to strengthen the contractions in the ventricles, so the heart is able to pump more blood with each heartbeat. In the past, digoxin preparations were used much more than they currently are. Newer drugs are often prescribed, although some patients are still prescribed this drug. Although listed in this chapter, see Chapter 14 for a full discussion of the actions, side effects, and other issues related to digoxin therapy. Be sure to consult a reliable drug reference for more information about digoxin.

DRUGS FOR TACHYDYSRHYTHMIAS

A *tachydysrhythmia* is an abnormally rapid heart rhythm. Drugs used to treat rapid abnormal heart rhythms work in one of three ways. They may reduce automaticity of the heart muscle cells, slow down conduction of electrical impulses through the heart, or prolong the refractory period of heart cells. Several classes of drugs are used to treat these rapid dysrhythmias (Table 15.2). The drugs are classified by the way they work. Some drugs have characteristics of more than one classification.

Goals of treatment with these drugs include preventing and relieving symptoms, prolonging life, and suppressing abnormal rhythms. Recent trends in the treatment of these heart rhythms include a decrease in the use of class I drugs and an increase in the use of class II and III drugs because there are more side effects with class I drugs.

Class I: Sodium Channel Blockers

Sodium channel blockers are a class of drugs that act by inhibiting sodium movement through cell membranes into cardiac muscle cells. This results in slowing of the heart rate, reducing cell excitability, and reducing speed of conduction. There are three subclasses of sodium channel blocker drugs (Ia, Ib, and Ic). Different subclasses are used to treat different tachydysrhythmias.

Class Ia sodium channel blockers

How class Ia drugs work. This group of drugs is used to treat patients who have symptoms associated with premature ventricular contractions (PVCs), supraventricular tachycardia (SVT), and ventricular tachycardia (VT). Another use of these drugs is to prevent the occurrence of ventricular fibrillation (VF).

Class Ia drugs decrease the excitability of the heart muscle cells and slow the conduction of electrical impulses through the heart. Together these actions slow the

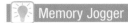

Memory Jogger

The three ways that drugs work to treat rapid abnormal heart rhythms are by:
- Reducing automaticity of the heart muscle cells.
- Slowing down conduction of electrical impulses through the heart.
- Prolonging the refractory period of heart cells.

Table **15.2**	Classes of Common Antidysrhythmic Drugs for Tachydysrhythmias
CLASS	**PURPOSE**
Class I: Sodium Channel Blockers	
Class Ia	Treat symptomatic PVCs, SVT, VT; prevent VF
Class Ib	Treat symptomatic PVCs, VT; prevent VF
Class Ic	Treat life-threatening VT or VF and SVT unresponsive to other drugs
Class I: Miscellaneous	Treat life-threatening ventricular dysrhythmias
Class II: Beta blockers	Treat SVT
Class III: Potassium channel blockers	Treat VT, VF; conversion of A fib and A flutter to sinus rhythm; maintain sinus rhythm
Class IV: Calcium channel blockers	Treat SVT
Unclassified	
Adenosine	Treat SVT
Magnesium sulfate	Treat torsades de pointes

A fib, Atrial fibrillation; *A flutter,* atrial flutter; *PVC,* premature ventricular contraction; *SVT,* supraventricular tachycardia; *VF,* ventricular fibrillation; *VT,* ventricular tachycardia.

heart rate and make the rhythm more regular. Procainamide may also decrease the strength of heart contractions. Common doses of class Ia drugs are listed in the following table. Be sure to consult a reliable drug reference for information about any specific class Ia antidysrhythmic drug.

Adult Dosages for Commonly Prescribed Class Ia Sodium Channel Blockers

Drug Category	Drug Name	Usual Maintenance Dose
Class Ia Sodium Channel Blockers	quinidine (Quinaglute, Quinora)	200–600 mg orally every 6–8 hr Extended release: 300 to 600 mg orally every 8 to 12 hr
	procainamide (Pronestyl, Pronestyl SR, Procanbid)	IV: Loading dose 15 to 17 mg/kg as an IV infusion, infused at a rate of 20 to 30 mg/minute. Maintenance dose 1–4 mg/min as a continuous IV infusion. Usual initial maintenance dose is about 50 mg/kg/day IM: 50 mg/kg/day IM, given in divided doses every 3–6 hr
	disopyramide (Norpace, Norpace CR)	100–200 mg orally every 6 hr Extended release: 200–400 mg orally every 12 hr

Intended responses of class Ia drugs
- Heart rate is decreased.
- Abnormal supraventricular and ventricular rhythms are decreased.
- Heart rhythm is normal and regular.
- Cardiac output is increased.

Common side effects of class Ia drugs. Common side effects include hypotension, loss of appetite, abdominal cramping, diarrhea, and nausea. As many as 30% to 50% of patients develop gastrointestinal side effects while taking these drugs. Disopyramide also commonly causes constipation, dry mouth, urinary retention, and urinary hesitation.

Possible adverse effects of class Ia drugs. Life-threatening adverse effects vary with the drug prescribed. Patients taking quinidine may become hypotensive or develop an abnormal life-threatening ventricular rhythm called *torsades de pointes*. Other life-threatening effects of procainamide include seizures, heart block, asystole, and decreased white blood cell count with increased risk for infection. Disopyramide has been known to cause heart failure.

Allergic reactions to class Ia antidysrhythmic drugs are rare but serious. Signs of allergic reaction include fever, neutropenia, Raynaud's syndrome (ice-cold hands), muscle aches, skin rashes, and blood vessel inflammation in the fingers.

⭐ **Priority actions to take *before* giving class Ia drugs.** In addition to the general priority actions to take before giving any antidysrhythmic drugs (p. 269), remember that although oral forms of these drugs are best absorbed on an empty stomach and with a full glass of water, if the patient develops gastrointestinal problems, the nurse may need to give them with food.

If the patient being started on disopyramide has been taking quinidine, wait 6 to 12 hours after the last dose of quinidine before beginning disopyramide. If immediate-release procainamide was being used, wait 6 hours after the last dose of procainamide to begin disopyramide because these medicines may interact and cause very harmful effects such as irregular rhythms. Check a baseline weight.

⭐ **Priority actions to take *after* giving class Ia drugs.** In addition to the general priority actions to take after giving any antidysrhythmic drug (p. 269), monitor intake and output because these drugs may cause or worsen urine retention. Also monitor daily weights. For the patient taking disopyramide, watch for signs of heart failure such

Do Not Confuse

quinidine *with* **quinine**

An order for quinidine may be confused with quinine. Quinidine is a class Ia antidysrhythmic drug, whereas quinine is an antimalarial drug.

QSEN: Safety

Common Side Effects

Class Ia Sodium Channel Blockers

Loss of appetite, Abdominal cramping, Diarrhea, Nausea   Hypotension

Critical Point for Safety

When patients develop gastrointestinal (GI) symptoms, give class Ia drugs with food to help reduce the symptoms.

QSEN: Safety

1+ Trace
A barely perceptible pit (2 mm)

2+ Mild
A deeper pit, with fairly normal contours, that rebounds in 10–15 s (4 mm)

3+ Moderate
A deep pit; may last for 30 s to more than 1 min (6 mm)

4+ Severe
An even deeper pit, with severe edema that may last as long as 2–5 min before rebounding (8 mm)

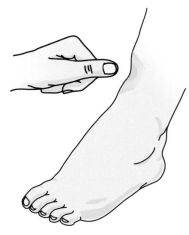

FIG. 15.6 Pitting edema scale.

> **⬢ Critical Point for Safety**
>
> Monitor patient weight as well as intake and output because class Ia antidysrhythmic drugs can cause or worsen urinary retention.
>
> QSEN: Safety

as ankle swelling (Figure 15.6) or weight gain, shortness of breath, and crackles when you listen to the lungs with a stethoscope.

Ask the patient about stomach upset or diarrhea. Remind the patient taking quinidine to call for help before getting up and to change positions slowly because of the potential for hypotension (low blood pressure) and increased risk for falls.

If he or she is also taking digoxin, watch for signs of digoxin toxicity because these drugs may lead to increased blood level of digoxin by as much as 50%. Indications of early *digoxin toxicity* include loss of appetite, nausea, vomiting, diarrhea, or vision problems. Other signs include changes in heart rate or rhythm (irregular or slow), palpitations, or fainting.

⭐ **Teaching priorities for patients taking class Ia drugs.** In addition to the general teaching priorities related to antidysrhythmic drugs (p. 269), include these teaching points and precautions:

- Monitor your urine output and to check and record your weight on a daily basis.
- Report decreased urine output or a weight gain of more than 2 pounds a day to your prescriber.
- Check your ankles for swelling as demonstrated by the nurse (see Figure 15.6), and report any swelling or shortness of breath to your prescriber. Increased weight gain, ankle swelling, and shortness of breath are signs of worsening heart failure.
- Take the drug at the same time every day and exactly as prescribed because the blood level of these drugs must be maintained to achieve the expected actions.
- Disopyramide can cause increased sun sensitivity (photosensitivity). To avoid exposure to sunlight, wear protective sun block and clothing.
- If you are taking quinidine, avoid high-alkaline ash foods (such as citrus fruits; milk; and vegetables such as broccoli, cabbage, and carrots), because these foods can affect the excretion of quinidine and may lead to toxic levels of this drug.
- Avoid the herb St. John's wort while taking quinidine because it can cause a decreased blood level of this drug.

> **⬢ Critical Point for Safety**
>
> Teach patients taking quinidine to avoid large amounts of high-alkaline ash foods because they affect excretion of the drug and can lead to drug toxicity.
>
> QSEN: Safety

> **⬢ Critical Point for Safety**
>
> The herb St. John's wort should not be taken with quinidine because it can cause a decreased blood level of quinidine.
>
> QSEN: Safety

Life span considerations for class Ia drugs

Considerations for pregnancy and lactation. Class Ia drugs have a low to moderate likelihood of increasing the risk for birth defects or fetal harm and are generally not considered safe for use during pregnancy or breastfeeding.

Considerations for older adults. Older adults may eliminate class Ia drugs more slowly and are at higher risk for side effects and toxicity.

Class Ib sodium channel blockers

How class Ib drugs work. Class Ib antidysrhythmic drugs are used to treat ventricular tachycardia and PVCs that cause patient symptoms. They are also used to prevent ventricular fibrillation, a life-threatening dysrhythmia.

Most of these drugs inhibit the ability of the ventricles to contract prematurely. This decreases the number of PVCs and episodes of ventricular tachycardia. In an emergency setting, amiodarone (Cordarone) is the first-line drug prescribed for ventricular tachycardia, followed by lidocaine (Xylocaine).

Lidocaine is only given intravenously or by airway inhalation (ET tube—remember "NAVEL") because, when given by mouth, the liver destroys most of the drug, making it ineffective. Lidocaine may be given intramuscularly in an emergency situation if an IV line is not available.

Common doses of class Ib drugs are listed in the following table. Be sure to consult a reliable drug resource for information about a specific class Ib antidysrhythmic drug.

Adult Dosages for Commonly Prescribed Class Ib Sodium Channel Blockers

Drug Category	Drug Name	Usual Maintenance Dose
Class Ib Sodium Channel Blockers	lidocaine ❶ (Xylocaine)	1–1.5 mg/kg/dose IV load then 1–4 mg/min by continuous infusion Endotracheal dosage for adults: 2–4 mg/kg/dose via ET tube
	mexiletine (Mexitil)	200–400 mg orally every 8 hr (may give loading dose of 400 mg). Max: 1200 mg/day
	phenytoin (Dilantin, Phenytek)	100 mg IV every 5 min as needed until desired effect of controlling the dysrhythmia or adverse events limit tolerance. Max: 1000 mg IV
	tocainide (Tonocard)	1200–1800 mg orally per day in divided doses every 8 hr, up to 2400 mg/day

❶ High-alert drug.

Intended responses of class Ib drugs
- Number of PVCs is decreased.
- Risk for ventricular tachycardia is decreased.
- Heart rhythm is regular and normal.
- Cardiac output is increased.

Common side effects of class Ib drugs. Common side effects include confusion and drowsiness. IV lidocaine may cause stinging at the IV site. Common side effects of mexiletine and tocainide include dizziness, tremors, nervousness, nausea, vomiting, and heartburn. A patient may also have visual disturbances, vertigo, or ringing in the ears (tinnitus). Dizziness and falls are more likely with older adults.

Possible adverse effects of class Ib drugs. A life-threatening adverse effect of lidocaine is cardiac arrest. Dysrhythmias may worsen with mexiletine and tocainide. A patient may develop pneumonitis, pulmonary fibrosis, or pulmonary edema while taking tocainide. Decreased white blood cell count (*neutropenia*) with increased risk for infection is an adverse effect of both tocainide and phenytoin. Two additional adverse effects of phenytoin are aplastic anemia and Stevens-Johnson syndrome, a skin disorder resulting from an allergic reaction to drugs, infections, or illness. See Chapter 1 and Figure 1.5 for more information about this syndrome.

⭐ **Priority actions to take *before* giving class Ib drugs.** In addition to the general priority actions to take before giving any antidysrhythmic drug (p. 269), ask specifically about herbal preparation use. St. John's wort may decrease the level of lidocaine in the blood and reduce its effectiveness.

To monitor for drug side effects, ask patients if they have ever had any problems with tremors, dizziness, light-headedness, visual problems, or ringing in the ears. Assess for baseline level of consciousness because IV lidocaine may cause confusion in older patients.

For IV drugs, be sure to check the IV site for patency and signs of infection. Ask the patient about stinging or discomfort at the IV site.

Common Side Effects

Class Ib Sodium Channel Blockers

Drowsiness

Tremors

Dizziness

Nausea, Vomiting, Heartburn (dyspepsia)

Tinnitus

Confusion

⭐ **Priority actions to take *after* giving class ib drugs.** In addition to the general priority actions to take after giving any antidysrhythmic drug (p. 269), tell the patient to report any chest pain or shortness of breath immediately. Watch for side effects, including confusion, tremors, dizziness, light-headedness, visual difficulties, and tinnitus (ringing in the ears).

Ask about any shortness of breath and listen to the patient's lungs with a stethoscope for crackles, a sign of heart failure. Assess the IV site for patency and any signs of infection. Ask whether the patient feels any stinging or burning at the IV site. Also ask about numbness, which can be caused by lidocaine and may mask the signs of IV infiltration.

With older adults, check for signs of confusion and other side effects because they are more sensitive to the effects of these drugs. Confusion may be a sign of lidocaine toxicity in these patients. Heart rate changes include decreased heart rate and asystole with hypotension and shock.

⭐ **Teaching priorities for patients taking class Ib drugs.** In addition to the general precautions related to antidysrhythmic therapy (p. 269), include these teaching points and precautions:

- Change positions slowly and hold on to handrails when using stairs to reduce the risk of falling.
- Have your family members assess you for confusion or any changes in level of cognition and report changes to the prescriber.
- Report any of the following symptoms to the prescriber immediately:
  - Irregular rhythms
  - Heart rates less than 60 beats per minute or more than 100 beats per minute
  - Chest pain
  - Shortness of breath
  - Wheezing

Life span considerations for class Ib drugs

Considerations for pregnancy and lactation. Class Ib drugs should not be used during pregnancy or breastfeeding because they cross the placenta and enter breast milk. All class 1b drugs have a moderate likelihood of increasing the risk for birth defects or fetal harm. Phenytoin has a moderate to high likelihood of increasing the risk for birth defects or fetal harm.

Considerations for older adults. Older adults are more likely to experience dizziness and falls while taking class Ib drugs. In addition, older adults are more likely to become confused.

Class Ic sodium channel blockers

How class Ic drugs work. Class Ic antidysrhythmic drugs are used to treat life-threatening ventricular tachycardia or fibrillation and supraventricular tachycardia that does not go away when other drugs are used.

Flecainide (Tambocor) and propafenone (Rythmol) are oral drugs given to adults to slow the electrical impulse conduction of the heart. Common doses of class Ic drugs are listed in the following table. Be sure to consult a reliable drug resource for information about any specific class Ic antidysrhythmic drug.

Adult Dosages for Commonly Prescribed Class Ic Sodium Channel Blockers

Drug Category	Drug Name	Usual Maintenance Dose
Class Ic Sodium Channel Blockers	flecainide (Tambocor)	100–150 mg orally every 12 hr. Max: 400 mg/day
	propafenone (Rythmol, Rhythmol SR)	150–300 mg orally every 8 hr SR: 225–425 mg orally every 12 hr

Intended responses of class Ic drugs
- Episodes of ventricular and supraventricular dysrhythmias are decreased.
- Cardiac output is increased.

- Symptoms are decreased.
- Heart rhythm is normal and regular.

Common side effects of class Ic drugs. Common side effects of class Ic antidysrhythmic drugs include dizziness, conduction system abnormalities leading to heart blocks, altered sense of taste, constipation, nausea, and vomiting. Patients taking flecainide may also have blurred vision and difficulty focusing. Side effects are more likely to occur with higher doses of these drugs.

Possible adverse effects of class Ic drugs. Adverse life-threatening effects of class Ic drugs include supraventricular and ventricular dysrhythmias such as heart blocks and ventricular tachycardia.

 Priority actions to take *before* giving class Ic drugs. In addition to the general priority actions to take before giving any antidysrhythmic drug (p. 269), check whether the patient has a history of bronchospasm with asthma or COPD because propafenone's action on beta adrenergic receptors can induce bronchospasms.

 Priority actions to take *after* giving class Ic drugs. In addition to the general priority actions to take after giving any antidysrhythmic drug (p. 269), ask the patient about dizziness, altered taste sensation, constipation, nausea, vomiting, and vision changes, which are indications of drug toxicity. Report any of these symptoms to the prescriber immediately.

 Teaching priorities for patients taking class Ic drugs. In addition to the general teaching priorities about any antidysrhythmic drug (p. 269), include these teaching points and precautions:

- Report any visual disturbances or other symptoms, including fever, sore throat, chills, unusual bleeding or bruising, chest pain, shortness of breath, excessive sweating (diaphoresis), or palpitations, to your prescriber at once. These symptoms may indicate toxicity or life-threatening dysrhythmias.
- Change positions slowly and hold on to handrails when using stairs to reduce the risk for falls.
- Report any liver or kidney problems to the prescriber immediately.

Life span considerations for class Ic drugs

Considerations for pregnancy and lactation. Class Ic drugs have a low to moderate likelihood of increasing the risk for birth defects or fetal harm. They should be used during pregnancy only when the potential benefit outweighs the risk to the fetus. It is not known whether class Ic drugs are excreted in breast milk. Because of possible serious adverse reactions in nursing infants, a different method of infant feeding should be considered.

Considerations for older adults. A slight increase in the incidence of dizziness has been seen in older adults. Because of the possible increased risk of liver and kidney problems in older adults, class Ic drugs should be used with caution in this group.

Class II: Beta Blockers

How beta blockers work. **Beta blockers** are used to treat supraventricular tachycardia (SVT). These drugs block the effects of epinephrine (adrenaline) on the heart. They decrease the heart rate and the force of heart contractions, which results in a decrease in blood pressure. Beta blockers are often used to slow the rate of ventricular contractions with supraventricular tachycardia, including rapid atrial fibrillation or flutter. As a result, the heart does not work as hard and requires less oxygen. Cardioselective beta blockers work only on the cardiovascular system. Noncardioselective beta blockers have systemic effects, especially on the respiratory system. Although listed in this chapter, see Chapter 13 for a full discussion of the actions, side effects, and other issues related to beta blocker drug therapy.

When a beta blocker is prescribed for a patient with kidney damage, a lower dose of the drug is ordered, or the time between doses is increased. An older adult patient may also be started on a lower drug dose.

Common Side Effects

Class Ic Sodium Channel Blockers

Taste changes

Blurred vision

Constipation, Nausea/ Vomiting

Dizziness

Critical Point for Safety

Side effects of class Ic antidysrhythmic drugs are more likely to occur as the dosage increases.

QSEN: Safety

Critical Point for Safety

Always ask older adults about liver or kidney problems because class Ic antidysrhythmic drug doses may be lower in these patients.

QSEN: Safety

Memory Jogger

Beta blockers can work on the cardiovascular system (cardioselective) or have systemic effects (noncardioselective).

Common doses of class II beta blockers approved for use with dysrhythmias are listed in the following table. Be sure to consult a reliable drug resource for information about a specific class II beta blocker antidysrhythmic drug. See Chapters 13 and 14 for additional information about beta blockers.

Adult Dosages for Commonly Prescribed Beta Blockers

Drug Category	Drug Name	Usual Maintenance Dose
Selective Beta Blockers	acebutolol ❶ (Sectral)	400–1200 mg/day orally, given in 2–3 divided doses *Special Considerations:* **When discontinued, this drug should be gradually decreased over 2 weeks**
	esmolol ❶ (Brevibloc)	IV 25–200 mcg/kg/min. Max: 300 mcg/kg/min
Nonselective Beta Blockers	propranolol ❶ (Inderal, Inderal LA, Inderal CR)	1–3 mg IV, given at a rate no faster than 1 mg/min 10–40 mg orally 3–4 times daily
	sotalol ❶ (Betapace)	80–120 mg orally every 12 hr

❶ High-alert drug.

Class III: Potassium Channel Blockers

How class III potassium channel blockers work. Class III antidysrhythmic drugs are **potassium channel blockers,** a class of drugs that act by inhibition of potassium movement through cell membranes. Blocking potassium channels lengthens the duration of action potentials. They are used to treat ventricular tachycardia and ventricular fibrillation, convert atrial fibrillation or flutter to normal sinus rhythm, and maintain normal sinus rhythm. Amiodarone (Cordarone) given intravenously is used to slow conduction through the AV node with atrial fibrillation and control ventricular tachycardia and fibrillation. Oral amiodarone is used to prevent recurrence of ventricular tachycardia and fibrillation and to maintain a normal sinus rhythm after conversion from atrial fibrillation or flutter. Dofetilide (Tikosyn) is given orally to keep a patient in normal sinus rhythm after conversion from atrial fibrillation. Ibutilide (Corvert) is given intravenously and makes cardioversion of a patient with atrial fibrillation or flutter to normal sinus rhythm more likely to be successful.

Common dosages of class III potassium channel blockers approved for use with dysrhythmias are listed in the following table. Be sure to consult a reliable drug reference for information about any specific class III potassium channel blocker antidysrhythmic drug.

Adult Dosages for Commonly Prescribed Class III Potassium Channel Blockers

Drug Category	Drug Name	Usual Maintenance Dose
Class III Potassium Channel Blockers	amiodarone (Cordarone, Nexterone, Pacerone)	200–400 mg orally daily in 1 or 2 divided doses IV: initial IV rapid infusion of 150 mg over 10 min then continuous infusion of 1 mg/min for the next 6 hr; maintenance IV infusion of 0.5 mg/min
	dofetilide ❶ (Tikosyn)	125–500 mcg orally twice daily *individualized* based on kidney function with maximum 1000 mcg/day orally *Special Considerations:* **Patient must be on cardiac monitor for first 72 hr on this drug; patient with atrial fibrillation should be anticoagulated**
	ibutilide (Corvert)	Adults weighing 60 kg or more: 1 mg IV over 10 min Adults weighing less than 60 kg: 0.01 mg/kg IV over 10 min Dose may be repeated **once** after 10 min if necessary: Maximum dose 2 mg IV over 20 min
	sotalol ❶ (Betapace)[a]	80–120 mg orally every 12 hr

❶ High-alert drug.

[a]Sotalol is a beta blocker but is also considered a class III antidysrhythmic drug.

Intended responses of class III drugs

- Blood vessel constriction is decreased.
- Blood flow to coronary arteries and heart muscle is increased.
- Electrical impulse conduction in all heart muscle tissues is slowed.
- Heart rate is decreased.
- Strength of contractions in the left ventricle is decreased.
- Success of cardioversion to normal sinus rhythm (ibutilide) is increased.
- Normal heart rhythm and rate (oral amiodarone and dofetilide) are maintained.

Common side effects of class III drugs. Common side effects of class III potassium channel blockers include dizziness, fatigue, malaise, bradycardia, hypotension (especially for IV drugs), loss of appetite, constipation, nausea, vomiting, unsteady gait (ataxia), involuntary movement, numbness and tingling, poor coordination, and tremor. Side effects unique to amiodarone include photosensitivity, hypothyroidism, peripheral neuropathy, and microdeposits on the corneas. Amiodarone and sotalol also can cause changes in taste sensation.

Hyperthyroidism may occur with amiodarone. Thyroid problems are more likely to occur during the first few weeks of treatment. A patient who is taking amiodarone for a long period may develop blue discoloration of the face, neck, and arms.

Possible adverse effects of class III drugs. Several potential life-threatening effects are associated with amiodarone, including adult respiratory distress syndrome (ARDS), pulmonary fibrosis, heart failure, worsening of heart dysrhythmias, decreased liver function, and toxic epidermal necrolysis. Toxic epidermal necrolysis is a rare but life-threatening skin disorder that is caused by an allergic reaction.

With dofetilide, patients also may experience chest pain or life-threatening ventricular dysrhythmias (e.g., torsades de pointes).

 Priority actions to take before giving class III drugs. In addition to the general priority actions to take before giving any antidysrhythmic drug (p. 269), if the patient is to receive an IV drug, check the site for patency and signs of infection. Ask if the patient has a history of renal problems because dofetilide is eliminated through the kidneys. For a patient newly prescribed dofetilide, place him or her on a cardiac monitor for at least 72 hours because of the risk for the life-threatening ventricular dysrhythmia torsades de pointes.

 Priority actions to take after giving class III drugs. In addition to the general priority actions to take after giving any antidysrhythmic drug (p. 269), continue to check the IV line for patency and signs of infection. Be sure to monitor blood pressure when a patient is receiving IV amiodarone (Cordarone) because of the risk for hypotension.

Watch for signs of pulmonary problems such as ARDS (including crackles when you listen to the lungs with a stethoscope), difficulty breathing, fatigue, cough, and fever.

Look for signs of thyroid problems, including weight gain; lethargy; and swelling in the hands, feet, or around the eyes. Report any of these signs to the prescriber immediately.

Make sure that any follow-up laboratory tests (e.g., liver, kidney, and thyroid function tests) and ECGs are completed. Keep the patient newly prescribed dofetilide on a cardiac monitor for 72 hours and regularly document the heart rate and rhythm.

 Teaching priorities for patients taking class III drugs. In addition to the teaching priorities related to antidysrhythmic drugs (p. 269), include these teaching points and precautions:

- If you are taking amiodarone you may need to wear dark glasses when going outside because of the potential for increased sensitivity to light.

Common Side Effects

Class III Potassium Channel Blockers

Fatigue

Hypotension

Bradycardia

Nausea/Vomiting, Anorexia, Constipation

Tremors

Dizziness

⭐ **Critical Point for Safety**

Be sure to monitor the respiratory status of patients taking amiodarone because ARDS and pulmonary fibrosis are possible adverse effects of this drug.

QSEN: Safety

⭐ **Critical Point for Safety**

Dosing of dofetilide must be done very carefully because it can cause serious cardiac dysrhythmias such as ventricular tachycardia (e.g., torsades de pointes).

QSEN: Safety

⭐ **Critical Point for Safety**

Monitor for signs of thyroid problems such as changes in heart rate, which are more likely to occur during the first few weeks of treatment with amiodarone (Cordarone).

QSEN: Safety

- Wear protective clothing and a sunscreen barrier for increased sun sensitivity (photosensitivity) while taking these drugs.
- Side effects may not appear for several days or weeks.
- Remember that long-term use of amiodarone may cause the development of a bluish discoloration of the face, neck, and arms. This side effect is reversible and will disappear over several months.
- You will need eye examinations every 6 to 12 months to determine if corneal microdeposits or other eye changes have occurred. These changes may not necessarily be apparent during the early stages.
- Report any persistent change in the rate or ease of breathing to your prescriber as soon as possible because the drug may cause serious lung problems.
- Take your prescribed drug exactly as prescribed.
- If you are a male patient, you should immediately report any pain or swelling in the scrotum to your prescriber, because your drug dosage of amiodarone may need to be decreased.
- Notify your prescriber for any signs of adverse effects to these drugs.

Life span considerations for class III drugs

Considerations for pregnancy and lactation. Potassium channel blockers have a moderate to high likelihood of increasing the risk for birth defects or fetal harm. Pregnant women should not take amiodarone because it can harm the fetus. Women who are breastfeeding should not use these drugs, and if the treatment is necessary, breastfeeding should be discontinued.

Class IV: Calcium Channel Blockers

How class IV calcium channel blockers work. Class IV antidysrhythmic drugs include the **calcium channel blockers** diltiazem (Cardizem) and verapamil (Calan, Isoptin). They are used primarily for the treatment of supraventricular tachycardia. As antidysrhythmic drugs, they act by slowing conduction through the SA and AV nodes of the conduction system of the heart, leading to a decreased heart rate. When these drugs are prescribed for older adults or patients with hepatic (liver) or renal (kidney) impairment, lower initial dosages are used.

Common dosages of class IV calcium channel blockers approved for use with dysrhythmias are listed in the following table. Be sure to consult a reliable drug resource for information about any specific class IV calcium channel blocker antidysrhythmic drug. Although listed in this chapter, see Chapter 13 for a full discussion of the actions, side effects, and other issues related to calcium channel blocker drug therapy.

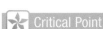
Critical Point for Safety

Male patients may experience pain or swelling in the scrotum while taking amiodarone (Cordarone), which should be reported to the prescriber immediately.

QSEN: Safety

Adult Dosages for Commonly Prescribed Class IV Calcium Channel Blockers

Drug Category	Drug Name	Usual Maintenance Dose
Class IV Calcium Channel Blockers	diltiazem (Cardizem)	30–60 mg orally 3–4 times daily Slow-release capsules 60–120 mg orally twice daily; extended-release capsules 240–360 mg orally once daily IV: 0.25 mg/kg over 2 min; second dose 0.35 mg/kg may be given after 15 min if needed; follow with continuous infusion 5–15 mg/hr for up to 24 hr
	verapamil (Calan, Calan SR, Isoptin, Isoptin SR)	240–480 mg/day orally, given in 3–4 divided doses IV: 5–10 mg over 2 min; may give additional 10 mg after 30 min if needed

Unclassified Antidysrhythmic Drugs
Adenosine

How adenosine works. Adenosine (Adenocard) is a drug administered intravenously for supraventricular tachycardia (SVT). Adenosine can help identify the rhythm, and certain SVT rhythms can be successfully terminated with adenosine. Its action is similar to that of calcium channel blockers. It slows electrical impulse conduction through the AV node to help restore a patient to a normal sinus rhythm. Adenosine is an IV drug given as a *rapid* IV bolus injection. When given slowly, adenosine is eliminated from the body before it can reach the heart and act to slow the rhythm. After giving adenosine, there will be a very brief period of asystole (10 to 20 seconds), then the heart will resume a normal rhythm. Be sure to consult a reliable drug resource for specific information about adenosine.

Adult Dosages for Commonly Prescribed Adenosine

Drug Category	Drug Name	Usual Maintenance Dose
Unclassified	adenosine (Adenocard)	6 mg IV given rapidly over 1–2 seconds; flush with normal saline and elevate arm after giving drug IV push; second and third doses of 12 mg can be given if necessary

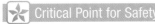

Critical Point for Safety

Always give IV adenosine (Adenocard) **rapidly** over 1 to 2 seconds.

QSEN: Safety

Common Side Effects

Vasodilators

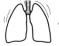

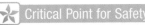

Shortness of breath   Dysrhythmias   Flushing

Critical Point for Safety

Always have emergency equipment, including the crash cart and defibrillator, at the bedside before giving an IV dose of adenosine.

QSEN: Safety

Intended responses of adenosine
- Impulse conduction through the AV node is slower.
- Heart rate is decreased.
- Supraventricular tachycardia is terminated.
- Heart rhythm is normal and regular.

Common side effects of adenosine. Common side effects of adenosine include facial flushing, shortness of breath, and transient dysrhythmias such as atrial fibrillation and atrial flutter.

Possible adverse effects of adenosine. Allergic reactions are rare. Adenosine should **not** be used with heart block unless the patient has an artificial pacemaker in place because it may lead to asystole.

Fatal cardiac arrest, sustained ventricular tachycardia, and nonfatal myocardial infarction have been reported after giving injections of adenosine. Patients with unstable angina may be at greater risk. Emergency equipment must be available at the bedside before this drug is given.

⭐ **Priority actions to take *before* giving adenosine.** In addition to the general priority actions to take before giving any antidysrhythmic drug (p. 269), tell the patient that there will be a brief period of asystole that may feel like a "mule kick" to the chest before the heart goes back into a normal rhythm.

Be sure that a physician is at the bedside. Bring emergency equipment to the bedside before giving this drug. Check the IV line for patency and any signs of infection. Draw the bolus up into a syringe and remember that it must be given by IV push *rapidly* over 1 to 2 seconds.

⭐ **Priority actions to take *after* giving adenosine.** In addition to the general priority actions to take after giving any antidysrhythmic drug (p. 269), always stay with the patient until the period of asystole is over and then check blood pressure every 15 to 30 minutes immediately after adenosine has been given. Be sure to check the heart monitor for changes in heart rhythm. Monitor for any side effects or adverse effects.

⭐ **Teaching priorities for patients taking adenosine.** In addition to the general teaching priorities related to any antidysrhythmic drug (p. 269), include these teaching points and precautions:
- The purpose of this drug is to quickly get your heart back into a normal rhythm.
- Ask for help when getting up and change positions slowly because doses of 12 mg or more can cause hypotension.
- Report any facial flushing, shortness of breath, or dizziness immediately.

Life span considerations for adenosine

Considerations for pregnancy and lactation. Adenosine has a low to moderate likelihood of increasing the risk for birth defects or fetal harm and should not be used during pregnancy.

Magnesium sulfate

How magnesium sulfate works. Magnesium sulfate is a major mineral and the fourth most abundant in the human body. It helps the heart rhythm remain steady. Magnesium sulfate is used intravenously to prevent the ventricular dysrhythmia *torsades de pointes* from returning after a patient has been defibrillated (given an electric shock) to return to a normal rhythm. An IV magnesium sulfate bolus can sometimes eliminate torsades de pointes in a patient who is not symptomatic. A normal level of magnesium in the blood keeps the heart muscle from becoming overexcited and reduces the risk for this life-threatening dysrhythmia. The common dose of magnesium sulfate used is listed in the following table. Although listed in this chapter, see Chapter 14 for a full discussion of the actions, side effects, and other issues related to magnesium sulfate therapy. Be sure to consult a reliable drug resource for more specific information about magnesium sulfate.

Adult Dosages for Commonly Prescribed Magnesium

Drug Category	Drug Name	Usual Maintenance Dose
Unclassified	magnesium sulfate ❶	1–2 g IV diluted with 10 mL of D_5W solution; give over 30 s ***Special Considerations:* Patient should be on cardiac monitor when receiving this drug**

❶ High-alert drug.

Other Drugs Used to Treat Dysrhythmias

Anticoagulants such as heparin and warfarin (Coumadin) are prescribed for rhythms when the patient is at increased risk for blood clots such as atrial fibrillation or flutter. For more information on these drugs, see Chapter 17.

Get Ready for the NCLEX® Examination!

Key Points

- The normal pacemaker of the heart is the SA node, which initiates 60 to 100 electrical impulses per minute to the heart.
- Dysrhythmias are abnormal heart rhythms.
- Some patients with symptoms do *not* have serious dysrhythmias, whereas others with *no* symptoms may have life-threatening dysrhythmias.
- Ventricular fibrillation causes death within minutes if not treated.
- Over-the-counter cough and cold drugs that contain pseudoephedrine (Sudafed) can cause abnormal rapid heart rhythms.
- Always check a patient's blood pressure, as well as their heart rate, and heart rhythm for a full minute before and after giving an antidysrhythmic drug.
- Always check IV sites for patency and signs of infection before and after a patient is given an IV antidysrhythmic drug.
- Teach patients taking antidysrhythmic drugs to check and record their heart rate and rhythm every day and to report any abnormal findings to their prescriber.
- A patient with liver or kidney problems needs lower doses of most antidysrhythmic drugs to avoid drug overdose and drug toxicity.

- Check patients for signs of heart failure after receiving antidysrhythmic drugs. Check daily weights, listen for crackles in the lungs, and assess for swelling.
- An older adult patient may need decreased doses of antidysrhythmic drugs because of increased sensitivity and age-related body changes.
- Do not give large doses of atropine to older adults because they are more sensitive to its effects and may experience confusion.
- Administering a dose of atropine less than 0.5 mg may make bradycardia worse (paradoxical bradycardia).
- When patients develop gastrointestinal (GI) symptoms, give class Ia drugs with food to help reduce the symptoms.
- Monitor patient weight as well as intake and output because class Ia antidysrhythmic drugs can cause urinary retention.
- Teach patients taking quinidine to avoid large amounts of high-alkaline ash foods (e.g., citrus fruit, milk, broccoli, cabbage, carrots) because they affect excretion of the drug and can lead to drug toxicity.
- Lidocaine (Xylocaine) should never be used for patients with severe heart block dysrhythmias, because the normal heart pacemaker is not functioning and this can lead to cardiac arrest.

- Ask patients receiving IV lidocaine about any numbness at the IV site because this can mask signs of IV infiltration.
- Always ask older adults about liver or kidney problems because class Ic antidysrhythmic drug doses may be lower in these patients.
- Be sure to monitor the respiratory status of patients taking amiodarone because ARDS and pulmonary fibrosis are possible adverse effects of this drug.
- Monitor for signs of thyroid problems such as changes in heart rate, which are more likely to occur during the first few weeks of treatment with amiodarone (Cordarone).
- Male patients may experience pain or swelling in the scrotum while taking amiodarone (Cordarone), which should be reported to the prescriber immediately.
- Adenosine must always be given by IV push rapidly over 1 to 2 seconds to be effective.

- Always have emergency equipment brought to the bedside before giving IV adenosine because of the risk of dysrhythmias and cardiac arrest.
- Magnesium sulfate is given to prevent the ventricular dysrhythmia torsades de pointes from returning after the patient's rhythm has been returned to a normal sinus rhythm.
- Anticoagulants are prescribed for abnormal heart rhythms with increased risk for clot formation such as atrial fibrillation or atrial flutter.

Additional Learning Resources

🌐 Be sure to visit your Evolve website (http://evolve.elsevier.com/Workman/pharmacology/) for additional online resources.

SG Go to your Study Guide for additional learning activities to help you master this chapter content.

Review Questions

See *Answers to In-Text Review Questions* in the back of the book for answers to these questions.

1. A patient's heart rate is regular at 68 beats per minute and the electrocardiogram (ECG) tracing shows P waves before every QRS complex. Which tissue does the nurse suspect is likely acting as the pacemaker of the heart?

   A. SA node
   B. AV node
   C. Bundle of His
   D. Purkinje fibers

2. A patient whose heart rate is 52 beats per minute reports feeling dizzy and light-headed. What is the nurse's **best first** action?

   A. Starting an IV line
   B. Asking if the patient has experienced this before
   C. Notifying the prescriber immediately
   D. Assessing the patient's blood pressure

3. A patient given atropine intravenously as a one-time dose for bradycardia now reports a very dry mouth. What is the nurse's **best response**?

   A. Notifying the prescriber immediately
   B. Documenting the report as the only action
   C. Reassuring the patient that this is a normal drug response
   D. Offering the patient the opportunity to brush his or her teeth and rinse the mouth

4. Which antidysrhythmic drugs may be given by the endotracheal tube route? **Select all that apply.**

   A. atropine
   B. digoxin
   C. epinephrine
   D. lidocaine
   E. procainamide
   F. naloxone

5. Nausea, vomiting, and an irregular heart rate develop in a patient who takes oral digoxin every morning. What is the nurse's **best** action?

   A. Giving prescribed diphenhydramine as needed
   B. Checking the laboratory results for a digoxin level

   C. Assessing the apical pulse for a full minute
   D. Interpreting the patient's cardiac monitor rhythm strip

6. A patient asks the nurse why an intravenous (IV) line must be used to receive the antidysrhythmic drug lidocaine. What is the nurse's **best response**?

   A. "The drug companies have not developed an oral form of this drug."
   B. "This drug can also be given by endotracheal tube in the ICU."
   C. "The drug in oral form would be destroyed by the liver, making it ineffective."
   D. "Your heart rate problem could become more severe, so it is important to give the drug by the fastest route."

7. An older adult patient with frequent premature ventricular contractions (PVCs) is receiving intravenous (IV) lidocaine by continuous infusion. The patient becomes confused and sees insects on the walls. What is the nurse's **best** action?

   A. Reorienting the patient to person, place, and time
   B. Asking the patient's family about alcohol use or abuse
   C. Checking the patient's chart for a history of dementia
   D. Notifying the prescriber immediately

8. A patient is to receive propafenone. What **important** question does the nurse ask the patient before giving the first dose?

   A. "Do you have any hearing problems?"
   B. "Are you having difficulty reading?"
   C. "Have you ever had a problem with bronchospasm?"
   D. "What other problems are being treated by your prescriber?"

9. Which laboratory result for a patient receiving sotalol does the nurse **immediately** report to the prescriber?

   A. Creatinine 2.4 mg/dL
   B. Potassium (K) 3.4 mEq/L
   C. Sodium (Na) 147 mEq/L
   D. Blood urea nitrogen (BUN) 21 mg/dL

10. A patient who has a history of depression is prescribed propranolol. Which precaution is **most important** for the nurse to teach the patient?

   A. "You may become more excitable and active while you are taking propranolol."

B. "While taking propranolol you may notice that your depression gets worse."

C. "Stop taking propranolol whenever you experience depression symptoms."

D. "Propranolol may cause difficulty with the ability to perform sexually."

11. A patient is prescribed an oral loading dose of amiodarone 1600 mg. Amiodarone is available in 400-mg tablets. How many tablets does the nurse give?

A. 2

B. 4

C. 6

D. 8

12. A patient prescribed amiodarone tells the nurse that his scrotum is swollen and painful. What is the nurse's **best** action?

A. Instructing the patient that this side effect is reversible and will go away over several months

B. Documenting this expected side effect as the only action

C. Supporting the patient's scrotum on a pillow

D. Holding the drug and notifying the prescriber immediately

Clinical Judgment

1. Which intended effects and common side effects will the nurse expect to assess for after a patient with supraventricular tachycardia is given an IV dose of adenosine? **Select all that apply.**

A. Increased heart rate

B. Chest pain

C. Shortness of breath

D. Wheezing

E. Facial flushing

F. Ankle swelling

G. Increased risk for ventricular fibrillation

H. Normal and regular heart rate

I. Increased number of premature ventricular contractions

J. Transient atrial dysrhythmias

2. The nurse is providing care for a 53-year-old patient with a 4-year history of symptomatic rapid atrial fibrillation. The patient has experienced five cardioversion attempts and two ablations that have not successfully managed to control the dysrhythmia. The patient's prescriber has tried controlling the dysrhythmia with beta blockers and digoxin without success. He is to be prescribed dofetilde, 250 mcg orally twice a day. Which actions or teaching points are relevant, less relevant, or not relevant for the nurse to include when teaching the patient about the care involved with implementation of administration of this drug? **Use an X to indicate which information is Relevant, Less Relevant, or Not Relevant.**

ACTION/TEACHING POINT	RELEVANT	LESS RELEVANT	NOT RELEVANT
Informing the patient of the increased risk for torsades de pointes			
Explaining that dofetilde is used to treat all tachydysrhythmias			
Placing the patient on a cardiac monitor for 72 hr			
Documenting the patient's heart rhythm every 2 hr			
Inserting a urinary catheter to monitor urine output for 3 days			
Instructing the patient to report any chest pain			
Instructing the patient to drink at least 2 L of fluid daily			
Asking if the patient has a history of kidney problems			
Checking laboratory kidney function test results			
Inserting an IV catheter to give the drug IV			

Drug Therapy for High Blood Lipids

Learning Objectives

The content presented in this chapter should help you to:

1. Explain how antihyperlipidemic drugs work to lower blood lipid levels.
2. Describe the common names, actions, usual adult dosages, possible side effects, and adverse effects of statins, bile acid sequestrants, cholesterol absorption inhibitors, and fibrate drugs.
3. Discuss the priority actions to take before and after giving drugs to lower blood lipid levels.
4. Prioritize essential information to teach patients taking drugs to lower blood lipid levels.
5. Describe life span considerations for drugs to lower blood lipid levels.
6. List the common names, actions, usual adult dosages, possible side effects, and adverse effects of nicotinic acid.
7. Discuss the priority actions to take before and after giving nicotinic acid.
8. Prioritize essential information to teach patients nicotinic acid.
9. Describe life span considerations for nicotinic acid.

Key Terms

antihyperlipidemics (ăn-tī-hī-pŭr-lĭp-DĒ-mĭks) (p. 287) Drugs that work against high levels of lipids (fats) in the blood.

bile acid sequestrants (BĪ-ŭl ĂS-ĭd sĕ-KWĔS-trĕnts) (p. 290) Cholesterol-lowering drugs that bind with cholesterol-containing bile acids in the intestines and remove them via bowel movements.

cholesterol absorption inhibitors (kō-LĔS-tŭr-ŏl ăb-SŌRP-shŭn ĭn-HĬB-ĭ-tŭrz) (p. 291) Cholesterol-lowering drugs that prevent the uptake of cholesterol from the small intestine into the circulatory system.

fibrates (FĪ-brāts) (p. 293) Lipid-lowering drugs that are used primarily to lower triglycerides and, to less extent, low-density lipoprotein (LDL) ("bad") cholesterol.

nicotinic acid (nĭ-kō-TĬN-ĭk ĂS-ĭd) (p. 294) Special type of vitamin B that helps to decrease blood cholesterol levels.

statins (STĂ-tĭnz) (p. 288) A class of drugs used to lower LDL ("bad") cholesterol and triglycerides by inhibiting their production by the body.

REVIEW OF RELATED PHYSIOLOGY AND PATHOPHYSIOLOGY

Cholesterol is a fatty, waxy material that the body needs to function. It is present in cell membranes everywhere in the body. It is used to produce hormones, vitamin D, and bile acids that help digest fat. A person needs some cholesterol for important body functions. Cholesterol is produced by the liver, and it is in the foods that you eat (Figure 16.1). However, your body needs only a small amount of cholesterol; too much in the bloodstream contributes to the development of narrowed arteries such as atherosclerosis and coronary artery disease. The chemical form of most fats in foods and the human body is *triglycerides*. Both cholesterol and triglycerides are present in the blood, making up the plasma lipids.

A high level of blood fats (plasma lipoproteins) is called *hyperlipidemia*. Table 16.1 lists the normal values for a patient's lipid profile. A high level of triglycerides in the blood is called *hypertriglyceridemia*. Chronic hyperlipidemia can lead to many health problems, including:

- Atherosclerosis
- Coronary artery disease (angina, heart attack)
- Hypertension
- Pancreatitis
- Peripheral vascular disease, which leads to organ damage or impairment

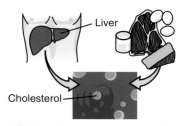

FIG. 16.1 Cholesterol is produced by the liver, but it is also consumed in meat and dairy products.

Table **16.1**	Lipid Profile Normal Values	
TYPE OF LIPID	**NORMAL VALUE**
Total cholesterol	<200 mg/dL
Low-density lipoprotein (LDL)	60–180 mg/dL
Very-low-density lipoprotein (VLDL)	25%–50%
High-density lipoprotein (HDL)	Male: >45 mg/dL Female: >55 mg/dL
Triglycerides	Male: 40–160 mg/dL
	Female: 35–135 mg/dL

- Stroke
- Xanthomas (skin atheromas—abnormal fat deposits)

CORONARY ARTERY DISEASE

The coronary arteries supply blood, oxygen, and nutrients to the heart muscle (myocardium) (Animation 16.1). Atherosclerosis, a major contributor to development of coronary artery disease, begins by forming a fatty streak on an arterial wall, leading to fat buildup (plaques). Fat buildup in the walls of coronary arteries can result in partial or complete blockage of blood flow to the heart muscle (Figure 16.2). The main lipids involved are cholesterol and triglycerides. Partial blockage in the coronary arteries can result in chest pain *(angina)*; complete blockage can result in heart attack *(myocardial infarction)*. Table 16.2 summarizes lipid levels related to the risk of developing coronary artery disease (CAD).

FAMILIAL HYPERLIPIDEMIA

Some people develop high blood fat levels that are related to genetic or inherited factors. This is called *familial hyperlipidemia* or sometimes *familial hypercholesterolemia*. The liver makes too much cholesterol and other fats, which lead to increased levels of fats in the blood and the development of atherosclerosis. The reason for this condition is not completely clear; however, it tends to occur in families. For people who have a genetic factor leading to hyperlipidemia, simply reducing fatty foods does not help lower blood lipid levels and antilipidemic drugs (lipid-lowering drugs) are prescribed to lower them.

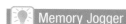
Memory Jogger

High blood lipid levels may result from genetic factors (familial hyperlipidemia).

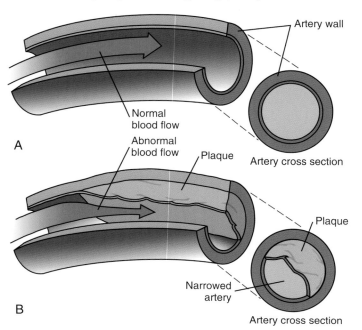

FIG. 16.2 Cholesterol can form plaques that narrow arteries. (A) Normal, clean artery. (B) Artery with plaque formation.

Table 16.2	Lipid Values and Risk for Coronary Artery Disease	
LIPID	**VALUE (mg/dL)**	**RISK FOR CORONARY ARTERY DISEASE**
Total cholesterol	<200	Low
	200–239	Borderline high
	>239	High
HDL ("good" cholesterol)	>35	Low
	<35	High
LDL ("bad" cholesterol)	<129	Low
	130–159	Borderline high
	>159	High
Triglycerides	<200	Low
	201–399	Borderline high
	400–1000	High
	>1000	Very high

HDL, High-density lipoprotein; *LDL,* low-density lipoprotein.

Antihyperlipidemic drugs, also called lipid-lowering drugs, work to decrease the levels of lipids in the blood. Some lipid-lowering drugs work to decrease the production of cholesterol in the body and increase the ability of the liver to remove the "bad" cholesterol *(low-density lipoprotein [LDL]).* Others reduce the amount of fat from food that the body absorbs. Still others bind with cholesterol-containing bile acids in the intestines and promote cholesterol loss in the stool. These drugs along with diet changes (e.g., decreased intake of fat) are used to reduce the amount of certain fats and cholesterol in the blood. While a person is taking a lipid-lowering drug, regular exercise (e.g., walking, swimming) helps to increase the level of *high-density lipoproteins (HDLs),* or the "good" cholesterol.

 Memory Jogger

Low-density lipoprotein (LDL) = "bad" cholesterol

High-density lipoprotein (HDL) = "good" cholesterol

GENERAL ISSUES FOR LIPID-LOWERING DRUGS

When lifestyle changes such as reduced-fat diets, increased exercise, smoking cessation, and weight loss fail to decrease high blood lipid levels, lipid-lowering drugs are most often used to treat high blood lipid levels. If these changes do not result in lower blood lipid levels, patients remain at risk for development of heart disease, especially in the presence of other risk factors such as high blood pressure (hypertension) and diabetes.

Lipid-lowering drugs may be prescribed for high total cholesterol or triglyceride levels, high levels of LDLs ("bad" cholesterol), or low levels of HDLs ("good" cholesterol). Some health problems for which these drugs are prescribed include:

 Memory Jogger

Lipid-lowering drugs are often used when lifestyle changes fail to treat high blood lipid levels.

- Coronary artery disease (heart disease)
- Hypertension
- Stroke

Several classes of drugs affect blood lipid levels. Each class has both common and different actions and effects. Responsibilities for the common actions and effects are listed in the following paragraphs. Specific responsibilities related to specific drugs are listed with the discussion of each lipid-lowering drug class.

✪ PRIORITY ACTIONS TO TAKE *BEFORE* GIVING ANY LIPID-LOWERING DRUG

Before giving any lipid-lowering drug, obtain a complete list of drugs that the patient is currently taking, including herbal and over-the-counter drugs. Ask women of childbearing age if they are pregnant, planning to become pregnant, or breastfeeding, because adequate lipids are important in prenatal life and during early childhood for good brain development. Check patient histories for liver or muscle problems.

Before giving the first dose, be sure that the patient has baseline blood lipid and liver function tests drawn. Check his or her lipid blood tests *(lipid profile)* (see Table 16.1) and liver function tests (see Table 1.4 in Chapter 1). Notify the prescriber about any abnormal results.

Critical Point for Safety

Be sure to monitor liver function blood test results because most lipid-lowering drugs can cause liver damage (hepatotoxicity).

QSEN: Safety

 Critical Point for Safety

Instruct patients to fast (no eating or drinking) for at least 8 hours before a lipid profile blood test is obtained for results to be accurate.

QSEN: Safety

 Memory Jogger

All lipid-lowering drugs reduce high blood lipid levels, but they do **not** cure the problem; treatment is long term, and these drugs must be taken even after blood fat levels are normal.

 Memory Jogger

The five types of lipid-lowering drugs are:
- Statins
- Bile acid sequestrants
- Cholesterol absorption inhibitors
- Fibrates
- Nicotinic acid

⊛ PRIORITY ACTIONS TO TAKE *AFTER* GIVING ANY LIPID-LOWERING DRUG

After giving any lipid-lowering drug, be sure to notify the prescriber if liver function laboratory tests are elevated. Ask patients about symptoms of muscle damage such as soreness, pain, or weakness because some lipid-lowering drugs can reduce muscle function. Assess patients for signs of liver damage, including jaundice, dark urine, or light-colored stools.

⊛ TEACHING PRIORITIES FOR PATIENTS TAKING LIPID-LOWERING DRUGS

- Be sure to continue lifestyle changes that help lower cholesterol such as a low-fat diet, exercise, and weight control.
- Check with your prescriber before using any over-the-counter drugs.
- Avoid eating or drinking for 8 hours before having follow-up laboratory tests drawn (lipid profile, liver function tests), because these test results can be changed by substances in some foods and fluids. Remember that these blood tests must be repeated every 3 to 6 months to monitor the effectiveness of your prescribed lipid-lowering drugs.
- If you are a female patient of childbearing years, inform your prescriber if you are pregnant, plan to become pregnant, or are at risk of becoming pregnant.
- Remember that all lipid-lowering drugs reduce high blood lipid levels but that they do **not** cure the problem. Treatment is long term, and these drugs must be taken even after blood lipid levels are normal.
- Take the drug exactly as prescribed because this ensures the best result.
- Report signs and symptoms of decreased liver function, muscle problems, or changes in urine output to your prescriber.

TYPES OF LIPID-LOWERING DRUGS

There are five main types of lipid-lowering drugs. The group most commonly used is the "statins" (HMG CoA reductase inhibitors). They control the rate of cholesterol produced by the liver. The other drug types include bile acid sequestrants, cholesterol absorption inhibitors, fibrates, and nicotinic acid.

STATINS

How Statins Work

Statins inhibit HMG CoA reductase (HMGCR 3-hydroxy-3-methylglutaryl-CoA reductase), an enzyme that controls cholesterol production in the liver. They lower blood lipid levels by slowing the production of cholesterol and increasing the ability of the liver to remove LDL cholesterol from the blood. Statins are the most effective group of these drugs for lowering LDL cholesterol. Short-acting statins (e.g., lovastatin, simvastatin) work best when taken in the evening. Long-acting statins (e.g., atorvastatin, rosuvastatin) work well when taken either in the morning or evening. Be sure to consult a reliable drug resource for more information on any specific statin.

Adult Dosages for Commonly Prescribed Statins

Drug Category	Drug Name	Usual Maintenance Dose
Statins: Long Acting	atorvastatin (Lipitor)	10–80 mg orally once daily—May be taken at any time during the day without regard to meals
	fluvastatin (Lescol, Lescol XL)	20–40 mg orally once daily at bedtime or twice daily extended-release (XL)—20—80 mg once daily
	pitavastatin (Livalo, NIKITA, Zypitamag)	2–4 mg orally once daily. Max: 40 mg/day
	rosuvastatin (Crestor, Ezallor)	5–40 mg orally once daily **Special Considerations: Start with low dose of 5 mg/day**
Statins: Short Acting	lovastatin (Altoprev, Mevacor)	20–80 mg orally once daily with evening meal or in 2 divided doses
	pravastatin (Pravachol)	10–80 mg orally once daily
	simvastatin (FloLipid, Zocor)	5–40 mg orally once daily in the evening

Intended Responses of Statins
- Total cholesterol is decreased.
- Triglycerides are decreased.
- LDL is decreased.

Common Side Effects of Statins
Statins rarely have side effects. Upset stomach, gas, constipation, abdominal pain, and cramps may occur. These symptoms are usually mild and disappear as the body adjusts to the drug. Other side effects include musculoskeletal discomfort and liver problems.

Possible Adverse Effects of Statins
Patients may develop *rhabdomyolysis* (muscle breakdown). Signs and symptoms of rhabdomyolysis include general muscle soreness, muscle pain and weakness, vomiting, stomach pain, and brown urine. The urine turns brown because small reddish-brown pieces of broken-down muscle are removed from the body through the urine.

Statins may cause decreased liver function. Because of this danger, the prescriber monitors liver function tests regularly (every 3 to 6 months). These tests are important because early, mild liver problems do not cause symptoms. Late symptoms of liver disease include yellowing (*jaundice*) of the skin, whites of the eyes, and roof of the mouth; pain over the liver on the right side just below the ribs; darkened urine; and pale gray-colored stools. The bile and bilirubin made by the liver normally leave the body in the stool, giving stool a medium-to-dark brown color. When the liver is not working well, these products do not reach the stool, so the stool becomes a light gray or green instead of brown. The bilirubin then enters the urine, turning it dark, and gets into skin and mucous membranes, turning them yellow.

✪ Priority Actions to Take *Before* Giving Statins
In addition to the general priority actions to take before giving any lipid-lowering drug (p. 287), check the patient's baseline kidney function tests (blood urea nitrogen [BUN] and creatinine) because kidney failure can be a side effect of rhabdomyolysis. See Table 1.5 in Chapter 1 for normal values of kidney function tests.

Ask patients about their alcohol consumption. Statins should not be given to patients who consume more than two alcoholic drinks per day, because drinking alcohol puts even more stress on the liver.

✪ Priority Actions to Take *After* Giving Statins
In addition to the general priority actions to take after giving any lipid-lowering drug (p. 288), regularly assess the patient for signs and symptoms of decreased liver function or muscle breakdown, including constant fatigue, itchy skin, general weakness, and jaundice (yellowish color of the skin and sclera). Report these signs and symptoms to the prescriber immediately.

Be sure to monitor the patient's urine output. Renal failure can occur if rhabdomyolysis develops, because protein released from broken-down muscle can block urine flow through the kidneys. Continue to check the patient's BUN and creatinine levels.

✪ Teaching Priorities for Patients Taking Statins
In addition to the general precautions related to taking any lipid-lowering drug (p. 288), include these teaching points and precautions:
- Take your prescribed drug exactly as directed. Some statins should be taken in the evening (e.g., short acting), some once a day without regard for meals (e.g., long acting), and some may be taken twice a day.
- If you are an older adult contact your prescriber if you notice any new muscle weakness, muscle aches, or joint aches. Do not assume that muscle ache or weakness is related to aging. It could be an indication of the adverse reaction rhabdomyolysis.
- Do not drink grapefruit juice or eat grapefruit, because these foods contain an enzyme that interferes with statin activity.

 Memory Jogger

The generic names of HMG CoA reductase inhibitors ("statins") all end in "-statin" (e.g., atorvastatin, rosuvastatin, simvastatin).

 Do Not Confuse

Zocor *with* Cozaar
An order for Zocor may be confused with Cozaar. Zocor is a lipid-lowering statin, whereas Cozaar is a blood pressure–lowering angiotensin II receptor antagonist.

QSEN: Safety

Common Side Effects

Statins

Abdominal discomfort

Liver problems

Musculoskeletal discomfort

 Critical Point for Safety

After a patient begins taking a statin drug, be sure to monitor for signs of rhabdomyolysis such as general muscle soreness or pain and vomiting, stomach pain, and brown urine.

QSEN: Safety

Life Span Considerations for Statins

Pediatric considerations. Statin use in older children is rare but may be prescribed for children with familial hypercholesterolemia.

Considerations for pregnancy and lactation. Statins drugs have a high likelihood of increasing the risk for birth defects or fetal damage. They should not be given to women who are pregnant, plan to become pregnant, or are breastfeeding. Statins decrease the amount of fat in the body. Fat is essential to brain development in the fetus and infant. When there is not enough fat in the body during pregnancy and infancy, the fetus can suffer poor brain development and mental retardation.

Considerations for older adults. Statin drugs are safe for use in older adults if there is no history of muscle problems (myopathy) or liver disease.

BILE ACID SEQUESTRANTS

How Bile Acid Sequestrants Work

The class of lipid-lowering drugs called **bile acid sequestrants** helps the body absorb less dietary cholesterol so that more cholesterol gets excreted. The drugs are taken by mouth and work directly on dietary fats in the intestine. They bind with cholesterol in the intestine, preventing the fats from being absorbed into the blood. This action then eliminates the cholesterol from the body through the stool. Be sure to check a reliable drug resource for more information on any specific bile acid sequestrant drug.

Adult Dosages for Commonly Prescribed Bile Acid Sequestrants

Drug Category	Drug Name	Usual Maintenance Dose
Bile Acid Sequestrants	cholestyramine (Lo-CHOLEST, Prevalite, Questran, Questran Light)	4–16 g orally in 2 divided doses with meals
	colesevelam (Welchol)	1.875 g PO twice daily or 3.75 g orally once daily. Oral suspension: One 3.75-g packet orally once daily. Dissolve each packet in 8 ounces of water, fruit juice, or diet soda, and administer with a meal
	colestipol (Colestid)	Granules: 5–20 g/day orally in 2–4 divided doses. Max 30 g/day Tablets: 2 g orally 1–2 times daily; may be increased monthly up to 16 g day in 1–2 doses

Intended Responses for Bile Acid Sequestrants
• LDL cholesterol level is decreased.
• HDL cholesterol level is increased.

Common Side Effects of Bile Acid Sequestrants
Side effects of bile acid sequestrants are rarely serious. The most common side effects are gastrointestinal symptoms, including constipation, bloating, nausea, vomiting, and gas.

Possible Adverse Effects of Bile Acid Sequestrants
Bile acid sequestrants decrease the ability of the body to absorb oral drugs. They also reduce intestinal absorption of fat-soluble vitamins (A, D, E, and K), so patients may need to take a daily vitamin supplement. Bile acid sequestrants may change the action of the anticoagulant warfarin (Coumadin) in two ways. They can decrease the absorption of vitamin K, which would intensify the effects of warfarin and increase

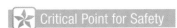
★ Critical Point for Safety

Women who are pregnant or breastfeeding should not take statin drugs.

QSEN: Safety

Common Side Effects
Bile Acid Sequestrants

Abdominal discomfort, Nausea/Vomiting, Constipation, Gas

the risk for bleeding. Bile acid sequestrants can also directly bind warfarin in the intestinal tract and cause its rapid elimination. This inactivates the activity of warfarin and increases the risk of clot formation. Therefore it is always important to monitor the international normalized ratio (INR) of a patient taking both warfarin and bile acid sequestrants.

Priority Actions to Take *Before* Giving Bile Acid Sequestrants

In addition to the general priority actions to take before giving any lipid-lowering drug (p. 287), do not give any bile acid sequestrants within 2 hours after giving any other oral drug, because these drugs can inhibit the absorption of other drugs.

Ask patients whether they are experiencing constipation. This is a very common side effect of the drug and can make the patient uncomfortable. Check whether the patient is prescribed warfarin (Coumadin).

Priority Actions to Take *After* Giving Bile Acid Sequestrants

In addition to the general priorities to take after giving any lipid-lowering drug (p. 288), after giving a bile acid sequestrant, assess the patient for gastrointestinal symptoms such as constipation, bloating, gas, nausea, or vomiting.

If the patient is also taking warfarin, monitor for signs of bleeding such as easy bruising, clammy skin, pale skin, dizziness, increased heart rate, decreased blood pressure, shortness of breath, or confusion. Monitor INRs for changes that are higher or lower than the patient's prescribed therapeutic range. Give vitamin supplements if prescribed.

Continue to monitor the patient for constipation.

Teaching Priorities for Patients Taking Bile Acid Sequestrants

In addition to the general teaching priorities related to taking any lipid-lowering drug (p. 288), include these teaching points and precautions:

- Take bile acid sequestrants with meals because they work by binding cholesterol present in your food while it is in the intestinal tract and prevent you from absorbing it.
- Do not to take other drugs for at least 2 hours before or 4 to 6 hours after bile acid sequestrants because bile acid sequestrants may interfere with absorption of other drugs.
- Mix the powder forms of bile acid sequestrants with 4 to 6 ounces of fruit juice or water.
- Drink at least 12 to 16 ounces of water when you take the tablet form of the drug to prevent stomach and intestinal problems such as bowel obstruction.
- Report any signs and symptoms of bowel obstruction, including abdominal pain, bloating, vomiting, and diarrhea or constipation to your prescriber.
- These drugs may be prescribed along with a statin drug to reduce cholesterol level further.

Life Span Considerations for Bile Acid Sequestrants

Pediatric considerations. Cholestyramine (Questran) and colestipol (Colestid) should be avoided in children because they can cause intestinal obstructions.

Considerations for pregnancy and lactation. Bile acid sequestrants have a low to moderate likelihood of increasing the risk for birth defects or fetal damage. The value of lowering cholesterol levels during pregnancy is controversial because the fetus needs a constant level of cholesterol for brain development.

CHOLESTEROL ABSORPTION INHIBITORS

How Cholesterol Absorption Inhibitors Work

Cholesterol absorption inhibitors are used when a low-fat, low-cholesterol diet does not control blood cholesterol levels. These drugs work to reduce the amount of cholesterol absorbed by the body. They are useful for patients who cannot take statin drugs because of side effects. They may also be used with statin drugs to increase the

 Critical Point for Safety

Always ask patients about constipation before administering bile acid sequestrants because these drugs can cause constipation.

QSEN: Safety

 Critical Point for Safety

When a patient is taking a bile acid sequestrant drug and warfarin, monitor for signs of bleeding.

QSEN: Safety

 Critical Point for Safety

Bile acid sequestrants should be taken 2 hr before or 2 hr after antacids for better absorption.

QSEN: Safety

cholesterol-lowering effects. Be sure to consult a reliable drug resource for more information on a specific cholesterol absorption inhibitor.

Adult Dosages for Commonly Prescribed Cholesterol Absorption Inhibitors

Drug Category	Drug Name	Usual Maintenance Dose
Cholesterol Absorption Inhibitors	ezetimibe (Zetia)	10 g orally once daily

Intended Responses for Cholesterol Absorption Inhibitors
- Level of LDL cholesterol is decreased.
- Level of total cholesterol is decreased.

Common Side Effects of Cholesterol Absorption Inhibitors
Common side effects of cholesterol absorption inhibitors include gastrointestinal discomforts such as stomach pain and diarrhea. Other common side effects include fatigue, back pain, joint pain, rash, and sinusitis.

Fenofibrate (Tricor), gemfibrozil (Lopid), and cyclosporine increase blood levels of ezetimibe (Zetia).

Possible Adverse Effects of Cholesterol Absorption Inhibitors
Angioedema is a rare adverse effect of ezetimibe. Angioedema is swelling beneath the skin, usually around the eyes, nose, and lips, caused by blood vessel dilation (see Figure 1.6 in Chapter 1). Swelling may be life threatening when it affects the airways.

⊛ Priority Actions to Take *Before* Giving Cholesterol Absorption Inhibitors
In addition to the general priority actions to take before giving any lipid-lowering drug (p. 287), ask if the patient has a history of liver disease or muscle disorders. Also check his or her liver function tests (Table 1.4 in Chapter 1) because the use of this drug may worsen liver disease when prescribed with a statin drug.

⊛ Priority Actions to Take *After* Giving Cholesterol Absorption Inhibitors
In addition to the general priority actions to take after giving any lipid-lowering drug (p. 288), check the patient for signs of decreased liver function such as decreased appetite, fatigue, jaundice, weakness, or muscle problems, including aches and pains. Monitor for fatigue or abdominal pain.

Monitor the patient for facial swelling, which may be an indicator of the adverse effect of angioedema. If this problem develops, hold the next dose and notify the prescriber immediately.

⊛ Priority Teaching for Patients Taking Cholesterol Absorption Inhibitors
In addition to the general teaching priorities for patients taking any antihyperlipidemic drug (p. 288), include these teaching points and precautions:
- Report any muscle pain, tenderness, or weakness to your prescriber.
- Take the drug once a day at the same time every day. Not only does this habit help you to remember to take the drug, but it also can help make the timing of any intestinal symptoms from the drug more predictable.
- If you are prescribed to take a statin or bile acid sequestrant drug, your cholesterol absorption inhibitor can be taken at the same time as a statin drug but should be taken at least 2 hours before or 4 hours after a bile acid sequestrants.
- You should go to the nearest emergency department or call 911 if you develop swelling of the face or tongue or start to have difficulty breathing or swallowing. These are signs of angioedema, a serious adverse reaction.

Life Span Considerations for Cholesterol Absorption Inhibitors
Considerations for pregnancy and lactation. Ezetimibe has a moderate likelihood of increasing the risk for birth defects or fetal damage, and safe use of this drug during pregnancy has not been established. During breastfeeding, this drug should only be

---

Common Side Effects
Cholesterol Absorption Inhibitors

Abdominal discomfort,
Diarrhea

Fatigue

Joint pain

Rash

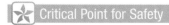
Critical Point for Safety

Teach patients to go to the nearest emergency department or call 911 if swelling of the face or tongue occurs or if they develop difficulty breathing or swallowing.

QSEN: Safety

used if the benefits outweigh possible risks to the infant because it is not known if ezetimibe passes into breast milk.

FIBRATES

How Fibrates Work

Fibrates activate cell lipid receptors that bind to and collect cholesterol and other lipids from the blood and break them down for elimination. The main effects of fibrates are to decrease blood triglyceride levels and cause a mild increase in HDL ("good" cholesterol). These drugs decrease liver production of triglycerides and increase the use of triglycerides by the fat tissues for metabolism. Fibrates are the best class of these drugs for lowering triglyceride levels. They also increase cholesterol excretion in bile. Be sure to consult a reliable drug resource for more information on a specific fibrate drug.

Adult Dosages for Commonly Prescribed Fibrates

Drug Category	Drug Name	Usual Maintenance Dose
Fibrates	fenofibrate (Antara, Lipofen, Tricor)	**For severe hypertriglyceridemia:** Antara capsules: 30–90 mg orally once daily Lipofen capsules: 67–200 mg orally once daily Tricor tablets: 48 or 145 mg orally once daily **For primary hypercholesterolemia:** Antara: 90 mg orally once daily Lipofen: 150 mg orally once daily Tricor: 145 mg orally once daily
	gemfibrozil (Lopid)	600 mg orally twice daily *Special Considerations:* **Give 30 min before morning and evening meal**

Intended Responses of Fibrates

- Triglycerides are decreased.
- HDL cholesterol is mildly increased.

Common Side Effects of Fibrates

The side effects of fibrates are usually mild. The most common side effects are stomach upset and diarrhea. Other common side effects include gastrointestinal discomfort such as indigestion or heartburn (dyspepsia) and nausea. Patients may also experience muscle weakness, headache, pruritus, and rash.

Possible Adverse Effects of Fibrates

In the patient with kidney disease, fibrates may cause increased creatinine levels. Fibrates increase cholesterol loss in bile, which may lead to the development of cholesterol-based gallstones. Bleeding can also occur in the patient taking fibrates.

Gemfibrozil (Lopid) interferes with the breakdown of statin drugs, causing higher levels of statins in the blood. This can lead to statin side effects, such as muscle damage, muscle weakness, rhabdomyolysis, or liver damage.

⍟ Priority Actions to Take *Before* Giving Fibrates

In addition to the general priority actions to take before giving any lipid-lowering drug (p. 287), ask patients about a history of kidney, liver, or gallbladder disease. Check whether the patient is also prescribed warfarin. Check baseline kidney and liver functions tests (Tables 1.4 and 1.5 in Chapter 1).

⍟ Priority Actions to Take *After* Giving Fibrates

In addition to the general priority actions to take after giving any lipid-lowering drug (p. 288), monitor the patient for indications of kidney, liver, or gallbladder

Common Side Effects
Fibrates

Abdominal discomfort, Diarrhea

Musculoskeletal discomfort

Headache

Rash

⍟ **Critical Point for Safety**

Fibrates can increase the effectiveness of warfarin (Coumadin) by causing a prolonged prothrombin time, which can lead to excessive bleeding.

QSEN: Safety

disease such as changes in urine output, decreased appetite, fatigue, weakness, nausea, and vomiting.

If the patient is also taking warfarin (Coumadin), monitor for signs of bleeding such as easy bruising, clammy skin, paleness, dizziness, increased heart rate, decreased blood pressure, shortness of breath, and confusion.

Remind the patient that his or her prescriber will check liver and kidney function laboratory tests periodically.

⊛ Teaching Priorities for Patients Taking Fibrates

In addition to the general teaching priorities related to taking any lipid-lowering drug (p. 288), include these teaching points and precautions:

- Take fibrates 30 minutes before meals. These drugs are usually given before the morning and evening meals.
- Avoid heavy alcohol use (more than two drinks per day).
- Do **not** drink grapefruit juice or eat grapefruit with fibrates because these contain an enzyme that interferes with the drug's action.
- If you are also taking warfarin, be sure to report any signs or symptoms of bleeding to your prescriber (e.g., easy bruising, clammy skin, pale skin, dizziness, increased heart rate, decreased blood pressure, shortness of breath, or confusion).

Life Span Considerations for Fibrates

Considerations for pregnancy and lactation. Fibrates have a moderate likelihood of increasing the risk for birth defects or fetal damage. Fibrates can cross the placenta and affect fetal brain development.

Considerations for older adults. Older adults are more likely to be taking the drug warfarin (Coumadin) and are at greater risk for bleeding problems. In addition to assessing themselves for signs and symptoms of bleeding, it is important that the INR be tested as prescribed. Remind the older adult to keep all appointments for INR testing.

NICOTINIC ACID AGENTS

How Nicotinic Acid Agents Work

Nicotinic acid (niacin) is a special type of vitamin B that helps to decrease triglyceride, total cholesterol, and LDL cholesterol levels. It also helps to increase HDL cholesterol. Nicotinic acid is given in doses much higher than the normal daily requirement when it is used to lower cholesterol. The effects of niacin are well known. The drug action that leads to the lipid-lowering effect works by blocking the enzyme responsible for making cholesterol in the liver. Be sure to consult a reliable drug resource for more information about a specific form of niacin.

Adult Dosages for Commonly Prescribed Nicotinic Acid Agents

Drug Category	Drug Name	Usual Maintenance Dose
Nicotinic Acid Agents	niacin (Niacor) immediate-release	1.5–3 g/day orally, given in 2–3 divided doses, with or after meals ***Special Considerations:* Do not exceed 6 g daily**
	niacin (Niaspan, Slo-Niacin) extended-release	1000–2000 mg orally once daily at bedtime

Intended Responses of Nicotinic Acid Agents

- Total cholesterol level is decreased.
- Total triglyceride level is decreased.
- LDL cholesterol level is decreased.
- HDL cholesterol level is increased.

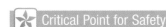

★ Critical Point for Safety

Patients should not drink grapefruit juice while taking fibrates because it interferes with the metabolism (breakdown) of fibrates in the body, making them less effective.

QSEN: Safety

Common Side Effects of Nicotinic Acid Agents

Nicotinic acid agents may cause many side effects. The most common are itching and nasal inflammation because the drug makes blood vessels dilate.

Other common side effects include gastrointestinal symptoms such as nausea, indigestion, gas, vomiting, diarrhea, and abdominal pain. The patient may also experience flushing (redness) and hot flashes, chills, dizziness, fainting, headaches, rapid heart rate (tachycardia), shortness of breath (dyspnea), sweating (diaphoresis), and swelling caused by fluid retention.

Possible Adverse Effects of Nicotinic Acid Agents

Liver problems, including toxicity, can occur, although liver failure is rare. Gout (painful swelling and redness of the toes, feet, or ankles) can occur because of a buildup of excess uric acid and calcium. Other adverse effects can include high blood sugar (hyperglycemia) and stomach ulcer flare-up. Nicotinic acid preparations are contraindicated for people who have hypertension, peptic ulcer disease, or any other active bleeding.

⊛ Priority Actions to Take *Before* Giving Nicotinic Acid Agents

In addition to the general priority actions taken before giving any lipid-lowering drug (p. 287), obtain baseline vital signs, including blood pressure and heart rate. Also check a baseline blood sugar level for patients with diabetes. Be sure to check baseline liver function tests (Table 1.4 in Chapter 1) such as AST and ALT.

To prevent common side effects such as flushing and hot flashes, give aspirin 325 mg orally as prescribed, 15 to 60 minutes before administering nicotinic acid.

Find out whether patients have a history of liver disease or diabetes. Ask them about their usual alcohol intake. Also ask if they have ever had gout.

⊛ Priority Actions to Take *After* Giving Nicotinic Acid Agents

In addition to the general priority actions taken after giving any lipid-lowering drug (p. 288), follow these specific responsibilities after giving nicotinic acid agents.

Notify the prescriber if liver function laboratory tests are elevated or if elevations of these tests are associated with nausea, vomiting, or weakness. Liver function tests that are three times the upper limits of normal indicate that the drug may need to be discontinued. (See Table 1.4 in Chapter 1 for normal liver function ranges.)

Check the patient's heart rate and blood pressure, and notify the prescriber about any changes. Flushing or hot flashes can be reduced by the use of aspirin or nonsteroidal antiinflammatory drugs (NSAIDs) 15 to 60 minutes before taking nicotinic acid or by taking nicotinic acid during or after meals. Monitor blood glucose levels regularly for patients with diabetes, because nicotinic acid can increase serum glucose levels.

⊛ Priority Teaching for Patients Taking Nicotinic Acid Agents

In addition to the general priority teaching related to taking any antihyperlipidemic drug (p. 288), include these teaching points and precautions:

- Nicotinic acid dosage is usually started low and gradually increased.
- Notify your prescriber for any side effects or signs and symptoms of adverse effects to nicotinic acid.
- If you are also prescribed a statin drug, be sure to notify your prescriber about any muscle pain, tenderness, or weakness.
- Take nicotinic acid agents with meals or snacks to decrease any gastrointestinal side effects.
- If you are also prescribed a bile acid sequestrants with a nicotinic acid agent, be sure to take these drugs 4 to 6 hours apart.
- If your prescriber agrees, take a 325-mg aspirin tablet 15 to 60 minutes before the drug to prevent flushing or hot flashes.
- Do not substitute a sustained-release form of the drug for an immediate-release form. Extended-release forms of the drug should be swallowed whole and never crushed or chewed.

Common Side Effects
Nicotinic Acid Agents

Itchiness

Abdominal discomfort

Headache

Tachycardia

Dizziness

Nasal inflammation

 Critical Point for Safety

If prescribed, give aspirin 325 mg 15–60 min before nicotinic acid to prevent flushing and hot flashes.

QSEN: Safety

 Critical Point for Safety

Monitor glucose levels regularly for a patient with diabetes, because nicotinic acid agents can increase serum glucose levels.

QSEN: Safety

 Critical Point for Safety

Extended-release forms of nicotinic acid drugs should never be crushed or mixed with water because crushing the drug causes immediate release of the entire drug dose and could lead to an overdose.

QSEN: Safety

- If you have diabetes, remember that nicotinic acid may increase blood glucose levels. Doses of the drugs prescribed to control your blood glucose may need to be increased.
- Before any surgery or dental work, your surgeon or dentist should be notified that you are taking a nicotinic acid agent, because this drug can slow the clotting process and excessive bleeding can occur. These problems are made worse if you are also taking aspirin or an NSAID daily along with a nicotinic acid agent.

Life Span Considerations for Nicotinic Acid Agents

Considerations for pregnancy and lactation. Nicotinic acid has a moderate likelihood of increasing the risk for birth defects or fetal damage. It is secreted in breast milk. If a woman plans to breastfeed, she should avoid breastfeeding or discontinue the nicotinic acid agent to prevent the newborn from receiving large amounts of nicotinic acid.

Get Ready for the NCLEX® Examination!

Key Points

- Low-density lipoproteins (LDLs) are the "bad" lipids, and high-density lipoproteins (HDLs) are the "good" protective lipids.
- Hyperlipidemia (high level of fats in the blood) can lead to cardiovascular disease.
- Familial hyperlipidemia is a form of high blood fat that is related to genetic or inherited factors.
- Be sure to monitor liver function blood test results because most antihyperlipidemic drugs can cause liver damage (hepatotoxicity).
- Instruct patients to fast (no eating or drinking) for at least 8 hours before a lipid profile blood test is obtained.
- All lipid-lowering drugs reduce high blood lipid levels, but they do not cure the problem; treatment is long term, and these drugs must be taken even after blood fat levels are normal.
- The major types of lipid-lowering drugs include statins, bile acid sequestrants, cholesterol absorption inhibitors, nicotinic acid agents, and fibrates.
- Lipid-lowering drugs should not be given if a woman is pregnant or plans to become pregnant.
- Muscle breakdown (rhabdomyolysis) is a rare but serious adverse effect of statin drugs that can lead to kidney failure.
- After a patient begins taking a statin drug, be sure to monitor for signs of rhabdomyolysis such as general muscle soreness or pain.
- Bile acid sequestrants can increase the action of warfarin (Coumadin) and cause excessive bleeding.
- If administering a bile acid sequestrant to a patient taking warfarin (Coumadin), be prepared to administer vitamin K, the antidote for warfarin.
- Bile acid sequestrants should be taken 2 hours before or 2 hours after antacids for better absorption.

- Teach patients to go to the nearest emergency department or call 911 if swelling of the face or tongue occurs.
- Fibrates can increase the effectiveness of warfarin (Coumadin) by causing a prolonged prothrombin time, which can lead to excessive bleeding.
- Patients should not drink grapefruit juice or eat grapefruit while taking fibrates because it interferes with the metabolism (breakdown) of fibrates in the body, making them less effective.
- Fibrates increase cholesterol excretion in bile, predisposing patients to gallstone formation.
- Extended-release forms of lipid-lowering drugs (e.g., niacin [Niaspan]) should not be crushed or given by feeding tube.
- Immediate-release forms of lipid-lowering drugs (e.g., niacin [Niacor]) should not be substituted for extended-release drugs.
- If prescribed, give aspirin 325 mg 15 to 60 minutes before nicotinic acid to prevent flushing and hot flashes.
- Gastrointestinal symptoms can be decreased by giving nicotinic acid agents with food.
- Extended-release forms of these drugs should never be crushed or mixed with water because crushing the drug causes immediate release of the entire drug dose and could lead to an overdose.

Additional Learning Resources

🌐 Be sure to visit your Evolve website (http://evolve.elsevier.com/Workman/pharmacology/) for additional online resources.

SG Go to your Study Guide for additional learning activities to help you master this chapter content.

Review Questions

See *Answers to In-Text Review Questions* in the back of the book for answers to these questions.

1. A patient with high blood lipids asks the nurse why the lipid profile did not improve after 3 months following a low-fat diet. What is the nurse's **best** response?

   A. "You may need to follow a no-fat diet to improve your lipid profile."
   B. "You must follow a low-fat diet for at least 6 months to see improvement."
   C. "You will definitely need to be prescribed a drug to see improvement."
   D. "You may have a genetic factor that is causing your high blood lipid levels."

2. Which statement by a patient who has been prescribed an antihyperlipidemic drug indicates to the nurse the need for additional teaching?

   A. "Once my lipid profile levels are normal, I will no longer need to take the drug."
   B. "Taking this drug will decrease my risk for having a heart attack."
   C. "My goal is to increase my HDL cholesterol and decrease my LDL cholesterol."
   D. "I will continue walking and watching the fat in my diet while I'm taking this drug."

3. A patient has been prescribed an antihyperlipidemic drug. Which laboratory value does the nurse report to the prescriber?

   A. Total cholesterol 198 mg/dL
   B. Triglycerides 135 mg/dL
   C. Low-density lipoprotein (LDL) 195 mg/dL
   D. High-density lipoprotein (HDL) 60 mg/dL

4. Which health problems does the nurse teach a patient can be caused by chronic hyperlipidemia? **Select all that apply.**

   A. Hypertension
   B. Pancreatitis
   C. Peptic ulcer disease
   D. Xanthoma
   E. Diabetes mellitus
   F. Gastrointestinal reflux

5. A patient prescribed atorvastatin reports all of the following problems or changes since starting this drug. Which problem or change does the nurse report to the prescriber **immediately**?

   A. Abdominal cramps and bloating
   B. Muscle aches and weakness
   C. Urinating more at night
   D. Loss of taste for sweet or salty foods

6. A patient who has been prescribed lovastatin and now has rhabdomyolysis asks the nurse why all urine must be saved for intake and output measurements. What is the nurse's **best** response?

   A. "All patients on this unit have orders for strict intake and output measurements."
   B. "Intake and output measurements are important indicators of how well your kidneys are functioning."
   C. "A side effect of this drug can be blockage of urine flow through the kidneys and decreased urine output."
   D. "Sometimes this drug can cause the kidneys to make extra urine resulting in increased urine output and dehydration."

7. How does the nurse **best** explain to a patient why the most common side effects of any bile acid sequestrant include bloating, abdominal discomfort, and constipation?

   A. "Many patients are lactose intolerant and these drugs contain lactose."
   B. "Bile acid sequestrants exert their effects directly in the intestinal tract."
   C. "The action of bile acid sequestrants on the liver releases bile into the intestinal tract."
   D. "These drugs inhibit the absorption of dietary fiber, increasing its concentration and effects in the intestinal tract."

8. Which laboratory blood value is **most important** for the nurse to monitor when a patient is prescribed both colestipol and warfarin?

   A. Hematocrit
   B. Hemoglobin
   C. Red blood cell (RBC) count
   D. International normalized ratio (INR)

9. A patient who is prescribed ezetimibe has developed swelling around the eyes, nose, and lips. What is the nurse's **best first** action at this time?

   A. Elevating the head of the bed.
   B. Notifying the prescriber.
   C. Assessing the patient's airway.
   D. Checking the patient's blood pressure.

10. A patient who has been taking niacin daily for 1 week reports intense itching. What is the nurse's **best** response?

    A. "This is a common side effect and many people can control it by taking aspirin."
    B. "Stop taking the drug and talk with your prescriber as soon as possible."
    C. "Unless your skin forms blisters or peels, continue to take the drug."
    D. "Do you have any other drug or other allergies?"

11. A patient is prescribed niacin (Niaspan). The pharmacy sends niacin (Niacor). What is the nurse's **best** action?

    A. Holding the drug and contacting the prescriber.
    B. Giving the Niacor in place of the Niaspan.
    C. Asking the pharmacy to send the patient's ordered Niaspan.
    D. Checking the patient's chart to find out if he or she takes Niacor at home.

12. A patient who is prescribed gemfibrozil is also taking warfarin. What is the **most important** nursing action for this patient?

    A. Monitoring liver function tests.
    B. Keeping an accurate record of urine output.
    C. Giving the drug 30 minutes before meals.
    D. Checking the patient for signs of bleeding.

Clinical Judgment

1. The risks of which health problem(s) can be reduced when blood levels of low-density lipoprotein (LDL) cholesterol are controlled and kept within the normal range? **Select all that apply.**

    A. Angina
    B. Asthma
    C. Colitis
    D. Heart attack
    E. High blood pressure
    F. Parkinson disease
    G. Stroke
    H. Peripheral vascular disease
    I. Cystitis
    J. Pancreatitis

2. A 57-year-old patient with familial hypercholesterolemia is prescribed simvastatin 20 mg orally once daily for elevated low-density cholesterol that did not improve with exercise and a low-fat diet. The nurse has taught the patient about this drug and is assessing what the patient has learned. Which statements by the patient indicate that the patient understands the teaching or requires further teaching? **Use an X to indicate which patient statement about issues related to this therapy is either Understood or Requires Further Teaching.**

PATIENT STATEMENT	UNDERSTOOD TEACHING	REQUIRES FURTHER TEACHING
"Simvastatin will help my body eliminate cholesterol through my bowels."		
"I will take my simvastatin once a day in the evening before I go to bed."		
"I will immediately get in touch with my prescriber if I start having pain in my leg muscles."		
"When my prescriber sends me to the laboratory for a lipid profile, I will have it done right after breakfast."		
"I will continue to watch what I eat and get some exercise while taking this drug."		
"Once my cholesterol is back to normal, I will no longer need to take the simvastatin."		
"If I get an upset stomach with gas and abdominal pain or cramps, I will stop taking this medicine."		
"If I notice any yellowing or my eyes or skin, I will contact my prescribed right away."		

Drugs That Affect Blood Clotting

Learning Objectives

The content presented in this chapter should help you to:

1. Explain the names, actions, usual adult dosages, possible side effects, and adverse effects of drug therapy to manage excessive or inappropriate clotting.
2. Describe priority actions to take before and after giving drug therapy to manage excessive or inappropriate clotting.
3. Prioritize essential information to teach patients taking drugs to manage excessive or inappropriate clotting.
4. Describe appropriate life span considerations for drugs to manage excessive or inappropriate clotting.

5. Explain the names, actions, usual adult dosages, possible side effects, and adverse effects of common drugs that improve clotting.
6. Describe priority actions to take before and after giving drugs that improve clotting.
7. Prioritize essential information to teach patients taking drugs that improve clotting.
8. Explain appropriate life span considerations for drugs that improve clotting.

Key Terms

anticoagulants (ăn-tē-kō-ĂG-yū-lĕntz) (p. 302) Drugs used to prevent clot formation or to prevent a clot that has already formed from getting bigger.

antiplatelet drugs (ăn-tē-PLĀT-lĕt DRŬGZ) (p. 309) Drugs that interfere with blood clotting by either inhibiting cyclooxygenase (COX) formation of thromboxane A2 in platelets or by preventing the activation of platelets. Both types of actions prevent platelets from sticking together and clumping *(aggregation)*. Also known as platelet inhibitors.

colony-stimulating factors (CSFs) (cŏl-ŏn-Ē STĬM-yū-lāt-ĭng FĂK-tŏrz) (p. 313) Drugs that are able to increase the production of all types of blood cells by stimulating the bone marrow, which is the primary source of all blood cells.

erythropoiesis-stimulating agents (ESAs) (ĕ-RĬTH-rō-poy-Ē-sis STĬM-yū-lāt-ĭng Ā-gĕntz) (p. 314) Drugs from the colony-stimulating class that most specifically increase the production of red blood cells in the bone marrow.

thrombin inhibitors (THRŎM-bĭn ĭn-HĬB-ĭ-tŭrz) (p. 304) Drugs that interfere with blood clotting by directly or indirectly blocking

the action of thrombin, which converts fibrinogen to fibrin to form clots.

thrombin receptor inhibitors (THRŎM-bĭn rē-SĔP-TŬR ĭn-HĬB-ĭ-tŭrz) (p. 310) A new class of antiplatelet drugs that work by strongly blocking the thrombin receptor on platelets, which disrupts the action of thrombin in promoting platelet activation and aggregation.

thrombolytic agents (thrŏm-bō-LĬT-ĭk Ā-gĕntz) (p. 302) A drug class that breaks down clots that have already formed. Also known as *fibrinolytics*.

thrombopoiesis-stimulating agents (TSAs) (THRŎM-bō-poy-Ē-sis STĬM-yū-lāt-ĭng Ā-gĕntz) (p. 314) Drugs from the colony-stimulating factor class that specifically increase the production of platelets in the bone marrow.

vitamin K antagonist (VKA) (VĪ-tă-mĭn K ăn-TĂG-ŏn-ĭst) (p. 307) A drug class that decreases the active form of vitamin K, which is an essential component in liver activation of four clotting factors.

REVIEW OF RELATED PHYSIOLOGY AND PATHOPHYSIOLOGY FOR EXCESSIVE OR INAPPROPRIATE BLOOD CLOTTING

Maintaining blood circulation in its liquid form is essential for life by promoting blood flow (perfusion) to all tissues for the purposes of providing oxygen and removing waste products. In order to maintain this continuous circulation, the hematologic system has actions that form clots when and where they are needed to plug blood vessel leaks and prevent hemorrhage with excessive blood loss. These are *proclotting* forces. At the same time, the hematologic system has *anticlotting* forces or actions that prevent clots from forming when and where they are not needed or that prevent clots from remaining in place too long. Thus, maintaining continuous circulation requires balancing proclotting forces with anticlotting forces so that neither excessive bleeding nor circulatory interruption from inappropriate blood clotting occurs.

NORMAL CLOT FORMATION

When a person is injured or wounded, the body protects itself from excessive bleeding and hemorrhage by allowing part of the blood to convert from a liquid to a solid form, known as a clot. This well-organized and rapid process allows small cellular components (*platelets*) and other proteins (*clotting factors*) in the plasma to stick together and form a clot. A critical point in the process begins with an enzyme called *thrombin* that, when activated, acts on the protein fibrinogen, converting it into fibrin, which then creates threads that make the plasma sticky and able to form a clot. Activated platelets stick and clump together (*aggregate*) to create the initial plug that helps to stop bleeding. This process of cellular reactions is called the *clotting* or *coagulation cascade* (Figure 17.1) (Animation 17.1). In order for normal clotting to occur

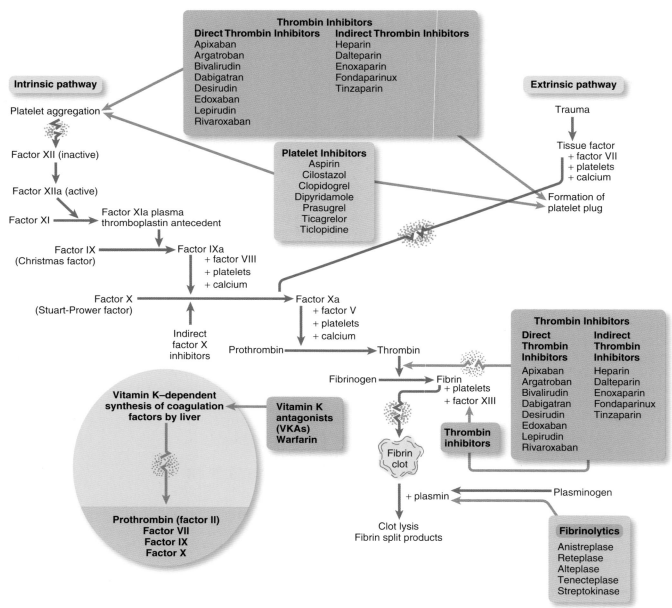

FIG. 17.1 The clotting cascade. *RBC,* Red blood cell. (From Ignatavicius, D., Workman, M. L., Rebar, C., & Heimgartner, N. [2021]. *Medical-surgical nursing: Concepts for interprofessional collaborative care* [10th ed.]. St. Louis: Elsevier.)

when it is needed, the person must have adequate amounts of all protein-based clotting factors, platelets, and calcium. The cascade has two pathways, the intrinsic and the extrinsic, which are started by different events. The two pathways merge into a final common pathway for actual blood clotting. The extrinsic pathway is the normal defensive response to vascular injury and helps prevent hemorrhage. Think of the extrinsic pathway as a "short-cut" to the final formation of a fibrin clot. On the other hand, activation of the intrinsic pathway is not a normal defensive response and is most responsible for abnormal or inappropriate clotting. The factors and actions of the common pathway are the most powerful of the proclotting forces.

ABNORMAL CLOT FORMATION

Thrombosis

Thrombosis occurs when a clot (*thrombus*) forms in the vascular system when it is not needed to prevent hemorrhage as a result of vascular injury. This process is often triggered by atherosclerotic plaques that narrow and damage blood vessels. When a thrombus develops in a coronary artery and blocks the blood supply to a part of the heart muscle, a heart attack (*myocardial infarction*) occurs. If a clot forms in an artery in the brain, it can result in a stroke. A clot in a deep vein such as a leg vein is a *venous thromboembolism*, or VTE, also known as *deep vein thrombosis (DVT)*. A clot that forms a VTE may also break off, forming an embolus that travels through the bloodstream to another part of the body such as the brain or lungs.

Embolus

As stated above, an *embolus* (embolism) is a clot that travels through the bloodstream until it lodges in a blood vessel and blocks it. An embolus can be a clump of bacteria, fat, or air, but it is most often a blood clot or portion of a clot. An embolus that travels to the brain can cause a stroke. An embolus in the lung is called a *pulmonary embolism*, which can cause severe, life-threatening problems in the respiratory system.

Thromboembolic Events

Thromboembolic events are always potentially life threatening if not managed properly. Although some people are at greater risk for these events than others, even temporary conditions can increase the risk. The three major factors that lead to thromboembolic events are conditions that (1) physically impair blood flow, (2) increase the blood's proclotting forces, and (3) damage blood vessel linings. Common conditions or problems that increase the risk for inappropriate or excessive clotting are listed in Box 17.1.

TYPES OF DRUGS USED TO PREVENT EXCESSIVE OR INAPPROPRIATE CLOTTING

Inappropriate blood clotting with thromboembolism formation can cause extensive tissue damage when perfusion is disrupted and oxygen does not reach tissues and organs. To prevent these life- and limb-threatening events, prescribers manage the problems with anticoagulants or thrombolytics. Figure 17.1 shows where in the blood clotting cascade different types of anticoagulants and thrombolytic agents

 Memory Jogger

The extrinsic pathway leads to normal defensive blood clotting, and the intrinsic pathway is started by abnormal conditions or events that lead to excessive or inappropriate blood clotting. However, because the factors and actions of the common pathway are the most powerful, therapies to manage inappropriate blood clotting always interfere with normal defensive clotting to some degree.

 Memory Jogger

A *thrombus* is a clot forming within a blood vessel of a tissue or organ that remains where it formed and usually disrupts circulation to some degree. An *embolus* is a clot that travels from its initial site of formation and lodges elsewhere to disrupt circulation. The larger the thrombus or embolus, the greater the disruption of circulation, perfusion, and oxygenation.

Box **17.1**   **Risk Factors for Thromboembolic Events**

- Major surgery (trauma, coronary artery bypass, abdominal or neurosurgery)
- Major orthopedic surgery (hip, pelvis, femur)
- History of cancer
- Age (>40 years)
- Previous venous thromboembolism
- Varicose veins
- Pregnancy
- Estrogen-based contraceptives
- Heart failure
- Immobility, especially prolonged bed rest
- Spinal cord injury
- Obesity
- Nicotine use, especially cigarette smoking or vaping

Table **17.1**	Normal and Therapeutic Coagulation Values	
TEST	**NORMAL RANGE**	**THERAPEUTIC RANGE**[a]
Prothrombin time (PT)	11.0–12.5 seconds	1.5–2 times the control value
Activated partial thromboplastin time (aPTT)	30–40 seconds	1.5–2.5 times the control value
International normalized ratio (INR)	0.8–1.2	2.0–3.0

[a]Therapeutic ranges for an individual patient may be greater depending on the severity of the condition and other patient factors.
Information from Pagana, K., & Pagana T. (2018). *Mosby's manual of diagnostic and laboratory tests* (6th ed.). St. Louis: Elsevier.

disrupt the clotting process. Although each anticlotting drug category has a primary area within the blood clotting cascade where it exerts effects, most anticlotting drugs also have some lesser effects in other areas of the cascade. Drug dosage and therapy with these drugs is guided by coagulation laboratory values (Table 17.1).

Anticoagulant drugs are used to reduce clot formation or to prevent an existing, already formed clot from becoming bigger. These drugs are sometimes called "blood thinners," but they do not actually thin the blood. Common conditions for which anticoagulants are prescribed include preventing clots from forming after a heart valve replacement, reducing the risk for stroke or heart attack, and preventing VTEs. They are often used during open heart surgery to prevent clots from forming. These drugs may also be prescribed to prevent clots in patients who are on bed rest for a long period and for patients with heart dysrhythmias such as atrial fibrillation (*A-fib*). Atrial fibrillation is an abnormal heart rhythm in which the atria do not contract effectively, leading to a high risk for clots forming in the atrial chambers of the heart. These clots may then break off and travel to other areas of the body, especially in the brain, as emboli.

When a clot already exists, a thrombolytic agent may be prescribed to dissolve it. **Thrombolytic agents** are able to break down the components of a formed clot. Other names for drugs in this category are *fibrinolytics* or sometimes "clot busters." They help to prevent death and additional tissue damage for patients with heart attack, stroke, pulmonary embolism, and other clot-related problems.

GENERAL ISSUES FOR ALL DRUGS TO MANAGE EXCESSIVE OR INAPPROPRIATE CLOTTING

Intended Responses for All Anticoagulant Drugs
- Clotting time is increased.
- Clot formation is decreased.
- Existing clots do not become larger.
- Thrombolytic events are prevented.
- Blood flow and oxygenation are maintained.

Several classes of drugs affect blood clotting. Each class has both unique and common actions and effects. Responsibilities for these common actions and effects are listed in the following paragraphs. Specific responsibilities are listed with each individual class.

⊗ Priority Actions to Take *Before* Giving Any Drug to Manage Excessive or Inappropriate Clotting

Obtain a complete list of current drugs that the patient is taking, including over-the-counter and herbal preparations, especially aspirin or aspirin-containing products, gingko biloba, and St. John's wort. All of these substances can worsen excessive bleeding. Check the heart rate and blood pressure. Also check the patient's baseline coagulation laboratory results.

When giving a drug that interferes with clotting and that has an antidote, be sure the antidote is available. Excessive bleeding and hemorrhage can occur quickly with some of these drugs, and having the antidote available can prevent harm.

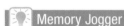
Memory Jogger

Anticoagulant drugs do not "thin" the blood or dissolve existing clots but can reduce the number of new clots that form and prevent existing clots from becoming larger.

Critical Point for Safety

With the exception of aspirin, *all* drugs used to reduce blood clotting or to break up existing clots are *high-alert* drugs and can cause harm if given to a patient in error. When possible, always check the order for a high-alert drug with another licensed health care professional or pharmacist.

QSEN: Safety

Ask female patients of childbearing age if they are pregnant, breastfeeding, or planning to become pregnant. These drugs cross the placenta and can cause excessive bleeding or death to an unborn baby. Also determine whether the patient has had a baby, a miscarriage, or an abortion within the past 24 hours. These bleeding conditions are made worse by drugs that disrupt blood clotting, which can lead to serious and possibly life-threatening hemorrhage.

Ask if the patient has a history of bleeding problems. Check the patient for any bruising or petechiae and ask whether he or she bruises easily. Ask if he or she is currently taking any drugs by injection.

⊛ Priority Actions to Take *After* Giving Any Drug to Manage Excessive or Inappropriate Clotting

Check patients frequently for signs of bleeding or allergic reaction. Hemorrhage is a risk with all anticlotting drugs and may be life threatening. Signs of bleeding include abdominal swelling or pain, back pain, bloody urine, bloody stools (black and tarry), constipation, coughing up blood, dizziness, headaches, joint pain, and vomiting emesis that looks like coffee grounds.

Recheck the patient's blood pressure, heart rate, and pulse oximetry. Watch for changes that may indicate bleeding such as a decrease in blood pressure (less than 90/60 mm Hg), an increase in heart rate (more than 100 beats/min), or a decrease in oxygen saturation 3% to 5% below the patient's baseline. Notify the prescriber immediately if the patient develops any signs or symptoms of bleeding.

Avoid giving intramuscular (IM) or intravenous (IV) injections. If you must give an IM or IV drug, hold pressure over the site for at least 5 minutes after administration. Use the smallest gauge needle possible if you must give an IM injection.

Make sure that follow-up coagulation laboratory values are drawn and be sure to check these values because they are often used to determine the drug dose that is prescribed. Also, check patient's red blood cell counts and platelet counts to monitor for bleeding.

 Critical Point for Safety

Hold pressure on an IM or IV site for at least 5 minutes when a patient is taking drugs that reduce clotting.

QSEN: Safety

⊛ Teaching Priorities for Patients Taking Any Drug to Manage Excessive or Inappropriate Clotting

- Always keep appointments for regular follow-up and blood tests that measure blood clotting.
- Take the drug exactly as prescribed and keep a record of each dose to prevent mistakes.
- If you miss a dose, take it as soon as possible but **never** take a double dose because this could cause serious bleeding.
- Watch for signs of excessive bleeding, including bleeding from the gums while brushing your teeth, bleeding or oozing from cuts or wounds, bruising, and nosebleeds that are excessive and hard to control. Additional signs of more serious bleeding include paleness around the mouth and nailbeds, rapid heart and respiratory rates, sensation of light-headedness or dizziness, and thirst. If any of these signs are present, notify your prescriber immediately.
- Use a soft toothbrush and electric shaver to prevent injuring your gums or skin.
- Inform all your other health care providers, including dentists, about your use of these drugs before any surgery, dental work, or any invasive test/procedure.
- Avoid contact sports and activities that may cause injuries because they can cause internal bleeding. Some activities that can cause internal bleeding (especially in the kidneys) and bleeding into the joints include running, jogging, jumping for any reason, and high-impact exercise.
- If you fall and hit your head or your spine, contact your prescriber immediately because severe and deadly internal bleeding can occur in these tissues, and interventions to prevent permanent damage or death may be necessary.
- Obtain and wear a medical alert bracelet that states you are taking an anticlotting drug.

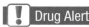

ANTICOAGULANT DRUGS

All anticoagulant drugs prevent or slow the formation of clots. For this reason, their use is prohibited in people who have conditions such as bleeding ulcers and for those who have had surgery or have delivered a baby within the previous 24 hours.

Thrombin Inhibitors

How thrombin inhibitors work. Thrombin inhibitor drugs interfere with blood clotting by directly or indirectly blocking the action of thrombin, which converts fibrinogen to fibrin to form clots. All thrombin inhibitors interfere with blood clotting in the common pathway for blood clotting. This means that they are able to reduce excessive or inappropriate clotting and also reduce normal blood clotting to some degree. They work by blocking the action of thrombin. Thrombin is an enzyme (clotting factor X) that when activated to clotting factor Xa converts fibrinogen into fibrin to form clots in the common blood pathway of the blood clotting cascade (see Figure 17.1). Some drugs are direct thrombin inhibitors and others work indirectly to reduce the amount of active thrombin present by increasing the activity of a protein known as antithrombin III. With more antithrombin III present, less thrombin is available to convert fibrinogen into fibrin and clot formation is reduced.

These drugs are most commonly used to prevent clots from forming in patients who have conditions that put them permanently at high risk such as nonvalvular atrial fibrillation (*A-fib*) and chronic heart failure. They may also be used temporarily (for a specified time period) such as after certain orthopedic surgeries or in patients who have actually had and were treated for a deep vein thrombosis or pulmonary embolism.

Direct thrombin inhibitors, also known as *DOACs* (direct oral anticoagulants), work by selectively blocking the active site of factor Xa both in its free form in the blood and when it is present in a clot. As a result, they both reduce formation of new clots and have a role in preventing existing clots from enlarging. Although these drugs do not have any direct action on the ability of platelets to aggregate, by reducing the available amount of thrombin, which does promote platelet aggregation, platelet action also is reduced indirectly in patients taking direct thrombin inhibitors.

Unlike heparin, therapy with direct thrombin inhibitors does **not** require monitoring with tests of coagulation. Parenteral direct thrombin inhibitors may be prescribed when heparin therapy has resulted in the complication of heparin-induced thrombocytopenia (HIT). The activity of the oral direct thrombin inhibitors is increased by regular consumption of grapefruit or grapefruit juice.

Indirect thrombin inhibitors are mostly natural and synthetic heparin and work mainly by increasing the activity of antithrombin III present in the blood. As a result, less thrombin is available to convert fibrinogen into fibrin and clot formation is reduced. These drugs have no effect on the thrombin present in clots. Heparins are all given parenterally. Original heparin is an animal product with a relatively large molecular weight. Because heparin has the most rapid onset of action of any of the thrombin inhibitors, it is usually the first drug used to treat clots that have formed outside of the heart and brain. Heparin may be given by IV or subcutaneous routes. IV heparin is usually given in the form of an IV push bolus followed by a continuous infusion. The bolus dose is usually based on the patient's weight; the infusion rate is based on and adjusted according to the patient's activated partial thromboplastin time (aPTT) laboratory results with a goal of keeping the aPTT within a therapeutic range to prevent clots from forming. Most often, the desired therapeutic range is an aPTT that is 1.5 to 2.5 times greater than the mean normal range (control value). However, an individual patient's therapeutic range may be extended to as high as 3.5 depending on the reason why the patient's blood clotting is being controlled.

Fractionated heparin may be synthetic or derived from natural heparin components and is a smaller molecule called low-molecular-weight heparin (LMWH). In addition, the fewer molecules present in LMWH reduce the risk for allergic reactions. Coagulation studies are not needed when LMWH is being used for prevention of excessive or inappropriate clotting. These drugs are given subcutaneously and patients often self-administer the injection at home.

The usual adult dosages for common thrombin inhibitors are listed in the table below. Check a reliable drug reference as a source for information about less common thrombin inhibitors.

Usual Adult Dosages for Common Thrombin Inhibitors

Drug Category	Drug Name	Usual Maintenance Dose
Direct Thrombin Inhibitors (Oral)	apixaban (Eliquis) ❶	2.5–5 mg orally twice daily
	dabigatran (Pradaxa) ❶	150 mg orally twice daily
	edoxaban (Savaysa) ❶	60 mg orally once daily
	rivaroxaban (Xarelto) ❶	20 mg orally once daily with food
Direct Thrombin Inhibitors (Parenteral)	argatroban (Acova) ❶	2 mcg/kg/min continuous IV infusion
	bivalirudin (Angiomax) ❶	IV bolus of 0.75 mg/kg followed by continuous IV infusion of 1.75 mg/kg/hr (angioplasty)
	desirudin (Iprivask) ❶	15 mg subcutaneously every 12 hr (surgical prophylaxis) 0.1 mg/kg IV bolus followed by 0.1 mg/kg/hr continuous IV infusion (acute coronary syndromes)
	lepirudin (Refludan) ❶	0.4 mg/kg IV bolus followed by 0.15 mg/kg/hr continuous IV infusion (acute coronary syndromes)
Indirect Thrombin Inhibitors	heparin ❶	80 units/kg IV bolus, then maintenance infusion of 18 units/kg/hr IV continuous infusion (DVT or PE treatment) 5000 units subcutaneously every 8–12 hr (DVT prophylaxis)
	fondaparinux (Artixa) ❶	2.5–5 mg once daily subcutaneously (DVT or PE prophylaxis)
Low-Molecular-Weight Heparins	daltaparin (Fragmin) ❶	150–200 units/kg/dose subcutaneously once daily (DVT or PE prophylaxis)
	enoxaparin (Lovenox) ❶	1 mg/kg/dose subcutaneously every 12 hr (DVT or PE treatment) 20–40 mg subcutaneously once daily or 30 mg subcutaneously every 12 hr (DVT or PE prophylaxis)
	tinzaparin (Innohep) ❶	175 units/kg subcutaneously once daily (DVT or PE treatment) for at least 6 days

❶ High-alert drug; *mcg*, Micrograms; *DVT*, Deep vein thrombosis; *PE*, Pulmonary embolism.

Common side effects of thrombin inhibitors. In addition to a risk for increased bleeding in response to injury, premenopausal female patients may develop heavy menstrual bleeding. Other side effects include increased blood potassium (hyperkalemia), thinning of the bones (osteoporosis), decreased number of platelets (thrombocytopenia), decreased aldosterone, blood clots in the spinal cord, and hair loss (alopecia) with prolonged use. *Rivaroxaban* is associated with digestive upsets and is recommended to be taken with food.

Possible adverse effects of thrombin inhibitors. Some patients develop allergic reactions (hypersensitivity) to these drugs. As described in Chapter 1, signs of allergic reaction include changes in skin color of the face, fast or irregular breathing, puffiness or swelling around the eyes, a lump in the throat, shortness of breath or difficulty breathing, chest tightness, wheezing, skin rash, hives, and itching.

Heparin-induced thrombocytopenia (HIT) is a low blood platelet count that can occur as a result of heparin use. It is an immune-mediated drug reaction in which heparin-dependent platelet-activating antibodies form and allow heparin to bind with platelet

Common Side Effects

Thrombin Inhibitors

Bleeding problems

Hyperkalemia

Hair loss

Stomach problems

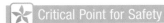

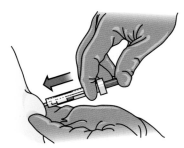

FIG. 17.2 Injection technique for low-molecular-weight heparin.

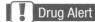

Drug Alert

Action/Intervention Alert

The antidote to heparin is IV protamine sulfate.

QSEN: Safety

Drug Alert

Action/Intervention Alert

To avoid losing any of the drug, do not expel the air bubble from a pre-filled syringe before injecting low-molecular-weight heparin.

QSEN: Safety

factor 4 (PF4). This response then creates a complex that activates the platelets, causing the formation of many microclots that use up circulating platelets leading to thrombocytopenia. HIT can occur in patients receiving any type of heparin, but it is most common with unfractionated heparin, especially among female patients who have been treated with heparin for longer than 1 week.

Heparin-induced skin necrosis is a rare but serious complication caused by subcutaneous heparin, most commonly seen on the abdomen where injection sites are located. In severe cases, surgery may be needed to remove necrotic skin.

⭐ ***Priority actions to take** before **giving thrombin inhibitors.*** In addition to the general responsibilities related to drug therapy to manage excessive or inappropriate clotting (p. 302), be sure to obtain an accurate patient weight before initiating bolus heparin therapy because the dose is weight-based. Ensure that the antidote to heparin, protamine sulfate, is readily available whenever a patient is receiving heparin therapy.

Give LMW heparin by deep subcutaneous injection with the patient lying down. To avoid losing any of the drug, do not expel the air bubble before injection. Insert the needle into a skinfold held between the thumb and forefinger (Figure 17.2) and do not aspirate before injection to avoid tissue damage. To avoid bruising, do not rub the injection site.

⭐ ***Priority actions to take** after **giving thrombin inhibitors.*** In addition to the general responsibilities related to anticoagulant therapy (p. 303), for patients receiving continuous IV heparin, adjust the flow rate based on the prescriber's orders, which are determined by the results of follow-up aPTT tests. Monitor the IV site for patency and signs of infection or phlebitis.

⭐ ***Teaching priorities for patients taking thrombin inhibitors.*** In addition to teaching patients about the general care needs and precautions related to drug therapy for excessive or inappropriate clotting (p. 303), include these teaching points and precautions:

- Do not take aspirin or aspirin-containing products while taking these drugs.
- Read the labels on both over-the-counter and prescription drugs to see if they contain aspirin.
- Do not to take ibuprofen or any other nonsteroidal antiinflammatory drug (NSAID) without asking your prescriber. Taking aspirin or NSAIDs while taking heparin greatly increases the risk for bleeding.
- Avoid eating grapefruit or drinking grapefruit juice because these products increase the activity of the oral forms of the direct thrombin inhibitors, which then increases the risk for excessive bleeding.
- If you are taking a direct thrombin inhibitor drug including apixaban (Eliquis), dabigatran (Pradaxa), edoxaban (Savaysa), or rivaroxiban (Xarelto), keep the tablets in the original container dispensed by the pharmacy because exposure to light degrades the drug. **Do not place these tablets in a daily pill organizer.**

Life span considerations for thrombin inhibitors

Considerations for pregnancy and lactation. Heparin has a low to moderate likelihood of increasing the risk for birth defects or fetal harm. It is the drug of choice when anticoagulation therapy is needed during pregnancy and breastfeeding. It may cause bleeding problems in the mother during the last trimester of pregnancy and during delivery of the baby. When heparin is needed during pregnancy, the prefilled syringes are used because these do not contain the preservative benzyl alcohol, which should be avoided during pregnancy. Heparin does not pass into breast milk, so it is safe to use while a mother is breastfeeding.

Considerations for older adults. Older adults are more sensitive to the effects of thrombin inhibitors and therefore are more likely to experience side effects such as bleeding. Because of this, older adults may require lower drug doses. Teach older adults to immediately apply cold compresses or ice packs to injection sites and to any injured areas to reduce bruising and bleeding.

Vitamin K Antagonists (VKAs)

How vitamin K antagonists work. Vitamin K antagonists (VKAs) are a class of drugs that decrease the active form of vitamin K in the intestinal tract. This vitamin is an essential component in liver activation of four clotting factors. In the presence of VKAs, production of the vitamin K-dependent clotting factors (clotting factors II, VII, IX, and X) in the liver is reduced. When the amounts of these critical clotting factors are reduced, anticoagulation results. The most commonly used VKA is warfarin (Coumadin, Jantoven), an oral agent. It is prescribed for adults and children to prevent forming of clots and emboli.

Most patients are started on warfarin before being taken off of heparin because the effects of VKAs take about 3 days to reduce clot formation. Patients may be prescribed heparin and warfarin together for a few days until the international normalized ratio (INR) is within the desired therapeutic range. Then the heparin is discontinued.

The international normalized ratio (INR) is a blood test used to monitor the effects of warfarin and determine an appropriate dose. Some patients may require higher or lower doses depending on other medical conditions and personal genetic factors affecting the drug's metabolism. The therapeutic range for the INR is usually between 2.0 and 3.0. If a patient has a mechanical heart valve, the therapeutic range is 2.5 to 3.5 because of the increased risk for clots forming on the valve. Warfarin is the only drug approved for use by patients who have a mechanical heart valve or who have atrial fibrillation (A-fib) caused by a heart valve problem.

In adults, the initial dose of warfarin is 2 to 15 mg orally once daily for 2 to 4 days, then adjusted based on INR laboratory test results. Because the dosage is based on each patient's personal response and INR levels, dosages vary greatly from one person to another and may vary for one person from week to week.

Common side effects of vitamin K antagonists. Excessive bleeding is the most common side effect of warfarin, and the drug has a Black Box Warning for this increased risk. Non-clotting-related side effects are less common but include headache, upset stomach, diarrhea, fever, and skin rash.

Possible adverse effects of vitamin K antagonists. In addition to excessive bleeding and hemorrhage, warfarin-induced skin necrosis (Figure 17.3) is a rare but serious complication that most often happens in women who are obese and going through menopause. It is associated with large doses of warfarin and usually occurs within 1 to 10 days of starting the drug. Management involves using high doses of IM or IV vitamin K as an antidote for warfarin and heparin for anticoagulation. Vitamin K should be readily available when a patient is taking warfarin.

Warfarin interacts with hundreds of other drugs, herbal supplements, and foods. Some of these interactions increase the action of warfarin and greatly increase the risk for bleeding at common therapeutic dosages. Other interactions reduce warfarin's activity, placing patients at increased risk for continued excessive or inappropriate clotting.

Genetic/genomic variation in metabolism of vitamin K antagonists. As described in Chapter 1, warfarin is metabolized for elimination primarily by several enzymes from the CYP enzyme system, and there are racial as well as ethnic variations in the presence of genetic variations affecting these and other enzymes associated with warfarin or vitamin K. A gene variation for one specific enzyme may be more common in people of one race, while a different gene variation for another specific enzyme is more common in people of another racial heritage. About 15% to 30% of white people and more than 50% of people of Asian heritage have small gene variations in specific metabolizing enzymes and metabolize warfarin more slowly. This

Memory Jogger

The normal INR range is 0.8–1.2; the therapeutic range is from 2.0 to 3.0 (or even up to 4.5), depending on the reason the person is prescribed to take this drug.

Common Side Effects

Warfarin

Bleeding problems   Headache   Stomach problems

Fever   Rash

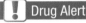

Drug Alert

Action/Intervention Alert

The antidote for warfarin is IM or IV vitamin K.

QSEN: Safety

Critical Point for Safety

Warfarin interacts with hundreds of drugs, herbal supplements, and foods. Thus, checking the patient's current drug list for any potential interactions is a critical nursing action.

QSEN: Safety

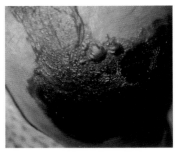

FIG. 17.3 Warfarin-induced skin necrosis. (From Hoffman, R., et al. [2008]. *Hematology: Basic principles and practice* [5th ed.]. Philadelphia: Churchill Livingstone.)

Critical Point for Safety

Because there is considerable genetic variation in the enzymes that activate and those that metabolize warfarin, closely monitor the INR of patients taking this drug to determine whether the expected results are being achieved. Report results that do not match the expected response to the prescriber for dosage adjustments.

QSEN: Safety

Drug Alert

Teaching Alert

Warn patients not to take any over-the-counter drugs (especially aspirin or aspirin-containing drugs) or herbal supplements without asking their prescriber first.

QSEN: Safety

Drug Alert

Teaching Alert

Remind patients that it takes several days after stopping warfarin for the body to recover its normal clotting ability.

QSEN: Safety

means that a warfarin dose remains in the patient's system longer, greatly increasing the risk for bleeding and other side effects. For people who are known to have such a gene mutation, warfarin dosages need to be much lower than those for the general population. Because the incidence of these variations is so common in people of Asian heritage, any person of Asian heritage who needs anticoagulation therapy should be started on very *low* dosages of warfarin and have his or her international normalized ratio (INR) monitored more frequently than people who do not have a known variation of these metabolizing enzyme genes. There are other variations in specific genes that result in either slower activity of warfarin or its more rapid elimination. Patients with these variations require *higher* dosages of warfarin to achieve the desired therapeutic response.

At the present time, genetic testing for such genetic/genomic variations before starting warfarin therapy is not commonly done because of economic and availability reasons. However, future genetic testing options specifically for genes affecting warfarin metabolism are being developed that are simple, accurate, and can easily be performed at the point-of-care. Nurses can help prevent problems by monitoring INR trends of patients receiving warfarin and reporting results that do not match the expected response to this therapy so the prescriber can use this information to make the appropriate dosage adjustments.

⭐ *Priority actions to take before giving vitamin K antagonists.* In addition to the general responsibilities related to anticoagulant therapy (p. 302), take these actions before beginning warfarin therapy:
- Ask what other prescribed drugs, over-the-counter drugs, herbal supplements, and vitamin supplements the patient takes on a daily or even occasional basis and ensure this information is included in the patient's medical record.
- Check the patient's INR laboratory results.
- Ensure that vitamin K, the antidote for warfarin, is readily available. A common brand of this antidote is phytonadione (AquaMEPHYTON).
- Find out whether the patient is following a vegetarian diet or eats a lot of green salads because some vegetables are rich in vitamin K (for example, green leafy vegetables) or drinks large amounts of green tea, which can decrease the action of warfarin. (Remember that vitamin K is the antidote for warfarin.)
- Ask female patients of childbearing age if they are pregnant or planning to become pregnant because warfarin can cause birth defects, bleeding, and death in an unborn baby.
- Ask female patients whether they use any oral or implanted estrogen-based contraceptive because these increase warfarin's activity and greatly increase the risk for bleeding even when dosages are at normal ranges.

⭐ *Priority actions to take after giving vitamin K antagonists.* In addition to the general responsibilities related to anticoagulant therapy (p. 303), tell the patient that an INR will be performed regularly to help adjust the dose of this drug. Remind him or her to avoid intermittent large amounts of foods rich in vitamin K (especially leafy green vegetables or large amounts of green tea) because they interfere with the action of warfarin.

Closely monitor the INR of patients taking this drug to determine whether the expected results are being achieved. Report results that do not match the expected response (either much higher or much lower) to the prescriber for dosage adjustments.

⭐ *Teaching priorities for patients taking vitamin K antagonists.* In addition to the general care needs and precautions related to anticoagulant therapy (p. 303), teach patients to maintain their current diet and to not attempt significant diet changes, such as an all-vegetarian or a "keto" diet. Abrupt changes in a person's diet can alter the INR results. It is important for patients to tell their prescriber if they have recently or are currently including large amounts of foods that are rich in vitamin K (such as liver, green leafy vegetables, broccoli, and cauliflower) in their diet because vitamin K interferes with the action of warfarin. Warn that alcohol can interfere with the action of warfarin, and advise patients to talk to their prescriber before drinking alcohol.

Life span considerations for vitamin K antagonists

Considerations for pregnancy and lactation. Warfarin is a *teratogen* (can cause birth defects) and has a high likelihood of causing fetal harm or death. For this reason, it is not prescribed during pregnancy. In addition, women who are of childbearing age are instructed to use two reliable methods of birth control while taking this drug.

Considerations for older adults. In addition to older adults being more sensitive to the effects of warfarin, they are at greater risk for inaccurate dosages and poor or unpredictable control of blood clotting. Warfarin tablets are small in physical size and the amount of drug per tablet is relatively low (e.g., 0.5, 1, 2 and 3 mg, etc.). Manufacturers use pastel colors to differentiate the dosage strength of the tablets and most have the mg amount visibly pressed into the pill. Also, the prescribed dosages may change for any patient from one day to the next based on INR responses. Thus, some patients have multiple containers with varying dosages of warfarin on hand and are often expected to change which tablets they take on some days. Not only do some older adults have less manual dexterity to handle the small pills, many also have difficulty distinguishing one color from another, especially when the pill colors are light and similar to each other (e.g., pink versus pale orange). Trying to read the mg number actually on the pill may also be difficult for older adults. These problems increase the risk for under-dosing, as well as overdosing. Both issues can have a severe negative impact on health.

Help patients understand that taking the exact dose prescribed is critically important to prevent health problems. Some suggestions that can assist older adults to safely self-administer changing dosages of warfarin include using a magnifying glass to be sure of a tablet's exact mg dose and preparing doses in an area where lighting is bright. Some older adults may have someone else mark the pharmacy container with the drug name and mg number per tablet with a heavy black marker.

Antiplatelet Drugs

Platelets are small, cell-like blood components that are formed from large megakaryocyte cells. As can be seen in Figure 17.1, platelets are essential components in the formation of clots at nearly every step in the blood clotting cascade (Animation 17.2). Therefore, altering or inhibiting the ability of platelets to become active and aggregate is an effective focus of drug therapy to prevent excessive or inappropriate blood clotting.

Platelets have an outer coating that prevents them from sticking together while they circulate in the blood so that clots do not form when they are not needed. They also have surface receptor sites for different substances such as thromboxane A_2 (TXA$_2$), adenosine diphosphate (ADP), thrombin, and fibrinogen. When these substances bind to their receptors, platelets are activated and can aggregate. In addition, when platelets are activated, they produce TXA$_2$ and ADP so they are self-stimulating to promote clotting. Three other substances, phosphodiesterase III (PDE III), prostacyclin, and adenosine, have the opposite effect on platelets to prevent activation and aggregation. Some antiplatelet drugs inhibit platelet aggregation and clotting by preventing TXA$_2$, ADP, and thrombin from binding to their receptors. Other antiplatelet drugs inhibit platelet aggregation by increasing the release of PDE III, prostacyclin, or adenosine.

How antiplatelet drugs work. Antiplatelet drugs, also known as platelet inhibitors, use different mechanisms to prevent platelets from clumping together (aggregating) to form harmful clots. These drugs are prescribed for prevention of clots in the brain and cardiovascular system. They are used to treat patients with coronary artery

Critical Point for Safety

Pregnancy is an absolute contraindication for warfarin use because it is highly likely to cause birth defects or fetal death.

QSEN: Safety

Memory Jogger

The four classes of antiplatelet drugs are:
- Thromboxane A₂ inhibitors
- Adenosine diphosphate (ADP) inhibitors
- Phosphodiesterase (PDE) III inhibitors
- Thrombin receptor inhibitors

Do Not Confuse

Ticlid *with* **Tequin**

A prescription for Ticlid may be confused with Tequin. Ticlid is a platelet inhibitor, whereas Tequin is a quinolone antibiotic used to treat infections.

QSEN: Safety

Drug Alert

Interaction Alert

Both grapefruit and cimetidine increase the action of vorapaxar and greatly increase bleeding risk. Instruct patients to avoid these products while taking vorapaxar.

QSEN: Safety

disease, heart attack, angina, stroke, transient ischemic attacks (TIAs), and peripheral artery disease (PAD).

Thromboxane A₂ inhibitors are powerful antiplatelet drugs. Aspirin is the most common thromboxane A₂ (TXA₂) inhibitor and works by irreversibly inhibiting the cyclooxygenase (COX) enzyme from making active TXA₂ in platelets. After a single dose of aspirin, clotting is reduced for at least 36 hours until a sufficient number of fresh platelets that have not been exposed to aspirin are released into circulation from the spleen. Aspirin comes in tablet, capsule, gum, and suppository forms. The aspirin dosage for the purpose of its antiplatelet activity is lower than for fever or pain reduction.

All other nonsteroidal antiinflammatory drugs (NSAIDs) also inhibit the production of TXA₂, but to a lesser degree than aspirin. Platelets recover the ability to clump within 8 hours after an NSAID is taken, making NSAIDs a poor antiplatelet drug.

ADP inhibitors have the main action of blocking the ADP receptor on platelets, preventing them from becoming activated. Drugs in this class include clopidogrel (Plavix), dipyridamole (Permole, Persantine), prasugrel (Effient), ticagrelor (Brilinta), and ticlopidine (Ticlid). Dipyridamole has several additional antiplatelet actions.

PDE III inhibitors work by preventing the breakdown of an internal compound in platelets known as cyclic AMP (cAMP) that helps prevent the activation of platelets. The most common drug in this class is cilostazol (Pletal).

Thrombin receptor inhibitors are a new class of antiplatelet drugs that work by strongly blocking the thrombin receptor on platelets, which disrupts the action of thrombin in promoting platelet activation and aggregation. The drug has limited activity and works best when given with a low dose of another antiplatelet drug. Currently, the only approved drug in this class is vorapaxar (Zontivity).

The usual adult dosages for common antiplatelet drugs are listed in the table below. Check a reliable drug reference for information about less common antiplatelet drugs.

Usual Adult Dosages for Common Antiplatelet Drugs

Drug Class	Drug Name	Usual Maintenance Dose
Thromboxane A₂ Inhibitors	aspirin	81–325 mg orally once daily
Adenosine Diphosphate (ADP) Inhibitors	clopidogrel (Plavix) ❶	75 mg orally once daily
	dipyridamole (Persantine) ❶	75–100 mg orally 4 times daily in conjunction with aspirin or warfarin therapy
	prasugrel (Effient) ❶	60 mg orally as a loading dose, then 10 mg orally once daily
	ticagrelor (Brilinta) ❶	60 mg orally twice daily plus aspirin 75–100 mg (e.g., 81 mg) orally once daily
	ticlopidine (Ticlid) ❶	250 mg orally twice daily
Phosphodiesterase III (PDE III) Inhibitors	cilostazol (Pletal) ❶	100 mg orally twice daily
Thrombin Receptor Inhibitors	vorapaxar (Zontivity) ❶	2.08 mg orally once daily with aspirin and/or clopidogrel ❶

❶ High-alert drug.

Common side effects of antiplatelet drugs. Common side effects of antiplatelet drugs include bleeding, headache, dizziness, and diarrhea.

Possible adverse effects of antiplatelet drugs. Adverse effects of salicylates (aspirin) are discussed in Chapter 10. As discussed in the general issues section, hemorrhage is the most common adverse effect and can be life threatening. Reduced blood counts, including platelets (*thrombocytopenia*) and red blood cells leading to anemia, are the second most common adverse effect of these drugs. Allergic reactions to these drugs, including rash and angioedema, but are not common.

⊛ *Priority actions to take before giving antiplatelet drugs.* In addition to the general responsibilities related to anticoagulant therapy (p. 302), check the patient's platelet count.

Antacids interfere with the absorption of antiplatelet drugs. Give antiplatelet drugs 2 hours after or 1 hour before giving antacids. Also give antiplatelet drugs with meals or just after eating to decrease side effects such as nausea and upset stomach.

⊛ *Priority actions to take after giving antiplatelet drugs.* Continue the general responsibilities related to anticoagulant therapy presented on p. 303.

⊛ *Teaching priorities for patients taking antiplatelet drugs.* In addition to the general care needs and precautions related to anticoagulant therapy (p. 303), teach patients these actions:
- Take antiplatelet drugs with food to decrease GI side effects.
- Avoid taking the drug with antacids because these reduce drug absorption.
- Depending on the condition for which you require these drugs, you may need to take them for the rest of your life to prevent clots from forming.
- Do not stop taking your antiplatelet drug unless your prescriber instructs you to do so.

Life span considerations for antiplatelet drugs
Considerations for pregnancy and lactation. Taking antiplatelet drugs during the last 2 weeks of pregnancy can cause bleeding problems in the baby before and after delivery. Antiplatelet drugs can be passed through breast milk to the baby. As discussed in Chapter 10, aspirin and other NSAIDs should not be taken during the last 3 months of pregnancy or while breastfeeding.

THROMBOLYTIC DRUGS

Thrombolytic drugs, also called *fibrinolytic drugs*, are drugs that dissolve clots that have already formed. This is why these drugs have the nickname "clot busters." They are prescribed for patients who have a heart attack, stroke, pulmonary embolism, or some other clot-related problem.

How Thrombolytic Drugs Work
Thrombolytic drugs are used to dissolve clots that form with myocardial infarction, thromboembolic strokes, and pulmonary embolism, although not every thrombolytic drug is approved for every indication. All thrombolytic drugs activate the body's normal plasminogen, which is inactive in body fluids and blood plasma, into its active form, plasmin. It is the active plasmin that is an enzyme and has the ability to bind to circulating fibrinogen, free fibrin, and the fibrin present in formed blood clots and dissolve them. The synthetic thrombolytics commonly used in North America are more selective in dissolving the fibrin within clots rather than acting on the circulating fibrin and fibrinogen (natural plasmin and an earlier drug, streptokinase, are not selective). In addition, all the thrombolytics degrade clotting factors V and VIII. As a result, these drugs break down existing clots and also can reduce or prevent new clots from forming.

The thrombolytics are most often administered by IV, usually in a setting with specially trained nurses (e.g., emergency department, cardiac catheterization lab, or intensive care unit). One drug, *reteplase*, is also approved for intra-arterial administration. For IV use, they may be given by a peripheral IV line or through a

 Critical Point for Safety

Streptokinase is **not** the thrombolytic of choice in the United States because it is less selective, causes more bleeding, and is derived from natural sources that make it more likely to cause an allergic reaction.

QSEN: Safety

long catheter that is guided to the clot. If started within 12 hours after the onset of symptoms for heart attack or 3 hours for stroke symptoms, thrombolytics can dissolve the clot that is blocking the artery and restore blood flow. This action may prevent or minimize tissue damage to the heart or brain. The sooner these drugs are begun, the more likely it is that they will achieve a positive result. In some situations (for example, certain types of heart attacks), thrombolytics are not used if more than 6 hours have passed since the symptoms began because tissue damage has already occurred, and at this point the drugs can cause more problems than they prevent.

The usual adult dosages for the most commonly used thrombolytics in the United States are listed in the table below. Check a reliable drug reference for information about less common thrombolytic drugs.

Usual Adult Dosages for Common Thrombolytic Drugs

Drug Name	Usual Therapeutic Dosages
alteplase (Activase) ❶	MI: 15 mg IV bolus, followed by 50 mg IV over next 30 min, and then 35 mg IV over the next 60 min Thromboembolic stroke: 0.9 mg/kg IV over 60 min with initial 10% of the total dose given as bolus over 1 min within 3 hr PE: 100 mg by IV infusion over 2 hr
reteplase (Retavase) ❶	MI: 10 units IV over 2 min followed by a second dose of 10 units IV 30 min after first dose Peripheral arterial thromboembolism: 0.125–0.5 units/hr IA
tenecteplase (TNKase) ❶	MI: 30–50 mg IV as a single bolus over 5 seconds

❶ High-alert drug; *IA*, Intra-arterial; *MI*, Myocardial infarction; *PE*, Pulmonary embolism.

Intended Responses of Thrombolytic Drugs

- Clotting time is increased.
- Existing clot is dissolved.
- Blood flow is restored in a blocked artery.
- Tissue damage is prevented or minimized.

Common Side Effects of Thrombolytic Drugs

The most common side effects of thrombolytic drugs include bleeding or oozing from cuts, gums, and wounds and around injection sites. Other common side effects include fever and low blood pressure.

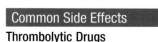

Common Side Effects
Thrombolytic Drugs

Bleeding problems   Fever   Hypotension

Possible Adverse Effects of Thrombolytic Drugs

Although allergic responses with the synthetic thrombolytics are less common than with streptokinase, they may still occur. Signs and symptoms of reactions may include shortness of breath, lump in the throat sensation, fever, chills, chest tightness, swelling, wheezing, skin rash, hives, or itching.

Hemorrhage is a major risk when patients receive thrombolytic therapy because the action of these drugs is to break down clots, and they also inhibit clotting factors V and VIII. They increase the risk for hemorrhagic stroke because of the increased risk for bleeding, which includes bleeding into the brain.

✪ Priority Actions to Take *Before* Giving Thrombolytic Drugs

In addition to the general responsibilities related to anticoagulant therapy (p. 302), determine whether the patient has experienced any of the events listed in Box 17.2 because they are absolute contraindications for thrombolytic therapy. With some other high-risk conditions, the prescriber weighs the pros and cons of the treatment before making a decision for each individual patient.

Box **17.2**   Absolute Contraindications for Thrombolytic Drugs

- Active internal bleeding
- Cerebrovascular processes:
  - Cranial neoplasm
  - Recent spinal or cerebral surgery
  - Recent stroke (within 2 months)
- Increased blood pressure greater than 200/120 mm Hg

- Known bleeding disorders
- Pregnancy or recent delivery (24 hr)
- Prolonged cardiopulmonary resuscitation
- Recent head trauma
- Suspected aortic dissection

Check the patient's coagulation laboratory study results. Make sure that all ordered laboratory tests have been completed and that the patient has an IV access.

⭐ Priority Actions to Take *After* Giving Thrombolytic Drugs

In addition to the general responsibilities related to anticoagulant therapy (p. 303), check the patient for any signs of bleeding at least every 2 hours and report these immediately. Ask the patient about headaches and monitor for changes in level of consciousness. Initially check the patient every 20 to 30 minutes, then every 1 to 2 hours, every 4 hours, every shift, and as needed.

Because of the risk for bleeding, do not give any injectable (intramuscular or subcutaneous) drugs to the patient. Do not start or remove IV lines. If a line must be removed, you will need to apply pressure to the site for at least 30 minutes.

Patients often also receive IV fluids, including anticoagulation with continuous heparin to prevent additional clots from forming. Make sure that these IV fluids are infusing at the correct rate and that the IV line is patent. Make sure that follow-up laboratory tests for coagulation are completed.

⭐ Teaching Priorities for Patients Receiving Thrombolytic Drugs

Thrombolytic drugs are only given in the hospital setting, so there are no priorities to teach patients about taking the drugs at home. However, the patient is an important partner in successful therapy and prevention of complications. Instruct patients to report any problems with their IV access sites such as bleeding, swelling, pain, or numbness or any of the indications of an allergic response listed under possible adverse events.

Instruct patients to report any unusual symptoms at once. Also tell them to report any arm or leg pain that seems to be getting worse.

Life Span Considerations for Thrombolytic Drugs

Considerations for pregnancy and lactation. Thrombolytic drugs have a moderate likelihood of increasing the risk for birth defects or fetal harm, especially during the first 5 months of pregnancy. Delivery of a baby, having had a miscarriage, or having had an abortion within the past 24 hours are absolute contraindications to giving these drugs.

DRUGS THAT IMPROVE BLOOD CLOTTING

COLONY-STIMULATING FACTORS

Many conditions can lower blood counts, including those cells that are important in blood clotting. The most common conditions that reduce blood cell counts include traditional cancer chemotherapy (reduces bone marrow production of all blood cell types) and chronic kidney disease (causes anemia and decreased red blood cell count [RBC]). Drugs generally known as **colony-stimulating factors (CSFs)** are able to increase the production of all types of blood cells by stimulating the bone marrow, which is the primary source of all blood cells. The bone marrow normally makes these blood components in response to naturally occurring hormones. For example,

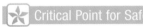

Critical Point for Safety

After a patient has received a thrombolytic drug, do not start or remove IV lines and do not give any unnecessary IM injections.

QSEN: Safety

Teaching Alert

Instruct patients to report any problems with IV access sites such as bleeding, swelling, pain, or numbness, and any signs or symptoms of an allergic response.

QSEN: Safety

when a person is *anemic* (has too few RBCs), the ability of the blood to carry oxygen is reduced, and tissues do not receive the normal amount of oxygen. When the kidney receives less oxygen, it secretes erythropoietin into the blood. This substance goes to the bone marrow and stimulates it to increase production of RBCs.

Subsets of CSFs are more specific and increase bone marrow production of just one blood cell type. Drugs that primarily increase RBC levels are known as **erythropoiesis-stimulating agents (ESAs)**, and those that increase platelet levels are known as **thrombopoiesis-stimulating agents (TSAs)**.

Specific Colony Stimulating Factors

How ESAs and TSAs work. ESAs and TSAs are similar to the naturally occurring hormones that trigger the bone marrow to produce more cells. ESAs make the bone marrow increase production of RBCs to the greatest extent, although they do increase all blood cell production to some degree. TSAs are more specific for stimulating the bone marrow to increase production of platelets, although the production of other cells also increases. ESAs are most often used for patients who have chronic kidney disease, are anemic from cancer chemotherapy, or need to increase RBC counts before surgery. TSAs are most often used for patients who have low platelet counts from cancer chemotherapy. Both types of drugs reduce the need for transfusion of blood and blood products.

The usual adult dosages for the most commonly used ESAs and TSAs are listed in the table below. Currently, these drugs are only available for parenteral administration. However, manufacturers are working on development of a transdermal delivery system. Check a reliable drug reference for information about the general colony-stimulating agents.

> **Memory Jogger**
>
> ESAs (erythropoiesis-stimulating agents) increase red blood cell (RBC) levels. TSAs (thrombopoiesis-stimulating agents) increase platelet levels. ESAs are less specific than the TSAs.

Usual Adult Dosages for Specific Colony-Stimulating Agents: ESAs and TSAs

Drug Class	Drug Name	Usual Therapeutic Dosages
Erythropoiesis-Stimulating Agents	darbopoetin alfa (Aranesp)	2.25 mcg/kg subcutaneously once weekly or 500 mcg every 3–4 weeks
	epoetin alfa (Epogen, Procrit, Retacrit)	50–100 units/kg IV or subcutaneously 3 times weekly until hemoglobin levels reach target range
Thrombopoiesis-Stimulating Agents	oprelvekin (Neumega)	50 mcg/kg subcutaneously once daily until the platelet count reaches 50,000/mm^3

Intended responses of ESAs and TSAs
- Specific blood cell levels are approaching normal.
- The need for transfusion therapy is reduced.
- The risk for excessive bleeding is reduced.

Common side effects of ESAs and TSAs. Because these drugs increase blood cell production, the blood becomes more *viscous* (thicker). This effect raises blood pressure, increases clot formation, and slows blood movement through small vessels. Other side effects include headaches, general body aches, flushing, fever, chills, and pain at the injection site.

Possible adverse effects of ESAs and TSAs. Because these agents, especially ESAs, increase blood viscosity and fluid retention, the patient is at risk for severe hypertension, blood clots, strokes, and heart attacks. In addition, certain types of cancer cells grow faster in the presence of these factors such as head and neck cancer cells, leukemias, and lymphomas. The basis of dosing for these drugs is to monitor individual

Common Side Effects

ESAs and TSAs

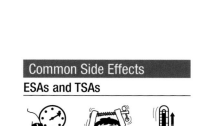

Hypertension   Headache   Fever

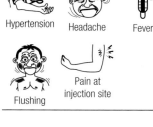

Flushing   Pain at injection site

patient hemoglobin or platelet levels to ensure that just enough cells are produced to avoid the need for transfusion.

⊛ *Priority actions to take **before** giving ESAs or TSAs.* If the patient is receiving a repeat dose of the drug, ask him or her if any allergic reactions or difficulty breathing occurred with a previous dose. If the patient has had such a response, notify the prescriber before giving the drug.

Check the patient's blood counts before therapy. If the platelet count is greater than 50,000/mm³ or if the hemoglobin level is at 12 g/dL (or higher), notify the prescriber before giving the drug.

Check the patient's blood pressure and use this value to monitor for drug-induced hypertension.

Follow the package directions for mixing and preparing the drug. Ensure that oprelvekin (Neumega) is administered only by deep subcutaneous injection and not intravenously or intradermally.

⊛ *Priority actions to take **after** giving ESAs or TSAs.* When giving the first IV dose of an ESA or TSA, check the patient every 20 minutes for any signs or symptoms of an allergic reaction (hives at the IV site, low blood pressure, rapid irregular pulse, swelling of the lips or lower face, the patient feeling a "lump in the throat"). If you suspect an allergic reaction, call the rapid response team and notify the prescriber.

Check the patient's blood pressure and complete blood count to determine the effectiveness of the drug and whether increased viscosity is occurring.

⊛ *Teaching priorities for patients receiving ESAs or TSAs*
- Weigh yourself daily and report a weight gain of more than 2 lb in a 24-hour period or 4 lb in a week to your prescriber.
- Immediately report any sign of a clot (swelling in one extremity, difference in skin color or temperature in one extremity, pain in one extremity) to your prescriber.
- Be sure to have blood tests done as often as prescribed.
- Go immediately to the emergency department or call 911 for chest pain, shortness of breath, change in level of consciousness, difficulty speaking, numbness or drooping of one side of the face, or blurred vision. These are signs of a heart attack or stroke.
- If you are self-administering the drug, use the technique you were taught for subcutaneous injection and how to monitor the site for problems.

Life span considerations for ESAs and TSAs

Considerations for pregnancy and lactation. The effects of ESAs and TSAs in human pregnancy are not known. Potential risks must be weighed against potential benefits for an individual patient.

Considerations for older adults. The increased viscosity of the blood is more likely to result in hypertension and increase the risk for congestive heart failure, pulmonary edema, heart attacks, and strokes. Older adults should be monitored more closely for blood cell responses, and the therapy should be stopped or decreased when hemoglobin levels approach 11 g/dL or if hypertension develops.

Critical Point for Safety

Monitor patients receiving the first dose of an ESA or TSA closely (at least every 20 minutes) for symptoms of an allergic reaction.

QSEN: Safety

Drug Alert

Teaching Alert

Teach patients to report signs of clot formation immediately (e.g., swelling in one extremity, pain in one extremity, a difference in temperature or color in one extremity).

QSEN: Safety

Get Ready for the NCLEX® Examination!

Key Points

- Clot formation is a normal, protective process that prevents blood loss.
- Abnormal and dangerous forms of clots include thrombi and emboli.
- Anticoagulant drugs prevent clots from forming or existing clots from getting bigger, and thrombolytic (fibrinolytic) agents ("clot busters") dissolve existing clots.
- With the exception of aspirin, *all* drugs used to reduce blood clotting or to break up existing clots are *high-alert drugs* and can cause harm if given to a patient in error.
- Hold firm pressure on an IM or IV site for at least 5 minutes when patient is taking or receiving a drug that reduces clotting.
- Initial IV doses of heparin are based on patient weight; the rate of the continuous infusion is based on the aPTT laboratory results.
- LMW heparins such as enoxaparin (Lovenox) do not require laboratory tests to guide therapy.
- Antidotes for heparin (protamine sulfate) and warfarin (vitamin K) must be readily available on the unit for patients receiving these drugs.
- Heparin therapy lasting longer than a week, especially with unfractionated heparin, can cause a drug reaction (heparin-induced thrombocytopenia) that activates platelets causing extensive microclot formation that depletes platelets and greatly increases the risk for bleeding. Closely monitor the platelet (thrombocyte) counts of patients on prolonged heparin therapy and remain alert for unusual bruising and bleeding.
- Dose prescription for warfarin is guided by the INR laboratory test. A common therapeutic INR goal is 2.0 to 3.0 (normal INR is 0.8 to 1.2).
- There is considerable genetic variation in the enzymes that activate and those that metabolize warfarin, and it is important to closely monitor the INR of patients taking this drug to determine whether the expected results are being achieved. Report results that do not match the expected response (either much higher or much lower) to the prescriber for dosage adjustments.

- Because warfarin interacts with hundreds of drugs, herbal supplements, and foods, always check the patient's current drug list (both prescribed and over-the-counter) for any potential interactions before beginning warfarin therapy.
- Warfarin is the *only* drug approved for use by patients who have a mechanical heart valve or who have atrial fibrillation (A-fib) caused by a heart valve problem.
- In addition to warfarin requiring several days of therapy before full anticoagulant effects are present, a return to normal clotting also requires several days after the drug is stopped.
- Pregnancy is an absolute contraindication for warfarin use because it is highly likely to cause birth defects or fetal death.
- A complete patient health history is very important before giving thrombolytic drugs because there are reasons the drugs may not be given (contraindications).
- The sooner thrombolytic drugs are given when symptoms of a thrombotic event have occurred, the more likely it is that the clot can be successfully dissolved.
- After a patient has received a thrombolytic drug, do not start or remove IV lines and do not give any unnecessary IM injections.
- Monitor patients receiving the first dose or an ESA or TSA closely (at least every 20 minutes) for symptoms of an allergic reaction.
- Teach patients taking an ESA or TSA to report signs of clot formation immediately (e.g., swelling in one extremity, pain in one extremity, a difference in temperature or color in one extremity).

Additional Learning Resources

🌐 Be sure to visit your Evolve website (http://evolve.elsevier.com/Workman/pharmacology/) for additional online resources.

SG Go to your study guide for additional learning activities to help you master this chapter content.

Review Questions

See *Answers to In-Text Review Questions* in the back of the book for answers to these questions.

1. **How are anticoagulant drugs and thrombolytic drugs different?**

    A. There is no difference; they both have the same actions.
    B. Anticoagulants prevent clots from forming, whereas thrombolytics can dissolve clots that have already formed.
    C. Thrombolytics must be administered intravenously while all anticoagulants are administered as oral agents.
    D. Anticoagulants prevent clots by actually thinning the blood whereas thrombolytics reduce platelet aggregation and do not affect blood thickness.

2. **Which drug or drug class used to prevent excessive or inappropriate clotting is not categorized as a high-alert drug?**

    A. Thrombin inhibitors
    B. Anticoagulants
    C. Thrombolytics
    D. Aspirin

3. **A patient who has been taking an anticoagulant daily for a year is now prescribed a one-time IM dose of an antibiotic. Which action will the nurse implement to reduce the patient's risk for bleeding?**

    A. Requesting an order for the antibiotic to be given intravenously
    B. Injecting the antibiotic into a site on the thigh instead of the arm
    C. Applying firm pressure to the injection site for at least 5 minutes
    D. Ensuring the site is maintained above the level of the heart for 10 minutes after the injection

4. A patient taking an oral anticoagulant drug every 12 hr at 9:00 a.m. and 9:00 p.m. reports that she forgot her morning dose and it is now 8:30 p.m. How will the nurse advise this patient?

A. "Take a double dose right now and skip the 9:00 p.m. dose."
B. "When you take your usual 9:00 p.m. dose tonight, also take a 325 mg aspirin."
C. "Take your 9:00 p.m. dose now and restart your regular two doses tomorrow."
D. "Go to the nearest emergency department to receive an injectable dose in addition to your usual oral dose."

5. A patient is admitted with a deep vein thrombosis in the right calf and is to receive heparin therapy with an IV bolus dose followed by continuous infusion. Which assessment is **most important** for the nurse to perform before the therapy is started?

A. Asking the patient whether she has any allergies to egg-based drugs
B. Inspecting the patient's body for the presence of bruising or petechiae
C. Comparing the circumference of the right calf with that of the left calf
D. Obtaining an accurate weight while the patient is wearing only a hospital gown

6. Which laboratory value indicates to the nurse that the patient may have developed heparin-induced thrombocytopenia (HIT)?

A. Elevated total white blood cell count
B. Decreased red blood cell count
C. Decreased platelet count
D. INR of 2.0

7. A patient newly prescribed an anticoagulant remarks that she believes she will have no trouble remembering when to take the drug because she has been using ginkgo biloba daily for a year and can take them at the same time. What is the nurse's best response?

A. "You will need to stop taking the ginkgo biloba because it decreases the effectiveness of anticoagulants, which will increase your risk for clots."
B. "You will need to stop taking the ginkgo biloba because it also interferes with blood clotting, which will increase your risk for excessive bleeding."
C. "Be sure to take the ginkgo biloba in the morning and your prescribed drug at night to avoid a possible interaction between the two."
D. "Keep vitamin K supplements at home at all times so you can take it whenever you notice an increase in bruising."

8. A patient who developed stroke symptoms 1 hour ago is in the emergency department. Which type of drug does the nurse expect to prepare to treat this problem?

A. Thrombolytic
B. Thrombin inhibitor
C. Antiplatelet drug
D. Warfarin

9. Which drug/agent does the nurse expect to be prescribed for a patient with a deep vein thrombosis (DVT) who is 5 months pregnant?

A. Aspirin
B. Warfarin
C. Heparin
D. Apixaban

10. The prescriber orders a patient to receive vorapaxar 2.08 orally along with 81 mg of aspirin. What is the nurse's **best** action?

A. Giving the vorapaxar and holding the dose of aspirin
B. Checking with the pharmacist before giving these drugs
C. Assessing the patient's most current laboratory coagulation test results
D. Reminding the prescriber that both aspirin and vorapaxar are both antiplatelet drugs

11. Which patient assessment finding indicates to the nurse that the oprelvekin therapy is effective?

A. INR is 3.0
B. Superficial bruises are fading
C. RBC count is above $250,000/mm^3$
D. Platelet count is above $60,000/mm^3$

12. A patient is prescribed to receive 10,000 units of heparin subcutaneously. The heparin on hand comes as 20,000 units in 1 mL. How may mL will the nurse prepare to give this patient?
_____ mL

Clinical Judgment

1 Which techniques are most appropriate for the nurse to use when administering low-molecular-weight heparin by prefilled syringe to a patient subcutaneously? **Select all that apply.**

A. Aspirating before injection
B. Expelling the air bubble before injecting
C. Inserting the needle at a 30-degree angle
D. Injecting into a pinched-up skinfold of tissue
E. Avoiding rubbing or massaging the site after injection
F. Injecting the drug as close to the umbilicus as possible
G. Ensuring that the drug is not given as an intradermal injection
H. Avoiding the thigh as an injection site

2. A 58-year-old woman is newly diagnosed with atrial fibrillation that is not associated with any heart valve problem and is prescribed to start taking apixaban (Eliquis) 5 mg twice daily. She also has type 2 diabetes, which is well controlled with oral antidiabetic drugs, and moderate hypertension for which she takes olmesartan (Benicar) daily. She has lost 40 lb over the past year by eating a low-fat, high-fiber diet with green salads every day. The nurse is developing a teaching plan with take-home instructions/precautions about these drugs. Use an X to indicate which instructions are Most Relevant, Not Relevant, or Potentially Harmful at this time for this patient with regard to direct-acting oral anticoagulant drug therapy

INSTRUCTION/PRECAUTION	MOST RELEVANT	NOT RELEVANT	POTENTIALLY HARMFUL
If you lose an additional 10 lb or more, report this to your prescriber because the dose will need to be reduced.			
Try to take the drug at the same time every day as close as possible to 12 hours apart.			
If you forget one dose, double the next dose.			
Switch to an electric shaver to shave your legs and other body hair.			
Do not take aspirin or NSAIDs while on this drug.			
If you develop swelling of the lips, tongue, and face, put ice on the swollen areas.			
Make and keep weekly laboratory appointments to have your INR measured.			
Keep the tablets in the container that came from the pharmacy rather than using a daily pill organizer.			
Avoid eating grapefruit or drinking grapefruit juice while on this drug.			
If you fall and hit your head or spine, contact your prescriber immediately.			

INR, International normalized ratio; NSAID, Nonsteroidal antiinflammatory drug.

Drug Therapy for Asthma and Other Respiratory Problems

18

Learning Objectives

The content presented in this chapter should help you to:

1. Describe the names, actions, usual adult dosages, possible side effects, and adverse effects of drug therapy to manage common, noninfectious respiratory problems.
2. Describe the priority actions to take before and after giving drug therapy to manage common, noninfectious respiratory problems.
3. Prioritize essential information to teach patients taking drug therapy to manage common, noninfectious respiratory problems.
4. Explain appropriate life span considerations for drug therapy to manage common, noninfectious respiratory problems.

5. List the names, actions, usual adult dosages, possible side effects, and adverse effects of drugs to treat pulmonary arterial hypertension and pulmonary fibrosis.
6. Describe the priority actions to take before and after giving drugs to treat pulmonary arterial hypertension and pulmonary fibrosis.
7. Prioritize essential information to teach patients taking drugs to treat pulmonary arterial hypertension and pulmonary fibrosis.

Key Terms

antiinflammatory drugs (ăn-tī-ĭn-FLĂM-ĕ-tōr-ē DRŬGZ) (p. 326) A class of drugs that prevents or limits inflammatory responses to injury or invasion.

beta₂-adrenergic agonists (BE-tă TU ăd-rĕn-ĔRJ-ĭk ĂG-ō-nĭsts) (p. 322) Drugs that bind to the beta₂-adrenergic receptors and act like adrenalin, causing an increase in the production of a substance that triggers pulmonary smooth muscle relaxation.

biologics (bīō LĂ jik) (p. 329) A class of complex antiinflammatory drugs derived from living sources that target specific inflammatory cells, components, or products to modify chronic disorders associated with inflammation and tissue damage.

bronchodilators (brŏn-kō-DĪ-lā-tŭr) (p. 322) Drugs that relax the smooth muscle around airways, causing the lumen centers to enlarge.

cholinergic antagonists (kō-lĭn-ĔRJ-ĭk ăn-TĂG-ō-nĭsts) (p. 322) Drugs that block the parasympathetic nervous system and

allow a person's natural epinephrine and norepinephrine to bind to smooth muscle receptors and cause bronchodilation.

corticosteroids (kōr-tĭ-kō-STĔR-ōydz) (p. 327) Drugs similar to natural cortisol that prevent or limit inflammation by slowing or stopping inflammatory mediator production.

endothelin-receptor antagonists (ĕn-dō-thē-lĭn rē-SĔP-tŏr ăn-TĂG-ō-nĭsts) (p. 332) Drugs that are able to block the endothelin-1 receptors on endothelial cells in blood vessels, resulting in blood vessel dilation.

mucolytics (myū-kō-LĬ-tĭk) (p. 331) Drugs that reduce the thickness of mucus, making it easier to move out of the airways.

prostanoids (prŏ-stăn-ōydz) (p. 332) A drug group composed of naturally occurring and synthetic agents with the main effect of dilating pulmonary blood vessels.

REVIEW OF RELATED PHYSIOLOGY AND PATHOPHYSIOLOGY OF COMMON RESPIRATORY DISORDERS

Oxygen (O₂) from the atmospheric air you breathe is an essential nutrient for all tissues and organs to live, grow, and perform their specific jobs. After entering the upper airway passages in the mouth and nose, this atmospheric air must travel through the entire lower airways in the lungs to the alveolar air sacs. Once in the alveoli, gases can be exchanged with O₂, diffusing into capillary blood to be carried to all tissues and organs. At the same time, the waste gas *carbon dioxide* (CO₂), generated by normal metabolism in all tissues and organs, moves from the blood into the alveoli so it can leave the body during exhalation.

 Memory Jogger

Atmospheric air entering the lungs is the **only** source of the essential nutrient oxygen. Any problem that interferes with oxygen intake or gas exchange adversely affects all tissues and organs.

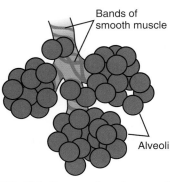

FIG. 18.2 Close-up view of one small airway with attached alveoli.

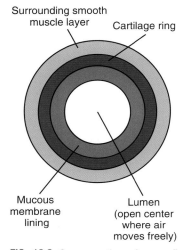

FIG. 18.3 Cross section of a small airway showing the tissue layers.

 Memory Jogger

Keeping airways open is critical for ensuring that oxygen reaches the lungs and gas exchange can occur.

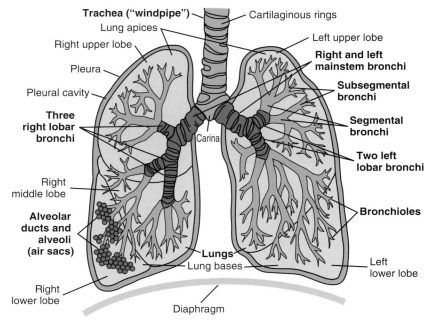

FIG. 18.1 Normal anatomy of the lungs.

Although any part of the airways and lungs can become infected, infection is not a respiratory-related *cause* of disease. Drugs for infection, including respiratory infections, are discussed in Chapters 6 through 8.

The major common health problems of the respiratory system are those that narrow the airways, such as asthma or chronic bronchitis, and diseases that destroy the alveoli, such as emphysema. Chronic obstructive pulmonary disease (COPD) is a respiratory disorder that is a combination of chronic bronchitis and emphysema. Other less common respiratory disorders that involve the lung tissue rather than the airways and result in impairment of gas exchange are pulmonary arterial hypertension (PAH) and pulmonary fibrosis. This chapter is focused on drug therapy for asthma, COPD, PAH, and pulmonary fibrosis.

Figure 18.1 shows the normal anatomy of the lungs, including the larger airways and the smaller airways leading to the alveoli. Figure 18.2 shows a close-up of one small airway with the alveoli attached. It is important for the airways to remain open for good airflow to and from the alveoli, where O_2 and CO_2 are exchanged. As shown in Figure 18.3, the airways have several layers around a hollow middle section. It is also important that the membranes of the alveoli remain thin enough to permit O_2 and CO_2 to diffuse through them. In addition, blood vessels in the lungs must remain mostly dilated, relatively thin, and have lower pressures to allow good blood flow through the lungs for proper gas exchange.

The open center of the hollow part of an airway is the *lumen*. Different health problems can make the lumens smaller or even close completely. The lumen center can be blocked by thick mucus and other substances. The mucous membranes lining the airway can swell when inflammation is present and obstruct the lumen. A layer of smooth muscle surrounds the outside of the airways. If this smooth muscle constricts tightly (*bronchoconstriction*), the airway lumen can narrow and even close.

ASTHMA

Asthma is a chronic disorder in which airway obstruction occurs intermittently from bronchoconstriction of the smooth muscles that surround the airways and from airway inflammation (Figure 18.4). Although the tissue conditions responsible for asthma are always present in susceptible individuals, symptoms occur in episodes or attacks (Animation 18.1). Between attacks, the airways are usually open and

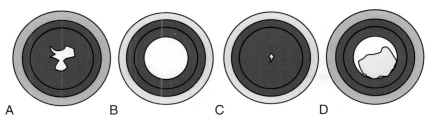

FIG. 18.4 Different causes of narrowed airways. (A) Mucosal swelling. (B) Constriction of smooth muscle. (C) Mucosal swelling and constriction of smooth muscle. (D) Mucus plug.

 Memory Jogger

The problems that narrow or block the airways include bronchoconstriction (smooth muscle tightening), which narrows the lumens from the outside of the airway, and inflammation, which causes swelling of the mucous membrane that obstructs the lumen inside the airways. Both problems are worse when mucus plugs also form within the lumens.

unobstructed. Thus, the problem is most often intermittent and reversible. Only the airways are affected, not the alveoli.

Inflammation of the mucous membranes lining the airways is a key event in triggering an asthma attack. It occurs in response to the presence of allergens: irritants such as cold air, dry air, or fine particles in the air; microorganisms; and aspirin. As described in Chapter 10, histamine, leukotrienes, and other inflammatory natural chemical mediators are released from inflammatory cells (neutrophils, eosinophils, and mast cells) into the mucous membranes. When this happens, blood vessels dilate, the tissue swells, and mucus increases. These same factors also cause bronchoconstriction. Asthma is most common in people who have excessive numbers and/or overactive inflammatory cells, especially eosinophils.

A patient with mild-to-moderate asthma has no symptoms between asthma attacks. Symptoms of an acute asthma attack are increased respiratory rate and a *wheeze*, which is a squeaky or snorelike sound made when air moves through narrowed airways (Animation 18.2). With inflammation, the patient also has increased coughing, which may be the major symptom in some people (known as *cough-variant asthma*). As breathing and gas exchange become less effective, blood O_2 levels decrease and blood CO_2 levels increase.

 Critical Point for Safety

When an asthma attack is so severe that oxygen levels become too low, the patient can die if interventions do not improve air movement.

QSEN: Safety

CHRONIC OBSTRUCTIVE PULMONARY DISEASE

Chronic obstructive pulmonary disease (COPD) is a combination of chronic bronchitis and emphysema. *Chronic bronchitis* is a **persistent** inflammation of the airways with swollen airway mucous membranes and enlargement of the mucus-producing cells. This creates large amounts of thick, sticky mucus that narrow the airways. As a result, moving air into and out of the lungs is more difficult (see Figure 18.4). In *emphysema* the normal elastic tissue in the alveoli becomes loose and flabby. Because exhalation depends on the recoil of the alveoli (just as the "stretch and recoil" of a full balloon helps it to deflate quickly), a loss of elastic tissue makes exhaling air more difficult. Both problems are progressive and become worse with time. The main risk factor for developing COPD is long-term cigarette smoking or vaping.

COPD is similar to asthma in terms of airway blockage. However, the symptoms of COPD *never* go away completely, although they can improve with drug therapy. The alveoli are damaged in COPD but *not* in asthma. Thick, sticky mucus is continuously produced in a patient with COPD.

Although most people with asthma do not develop COPD, a patient may have both disorders at the same time. In addition, people who have had severe, poorly controlled asthma for a long time have a higher risk for COPD development—even when they have never smoked.

TYPES OF DRUGS FOR ASTHMA AND COPD

When asthma is well controlled, the airway narrowing is temporary and reversible. With poor control, attacks become worse, happen more often, and can become so severe that death from lack of oxygen may occur during an attack. The goals of drug therapy for asthma are to improve airflow, reduce symptoms, and prevent active asthma attacks. Drug therapy for asthma management involves specifically selecting drugs from several categories for each patient.

Memory Jogger

Rescue (or reliever) drugs stop an active asthma attack or reduce its severity; controller drugs prevent an attack from starting.

Memory Jogger

Types of drugs for asthma treatment and prevention and COPD maintenance include:
- Bronchodilators
- Antiinflammatories
- Biologics
- Mucolytics

Memory Jogger

Inhaled short-acting beta₂-adrenergic agonists (SABAs) are rescue drugs because they provide rapid (but short-term) relief.

Critical Point for Safety

Controller drugs for prevention, such as long-acting beta₂-adrenergic agonists (LABAs), must be taken daily and exactly as prescribed, even on days when no symptoms are present, to be effective. They are **NOT** to be used in place of rescue drugs.

QSEN: Safety

Drug therapy for asthma is based on disease severity. Some patients may need drug therapy with a *rescue drug (reliever drug)* only during an asthma episode. Others need daily drugs as *prevention (controller drugs)* to keep asthma attacks from happening—or, at least, to reduce their frequency. Total therapy for best management involves the use of drugs that make the smooth muscle around the airways relax (*bronchodilators*) and antiinflammatory drugs.

Although COPD cannot be reversed, its progression can be slowed, and the symptoms reduced with proper drug therapy. Drug therapy for COPD is based on disease severity and the patient's responses to the drugs. Because the chronic bronchitis airway problems of COPD are similar to the airway changes that occur during an asthma attack, most of the drugs used to treat COPD are the same as those used to treat asthma. Drug dosages, frequency, and delivery mechanisms may differ, with the person who has COPD taking higher or more frequent doses.

The patient with asthma or chronic bronchitis can help manage his or her disease by assessing trigger activities and symptom severity daily. As a partner in long-term management, the patient learns to adjust prescribed drugs for inflammation and bronchospasms to prevent or relieve symptoms.

Airway narrowing with asthma and COPD has more than one cause, which often requires the use of more than one drug type. The main drugs usually prescribed for asthma and COPD are bronchodilators and antiinflammatories. Asthma management may also include biologics, and COPD management often includes mucolytics. More drugs for COPD are available as combination agents with two or more drugs.

Bronchodilators

Bronchodilators are drugs that relax the smooth muscles around airways, causing the lumen centers to enlarge for better airflow. Different types of bronchodilators work in several ways to relax smooth muscles in the airways, causing the lumen center to enlarge. They have no effect on inflammation. So when a patient's asthma or chronic bronchitis is caused by both bronchoconstriction and inflammation, at least two types of drug therapy are needed. Bronchodilators include beta₂-adrenergic agonists, cholinergic antagonists, and xanthines.

How bronchodilators work

Beta₂-adrenergic agonists. Natural adrenalin helps asthma by binding to beta₂-adrenergic receptors on bronchiolar smooth muscle, which then increases the production of *cyclic adenosine monophosphate (cAMP)* inside these muscle cells and triggers their relaxation. Drugs that mimic this action are beta₂-adrenergic agonists. Some are fast-acting with effects that last only a short time. These are known as short-acting beta₂-adrenergic agonists (SABAs) and are *rescue drugs* (or reliever drugs) because they provide rapid (but short-term) relief when an asthma attack begins. They are also useful when a patient is about to start an activity that is likely to induce an asthma attack. These drugs are used for COPD when the patient feels more breathless than usual. When inhaled, the drug is delivered directly to the lungs, and systemic effects are minimal (unless the agent is overused).

Long-acting beta₂-adrenergic agonists (LABAs) work in the same way as SABAs but need time to build up an effect. Therefore, LABAs are used to *prevent* an asthma attack because their effects last longer but have no value during an acute attack. For COPD, these drugs are taken daily to maintain open airways. The patient with COPD may use a nebulizer and mask for some of these drugs, rather than a handheld inhaler (Animation 18.3).

Cholinergic antagonists. Cholinergic antagonists, also known as *anticholinergic drugs*, block the parasympathetic nervous system. This blockade allows a person's natural epinephrine and norepinephrine to bind to smooth muscle receptors and bronchodilation results. These inhaled drugs also bind to mucous membrane receptors and decrease airway secretions. Like LABAs, they are *controller (prevention)* drugs and must be taken on a daily basis to prevent asthma attacks and reduce airway blockage in COPD. The patient with COPD is more likely to be prescribed a longer-acting cholinergic antagonist. These controller drugs are used to prevent an asthma attack but have no value during an acute attack.

Xanthines. Xanthines are powerful systemic drugs, such as theophylline, but have many side effects and adverse effects. For this reason, they are rarely used today. Check a drug reliable reference source for information about xanthines or methylxanthines.

Usual Adult Dosages for Common Bronchodilators

Drug Category	Drug Name	Usual Maintenance Dose
Short-Acting Beta₂-Agonists (SABAs)	albuterol (Accuneb, Proventil, Respirol, Ventolin, Volmax, VoSpire)	1–2 inhalations of 90 mcg every 3–4 hr by MDI
	levalbuterol (Xopenex)	2 inhalations of 45 mcg every 4–6 hr
Long-Acting Beta₂-Agonists (LABAs)	arformoterol (Brovana)	15 mcg (contents of one 2-mL vial) every 12 hr via nebulization
	formoterol (Foradil, Perforomist)	20 mcg (2-mL unit) by nebulizer 12 hr
	salmeterol (Serevent)	1 oral inhalation of 50 mcg every 12 hr by MDI
Cholinergic Antagonists	ipratropium (Atrovent)	2–4 puffs of 17 mcg/puff 3–4 times daily by MDI
	tiotropium (Spiriva)	2 puff (2.5 mcg/puff) once daily (MDI)
	aclidinium (TUDORZA PRESSAIR)[a]	1 puff (400 mcg) every 12 hr by DPI
Selected Bronchodilator Combination Agents[b]	BEVESPI	glycopyrronium/formoterol
	Duakir	aclidinium/formoterol
	STIOLTO	tiotropium/olodaterol

[a] Approved only for use with COPD, not asthma.

[b] Dosages vary.

DPI, Dry powder inhaler; *MDI,* Metered dose inhaler.

Intended responses of bronchodilators
- Pulmonary smooth muscles relax.
- Airway lumens widen, allowing air to move more freely into and out of the alveoli.
- Wheezing decreases or disappears.

Common side effects of bronchodilators. Most bronchodilator therapy for asthma and COPD is orally inhaled using inhalers or nebulizers. When taken as prescribed, inhaled bronchodilators have few side effects unless heavily used. Using an inhaler too often allows the drug to be absorbed through the mucous membranes of the mouth, throat, and respiratory linings and enter the bloodstream. Once a drug has entered the bloodstream, it can have systemic effects. Some of the systemic effects of bronchodilators include rapid heart rate, increased blood pressure, a feeling of nervousness, tremors, and difficulty sleeping. Inhaled drugs can dry the mouth and throat, and may leave a bad taste in the mouth.

Cholinergic antagonists cause some specific side effects if they reach the bloodstream. These effects include urinary retention, blurred vision, eye pain, nausea, constipation, dry mouth, and headache.

Adverse effects of bronchodilators. Some brands of inhaled bronchodilators contain preservatives that can cause minor-to-severe allergic reactions. Warn patients to check with their prescriber if a rash, chest pain, or lightheadedness occurs within a few minutes after using the inhaler. In addition, if a patient uses the inhaler more frequently than prescribed, enough of the drug can reach the blood and cause the blood vessels in the heart to constrict, leading to angina or a heart attack (myocardial infarction).

 Do Not Confuse

Xopenex *with* **Xanax**

An order for Xopenex may be confused with Xanax. Xopenex is an inhaled, short-acting bronchodilator, whereas Xanax is an oral benzodiazepine used to treat anxiety.

QSEN: Safety

 Memory Jogger

An easy way to remember the side effects of cholinergic antagonists is the rhyme "can't see, can't spit, can't pee, can't...poop."

Common Side Effects

Bronchodilators

Tachycardia   Hypertension   Dry mouth

Tremors

⚠ Drug Alert

Action/Intervention Alert

Assess for chest pain in the patient taking a bronchodilator. If any chest discomfort is present, notify the prescriber immediately.

QSEN: Safety

✪ *Priority actions to take* before *giving bronchodilators.* Many drugs for asthma and COPD are delivered using inhalers. The three types of inhalers (often called "puffers" by patients) are metered dose inhalers (MDIs), which deliver drugs as a fine liquid spray aerosol; dry powder inhalers (DPIs), which deliver drugs as a fine powder; and soft mist inhalers (SMIs) (also known as "slow moving inhalers"), which deliver drugs as a very fine soft mist. The MDIs use a propellent to become an aerosol and move the spray into the airways. Drug delivery with an MDI is best when a spacer is used (Figure 18.5). DPIs have no propellent and must be sucked into the airways during inhalation to reach the respiratory tract. SMIs have a mechanical spring-loaded device that creates an aerosol mist the patient sucks into the respiratory tract by inhalation. Neither DPIs nor SMIs uses a spacer for drug delivery.

Many patients have never used an oral inhaler or a spacer and may not know the correct technique. Others may have used an inhaler but do not use the correct technique. *Correct technique is critical for drug effectiveness.* Ask whether the patient has ever used an inhaler. If the answer is yes, ask him or her to demonstrate or describe the technique used. If the patient has not used an inhaler or a spacer, teach the correct technique. Box 18.1 describes teaching tips for using an aerosol (metered-dose) inhaler with a spacer.

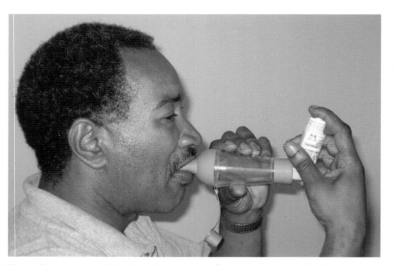

FIG. 18.5 Patient using an aerosol inhaler with a spacer. (From Ignatavicius, D., & Workman, M. L. [2016]. *Medical-surgical nursing: Patient-centered collaborative care* [8th ed.]. St. Louis: Elsevier.)

Box 18.1 Teaching Tips for Using an Aerosol Metered-Dose Inhaler with a Spacer

- Before each use, remove the caps from the inhaler and the spacer.
- Insert the mouthpiece of the inhaler into the non-mouthpiece end of the spacer.
- Shake the whole unit three or four times vigorously to mix the drug in the inhaler.
- Place the mouthpiece of the spacer into your mouth, over your tongue. Seal your lips around the mouthpiece.
- Press down firmly on the canister to release one dose of the drug into the spacer.
- Breathe in slowly and deeply. If the spacer makes a whistling sound, you are breathing in too fast.
- Remove the mouthpiece from your mouth, closing your lips immediately.
- Keep your lips closed and hold your breath for at least 10 seconds, then slowly breathe out.
- If you are prescribed to take two puffs, wait at least 1 minute before taking the second puff.
- Use the same technique for the second puff as you did for the first.
- When finished, remove the inhaler canister from the spacer.
- Replace the caps on the inhaler and the spacer.
- At least once each day, clean the plastic mouthpiece and the cap of the inhaler by thoroughly rinsing them in warm, running tap water.
- Clean the spacer and its mouthpiece at least weekly by thoroughly rinsing them in warm, running tap water.

The powder used in a DPI may already be loaded in the inhaler or may have to be placed in the inhaler each time it is used. The technique used with DPIs differs from that of standard aerosol inhalers (MDIs) because the powder must remain dry to be active. Box 18.2 describes teaching tips for how to use a DPI.

Soft mist inhalers are considered more effective because, upon activating the device, the mist forms a heavier cloud of particles that moves more slowly and allows the patient time to inhale it before the drug escapes through the nose. Also, the heavier particles are more likely to move deep into the airways. Spacers are not used. However, loading and activating the device may be more difficult than for other inhaler types, and the device is more expensive. Box 18.3 describes teaching tips for how to use an SMI.

Use a stethoscope to listen to the lungs of the patient before giving or having a patient use an inhaled bronchodilator. This information can be used to determine drug effectiveness by comparing it with the patient's breath sounds after therapy. Also, assess oxygen saturation with a pulse oximeter.

 Priority actions to take after *giving bronchodilators.* Assess the patient's breathing status after giving short-acting inhaler drugs to determine whether the drugs are effective. Breathing improvement—as measured by a slower respiratory rate, decreased or absent wheezes, and pulse oximetry values of 95% or higher—usually occurs within 5 minutes of inhalation of short-acting bronchodilators. Compare the patient's heart rate and blood pressure within 15 minutes after giving the drug to determine whether any systemic effects are present.

If a patient is to receive two or more drugs by inhaler for breathing problems, give the bronchodilator first and wait at least 5 minutes before giving the next drug. This action allows time for the bronchodilator to widen the airways so the next drug can be inhaled more deeply into the respiratory tract and be more effective.

> ### ⭐ Critical Point for Safety
>
> Within 5–15 min after administering an inhaled bronchodilator, ask about any chest pain. Immediately report severe tachycardia, a rapid rise in blood pressure, or chest pain/discomfort to the prescriber.
>
> QSEN: Safety

> ### ❗ Drug Alert
>
> **Administration Alert**
>
> When giving two or more inhalation drugs for asthma at the same time, give the bronchodilator first and wait at least 5 min before giving the second and third drugs.
>
> QSEN: Safety

Box 18.2   **Teaching Tips for Using a Dry Powder Inhaler**

For inhalers requiring loading:
First load the drug by:
- Turning the device to the next dose of drug or
- Inserting the capsule into the device or
- Inserting the disk or compartment into the device.

After loading the drug and for inhalers that do not require drug loading:
- Read your health care provider's instructions for how fast you should breathe for your particular inhaler.
- Place your lips over the mouthpiece and breathe in forcefully (there is no propellant in the inhaler; only your breath pulls the drug in).

- Remove the inhaler from your mouth as soon as you have inhaled completely and hold your breath for 10 seconds.
- Never exhale (breathe out) into your inhaler. Your breath will moisten the powder, causing it to clump and not be delivered accurately.
- Never wash or place the inhaler in water.
- Never shake your inhaler.
- Keep your inhaler in a dry place at room temperature.
- If the inhaler is preloaded, discard the inhaler after it is empty.
- Because the drug is a dry powder and there is no propellant, you may not feel, smell, or taste it as you inhale.

Box 18.3   **Teaching Tips for Using a Soft Mist Inhaler**

- Prepare the device according to the manufacturer's directions.
- Open the cap of the device.
- Breathe out slowly and completely.
- Place your lips around the mouthpiece.
- Be sure not to cover the air vents on the side of the device with your fingers.
- Take a slow, deep breath at the same time that you press the dose release button and inhale the mist.

- After you have inhaled completely, hold your breath for 10 seconds.
- Remove the inhaler from your mouth and recap it.
- Clean the inhaler at least once a week by wiping the inside and outside of the mouthpiece with a clean, damp cloth.

⭐ *Teaching priorities for patients taking bronchodilators.* When used with the correct technique and prescribed dosing, inhaled bronchodilators can be very effective in controlling or preventing an asthma attack. Teach patients to carry a short-acting beta agonist (SABA) inhaler with them at all times and ensure that it contains enough drugs to be effective. Most inhalers have a "counter" built into them that indicates the number of drug dosages remaining in the device (Figure 18.6). Instruct patients to be sure and refill the prescription whenever the counter indicates the number of remaining doses is less than what is needed for 5 days. Teach patients that if the short-acting inhaler is needed increasingly more often as a "rescue" from asthma attacks, notify the prescriber and discuss the need for other therapy options.

For best effectiveness, teach patients that long-acting beta-adrenergic agonists (LABAs) *must* be taken as prescribed—even when symptoms of asthma are not present—because these drugs are used to *prevent* an attack, not to stop an attack that has already started. Remind them **not** to use LABAs for rescue during an attack or when wheezing worsens, but to use a SABA. *Relying on LABAs or cholinergic antagonists during an attack can lead to worsening of symptoms and death.*

Often, patients do not get the full benefit of inhaled drug therapy because of incorrect device usage. When used incorrectly, the inhaled drug stays in the mouth and throat or exits through the nose without ever reaching the lower airways. Thus, ensuring that the patient uses the correct technique for the inhaler type is critical for drug dosages to reach the site of action.

Review the specific teaching tips in Boxes 18.1 to 18.3 with the patient for the correct technique to use with the inhaler type prescribed and demonstrate all steps. Have the patient perform a teach-back demonstration. Praise the patient when the correct steps are used, and reteach steps that are not correct. In addition to the personal demonstration, teach patients the correct techniques by using manufacturer-generated videos that show the recommended technique for the prescribed inhaler. Most videos are available online so the patient can have the correct technique reinforced at home as often as needed.

Life span considerations for bronchodilators

Pediatric considerations. Children under the age of 4 years often are not able to use an aerosol inhaler effectively. Usually, nebulized forms of the drug with a tight-fitting facemask are required. With beta$_2$-adrenergic agonists, children taking the drugs close to bedtime have difficulty sleeping.

Considerations for older adults. Older adults may be more sensitive to the cardiac and nervous system side effects of bronchodilators. Teach older patients to check their pulse rates before and after taking a bronchodilator. Tell them to report any new development of tremors or sleep difficulties to their prescriber. Instruct them to call the life squad or go to the nearest emergency department if chest pain occurs.

Older adults with cognitive problems or fine muscle coordination and strength issues may not be able to use an inhaler. Instead, the drugs may be delivered by nebulizer treatments.

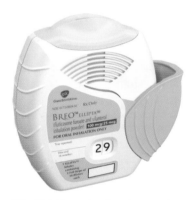

FIG. 18.6 Example of a dry powder inhaler with a counter (GlaxoSmithKline). (From Visovsky, C. G., et al. [2019]. *Introduction to clinical pharmacology* [9th ed.]. St. Louis: Elsevier.)

Inhaled General Antiinflammatory Drugs

Antiinflammatory drugs prevent or limit inflammatory responses to injury or invasion. Some are general and target nearly all inflammatory cells to some extent. Others are more specific for one type of inflammatory cell or cell product. These specific antiinflammatories are known as *biologics* and are discussed later in this chapter. The general antiinflammatories used as therapy for asthma and COPD are corticosteroids and mast cell stabilizers. *None of the antiinflammatory drugs directly induce bronchodilation; therefore, they are all controller drugs, not rescue drugs.* Specific information about oral and parenteral general antiinflammatories is presented in Chapter 10. Issues related to the inhaled forms of these drugs are presented in the following sections.

Inhaled general antiinflammatory drugs can be very effective in controlling or preventing an asthma attack and reducing the inflammation of chronic bronchitis

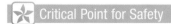

in COPD if used correctly. They carry a warning that the risk for death from asthma is increased when using these drugs. This is because the antiinflammatory drugs for respiratory problems may help prevent inflammation but do not cause bronchodilation.

How inhaled general antiinflammatories work. Corticosteroids work like natural cortisol, and they are the most powerful agents that slow or stop the production of most inflammatory mediators. When they enter inflammatory cells, corticosteroids bind to control points of protein synthesis in the cell and prevent the conversion of substances into active mediators that cause inflammation. Thus, they suppress both inflammatory responses and immune responses. Although oral corticosteroids may be used daily when asthma is severe and not well controlled, inhaled corticosteroids are much more commonly prescribed. During severe, life-threatening asthma attacks, corticosteroids may be given intravenously.

Mast cells are tissue inflammatory cells that contain the mediators histamine and leukotriene. Mast cell stabilizers work by preventing the membranes of mast cells from degranulating and releasing histamine and leukotriene. They do not stop the synthesis of these mediators, nor do they interact with them. These drugs help keep the mediators confined inside the mast cell where they do not induce inflammation.

An option for prevention therapy in people with asthma and COPD is the use of inhalers that combine a bronchodilator and a corticosteroid. Therapeutic effects, side effects, adverse effects, precautions, and patient education are the same for each drug individually.

Adult Dosages for Common Inhaled General Antiinflammatory Drugs

Drug Category	Drug Name	Usual Maintenance Dose
Inhaled Corticosteroids	beclomethasone (Qvar Redihaler)	1–2 puffs of 40 mcg twice daily by MDI
	budesonide (Pulmicort)	1–2 puffs of 180 mcg twice daily by DPI
	fluticasone (Flovent HFA, Flovent Diskus)	88–220 mcg twice daily by MDI (dosages per MDI vary—44 mcg, 110 mcg, 220 mcg)
	mometasone (Asmanex Twist-haler [DPI], Asmanex HFA [MDI])	1–2 puffs of 220 mcg once or twice daily by DPI or 2 puffs of 100 mcg once or twice daily by MDI
Mast Cell Stabilizers	cromolyn sodium (generic only)	20 mg (via nebulizer) 3–4 times daily
Selected Antiinflammatory/ Bronchodilator Combination Agents[a]	Advair Diskus	fluticasone/salmeterol
	Breo	fluticasone/vilanterol
	Dulera	mometasone/formoterol
	Symbicort	budesonide/formoterol
	Breztri Aerosphere[b]	budesonide/glycopyrronium/formoterol
	Trelegy Ellipta[b]	fluticasone/umeclidinium/vilanterol

[a]Dosages vary.
[b]Approved only for use with COPD, not asthma.
DPI, dry powder inhaler; *MDI,* metered dose inhaler.

Intended responses of inhaled general antiinflammatories
- Swelling of pulmonary mucous membranes is reduced.
- Pulmonary secretions are reduced.
- Airway lumens open, allowing air to move more freely into and out of the alveoli.
- Wheezing and coughing decrease or disappear.

Common side effects of inhaled general antiinflammatories. Side effects of inhaled antiinflammatories and inhaled mast cell stabilizers are local and include cough, bad

Common Side Effects

Inhaled General Antiinflammatories

Cough

Dry mouth, Taste changes

taste, mouth dryness, and an increased risk for oral infection—specifically, a candida fungal infection known as "thrush." Mast cell stabilizers also may cause nausea and vomiting.

Adverse effects of inhaled general antiinflammatories. The propellant and preservatives in drug mixtures delivered by metered dose inhalers can irritate tissues, causing the patient to cough severely or have bronchospasms temporarily.

When inhaled corticosteroids are used as prescribed, they have a low risk for any adverse effects. However, when heavily used, they can be absorbed into the bloodstream and cause adrenal gland suppression just as systemic corticosteroids do (see Chapter 10).

⊛ *Priority actions to take* before *giving inhaled general antiinflammatories.* Inspect the patient's mouth and throat to assess whether an infection or thrush is present. Thrush appears as white or cream-colored patches of a cottage cheese–like coating on the mucous membranes, roof of the mouth, and tongue.

If the patient also is receiving an inhaled bronchodilator, give the bronchodilator first and wait at least 5 minutes before giving the inhaled antiinflammatory. Giving the bronchodilator first allows the greatest widening effect on the airways so the antiinflammatory can be inhaled more deeply into the respiratory tract and be more effective.

Just as with inhaled bronchodilators, be sure the patient is using the correct technique for the inhaler type to ensure the greatest effectiveness (see Boxes 18.1 to 18.3).

⊛ *Priority actions to take* after *giving inhaled general antiinflammatories.* Assist the patient with brushing his or her teeth or rinsing with water or mouthwash to remove the drug from the oral cavity. This practice helps reduce the bad taste and mouth dryness, as well as decreases the risk for thrush and other oral infections.

⊛ *Teaching priorities for patients taking inhaled general antiinflammatories.* Inhaled general antiinflammatory drugs are commonly prescribed for asthma and COPD. They can be very effective when used correctly. The following points are essential for patient and family education when inhaled general antiinflammatories are prescribed:

- Take the drug as directed by your prescriber and do not change the dose.
- If you also take an inhaled bronchodilator, use it first and wait at least 5 minutes before using the antiinflammatory inhaler.
- Do not use antiinflammatory drugs alone to stop or reduce bronchoconstriction.
- Follow the correct technique(s) recommended by the manufacturer for using your inhaler(s).
- After using your inhaler, brush your teeth or rinse your mouth with water to decrease dry mouth, bad taste, and reduce the risk for mouth infections.
- Get a new inhaler at least 5 days before the counter indicates the device contains no remaining doses.
- Clean your inhaler according to the manufacturer's directions.
- Check your gums, mouth, and throat daily in the mirror for increased redness or the presence of white/cream-colored patches that may indicate an infection.
- Use good oral hygiene at least three times a day to prevent oral infections.

Life span considerations for inhaled general antiinflammatories. Manipulation of an inhaler may be difficult for children under 4 years of age and older adults. These populations may need to receive inhaled general antiinflammatories by nebulizer. The risk for oral infections is greater in small children and older adults because of reduced immunity in these populations.

Biologics

A new form of specific antiinflammatory drugs are the biologics. As described in Chapter 11, **biologics** are a class of complex antiinflammatory drugs derived from living sources that target specific inflammatory cells, components, or products to modify chronic disorders associated with inflammation and tissue damage. Many are antibodies developed using mouse cells and then are "humanized" to eliminate the mouse proteins that are more likely to trigger allergic responses. Each antibody used as a drug binds to a specific inflammatory cell or cell product to prevent the cell or cell product from stimulating or continuing inflammatory responses. So, while all of them work similarly, each biologic has a different specific target or targets. Patients with a specific type of inflammatory condition vary with regard to which specific cell type is present in greater numbers and/or greater activity to cause the inflammation. Thus, not all biologics work equally in all patients with the same inflammatory condition. In addition, biologics are approved as "add-on" drugs, which means that traditional asthma therapy with inhaled bronchodilators and general antiinflammatories is prescribed for daily use and continues along with biologics.

The two inflammatory cell types most responsible for severe asthma are the eosinophils and the neutrophils. About 70% of people with moderate to severe asthma have excessive numbers of eosinophils. At this time, no specific biologics that target *only* neutrophil cells, components, or products have been developed and approved for use as an asthma treatment. Five biologics have been approved for use in managing moderate to severe asthma, and another two are in clinical trials. Although research is ongoing to determine whether biologics could be useful for the management of chronic bronchitis associated with COPD, none have yet been approved for this purpose.

 Memory Jogger

Any biologic works best in a person who has more of the specific target cells or cell products that start or promote the inflammation.

Adult Doses of Biologics for Management of Moderate to Severe Asthma

Drug Category	Drug Name	Usual Maintenance Dose
Interleukin-4 (IL-4) and Interleukin-13 (IL-13) Antagonists	dupilumab (Dupixent)	400 mg initially by subcutaneous injection, followed by 200–300 mg once every 2 weeks by subcutaneous injection
Interleukin-5 (IL-5) Antagonists	benralizumab (Fasenra)	30 mg subcutaneously initially and after 4 weeks, then once every 8 weeks
	mepolizumab (Nucala)	100 mg subcutaneously once every 4 weeks
	reslizumab (CINQAIR)	3 mg/kg IV infusion once every 4 weeks
Immunoglobulin E (IgE) Antagonists	omalizumab (Xolair)	300 mg subcutaneously every 4 weeks

How biologics for asthma work. The exemplar drug in the category of biologics for asthma management is benralizumab (Fasenra). Benralizumab is an antibody with strong binding powers for the interleukin-5 (IL-5) inflammatory mediator produced by eosinophils. (Recall from Chapter 11 that an antibody is a "Y-shaped" molecule in which the tips of the Y bind very tightly to specific protein sequences.) IL-5 promotes the growth and activation of eosinophils and causes the release of large amounts of additional inflammatory mediators from these cells. When the benralizumab antibodies bind to IL-5 molecules, fewer eosinophils are produced, and the remaining ones are made less active so that inflammation is greatly reduced.

Intended responses of biologics for asthma. Regardless of which biologic drug is used for asthma, the intended responses are:

- Swelling of pulmonary mucous membranes is reduced.
- Pulmonary secretions are reduced.

- Airway lumens open, allowing air to move more freely into and out of the alveoli.
- Wheezing and coughing decrease or disappear.

Common side effects of biologics for asthma. Biologics for asthma are given parenterally, most often subcutaneously. These drugs are only given at specific intervals ranging from every 2 weeks to every 8 weeks. The two most common side effects reported are headache and injection site reactions. The reduced inflammatory response also reduces immunity to some extent and increases the risk for infection.

Possible adverse effects of biologics for asthma. Patients receiving parenteral biologics for asthma are at risk for hypersensitivity (allergic) reactions (see Chapter 1). The reaction may occur the very first time the drug is administered; however, some patients may develop allergic reactions with subsequent doses because they develop antibodies against the drug. Allergic reactions may be as simple as a rash or as life-threatening as angioedema or anaphylaxis.

The reduced immunity resulting from these drugs increases the risk for worsening (*exacerbation*) of pre-existing infections, especially helminth infections (worms) and tuberculosis. In addition, patients taking these drugs may not get the full benefit from any vaccinations/immunizations they receive.

⭐ ***Priority actions to take*** *before* ***giving biologics for asthma.*** Because biologics reduce immunity, which increases the risk for new infections and reactivation of dormant infections, most manufacturers recommend that the patient be tested for tuberculosis a week before the first dose of a biologic is given and not to give the drug to anyone who has a positive tuberculosis test. Ask whether the patient currently has an infection or has ever been diagnosed with tuberculosis.

Have emergency equipment for anaphylaxis available in the room where the patient is located because the risk for allergic reactions is relatively high. As a result of this risk, only a licensed health care professional should give the injection, and a physician must be in the facility. Ask whether the patient has ever had a drug reaction.

Most biologics are given by subcutaneous injection, although some are given as an IV infusion. Allow the drug or prefilled syringe to reach room temperature before injection (about 30 minutes after removal from refrigeration) and inspect the liquid. Do not use if the drug is cloudy, discolored, or contains large particles. For subcutaneous injections, select an appropriate site such as the upper arm, thigh, or abdomen (except for a 2-inch area surrounding the umbilicus), and be sure the skin is intact. After cleansing the area, pinch up the skin, insert the needle at a 90-degree angle, and inject it subcutaneously.

⭐ ***Priority actions to take*** *after* ***giving biologics for asthma.*** Do not massage the site after injection. Ensure that the patient remains in the facility under observation for 30 to 60 minutes. Assess oxygenation and blood pressure every 5 to 10 minutes. Monitor for symptoms of an allergic reaction, such as swelling of the lips, tongue, or throat; difficulty breathing; chest tightness; drooling; decreased oxygen saturation; hypotension; or changes in consciousness or cognition. If any of these symptoms appear, call the physician or emergency response team immediately. If the drug is being infused, stop the infusion while maintaining IV access. Apply oxygen.

⭐ ***Teaching priorities for patients taking biologics for asthma***
- Teach patients and families the signs and symptoms of an allergic response because these may occur even several hours after the injection.
- Instruct patients to call 911 or go to the nearest emergency department if any symptoms of an allergic reaction occur.
- If the patient or family is determined to be appropriate for self-administration of the drug, teach whoever will be performing the injection how to select a site and the technique for giving the injection with a prefilled autoinjector.

- Teach patients and families the signs and symptoms of infection, and to notify the prescriber at the first indication of an infection.
- Instruct patients to keep all appointments for laboratory testing.
- Urge patients to avoid crowds and people who are ill.
- Remind patients that biologics are "add-on" drugs that do not replace their prescribed controller and rescue drugs.

Mucolytics

Mucolytics are drugs that reduce the thickness of mucus, making it easier to move out of the airways. Most people with COPD take a mucolytic drug daily to reduce the thickness of mucus, allowing the mucus to more easily move out of the airways. Patients with asthma may use mucolytics when increased thick secretions are a problem. With reduced mucus, airflow is improved.

Guaifenesin is a systemic mucolytic that is taken orally. Another mucolytic drug prescribed for a person with COPD is acetylcysteine. Mucus contains protein molecules and mucus molecules held tightly together. This drug works by breaking the connections that bind the protein and mucus molecules. As a result, the mucus becomes thinner and less sticky, which is easier to cough up and spit out.

Acetylcysteine is most commonly delivered with a nebulizer face mask and is also available as an oral drug for non-pulmonary problems. Typically, 1 to 10 mL of a 20% solution is placed in a medication nebulizer, and every 6 hours, the patient uses a mask to breathe in the mist containing the drug. The drug has few side effects but does have a very unpleasant odor. Some patients experience nausea and even vomiting from the smell.

REVIEW OF RELATED PHYSIOLOGY AND PATHOPHYSIOLOGY OF PULMONARY ARTERIAL HYPERTENSION AND PULMONARY FIBROSIS

Two additional serious respiratory problems that are managed by drug therapy are pulmonary arterial hypertension and pulmonary fibrosis. Although drug therapy does not currently result in a cure for either problem, it can reduce symptoms and prolong the life of a patient.

PULMONARY ARTERIAL HYPERTENSION

Pulmonary arterial hypertension (PAH) is a chronic problem in which all the blood vessels of the lungs, especially the pulmonary artery, severely constrict, resulting in reduced blood flow and higher pressures throughout the lungs. This problem makes the right side of the heart work much harder for good lung blood flow to allow adequate gas exchange and oxygenation. Over time, the increased pressures damage lung tissue, greatly reduce gas exchange, and cause a type of right-sided heart failure known as *cor pulmonale.* Heart failure is the most common cause of death along with severe hypoxia. Some people develop PAH after exposure to drugs such as fenfluramine/phentermine (Pondimin or "Fen-Phen") or dasatinib. For other people, there is no known cause, but genetic mutations in several inter-related genes that regulate blood vessel and connective tissue growth predispose the person to develop the problem when exposure to inhalation irritants also enhances the risk. The disorder is rare and occurs mostly in women between the ages of 20 and 40 years. Without treatment, death usually occurs within 2 years after diagnosis. Often, PAH is not diagnosed until late in the disease process when the lungs and heart have already been damaged extensively.

A key problem with PAH is an increase in the growth of smooth muscle cells in blood vessel walls and of endothelial cells lining the pulmonary blood vessels. The excess muscle constricts blood vessels, and the excess endothelial cells narrow the blood vessel lumens. Both problems increase the risk for clot formation inside these blood vessels, as well as increased lung pressures.

Drug therapy for PAH focuses on relaxing blood vessel smooth muscle, stopping the growth of excess blood vessel tissues, and preventing the formation of clots in these vessels. Dosages and delivery methods vary with the stage of disease and degree of lung and heart damage. Drug therapy with prostanoids, endothelin-receptor antagonists, and guanylate cyclase stimulators can reduce pulmonary pressures and slow the development of heart failure by dilating pulmonary vessels and preventing clot formation.

Adult Dosages for Drugs to Manage Pulmonary Arterial Hypertension

Drug Category	Drug Name	Usual Maintenance Dose
Prostanoids	epoprostenol (Flolan, Veletri)	Variable; most common is 5 ng/kg/min continuous IV infusion
	treprostinil (Remodulin, Tyvaso)	Remodulin: 1.25–2.5 ng/kg/min by continuous IV or subcutaneous infusion or 0.125 mg orally every 8 hr, or 0.25 mg orally every 12 hr Tyvaso: Oral inhalation 16 mcg every 6 hr
	iloprost (Ventavis)	5 mcg by nebulizer inhaler 6–9 times daily
Endothelin-Receptor Antagonists	ambrisentan (Letairis)	10 mg orally once daily
	bosentan (Tracleer)	Initially, 62.5 orally every 12 hr for 4 weeks, then 125 mg orally every 12 hr
	macitentan (Opsumit)	10 mg orally once daily
Guanylate Cyclase Stimulators	riociguat (Adempas)	1–2.5 mg orally every 8 hr

Administration Alert

It is critical that drugs for PAH given by continuous infusion are **never** interrupted. Even an interruption of only minutes increases the risk for death. In addition, no other drugs are to be administered through the same line as these drugs.

QSEN: Safety

How Drugs for PAH Work

Prostanoids. Prostanoids include natural and synthetic prostacyclin agents, which act as prostaglandins receptor agonists. These drugs inhibit thromboxane A_2 and increase the amount of cyclic adenosine monophosphate (cAMP) in blood vessel smooth muscle. The overall result of this action is dilation of lung blood vessels, decreased resistance in lung blood vessels, and increased blood return from the lungs to the left side of the heart with increased cardiac output. The main drugs in this class include epoprostenol, iloprost, and treprostinil. Epoprostenol is given as a continuous IV infusion. One treprostinil (Remodulin) can be given intravenously or subcutaneously and, after the establishment of a successful and well-tolerated dose, an oral tablet. The other approved treprostinil (Tyvaso) is an inhaled agent. Iloprost (Ventavis) is an inhaled drug given by a nebulizer.

Endothelin-receptor antagonists. Endothelin is a circulating protein that binds to blood vessel endothelin receptors and causes vasoconstriction. Endothelin-receptor antagonists are drugs that block endothelin receptors to increase blood vessel dilation and prevent the overgrowth of blood vessel cells. Two drugs in this class, bosentan and macitentan, block two types of endothelin receptors and cause more systemic vasodilation. Another drug in this class, ambrisentan, strongly and selectively blocks the endothelin-A receptor on lung blood vessel cells, resulting in greater pulmonary vasodilation. All endothelin receptor antagonists are most effective when used earlier in the disease process and when combined with phosphodiesterase 5 inhibitor therapy, which are drugs most commonly used for erectile dysfunction (see Chapter 28 for a discussion of all issues related to phosphodiesterase 5 inhibitor drug therapy).

Guanylate cyclase stimulators. Nitric oxide (NO) is a powerful blood vessel dilator that works by binding to its receptor (soluble guanylate cyclase [sGC]) and increasing the amount of cyclic guanosine monophosphate (cGMP) in the smooth muscles of pulmonary blood vessels. Guanylate cyclase stimulators help NO bind better to its receptor and greatly increase the amount of cGMP available to induce lung blood vessel smooth muscle relaxation.

Supportive drug therapy. When PAH has progressed to the point that heart function is affected, a variety of drugs for heart failure may be used. These include digoxin, diuretics, and calcium channel blockers (see Chapter 14 for more information on drug failure for heart failure).

Warfarin therapy is used to reduce blood clots (see Chapter 17 for a discussion of issues related to warfarin therapy).

Intended Responses of Drugs for PAH
- Improved blood flow through the lungs
- Reduced pulmonary pressures
- Reduced breathlessness
- Improved cardiac output

Common Side Effects of Drugs for PAH
The most common side effects of drugs for PAH in all three categories are headache, severe hypotension, dizziness, and flushing. Less common side effects include nausea and vomiting. Heartburn and acid reflux are reported with guanylate cyclase stimulators.

Possible Adverse Effects of Drugs for PAH
A major adverse effect of prostanoids and guanylate cyclase stimulators is severe bleeding. A major adverse effect of the endothelin-receptor antagonists is elevated liver enzymes. All drugs for PAH can cause bone marrow suppression with anemia and low white blood cell counts.

All drugs for PAH increase the risk for birth defects and are contraindicated for women who are pregnant or breastfeeding. Instruct women who are of childbearing age and those sexually active with male partners to use two reliable methods of contraception while taking these drugs. All drugs for PAH are associated with liver toxicity to varying degrees, and patients should avoid drinking alcoholic beverages while taking any of them. Teach patients the indications of liver problems (e.g., jaundice, nausea, pain or tenderness in the upper right abdominal quadrant, dark urine).

⭐ Priority Actions to Take *Before* Giving Drugs for PAH
Before giving any drug for PAH, check the patient's blood pressure because all drugs prescribed for PAH can cause severe systemic hypotension. Also assess the patient's respiratory and cardiac status to use as a baseline for determining when an increased dose may be needed.

With parenteral prostanoids, inspect the vial for discoloration or the presence of particles. If either is present, discard the vial and open a new one. Always administer the IV preparation of the product using an appropriate pump infusing into a central line. The central line IV setup provides an access for organisms to enter the bloodstream directly. Use strict aseptic technique to avoid introducing organisms into the patient's bloodstream. Additionally, the line dedicated to prostanoid therapy is never to be used to give any other drugs. If another IV drug is prescribed, it must be given through a completely separate intravenous system. With oral forms of prostanoids, do not split or crush the tablets.

Because all drugs for PAH can cause birth defects, ensure that female patients of childbearing age have a negative pregnancy test before starting these drugs. Sexually active women with male partners should use two reliable forms of contraception.

⭐ Priority Actions to Take *After* Giving Drugs for PAH
With the parenteral forms of these drugs, do not use the IV line to give any other parenteral drugs. Ensure that there are no interruptions of continuous parenteral therapy. Ensure that all oral, parenteral, and inhaled drugs to treat PAH are given on time.

The most appropriate monitoring for the effectiveness of all of these drugs is by assessing arterial blood gas (ABG) levels. Ensure that these are ordered on a regular

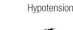

Common Side Effects
All Drugs for PAH

Headache   Hypotension

Dizziness   Flushing

 Critical Point for Safety

All drugs for PAH can cause birth defects or fetal death and must be avoided during pregnancy and breastfeeding. A negative pregnancy test is required before starting these drugs.

QSEN: Safety

⚠ Drug Alert

Administration Alert

A major complication of continuous IV infusion is the development of sepsis and septic shock because the IV line is a direct link to the bloodstream. Use sterile technique whenever working with the IV line and always monitor the patient for signs and symptoms of infection.

QSEN: Safety

basis, and monitor the results as soon as they are known. Report changes to the prescriber as soon as possible. Continue to monitor the respiratory and cardiac status at least every 4 hours.

With the prostanoids, which can cause bleeding, ensure that bleeding times are assessed using the international normalized ratio (INR). Bleeding risk is higher for patients who are also taking warfarin therapy. Immediately report results higher than 3 to the prescriber. For all drugs to treat PAH, examine the complete blood count for reduced red blood cell (RBC) and white blood cell (WBC) counts. Also, monitor hematocrit and hemoglobin levels.

With parenteral agents given through a central line, assess the patient every shift for signs and symptoms of infection and sepsis. If present, immediately report these to the prescriber. Ensure that the liver enzyme levels of patients taking an endothelin-receptor antagonist are drawn on a regular basis. Assess the patient for any signs of jaundice and pain in the right upper abdominal quadrant.

⊛ Teaching Priorities for Patients Taking Drugs for PAH

- Teach patients taking continuous parenteral therapy for PAH to not stop the therapy, and to avoid any interruptions in therapy because of the associated risk for death.
- Stress the importance of taking all prescribed drugs on time, exactly as prescribed, and not to skip or delay doses.
- Remind patients to always have an adequate supply of the drug or drugs on hand.
- Teach patients using parenteral therapy how to self-administer the drugs and work the pump **using strict aseptic technique**.
- Instruct patients to notify the prescriber or go to the emergency department at the first sign of infection (e.g., fever, chills, purulent drainage, cough, increased sputum production).
- Instruct all patients to notify the prescriber or go to the emergency department immediately if any of these problems occur: increased and persistent shortness of breath, chest pain, swelling of the feet and legs, and/or sudden weight gain.
- Instruct patients taking oral drugs to not split, crush, or chew the tablets.
- Remind female patients of childbearing age who are taking endothelin-receptor antagonists and who have male sexual partners to use two reliable forms of contraception, as well as to undergo monthly pregnancy testing.
- Teach patients taking endothelin-receptor antagonists to report liver impairment symptoms (persistent jaundice, right upper abdominal pain, dark urine, pale stools) to the prescriber.
- Instruct patients to keep all follow-up appointments for blood tests to monitor effectiveness and identify complications early.

Life Span Considerations for Drugs for PAH

The prostanoids have a moderate likelihood of increasing the risk for birth defects or fetal damage. Although drugs with this pregnancy designation are usually not recommended for use during pregnancy, PAH is life threatening when not treated, and drug therapy must continue. Breastfeeding is not recommended while taking prostacyclin agents.

The endothelin-receptor antagonists and guanylate cyclase stimulators will cause birth defects and are not to be used during pregnancy or while breastfeeding.

PULMONARY FIBROSIS

Pulmonary fibrosis is a relatively common restrictive lung disease in which a previous lung injury causes inflammation of the lungs, leading to excessive cell division and replacement of normal lung cells with fibrotic scar tissue years after the initial injury. These changes thicken the alveoli and make gas exchange difficult. Most often, the patient is an older adult with a history of cigarette smoking, chronic exposure to inhalation irritants, or exposure to the drugs amiodarone, bleomycin, or ambrisentan. Most patients have progressive disease with few remission periods. Even with proper treatment, most patients usually survive only 1 to 2 years after diagnosis.

Drug therapy focuses on slowing the fibrotic process. Corticosteroids and other immunosuppressants are the mainstays of therapy. Immunosuppressant drugs include cytotoxic drugs, such as cyclophosphamide, azathioprine, chlorambucil, or methotrexate. See Chapter 10 for information regarding corticosteroid drug therapy. See Chapter 11 for information about other drugs to modulate the immune system.

A newer class of drugs used in addition to immunosuppressants are antifibrotic agents that can slow fibrous cell growth and scarring, which delays progression. Although neither drug is a cure nor life-extending, patients breathe more easily and have somewhat greater activity tolerance. The two approved drugs in this class are the oral biologic nintedanib (Ofev) and pirfenidone (Esbriet). Nintedanib is taken twice daily and pirfenidone is taken three times daily. Both drugs have many side effects and are hepatotoxic. In addition, neither drug should be taken during pregnancy or while breastfeeding. The cost of these drugs approaches $100,000 per year, which limits their use.

Get Ready for the NCLEX® Examination!

Key Points

- When an asthma attack is so severe that oxygen levels become too low, the patient can die if interventions do not improve air movement.
- Teach patients with asthma or COPD to take drugs exactly as prescribed, even when symptoms have not been present for days.
- Rescue or reliever drugs stop an active asthma attack or reduce its severity; controller drugs prevent an attack from starting.
- Teach patients with asthma to carry a short-acting adrenergic rescue inhaler at all times.
- Assess for chest pain in the patient taking a bronchodilator. If any chest discomfort is present, immediately notify the prescriber.
- When giving two or more inhalation drugs for asthma at the same time, administer the bronchodilator first and wait at least 5 minutes before giving the second and third drugs.
- Teach patients using dry powder inhalers not to wash the inhaler or exhale into it.
- Only short-acting beta$_2$-agonists (SABAs) are appropriate as rescue drugs.
- Inhaled corticosteroids reduce local immune responses and can lead to the development of oral thrush.
- Inhaled drugs for asthma and COPD have no benefit unless the patient uses the inhaler correctly.
- Any biologic for asthma works best in a person who has more of the specific target cells or cell products that start or promote the inflammation.

- The risk for allergic reactions to parenteral biologics for asthma increases with multiple doses over time.
- Mucolytic drugs only help reduce thick secretions and do not cause bronchodilation or reduced inflammation.
- Drug therapy for pulmonary arterial hypertension (PAH) should not be stopped, delayed, or interrupted.
- To reduce the risk for bloodstream infection and sepsis, use strict aseptic technique when working with continuous parenteral prostacyclin drug therapy.
- Never give any other drugs through the line in use for continuous prostacyclin therapy.
- Drugs for PAH can cause birth defects and are not to be used during pregnancy or lactation.
- Do not split or crush oral drugs for PAH.
- Prostanoids can cause severe bleeding.
- Endothelin-receptor antagonists are more liver toxic than are other drugs for PAH.

Additional Learning Resources

⊕ Be sure to visit your Evolve website (http://evolve.elsevier.com/Workman/pharmacology/) for additional online resources.

SG Go to your Study Guide for additional learning activities to help you master this chapter content.

Review Questions

See *Answers to In-Text Review Questions* in the back of the book for answers to these questions.

1. **How do mast cell stabilizers work to assist in asthma management?**

   A. Breaking the connection between protein molecules in respiratory mucus

   B. Inhibiting the synthesis of inflammatory mediators in mast cells

   C. Relaxing bronchial smooth muscles within the lower airways

   D. Preventing mast cells from releasing inflammatory mediators

2. The nurse will recognize which differences in common drug therapy for an adult patient who has chronic obstructive pulmonary disease (COPD) from that prescribed for adult patients with asthma? **Select all that apply.**

   A. Addition of mucolytics
   B. Absence of reliever drugs
   C. Daily use of nebulizer delivery
   D. Addition of cholinergic antagonists
   E. Controllers in combination of three drugs
   F. Increased use of interleukin 5 (IL-5) antagonists

3. For which activity or symptom would the nurse tell a patient with COPD to use a short-acting beta$_2$-adrenergic agonist?

   A. Right before going to bed for the night
   B. As soon as possible after arising in the morning
   C. Whenever he or she feels more breathless than usual
   D. Whenever coughing produces mucus that is thicker or stickier than usual

4. A patient with COPD who uses a tiotropium inhaler has all of the following symptoms. Which symptoms does the nurse recognize as possible side effects of this drug? **Select all that apply.**

   A. Cough
   B. Blurred vision
   C. Constipation
   D. Sleepiness
   E. Urinary retention
   F. Runny nose

5. A patient newly prescribed to use a soft mist inhaler (SMI) asks why a spacer is not used with this device. What is the nurse's best response?

   A. "The face mask used with the SMI takes the place of a spacer."
   B. "The SMI has a propellent that forces the drug forward, making a spacer unnecessary."
   C. "The particles in the mist are slow and heavy, giving you enough time to breathe it in."
   D. "All SMIs are a type of dry powder inhaler and must be 'sucked into' the lungs through the mouth."

6. Which precaution is **most** important for the nurse to teach a patient prescribed to take an oral prostanoid?

   A. "Do not chew or crush the tablet."
   B. "Take the drug with a meal or snack."

   C. "Remain in the upright position for an hour after taking the drug."
   D. "Do not take other medications for 1 hour before or 2 hours after taking this drug."

7. For which patient will the nurse expect the use of a nebulizer for self-administration of asthma management drugs to be prescribed rather than an inhaler?

   A. 25-year-old with diabetes and limited vision
   B. 45-year-old with severe arthritis of the hands
   C. 65-year-old with memory loss
   D. 85-year-old who lives alone and manages all aspects of self-care

8. A patient receiving IV reslizumab reports lip swelling and chest tightness during the infusion. What is the nurse's **best first action to prevent harm?**

   A. Notifying the prescriber immediately
   B. Stopping the infusion while maintaining IV access
   C. Measuring the patient's oxygen saturation and blood pressure
   D. Asking the patient whether these symptoms have occurred with previous doses

9. For which side effect will the nurse monitor a patient with pulmonary arterial hypertension (PAH) who is receiving endothelin receptor antagonist therapy?

   A. Increased clot formation
   B. Decreased urine output
   C. Shock and sepsis
   D. Hypotension

10. A patient is prescribed to receive 90 mcg of levalbuterol every 4 hours by oral inhalation. The available drug is levalbuterol 45 mcg/puff. How many total puffs will the nurse instruct this patient to take daily?

    A. 4 puffs
    B. 8 puffs
    C. 12 puffs
    D. 16 puffs

Clinical Judgment

A 34-year-old male patient has had severe asthma for many years. Over time, attacks have increased and, even though he faithfully takes his controller drugs, he has had to use his rescue inhaler many times each day. Recently he was found to have the type of asthma associated with a high number of eosinophils and is starting on benralizumab. The nurse has started a teaching plan about the therapy for this patient. He makes the following statements. **Use an X to indicate which patient statements about issues related to this therapy are either Understood or Requires Further Teaching.**

PATIENT STATEMENT	UNDERSTOOD	REQUIRES FURTHER TEACHING
"I am lucky that I have the eosinophilic type of asthma for this drug to work."		
"My wife is willing to learn how to give me those subcutaneous injections."		
"It will be great to take asthma drugs only once every 8 weeks instead of daily."		
"If I have a fever or any sign of infection, I will call my health care provider immediately."		
"I will use a condom whenever my wife and I have sex to limit her exposure to this drug."		
"If the injection site becomes red or sore, I will go to the emergency department immediately.		

2. **Which precautions are important for the nurse to teach a patient with asthma about the use of the short-acting beta$_2$-adrenergic agonist aerosol inhaler? Select all that apply.**

A. Carry the inhaler with you at all times
B. Report any chest pain to your prescriber immediately
C. The inhaler is most effective when used with a spacer
D. Breathe in as rapidly as possible while pressing on the canister
E. After inhaling, hold your breath for at least 10 seconds before exhaling
F. Avoid using the inhaler within 1 hour before or 2 hours after eating a meal
G. Clean the mouthpiece at least once daily by rinsing it in warm running water
H. Remember to take this drug twice daily even when symptoms of asthma are not present
I. Use the inhaler about 15 minutes before starting any activity that usually triggers your asthma
J. If you are sexually active with a male partner, be sure to use two reliable methods of birth control

19

Drug Therapy for Gastrointestinal Problems

http://evolve.elsevier.com/Workman/pharmacology/

Learning Objectives

The content presented in this chapter should help you to:

1. Describe the common names, actions, usual adult dosages, possible side effects, and adverse effects of antinausea and antiemetic drugs.
2. Discuss the priority actions to take before and after giving antinausea and antiemetic drugs.
3. Prioritize essential information to teach patients taking antinausea and antiemetic drugs.
4. Discuss life span considerations for antinausea drugs and antiemetic drugs.

5. Describe the common names, actions, usual adult dosages, possible side effects, and adverse effects of drugs for diarrhea and constipation.
6. Discuss the priority actions to take before and after giving drugs for diarrhea and constipation.
7. Prioritize essential information to teach patients taking drugs for diarrhea and constipation.
8. Discuss life span considerations for drugs for diarrhea and drugs for constipation.

Key Terms

5HT₃-receptor antagonists (rē-SĔP-tŏr ăn-TĂG-ŏ-nĭsts) (p. 340) Drugs that work in the brain's chemotrigger zone (vomiting center) to prevent nausea and vomiting caused by chemotherapy treatments.

adsorbent/absorbent drugs (ăd-SŌRB-ĕnt /ăb-SŌRB-ĕnt DRŬGZ) (p. 350) Drugs that remove substances that cause diarrhea from the body.

anticholinergic drugs (ăn-tĭ-kō-lĭn-ĔRJ-ĭk DRŬGZ) (p. 340) Drugs that inhibit pathways of the vomiting reflex; they stop intestinal cramping and inhibit vestibular input (balance and position) into the central nervous system (CNS).

antidiarrheal drugs (ăn-tē-dī-ŭ-RĒ-ŭl DRŬGZ) (p. 350) Drugs that relieve or control diarrhea or some of the symptoms that go along with diarrhea.

antiemetic drugs (ăn-tē-ĕ-MĔT-ĭk DRŬGZ) (p. 340) Drugs that prevent or control nausea and vomiting.

antihistamines (ăn-tĭ-HĬS-tă-mēnz) (p. 340) Drugs that work against nausea and vomiting caused by opiate drugs or motion; they block the action of histamine (a compound released in allergic inflammatory reactions) at the H₁ receptor sites.

antimotility drugs (ăn-tĭ-mō-TĬL-ĭ-tē DRŬGZ) (p. 350) Drugs that slow down peristalsis (movement) in the gastrointestinal (GI) tract, used to treat diarrhea.

antisecretory drugs (ăn-tĭ-sĕ-KRĒ-tŏr-ē DRŬGZ) (p. 350) Drugs that inhibit secretory actions in the GI tract, used to treat diarrhea

dopamine antagonists (DŌ-pă-mēn ăn-TĂG-ŏ-nĭsts) (p. 341) Drugs that directly block dopamine from binding to receptors in the brain's chemotrigger zone and in the intestinal tract, causing food to move more quickly through the GI tract.

laxatives (LĂK-să-tĭvz) (p. 345) Drugs used to produce bowel movements and relieve constipation.

lubricants (LOO-brĭ-kăntz) (p. 346) Oily or slippery substances that can help make bowel movements easier.

phenothiazines (FĒ-nō-thī-ŭ-zēnz) (p. 340) Drugs that block dopamine receptors in the chemotrigger zone of the brain; this action inhibits one or more of the vomiting reflex pathways

stool softeners (STOOL SŌF-ĕn-ĕrz) (p. 346) A laxative that adds fluid to stool, softening it to make bowel movements easier.

REVIEW OF RELATED PHYSIOLOGY AND PATHOPHYSIOLOGY FOR NAUSEA AND VOMITING

The gastrointestinal (GI) system begins at the mouth and ends at the anus (Animation 19.1). It is composed of a hollow tube that is about 25 feet long in an adult (Figure 19.1) and is also called the *digestive system* or the *alimentary canal*. Functions of the GI system include taking in fluids and nutrients (food), breaking down food into forms that the body can use, absorbing useful fluid and nutrients, and eliminating waste products.

The bowel is the lower part of the GI system (see Figure 19.1). Its roles include digesting the food we eat, absorbing the nutrients and fluids from digested foods, processing waste products, and expelling waste products that the body cannot use.

The small bowel is where parts of digested food that the body can use are absorbed. It sends waste products to the large bowel *(colon)*. The colon is the waste-processing and fluid-absorbing part of the bowel. Waste products have a consistency similar to that of pea soup when entering the colon. The large bowel absorbs fluids from waste products as they move through the colon and form stool *(feces)* (Figure 19.2). Depending on how long stool remains in the colon and how much water is absorbed, the consistency of stool may vary from soft and loose (watery diarrhea) to very hard lumps (constipation).

The rectum and left side of the colon are where stool is stored before a bowel movement occurs. Bowel movements are complex processes involving several different muscles and nerves located in the pelvic floor. In addition to parasympathetic nerve stimulation, mass movements *(peristalsis)* cause stool to enter the rectum (Figure 19.3). These movements can be triggered by food arriving in the stomach or by physical activity such as getting out of bed in the morning, which results in the sensation that the bowel needs to be emptied. When a person sits on the toilet to move the bowels, first the internal anal sphincter relaxes; then the external sphincter relaxes, and the bowel empties. Normal bowel function is different for every person. Bowel movements may occur anywhere between several times per day to several times a week. Consistency of bowel movements is more important than frequency. A person's stool should be soft enough to pass easily out of the bowel but should not be liquid.

Nausea and vomiting are defenses of the GI system and are signs of altered body function. *Nausea* is the unpleasant sensation of the need to vomit. *Vomiting (emesis)* is the forcing of stomach contents up through the esophagus and out the mouth. The process of vomiting consists of three phases: nausea, retching, and vomiting.

Nausea usually occurs before vomiting. It can be accompanied by cold sweats, pallor, increased salivation, loss of gastric tone, duodenal contractions, and reflux of intestinal contents into the stomach. It is often followed by retching. *Retching* involves labored respiratory movements against a closed throat, with contractions of the abdominal muscles, chest wall muscles, and diaphragm without vomiting. Vomiting does not always follow retching, but retching usually causes enough pressure buildup to lead to vomiting.

Vomiting results from powerful contractions of the abdominal and chest wall muscles, accompanied by lowering of the diaphragm and opening of the sphincter between the stomach and esophagus *(cardiac sphincter)*. It is a reflex, not a voluntary action that involves interactions among the nervous system, vestibular system, vomiting center of the brain, and receptors within the GI tract. The *vestibular apparatus* is the inner ear structures associated with balance and position sense. When balance or sense of position is upset, vomiting can occur. Tension receptors *(mechanoreceptors)* initiate vomiting because of distention and contraction such as with a bowel obstruction. Chemoreceptors are sensory nerve cells that respond to chemical stimuli such as poisonous substances *(toxins)* in the intestines. The mechanoreceptor and chemoreceptor stimuli are sent to the vomiting center in the brain (chemotrigger zone), which controls the act of vomiting (Figure 19.4).

The vomiting center located in the medulla is responsible for initiating the vomiting reflex. It combines the input from the GI tract, vestibular apparatus, and higher brain pressure centers for activation. Once activated, the vomiting center causes vomiting by stimulating the salivary and respiratory centers and the throat (pharyngeal), GI, and abdominal muscles.

There are many causes of nausea and vomiting (Table 19.1). When a person vomits, the body is often trying to remove harmful substances that were ingested. Other possible triggers include disgusting sights, smells, or memories. People often learn to avoid the stimuli that lead to nausea and vomiting because these responses are so unpleasant. Nausea and vomiting are common and severe side effects of chemotherapy.

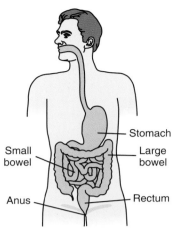

FIG. 19.1 The gastrointestinal system.

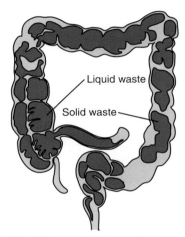

FIG. 19.2 Fluid is absorbed from the stool by the large bowel as it moves through the colon.

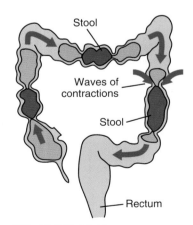

FIG. 19.3 Peristalsis: mass movements in the colon.

? Did You Know?

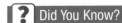

Food usually takes 1–3 days to be processed by the bowel; about 90% of that time is spent in the colon.

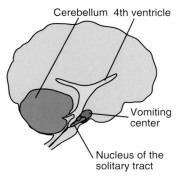

FIG. 19.4 The vomiting center.

Table 19.1	Causes of Nausea and Vomiting
CAUSE	**AGENTS**
Drug or treatment induced	Antibiotics Cancer chemotherapy Opiate drugs Radiation therapy
Labyrinth disorders	Ménière disease Motion
Endocrine system	Pregnancy
Infection	Gastroenteritis Viral labyrinthitis
Increased intracranial pressure	Hemorrhage Meningitis
Postoperative	Analgesics Anesthetics Procedural
Central nervous system	Anticipatory Bulimia nervosa Migraine

Nausea and vomiting are not only stressful to a person having these experiences; they can also create complications such as bleeding, aspiration pneumonia, dehydration, and reopening of surgical wounds, which can lead to longer hospital stays.

TYPES OF DRUGS FOR NAUSEA AND VOMITING

Antiemetic Drugs

How antiemetic drugs work. Antiemetic drugs control nausea and prevent vomiting. Nausea and vomiting often occur together, and the same drugs are prescribed for both problems. In addition to drugs, management of a patient with nausea and vomiting includes identifying and treating or eliminating the cause, controlling the symptoms, and correcting imbalances (e.g., electrolyte, fluid, and nutritional).

Antiemetic drugs include the phenothiazines, anticholinergics, antihistamines, $5HT_3$-receptor antagonists, and dopamine receptor antagonists. Each type of drugs affects different receptors, and some drugs affect several receptor sites. For example, $5HT_3$-receptor antagonists work against nausea and vomiting caused by chemotherapy treatments, whereas antihistamines work against nausea and vomiting caused by opiate drugs or motion. Multiple drugs may be used for nausea and vomiting because different drugs affect different parts of the vomiting reflex pathways.

The **phenothiazines** block dopamine receptors in the chemotrigger zone of the brain. This action inhibits one or more of the vomiting reflex pathways. The sedating effects help control the sensation of nausea.

Anticholinergic drugs inhibit other pathways of the vomiting reflex. They stop intestinal cramping and inhibit vestibular input (balance and position) into the central nervous system (CNS).

Antihistamines block the action of histamine (a compound released in allergic inflammatory reactions) at the H_1 receptor sites. They inhibit the same pathways as anticholinergic drugs and depress inner ear excitability, reducing vestibular stimulation. These different actions work together to control nausea and prevent vomiting.

The **$5HT_3$-receptor antagonists** bind to and block serotonin receptors in the intestinal tract and the chemotrigger zone of the brain. By blocking the receptors in both of these sites, at least two pathways of the vomiting reflex are interrupted. These drugs are commonly used to manage the nausea and vomiting resulting from cancer chemotherapy.

Dopamine antagonists directly block dopamine from binding to receptors in the chemotrigger zone and the intestinal tract. Food in the intestinal tract moves along more quickly and is less likely to stimulate responses that trigger the vomiting reflex.

Common names and doses of antiemetic drugs are listed in the following table. Be sure to consult a reliable drug resource for information on specific antiemetic drugs.

Adult Dosages for Commonly Prescribed Antiemetic Drugs

Drug Category	Drug Name	Usual Maintenance Dose
Phenothiazides	promethazine (Phenergan)	12.5–25 mg orally every 4–6 hr as needed 12.5–25 mg IM or IV every 4–6 hr as needed 12.5–25 mg rectally every 4–6 hr as needed
	prochlorperazine (Compazine)	5–10 mg orally 3–4 times daily Sustained release: 10 or 15 mg orally every 12 hr Rectal 25 mg twice a day IM or IV 5–10 mg every 3–4 hr as needed
Anticholinergics	scopolamine (L-hyoscine)	0.6–1 mg subcutaneously Transdermal patch: 1 patch delivers approximately 1 mg over 3 days
Antihistamines	cyclizine (Cyclivert, Marezine)	50 mg orally 30 min *before* travel and every 4–6 hr as needed
	meclizine (Antivert, Dramamine)	25–50 mg orally 1 hr *before* travel for motion sickness 25–100 mg orally per day for vertigo
5HT$_3$-Receptor Antagonists	granisetron (Kytril, granisol, sustol)	1 mg orally twice daily, begin 1 hr *before* chemotherapy; IV, 10 mcg/kg over 30 min, begin 30 min *before* chemotherapy
	ondansetron (Zofran)	8 mg orally twice daily on days of chemotherapy administration. Give first dose 30 min before chemotherapy. IV 10 mcg/kg over 15 min within 30 min *before* beginning chemotherapy.
Dopamine Antagonists	metoclopramide (Gimoti, Metozolv, Reglan)	10 mg orally, IV, or IM 4 times per day, given 30 min before meals and at bedtime 1–2 mg/kg IV infusion given 30 min *before* beginning chemotherapy and repeated every 2 hr for 2 doses, and then every 3 hr for 3 doses
	trimethobenzamide (Navogan, Tebamide, Tigan, Trimazide)	300 mg orally 3 to 4 times daily as needed; 200 mg 3–4 times daily IM or rectally daily as needed

IM, Intramuscular; *IV,* intravenous.

Intended responses of antiemetic drugs
- Vomiting reflex is inhibited.
- Vomiting reflex pathways are interrupted or disrupted.
- Patient is sedated.
- Nausea is relieved.
- Vomiting is prevented.

Common side effects of antiemetic drugs. Common side effects of antiemetic drugs vary with the prescribed drug. The most common side effects are listed in the following table. Be sure to consult a drug resource for additional information on any specific antiemetic drug.

Critical Point for Safety

To prevent nausea and vomiting associated with a specific trigger such as cancer chemotherapy or motion, give antiemetics before the triggering events occur and during the time the person usually has these responses.

QSEN: Safety

Critical Point for Safety

Ask patients about a history of depression. Metoclopramide (Reglan) can cause mild-to-severe depression and should not be prescribed for patients with a history of depression.

QSEN: Safety

Do Not Confuse

Antivert *with* Axert

An order for Antivert may be confused with Axert. Antivert is an antihistamine used for nausea, vomiting, and dizziness from motion sickness and for vertigo associated with diseases affecting the inner ear vestibular apparatus. Axert is a vascular headache suppressant used to treat migraine headaches.

QSEN: Safety

Common Side Effects of Antiemetic Drugs

Drug	Common Side Effects
cyclizine (Marezine)	Drowsiness, dry mouth, hypotension
meclizine (Antivert)	Drowsiness
metoclopramide (Reglan)	Drowsiness, fatigue, increased depression, restlessness
prochlorperazine (Compazine)	Blurred vision, constipation, dizziness, dry eyes, dry mouth, involuntary muscle spasms, jitteriness, mouth puckering
promethazine (Phenergan)	Confusion, disorientation, dizziness, dry mouth, nausea, vomiting, rash
ondansetron (Zofran)	Abdominal pain, constipation, fatigue, headache
granisetron (Kytril)	Headache, constipation, loss of energy
scopolamine (L-hyoscine)	Blurred vision, constipation, dilated pupils, dizziness, drowsiness, dry mouth, lightheadedness, rash, urinary retention
trimethobenzamide (Tigan)	Blurred vision, diarrhea, drowsiness, cramps, headache, hypotension, rectal irritation with suppositories

Common Side Effects
Antiemetic Drugs

Dizziness

Drowsiness, Fatigue

Headache

Blurred vision

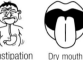
Constipation

Dry mouth

Additional side effects include insomnia; diplopia (double vision); tinnitus (ringing in the ears); hypertension; photosensitivity; electrocardiogram (ECG) changes such as tachycardia, bradycardia, and supraventricular tachycardia (SVT); pink or reddish-brown urine; urinary retention; anxiety; and depression.

Possible adverse effects of antiemetic drugs. Adverse effects of antiemetic drugs also vary with the prescribed drug. Promethazine (Phenergan), prochlorperazine (Compazine), and metoclopramide (Reglan) can cause neuroleptic malignant syndrome, a rare and life-threatening side effect in which dangerously high body temperatures can occur. Without prompt and expert treatment, this condition can be fatal in as many as 20% of those who develop it. Signs and symptoms include fever, respiratory distress, tachycardia, seizures, diaphoresis, blood pressure changes, pallor, fatigue, severe muscle stiffness, and loss of bladder control.

Trimethobenzamide (Tigan) may cause coma and seizures. Promethazine (Phenergan) and metoclopramide (Reglan) can cause *tardive dyskinesia*, a chronic disorder of the nervous system. Signs and symptoms include uncontrolled rhythmic movement of the mouth, face, or extremities; lip smacking or puckering; puffing of cheeks; uncontrolled chewing; and rapid or wormlike movements of the tongue. This adverse effect usually occurs after a year or more of continued use of these drugs and is often irreversible. If diagnosed early, tardive dyskinesia may be reversed by stopping the drug.

Promethazine (Phenergan) and prochlorperazine (Compazine) may cause *neutropenia*, a decrease in the number of neutrophils (white blood cells), putting the patient at higher risk for infections. When given by intravenous (IV) push, undiluted promethazine has been associated with severe tissue necrosis.

Respiratory depression (decreased drive for breathing) is a life-threatening effect that can occur with cyclizine (Marezine), promethazine (Phenergan), and scopolamine (L-hyoscine).

⭐ ***Priority actions to take*** before ***giving antiemetic drugs.*** Check the patient's body temperature, blood pressure, and heart rate and rhythm. Also check his or her baseline respiratory rate and level of consciousness. Obtain a baseline weight, and check electrolyte laboratory values. Ask the patient about nausea and vomiting. Ask about any possible causes, allergies, or reactions such as motion sickness.

Use your stethoscope to listen for active bowel sounds in the patient's abdomen. Look for abdominal distention. Ask about the patient's usual diet and fluid intake, bowel movements, constipation, or difficulty swallowing.

Obtain a complete list of drugs the patient is currently taking, including over-the-counter and herbal drugs. Ask whether the patient who is prescribed metoclopramide (Reglan) has experienced depression in the past. If so, notify the prescriber before giving the drug.

If a drug is to be given intravenously, be sure to dilute it first to decrease the risk of tissue necrosis.

⊛ *Priority actions to take after giving antiemetic drugs.* Keep track of any episodes of nausea or vomiting to determine the effectiveness of these drugs.

Because ECG changes and dysrhythmias may occur, recheck the patient's blood pressure, heart rate and rhythm, and respiratory rate. Check the patient's temperature with each set of vital signs, and monitor for any signs of infection (e.g., WBC values).

Obtain daily weights using the same scale and the same amount of clothing at the same time each day. Ask the patient about nausea and vomiting at least every shift. Continue to listen for active bowel sounds and assess for abdominal distention.

Immediately report any signs of respiratory depression to the prescriber. Instruct the patient to call for help getting out of bed, and ensure that the call light is within easy reach. Watch for signs of side effects or adverse effects, especially malignant neuroleptic syndrome and tardive dyskinesia. Report any signs immediately to the prescriber.

Check the patient's level of consciousness, and watch for sedation effects, especially with older adults.

Some antiemetic drugs (e.g., cyclizine [Marezine], prochlorperazine [Compazine], promethazine [Phenergan], and scopolamine [L-hyoscine]) may cause hypotension or dizziness. Instruct the patient to change positions slowly and call for help when getting out of bed. Be sure that the call light is within easy reach.

Keep track of intake and output (both food and fluid). Ask about GI upset. If these drugs cause GI symptoms, give them with food, milk, or a full glass of water.

Watch for signs of depression in patients taking metoclopramide (Reglan) because this drug may cause mild-to-severe depression. Notify the prescriber immediately because a different drug may be needed to treat the nausea and vomiting.

⊛ *Teaching priorities for patients taking antiemetic drugs*
- Avoid driving or operating heavy or dangerous equipment because of dizziness and drowsiness.
- Get up slowly from bed or a chair because of hypotension and dizziness.
- Use sunscreen, wear protective clothing, and avoid tanning beds because of sun sensitivity.
- Report any signs and symptoms of malignant neuroleptic syndrome (e.g., fever, respiratory distress, tachycardia, seizures, diaphoresis, blood pressure changes, pallor, fatigue, severe muscle stiffness, loss of bladder control) and tardive dyskinesia (e.g., uncontrolled rhythmic movement of the mouth, face, or extremities; lip smacking or puckering; puffing of cheeks; uncontrolled chewing; rapid or worm-like movements of the tongue) to your prescriber.
- Check your body temperature every day, and report abnormal values as well as signs and symptoms of infection (e.g., fever, chills or sweating, redness, swelling) to your prescriber.
- Remember that prochlorperazine (Compazine) may cause your urine to change color to pink or reddish-brown. This condition is temporary and disappears within days after the drug is discontinued.
- For best control of nausea or vomiting, take antiemetic drugs before events that usually cause nausea.
- Consult with your prescriber before taking over-the-counter drugs.
- Avoid using CNS depressants such as alcohol, antihistamines, sedatives, tranquilizers, or sleeping drugs while taking antiemetic drugs because these drugs make drowsiness worse.
- Use of a mild analgesic such as acetaminophen for relief from headaches.

Critical Point for Safety

Before giving an antiemetic drug, always observe the abdomen for distention and listen for active bowel sounds.

QSEN: Safety

Critical Point for Safety

Carefully monitor respiratory status and rate while patients are taking the antiemetic drugs cyclizine (Marezine), promethazine (Phenergan), and scopolamine (L-hyoscine).

QSEN: Safety

Memory Jogger

Prochlorperazine (Compazine) may cause urine to change color to pink or reddish-brown. This is temporary and disappears within days after the drug is discontinued.

Critical Point for Safety

To prevent nausea and vomiting from cancer chemotherapy, teach patients to take antiemetic drugs 30 min *before* meals.

QSEN: Safety

Critical Point for Safety

To prevent nausea from motion sickness, teach patients to take antiemetic drugs at least 30 min, but preferably 1–2 hr, *before* activities that cause nausea.

QSEN: Safety

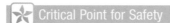
• Use frequent mouth rinses and oral care to manage dry mouth. If long-term use of these drugs is planned, see your dentist regularly to prevent dental disorders.
• Take a missed dose of the drug as soon as possible but do **not** take double doses.

Life span considerations for antiemetic drugs

Pediatric considerations. Unintentional overdoses of metoclopramide (Reglan) have occurred with infants and children. Teach parents how to read the drug label and correctly give this drug to a child.

Children may have muscle spasms of the jaw, neck, and back along with jerky movements of the head and face while taking metoclopramide. Balance disturbance is more likely to occur in children with high doses of antiemetic drugs used for cancer chemotherapy.

Considerations for pregnancy and lactation. Most of these drugs have a low to moderate likelihood of increasing the risk for birth defects or fetal harm. A woman should check with her prescriber before taking these drugs if she is pregnant, planning to get pregnant, or breastfeeding. Some of these drugs, such as metoclopramide, pass into breast milk and should be avoided while breastfeeding.

Considerations for older adults. Older adults are more likely to experience side effects such as acute confusion and dizziness. They may develop a shuffling walk, trembling, and shaking of the hands after taking metoclopramide over a long period of time. They are more likely to develop CNS effects of scopolamine (L-hyoscine) such as confusion, memory loss, unusual excitement, and heat-related disorders. Older adults are also more likely to experience symptoms of balance disturbance with high doses of antiemetic drugs used for cancer chemotherapy and may need lower doses of these drugs.

REVIEW OF RELATED PHYSIOLOGY AND PATHOPHYSIOLOGY FOR CONSTIPATION

Constipation occurs when a person has fewer than three bowel movements a week. Stools become very hard, dry, and difficult to eliminate. Having a bowel movement can be uncomfortable, even painful because of straining, bloating, and having a full bowel. Constipation may also include straining or pushing for longer than 10 minutes when trying to have a bowel movement. Figure 19.5 summarizes how constipation occurs.

Constipation is a symptom, not a disease, usually indicating some other health problem. Just about everyone experiences constipation at some time in his or her life, often because of poor diet. Most episodes of constipation are temporary and are not serious.

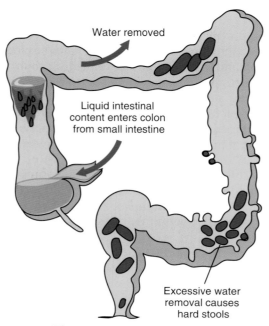

FIG. 19.5 How constipation occurs.

Box **19.1**   **Common Causes of Constipation**

- Abuse of laxatives
- Bowel diseases (e.g., irritable bowel syndrome, cancer)
- Changes in life (e.g., pregnancy, aging, travel)
- Dehydration
- Drugs
- Ignoring the urge to have a bowel movement

- Lack of physical activity
- Medical problems (e.g., hypothyroidism, cystic fibrosis, stroke)
- Mental problems such as depression
- Milk
- Not enough fiber in the diet
- Problems with the colon or rectum
- Problems with intestinal function

Table **19.2**   **Drug Categories That Cause Constipation**

CATEGORY	EXAMPLES
Antacids	Drugs containing magnesium
Anticholinergics	amitriptyline, carbidopa-levodopa, dicyclomine, levodopa, nortriptyline, propantheline
Anticonvulsants	phenytoin, valproic acid
Antidepressants	amitriptyline, imipramine, phenelzine
Antihypertensives	clonidine, methyldopa
Antipsychotics	haloperidol, risperidone
Bile acid sequestrants	cholestyramine, colestipol
Calcium channel blockers	diltiazem, nifedipine, verapamil
Calcium supplements	calcium carbonate, PhosCal
Iron supplements	Iron aid (vitamin C, vitamin B_{12}, folic acid), chelated iron
Opiates	oxycodone/acetaminophen, propoxyphene napsylate and acetaminophen, drugs containing morphine or codeine

The most common causes of constipation are low-fiber diet, lack of physical activity, not taking in enough fluid, and delaying going to the bathroom when the urge to have a bowel movement is felt (Box 19.1). Stress, travel, and other changes in bowel habits can lead to constipation. Misuse of laxatives can cause constipation because the body becomes dependent on these drugs, needing higher and higher doses until the bowel no longer works. Bowel diseases, pregnancy, medical illnesses, mental health problems, neurologic problems, and many drugs may also cause constipation (Table 19.2). Drugs may cause constipation by affecting nerve and muscle activity of the colon or binding intestinal fluids. Children often develop constipation when holding back having a bowel movement if they are not yet ready for or are afraid of toilet training.

Mild constipation is usually not serious. However, if symptoms are severe, last more than 3 weeks, or if complications such as bleeding occur, a health care provider should be consulted. Constipation that does not respond to self-treatment and constipation that occurs with rectal bleeding, abnormal pain and cramps, nausea and vomiting, and weight loss should also be reported. Patients with severe constipation should be referred to their health care provider to rule out colon cancer. A health care provider should be consulted whenever constipation occurs during pregnancy or breastfeeding.

TYPES OF DRUGS FOR CONSTIPATION

Laxatives, Lubricants, and Stool Softeners

How drugs for constipation work. Many people buy over-the-counter (OTC) drugs to self-treat constipation. The purpose of drugs for constipation is to help the body eliminate hard stools. Products that are available include bulk-forming laxatives, stool softeners, lubricants, saline laxatives, and stimulant laxatives. It is important to remember that **laxatives** (drugs used to produce bowel movements and relieve constipation) are not meant for long-term use and should not be used for longer than 1 week unless prescribed for longer. Long-term use of laxatives can cause other

 Memory Jogger

Signs and symptoms of constipation are:
- Fewer than three bowel movements a week
- Sudden decrease in frequency of bowel movements
- Stools that are harder than normal
- Bowels still feeling full after a bowel movement
- Bloated sensation

 Memory Jogger

Patients with severe constipation should be referred to a health care provider to rule out colon cancer.

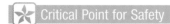

health problems. The exception is bulk-forming laxatives such as psyllium (Metamucil) that may be taken once a day to help avoid constipation. This drug is not absorbed from the intestines into the body and is safe for long-term use.

Bulk-forming drugs for constipation add bulk to the stool, which increases stool mass that stimulates peristalsis (Animation 19.2). This helps stool move through the bowel. These drugs may work in as little as 12 hours but can take as long as 3 days to be effective.

Emollient or **stool softener** drugs soften stool, allowing the stool to mix with fatty substances and making it easier to eliminate. Some drugs combine the softening effect with a stimulant to both soften the stool and increase peristalsis to eliminate stool. They usually work within 12 to 72 hours. Rectal suppositories usually work within 15 to 30 minutes.

Osmotic laxatives cause retention of fluid in the bowel, increasing the water content in stool; they may take 2 to 3 days to work. Drugs such as **lubricants** coat the surface of stool and help it hold water so the body can more easily expel it. *Stimulant laxatives* work by stimulating intestinal motility and secretion of water into the bowel; they usually take 6 to 12 hours to take effect but may take up to 72 hours. Senna is an over-the-counter (OTC) herbal preparation that contains sennosides that irritate the lining of the bowel, causing a stimulant laxative effect.

Common names and doses of drugs for constipation are listed in the following table. Be sure to consult a reliable drug resource for information on any specific constipation drugs.

Adult Dosages for Commonly Prescribed Drugs for Constipation

Drug Category	Drug Name	Usual Maintenance Dose
Bulk-Forming Drugs	methylcellulose (Citrucel)	1 heaping tablespoonful (2 g methylcellulose per 19 g powder) in at least 240 mL (8 oz) of water orally, given 1–3 times per day as needed 2 caplets (total 1 g methylcellulose) orally with at least 240 mL (8 oz) of liquid, up to 6 times per day as needed
	psyllium (Fiberall, Hydrocil, Metamucil)	1 rounded teaspoonful, tablespoonful, or premeasured packet in 240 mL of fluid orally, 1–3 times per day (contain 2 g of soluble dietary fiber per dose)
Emollients/Stool Softeners	docusate (Colace, Correctol, Surfak)	50–300 mg/day orally given in single or divided doses
Stimulants	bisacodyl (Dulcolax)	5–15 mg single oral dose 10 mg rectally
	senna (Ex-Lax)	1–2 tablets (8.6–17.2 mg sennosides) orally twice daily; 2 soft gel capsules (17.2 mg sennosides) orally at bedtime ***Special Considerations:* Senna is an OTC herbal preparation approved for use by the FDA**
Osmotic Laxatives	lactulose (Cephulac, Cholac, Constilac)	15–30 mL orally once daily, increasing to 60 mL orally once daily if needed
	lubiprostone (Amitiza)	24 mcg orally twice daily with food and water
	magnesium hydroxide (Dulcolax, Ex-Lax, Phillips' Milk of Magnesia)	15–60 mL orally once per day at bedtime, or the daily dose may be given in divided doses as directed by prescriber
	polyethylene glycol (GoLYTELY, MiraLax)	17 g orally mixed in 120–240 mL of appropriate fluid (e.g., water, juice, soda, coffee or tea) once daily
	sodium phosphate (Fleet Enema)	One 4.5-oz enema given rectally
Lubricants	castor oil (Purge, Emulsoil)	15–60 mL orally once daily as needed at bedtime
	glycerin suppository (Sani-Supp)	1 adult strength suppository (2 g) rectally once every 24 hr or as directed ***Special Considerations:* Hold in rectum 15 min; bowel movement should occur within 15 min to 1 hr**

FDA, US Food and Drug Administration; *OTC,* over-the-counter.

Intended responses of drugs for constipation

- Stool is softened.
- Stool is passed.
- Constipation is relieved and prevented.

Common side effects of drugs for constipation. Common side effects of drugs for constipation vary with the prescribed drug. The most common side effects are listed in the following table. Be sure to consult a reliable drug resource for additional information on any specific constipation drug.

Common Side Effects of Drugs for Constipation

Drug	Common Side Effects
Bulk-Forming Drugs	
psyllium (Metamucil)	Bronchospasm, GI cramps, intestinal or esophageal obstruction, nausea, vomiting
Emollients/Stool Softeners	
docusate (Colace, Surfak)	Mild GI cramps, throat irritation, rashes
Emollients Combined with Stimulants	
docusate sodium and casanthranol (Peri-Colace)	Diarrhea, skin rash, stomach cramps, throat irritation
Stimulants	
bisacodyl (Dulcolax)	Abdominal cramps, diarrhea, hypokalemia (low potassium), muscle weakness, nausea, rectal burning
senna (Ex-lax)	Abdominal cramps, stomach discomfort, diarrhea
Osmotic Laxatives	
lactulose (Cephulac, Cholac, Constilac)	Abdominal distention, belching, diarrhea, flatulence, GI cramps, hypoglycemia in patient with diabetes
lubiprostone (Amitiza)	Abdominal pain and distention, diarrhea, dizziness, dry mouth, gas, headache, nausea, peripheral swelling, reflux
magnesium hydroxide (Phillips' Milk of Magnesia)	Diarrhea, flushing, sweating
polyethylene glycol (MiraLax)	Abdominal bloating, cramping, flatulence (gas), nausea
sodium phosphate (Fleet Enema)	Abdominal bloating, abdominal pain, dizziness, electrolyte imbalances (hyperphosphatemia, hypocalcemia, hypokalemia, sodium retention), GI cramping, headache, nausea, vomiting
Lubricants	
castor oil (Purge, Emulsoil)	Belching, cramping, diarrhea, nausea
glycerin suppository (Sani-Supp)	Abdominal cramps, hyperemia (increased blood flow) of rectal mucosa, rectal discomfort

Possible adverse effects of drugs for constipation. Severe life-threatening adverse effects are rare with drugs for constipation. Psyllium (Metamucil) and docusate (Colace) may cause allergic reactions that include difficulty breathing, swelling and closing of the throat, swelling of lips and tongue, or hives.

Side effects of castor oil (Purge) that require medical attention include confusion, irregular heartbeat, muscle cramps, skin rash, and unusual tiredness or weakness.

Lactulose (Cephulac) and bulk-forming drugs containing sugar may cause hyperglycemia (high blood sugar) in patients with diabetes.

Bisacodyl (Dulcolax) may cause hypokalemia, which can lead to life-threatening dysrhythmias.

Fleet enemas are meant to be used occasionally and can cause electrolyte imbalances when used often.

 Do Not Confuse

Colace *with* Cozaar

An order for Colace may be confused with Cozaar. Colace is a stool softener, whereas Cozaar is an angiotensin II receptor antagonist used to manage high blood pressure.

QSEN: Safety

 Do Not Confuse

MiraLax *with* Mirapex

An order for MiraLax may be confused with Mirapex. MiraLax is an osmotic diuretic used to treat constipation, whereas Mirapex is a drug used to manage Parkinson disease.

QSEN: Safety

Common Side Effects

Drugs for Constipation

Diarrhea,
Abdominal cramps,
Abdominal distension,
Nausea

✪ *Priority actions to take* before *giving drugs for constipation.* Obtain a complete list of drugs that the patient is currently using, including over-the-counter and herbal drugs. Ask the patient about current bowel habits and the nature of his or her normal stools as well as use of laxatives. Check the abdomen for distention and bowel sounds. Obtain baseline vital signs and the patient's weight. If the patient has diabetes, obtain a baseline blood sugar using a fingerstick test.

Ask the patient about abdominal pain. Drugs for constipation should *not* be given to a patient experiencing undiagnosed abdominal pain or acute abdomen because these drugs increase peristalsis and the risk of bowel perforation.

Prepare a full glass (8 ounces) of fluid to give with oral drugs. If the patient is also taking antacids, give these drugs at least 1 hour before or after taking them. Be sure to lubricate suppositories before placing them in the rectum.

✪ *Priority actions to take* after *giving drugs for constipation.* Recheck the patient's abdomen for distention and bowel sounds. Monitor for bowel movements, and assess the quality and quantity of stools. Continue to monitor vital signs and patient weight.

Instruct the patient to report bowel movements and any drug side effects. Be sure to remind patients to drink at least 1500 to 2000 mL of fluid every day to prevent constipation recurrence.

✪ *Teaching priorities for patients taking drugs for constipation*
- Consume foods with increased bulk and drink enough fluids to prevent constipation.
- Exercise moderately to help prevent the side effect of constipation.
- Take oral drugs for constipation with 8 ounces of fluid to be sure the drugs are safe and effective.
- Keep a daily record of bowel movements, including the nature of your stools. Remember that normal bowel patterns vary from person to person and you need to determine your own normal pattern.
- Drink at least 1500 to 2000 mL of fluid every day to help prevent constipation from returning.
- Remember that most laxatives should be used only short term (except for bulk-forming drugs such as psyllium, which are safe to take every day).
- Notify your prescriber if constipation is not relieved or if rectal bleeding or signs of electrolyte imbalance such as muscle cramps or pain, weakness, or dizziness occur.
- Do not to take oral forms of these drugs within 1 hour of taking an antacid drug because antacids decrease absorption.
- Follow package directions for use of any laxative.

Life span considerations for drugs for constipation

Pediatric considerations. Doses of drugs for constipation given to children 6 to 12 years of age are generally half of the adult dose but should still be given with 8 ounces of fluid. Laxatives or enemas should not be given to children without specific instructions from the prescriber.

Considerations for pregnancy and lactation. Most drugs for constipation are considered safe for use during pregnancy and have a low likelihood of increasing the risk for birth defects or fetal harm. However, the prescriber must assess the benefits before ordering these drugs. Sodium phosphate (Fleet enema) and lubiprostone (Amitiza) have a moderate likelihood of increasing the risk for birth defects or fetal harm and should not be used.

Considerations for older adults. Constipation is common in older adults, and most constipation drugs are safe for them to use. Psyllium is safe for older adults to use on a daily basis to prevent constipation. Older patients often use laxatives for a longer period and at higher dosages than recommended, which places them at risk for diarrhea and fluid imbalance. Reinforce that increasing fluid intake often relieves constipation without the need for laxatives.

REVIEW OF RELATED PHYSIOLOGY AND PATHOPHYSIOLOGY FOR DIARRHEA

Diarrhea is an increase in the amount of water in bowel movements and in their volume and frequency. It is not a disease but is a symptom of another health problem. Diarrhea may occur suddenly and usually disappears in a few days even without treatment. It is a fairly common occurrence for all age groups, and most cases of diarrhea are not serious. However, in children, infants, and some older adults, diarrhea can cause dehydration fairly rapidly. It may be an acute, self-limiting occurrence, or it may be a severe, life-threatening illness because of fluid and electrolyte imbalances.

An imbalance between the absorption and secretion functions of the intestines can lead to diarrhea. Absorption is decreased, and secretion is increased (Figure 19.6). Acute diarrhea is three or more loose stools within a 24-hour period, continuing for less than 2 weeks. Most often acute diarrhea goes away within 72 hours. Diarrhea that lasts longer than 2 weeks is considered chronic; however, it may not always include frequent daily passing of loose, watery stools.

There are many causes of diarrhea (Box 19.2), but the most common cause is inflammation of the small bowel (*enteritis*). Most cases of infectious diarrhea are caused by viruses or bacteria taken in with contaminated food or water or with undercooked meat, poultry, fish, or eggs. Many drugs, including antibiotics, cardiac drugs, GI drugs, and neuropsychiatric drugs can cause diarrhea. Examples of these drugs are listed in Box 19.3. Other causes of diarrhea include radiation therapy, medical problems, gastrectomy, and nerve disorders. The four major classifications of diarrhea are osmotic, secretory, exudative, and motility disorder (Table 19.3).

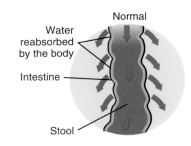

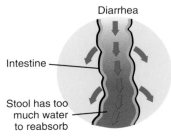

FIG. 19.6 Pathophysiology of diarrhea.

Box 19.2   Common Causes of Diarrhea

- Drugs (e.g., antibiotics, laxatives, chemotherapy)
- Food poisoning/traveler's diarrhea
- Gastrectomy (partial removal of the stomach)
- High-dose radiation therapy
- Medical conditions (e.g., malabsorption, inflammatory bowel diseases such as Crohn disease or ulcerative colitis, irritable bowel syndrome, celiac disease)
- Nerve disorders (autonomic neuropathy, diabetic neuropathy)
- Other infections (bacterial, parasites)
- Viral gastroenteritis (most common cause)
- Zollinger-Ellison syndrome

Memory Jogger

Signs and symptoms of diarrhea are:
- Frequent need to have a bowel movement
- Frequent loose, watery stools
- Abdominal pain and cramping
- Fever, chills, and generally feeling ill
- Weight loss

Box 19.3   Examples of Drugs That Can Cause Diarrhea

ANTIBIOTICS
- Ampicillin
- Broad-spectrum antibiotics
- Cephalosporins
- Clindamycin
- Erythromycin
- Sulfonamides
- Tetracycline

ANTIHYPERTENSIVE DRUGS
- Guanabenz
- Guanadrel
- Guanethidine
- Methyldopa
- Reserpine
- Angiotensin-converting enzyme inhibitors

CARDIAC DRUGS
- Beta-blockers
- Digoxin

- Diuretics
- Hydralazine
- Procainamide
- Quinidine

CHOLINERGICS
- Bethanechol
- Metoclopramide
- Neostigmine

GASTROINTESTINAL DRUGS
- Antacids
- Laxatives
- Misoprostol
- Olsalazine

HYPOLIPIDEMIC DRUGS
- Clofibrate
- Gemfibrozil
- Statin drugs

NEUROPSYCHIATRIC DRUGS
- Alprazolam
- Ethosuximide
- Fluoxetine
- L-dopa
- Lithium
- Valproic acid

MISCELLANEOUS
- Chemotherapy drugs
- Colchicine
- Nonsteroidal antiinflammatory drugs
- Theophylline
- Thyroid hormones

Table 19.3	Classifications of Diarrhea	
CLASSIFICATION	**MECHANISM**	**CAUSES**
Osmotic	Unabsorbed solutes	Lactose intolerance (lactose deficiency), magnesium antacid excess
Secretory	Increased secretion of electrolytes	*Escherichia coli* infections, ileal resection, thyroid cancer
Exudative	Defective colonic absorption, outpouring of mucus and/or blood	Ulcerative colitis, Crohn disease, shigellosis, leukemia
Motility disorder	Decreased contact time	Irritable bowel syndrome, diabetic neuropathy

TYPES OF DRUGS FOR DIARRHEA

Antimotility, Adsorbent/Absorbent, and Antisecretory Drugs

How antidiarrheal drugs work. Drugs for diarrhea (antidiarrheal drugs) are given to control diarrhea and some of the symptoms that occur with this condition. The three types of antidiarrheal drugs are antimotility drugs, adsorbent/absorbent drugs, and antisecretory drugs. The purpose of drugs prescribed for diarrhea is to correct the underlying problem and help the body control diarrhea and its uncomfortable symptoms. Goals of treatment include keeping the patient hydrated, treating the underlying cause, and relieving diarrhea. Be sure to watch for signs and symptoms of electrolyte imbalances that may be caused by diarrhea such as a low potassium level (*hypokalemia*).

When diarrhea is caused by an infection from bacteria or parasites, antidiarrheal drugs can make the condition worse. This is because the drugs prevent the body from eliminating the organisms causing the diarrhea. Antidiarrheal drugs are usually not given for this type of diarrhea. Treatment focuses on preventing dehydration and rehydration.

Drugs for diarrhea act in several ways. Antimotility drugs slow the movement of stool through the bowel, allowing more time for water and essential salts to be absorbed by the body. Adsorbent/absorbent drugs remove substances that cause diarrhea from the body. Antisecretory drugs decrease secretion of intestinal fluids and slow bacterial activity.

Common names and doses of drugs for diarrhea are listed in the following table. Be sure to consult a reliable drug resource for information on specific antidiarrheal drugs.

 Memory Jogger

Signs and symptoms of hypokalemia include cardiac dysrhythmias, muscle pain, general discomfort or irritability, weakness, and paralysis.

Memory Jogger

The three types of antidiarrheal drugs are:
- Antimotility drugs
- Adsorbent/absorbent drugs
- Antisecretory drugs

Adult Dosages for Commonly Drugs for Diarrhea

Drug Category	Drug Name	Usual Maintenance Dose
Antimotility Drugs	difenoxin with atropine (Motofen)	2 tablets (2 mg) orally, then 1 tablet (1 mg) after each loose stool or every 3–4 hr as needed **Special Considerations: Treatment should not extend beyond 48 hr**
	diphenoxylate with atropine (Lomotil, Lenox, Vi-Atro)	5 mg (2 tablets) orally 4 times per day; discontinue as soon as possible Oral solution: 5 mg (10 mL) orally 4 times per day **Special Considerations: Discontinue after 10 days if clinical improvement is not observed**
	loperamide (Imodium)	4 mg orally followed by 2 mg orally after each subsequent unformed stool **Special Considerations: Do not exceed 16 mg per day if prescribed; do not exceed 8 mg per day if over-the-counter**
	paregoric (Camphorated Opium Tincture)	5–10 mL orally after each unformed stool; may be given every 2 hr up to 4 times daily **Special Considerations: Each 5 mL contains 2 mg of anhydrous morphine; may be habit forming**
Adsorbent/ Absorbent Drugs	bismuth subsalicylate (Kaopectate, Kaopectolin)	524 mg (2 tablets) orally every 30–60 min, as needed Liquid: 524 mg (30 mL) orally every 30–60 min, as needed **Special Considerations: Do not exceed 8 doses per day**

Adult Dosages for Commonly Drugs for Diarrhea—cont'd

Drug Category	Drug Name	Usual Maintenance Dose
	calcium polycarbophil (FiberCon)	2 tablets (1250 mg calcium polycarbophil) orally 1–4 times daily as needed. Max: 8 tablets/day
Antisecretory Drugs	bismuth subsalicylate (Pepto-Bismol)	2 tablets or 30 mL orally every 30 min to 1 hr as needed ***Special Considerations:* Do not exceed 8 doses per day**

Intended responses of antidiarrheal drugs
- GI motility is decreased.
- Diarrhea is decreased.
- Fluid from bowel is reabsorbed.
- Secretion of fluids into the bowel is decreased.
- Activity of bacteria is decreased.
- Dehydration is prevented.

Common side effects of antidiarrheal drugs. Side effects of antidiarrheal drugs are uncommon in healthy adults and vary with the prescribed drug. The most common side effect is constipation. Additional side effects are listed in the following table. Be sure to consult a reliable drug reference for additional information on any specific antidiarrheal drug.

Common Side Effects of Antidiarrheal Drugs

Drug	Common Side Effects
bismuth subsalicylate (Kaopectate)	Constipation, bloating, feeling of fullness
bismuth subsalicylate (Pepto-Bismol)	Constipation, gray-black stools, impaction in infants and debilitated patients, tinnitus (ringing in the ears)
calcium polycarbophil (FiberCon)	Abdominal fullness, flatulence (gas), laxative dependence with long-term use
difenoxin with atropine (Motofen)	Blurred vision, constipation, confusion, dizziness, drowsiness, dry eyes, dry mouth, flushing, GI distress, headache, insomnia, nausea, nervousness, tachycardia, urinary retention, vomiting
diphenoxylate with atropine (Lomotil)	Blurred vision, constipation, confusion, dizziness, drowsiness, dry eyes, dry mouth, flushing, GI distress, headache, insomnia, nervousness, tachycardia, nausea, urinary retention, vomiting
loperamide (Imodium)	Abdominal pain/discomfort, allergic reactions, constipation, distention, dizziness, drowsiness, dry mouth, nausea, vomiting
paregoric (Camphorated Opium Tincture)	Abdominal pain, constipation, loss of appetite, nausea, vomiting

Possible adverse effects of antidiarrheal drugs. Adverse effects are rare with antidiarrheal drugs. Calcium polycarbophil (FiberCon) may cause intestinal obstruction.

A potential life-threatening adverse effect of antimotility drugs is *toxic megacolon*, which is a very inflated colon with abdominal distention (Figure 19.7). Other signs and symptoms of this condition include fever, abdominal pain, rapid heart rate, and dehydration. A patient with toxic megacolon may go into shock, and if this condition is not recognized and treated early, there is a risk for death.

⊛ **Priority actions to take before giving antidiarrheal drugs.** Obtain a complete list of drugs that the patient is currently using, including over-the-counter and herbal drugs. Ask patients to describe their experiences with diarrhea. Check the patient's baseline weight, and get a set of vital signs. Listen to the abdomen with your

---

 Memory Jogger

The most common side effect of antidiarrheal drugs is constipation.

Common Side Effects

Drugs for Diarrhea

Constipation, Abdominal discomfort   Dizziness

Dry mouth   Blurred vision

 Critical Point for Safety

After giving an antimotility drug, be sure to check the patient for abdominal distention, a sign of toxic megacolon.

QSEN: Safety

 Critical Point for Safety

Antidiarrheal drugs are not usually given when diarrhea is caused by bacteria or parasites because the drugs prevent the body from eliminating the organisms, which can cause the condition to worsen.

QSEN: Safety

 Critical Point for Safety

Bismuth subsalicylate (Pepto-Bismol) contains an aspirin-like drug. Watch for bleeding because this drug can also increase the effects of the anticoagulant warfarin (Coumadin).

QSEN: Safety

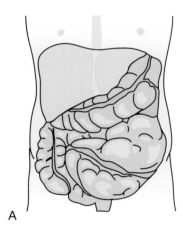

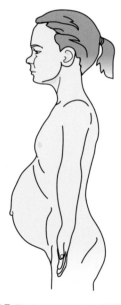

B

FIG. 19.7 Toxic megacolon. (A) Note the enlarged intestines. (B) Side view.

stethoscope for active bowel sounds, and check for abdominal distention. Observe the patient's skin turgor for signs of dehydration. When a patient is dehydrated, gently pinching and lifting the skin over the sternum, back of the hand, or arm will form a "tent." Use the sternum or forehead to test for tenting in the older adult because the skin on the back of hand may tent due to aging. The worse the dehydration, the longer the skin will take to return to its normal position. Ask patients about allergies or unusual reactions to aspirin or other drugs containing aspirin because bismuth subsalicylate (Pepto-Bismol) contains an aspirin-like drug. This drug may interact with and increase the effects of anticoagulant drugs such as warfarin (Coumadin). Determine whether the patient's diarrhea is caused by bacteria or parasites (e.g., send a stool sample to the lab).

⭐ *Priority actions to take* after *giving antidiarrheal drugs.* Reassess the abdomen for bowel sounds and distention. Watch for signs of toxic megacolon if the patient is taking an antimotility drug. If symptoms occur, notify the prescriber immediately.

Recheck and continue to monitor vital signs every 4 to 8 hours. Keep a record of how often the patient has diarrhea stools. Be sure to document the consistency, odor, and appearance of stools. Continue to monitor the skin turgor and encourage the patient to drink plenty of fluids to avoid dehydration. Check patient weights on a daily basis.

⭐ *Teaching priorities for patients taking antidiarrheal drugs*
- Take the drug exactly as ordered by your prescriber. Do not take double doses of these drugs because constipation may result.
- Because of possible dizziness or drowsiness, avoid driving or performing any activities that require alertness until you know how the drugs will affect you.
- Use frequent mouth rinses, mouth care, and sugarless gum or candy to relieve symptoms of dry mouth.
- If the prescribed drug is in a liquid form, shake the bottle well before measuring and taking it.
- Notify your prescriber if the diarrhea is not relieved in 2 days while taking antidiarrheal drugs, or if you develop a fever, abdominal pain, or abdominal distention.
- Also notify your prescriber if any blood or mucus appears in your stools.
- Avoid the use of alcohol and other CNS depressants while taking antidiarrheal drugs.
- Remember that bismuth subsalicylate (Pepto-Bismol) contains an aspirin-like drug and that additional aspirin should not be taken because it may cause ringing in the ears (tinnitus). Also be aware that this drug may turn your stool and the tongue gray-black.

Life span considerations for antidiarrheal drugs
Pediatric considerations. Children should not be given bismuth subsalicylate because it contains an aspirin-like drug and may cause Reye syndrome. This is a life-threatening condition that affects the liver and central nervous system (CNS), and it causes vomiting and confusion. This syndrome usually occurs soon after the onset of a viral illness if a child was treated with aspirin. Children are more sensitive to the drowsiness and dizziness caused by loperamide (Imodium). Bismuth subsalicylate (Kaopectate) and calcium polycarbophil (Fibercon) are not recommended for preschool children. Infants and children are at increased risk for dehydration with diarrhea.

Considerations for pregnancy and lactation. Women who are pregnant or breastfeeding should check with their prescriber before using any antidiarrheal drugs. They should also ask about replacing lost fluids because dehydration can cause a woman to go into early labor.

Considerations for older adults. Older adults are at higher risk for dehydration from diarrhea. Be sure that they receive adequate fluid replacement to prevent dehydration. Older adults (older than 60 years) should not use bismuth subsalicylate (Kaopectate) because they are more likely to experience side effects such as constipation.

Get Ready for the NCLEX® Examination!

Key Points

- Nausea and vomiting are distressing for patients and can cause significant clinical complications and extended hospital stays.
- There are many causes of nausea and vomiting involving several central and peripheral neurotransmitter pathways.
- Nausea and vomiting are GI defense mechanisms used to remove harmful substances from the body.
- When a patient has nausea and vomiting, be alert for electrolyte, fluid, and nutritional imbalances that must be corrected.
- Drugs for nausea and vomiting are prescribed to manage these symptoms, eliminate the causes, and correct electrolyte and nutritional imbalances.
- To prevent nausea and vomiting associated with a specific trigger such as cancer chemotherapy or motion, give antiemetics *before* the triggering events and during the time the person usually has these responses.
- Ask patients about a history of depression. Metoclopramide (Reglan) can cause mild-to-severe depression and should not be prescribed for patients with a history of depression.
- Prochlorperazine (Compazine) can cause a decrease in sweating, increasing the risk of overheating of the patient's body. Check body temperature every 4 to 8 hours while a patient is taking this drug.
- Before giving an antiemetic drug, always observe the abdomen for distention and listen for active bowel sounds.
- Always check a patient's respiratory status before and after giving drugs for nausea and vomiting because respiratory depression can be an adverse effect of some of these drugs.
- Neuroleptic malignant syndrome is a rare, life-threatening side effect of antiemetic drugs in which dangerously high body temperatures can occur. Be sure to monitor a patient's body temperature every 4 to 8 hours.
- Tardive dyskinesia is an adverse effect of the antiemetic drugs promethazine (Phenergan) and metoclopramide (Reglan). It occurs after a year or more of continuous use of these drugs. If it is not diagnosed early, it is not reversible.
- Teach patients taking antinausea drugs for motion sickness to take the drug 30 to 60 minutes before expected travel.
- A patient should not take CNS depressants while taking antiemetic drugs because they add to CNS-depressant effects, causing drowsiness and a decreased level of alertness.

- Normal bowel patterns vary widely from several times a day to several times a week.
- Constipation and diarrhea are symptoms, **not** diseases.
- The most common causes of constipation are poor diet and lack of exercise.
- Patients with severe constipation should be referred to a health care provider to rule out colon cancer.
- Most laxatives should not be taken for longer than 1 week, unless a patient is instructed to do so by the prescriber.
- Do not give constipation drugs if a patient has undiagnosed abdominal pain or acute abdomen because of the increased risk for bowel perforation.
- Always give drugs for constipation with 8 ounces of fluid.
- Teach older adults that increasing fluid intake often relieves constipation without the need for laxatives.
- Antidiarrheal drugs are **not** usually given when diarrhea is caused by bacteria or parasites because the drugs prevent the body from eliminating the organisms, which can cause the condition to worsen.
- A person with diarrhea is at high risk for dehydration because of fluid lost in the stool.
- After giving an antimotility drug for diarrhea such as loperamide (Imodium), be sure to check for signs of the life-threatening adverse effect toxic megacolon.
- Teach patients that antidiarrheal drugs should not be taken for more than 2 days unless instructed to do so by their prescriber.
- Bismuth subsalicylate (Pepto-Bismol) contains an aspirin-like drug. Watch for bleeding because this drug can also increase the effects of the anticoagulant warfarin (Coumadin).

Additional Learning Resources

⊕ Be sure to visit your Evolve website (http://evolve.elsevier.com/Workman/pharmacology/) for additional online resources.

SG Go to your Study Guide for additional learning activities to help you master this chapter content.

Review Questions

See *Answers to In-Text Review Questions* in the back of the book for answers to these questions.

1. When discussing normal bowel function with a patient, which statement is **most accurate** for the nurse use during this discussion?
   A. Bowel movements should occur once a day every day.
   B. Frequency of bowel movements is more important than their consistency.
   C. Bowel movements are very simple processes.
   D. Bowel movements should be soft and easily pass out of the bowel.

2. The nurse is teaching a patient about strategies to prevent constipation. Which point does the nurse make sure to include in the teaching plan?
   A. "You should drink plenty of fluids every day to prevent constipation."
   B. "Prevent the possibility of constipation by using a laxative on a daily basis."
   C. "Limiting physical activity can promote better bowel function."
   D. "Be sure to eat a diet that is low in fiber."

3. The nurse is instructing a patient about ways to help prevent the spread of diarrhea. Which point will the nurse include in the teaching plan?

   A. "When traveling internationally it is best to drink bottled water with ice cubes."
   B. "Be sure to wash your hands after using the bathroom or changing diapers."
   C. "Always wear clean gloves when handling raw meat or poultry."
   D. "Cut down on your fluid intake to decrease the number of diarrhea episodes."

4. A patient receiving chemotherapy who is prescribed ondansetron asks the nurse why the drug is given before meals. What is the nurse's **best** response?

   A. "Ondansetron is given 30 minutes before your meals to prevent nausea."
   B. "The purpose of this drug is to move food rapidly through your GI tract."
   C. "This drug works by preventing nausea caused by morphine given for your pain."
   D. "If this drug were given after your meals, you could become nauseated before it can exert its effects."

5. A patient prescribed metoclopramide tells the nurse that his abdomen is making gurgling sounds. What is the nurse's **best** action?

   A. Reassuring the patient that this is an expected effect of the drug
   B. Documenting this finding as the only action
   C. Holding the drug and notifying the prescriber
   D. Giving the drug and notifying the prescriber

6. The spouse of a patient who is prescribed promethazine as part of her antiemetic therapy with chemotherapy reports that after the last dose she did not remember the drive home. What is the nurse's **best** action?

   A. Thanking the spouse for reporting the problem, and documenting the adverse drug reaction
   B. Holding the dose of promethazine for this round of chemotherapy until the patient is seen by the prescriber
   C. Reassuring the patient and spouse that this is a normal response to the drug and reinforcing that the patient should not drive home
   D. Performing a mini-mental status exam and assessing the patient's pupillary reflexes before administering the promethazine

7. The nurse is administering a patient's first dose of cyclizine. What **safety** action does the nurse take for this patient?

   A. Instructing the patient to call for help when getting out of bed
   B. Raising all four side rails to the upright position
   C. Giving the patient a full glass of water with the medication
   D. Telling the patient to avoid eating for at least 2 hours

8. A patient reports taking an over-the-counter laxative for constipation daily for the past 3 weeks. What is the nurse's **best first** action?

   A. Reminding the patient about the importance of adequate fluid intake and exercise to prevent constipation
   B. Instructing the patient that these drugs should not be used for more than a week without consulting the prescriber

   C. Asking the patient about usual fluid intake and urinary and bowel habits, and having the patient describe the nature of stools
   D. Contacting the prescriber about an order for a stronger laxative because the one the patient is taking is not working

9. A patient reports taking psyllium with a full glass of water every morning to prevent constipation. What is the nurse's **best** action?

   A. Reminding the patient that over-the-counter laxatives should not be taken for more than 1 week
   B. Instructing the patient that long-term use of psyllium can cause health problems
   C. Holding the drug and notifying the prescriber immediately
   D. Documenting this information as the only action

10. Which patient laboratory value will the nurse monitor after giving a patient bisacodyl for constipation?

    A. Sodium
    B. Potassium
    C. Creatinine
    D. Blood urea nitrogen

11. A 79-year-old patient with nausea is prescribed scopolamine. Which nursing assessment determines whether he is experiencing a **serious** side effect?

    A. Checking capillary refill
    B. Measuring abdominal girth
    C. Evaluating handgrip strength
    D. Evaluating daily intake and output

12. A patient who is prescribed prochlorperazine for postoperative nausea and vomiting has all of the following changes. For which change will the nurse **immediately** contact the prescriber?

    A. Systolic blood pressure decrease of 12 mm Hg
    B. Increased sleepiness but arouses with light shaking
    C. Oral temperature increase of 2°F
    D. Urine color change from yellow to reddish-brown

13. Which teaching points does the nurse include when instructing a patient about how to take polyethylene glycol for constipation? **Select all that apply.**

    A. "Drink between 1500 and 2000 mL of fluids every day."
    B. "Avoid bulk foods such as whole grain bread and vegetables."
    C. "Use the bathroom right away when you feel the urge to have a bowel movement."
    D. "Try to get some regular exercise each day to prevent constipation."
    E. "Be sure to take the laxative when you have not eaten for at least 3 hours."
    F. "Notify your prescriber if your constipation is not relieved within a week."

14. A patient has been taking attapulgite for diarrhea over the past 4 days. What is the nurse's **best** action?

    A. Sending a stool specimen to the lab for analysis.
    B. Instructing the patient to notify nursing staff for all episodes of diarrhea and saving the stool for assessment.
    C. Checking the patient's blood pressure and heart rate.
    D. Teaching the patient that antidiarrheal drugs should not be taken for more than 2 days unless instructed to by their prescriber.

Clinical Judgment

1. Which topics does the nurse include when teaching a group of patients about antiemetic drugs? **Select all that apply.**

   A. "Get up slowly because of dizziness and hypotensive effects."
   B. "If you miss a dose, take a second dose when your next dose is due."
   C. "Because of sun sensitivity use sunscreen, and wear protective clothing."
   D. "The best way to manage nausea is to take the drug every morning before breakfast."
   E. "Drink plenty of fluids to prevent constipation."
   F. "To manage dry mouth, use frequent mouth rinses and oral care."
   G. "Consult with your prescriber before taking over-the-counter (OTC) drugs."
   H. "To prevent dental problems related to dry mouth, see your dentist every 2 months."
   I. "If you experience headache, take a mild analgesic such as acetaminophen but avoid aspirin."
   J. "If you have difficulty with sleeping, ask your prescriber about a sleeping pill."

2. An 84-year-old patient was admitted to the hospital with severe diarrhea over the past week which resulted in dehydration. The patient is prescribed loperamide 2 mg orally after each unformed stool. An IV is started, and intravenous fluids of normal saline are ordered to run at 100 mL per hour. **Use an X to indicate which actions are Most Relevant, Less Relevant, or Not Relevant at this time for this patient.**

INSTRUCTION	MOST RELEVANT	LESS RELEVANT	NOT RELEVANT
Weighing the patient every morning			
Inserting a urinary catheter for accurate intake and output			
Giving each loperamide dose with a meal of snack			
Listening for active bowel sounds every shift			
Checking the patient's skin turgor for tenting on the back of the hand			
Preparing a full glass of water to give with each dose of loperamide			
Placing call light within easy patient reach			
Assisting the patient up to the bathroom			
Sending a stool sample for bacteria and parasites			
Monitoring for changes in skin and mucous membranes			
Checking for signs of constipation			

Learning Objectives

The content presented in this chapter should help you to:

1. Discuss how different classes of drugs are used to treat peptic ulcer disease (PUD), gastroesophageal reflux disease (GERD), and inflammatory bowel diseases (IBD) (e.g., Crohn disease, ulcerative colitis).
2. Describe the common names, actions, usual adult dosages, possible side effects, and adverse effects of drugs for PUD, GERD, and IBD.

3. Discuss the priority actions to take before and after giving drugs for PUD, GERD, and IBD.
4. Prioritize essential information to teach patients taking drugs for PUD, GERD, and IBD.
5. Discuss life span considerations for drugs for PUD, GERD, and IBD.

Key Terms

aminosalicylates (ə-ME-nō-sə-lis-ə-lātz) (p. 364) A group of drugs that can help to control the symptoms of some inflammatory bowel diseases, such as ulcerative colitis and Crohn disease.

antacids (ănt-ĂS-ĭdz) (p. 363) Drugs that neutralize the acids produced by the stomach.

biologics (bīō LÄ jikz) (p. 364) A class of complex anti-inflammatory drugs derived from living sources that target specific inflammatory cells, components, or products to modify chronic disorders associated with inflammation and tissue damage (see Chapter 11).

corticosteroids (kŏr-tĭ-kō-STĚR-ōydz) (p. 364) Drugs similar to natural cortisol that prevent or limit inflammation by slowing or stopping inflammatory mediator production (see Chapter 10).

cytoprotective drugs (sī-tō-prō-TĚK-tĭv DRŬGZ) (p. 363) Drugs that decrease the acid content of the stomach by coating the stomach mucosa and reducing the risk of developing ulcers.

histamine H₂ blockers (HĬS-tă-mēn BLŎ-kŭrz) (p. 363) Drugs that treat the gastric effects of histamine in cases of peptic ulcers, gastritis, and GERD by blocking the effects of histamine on the receptor site known as H2.

immunomodulators (ĬM-ū-nō-MOD-u-lā-tərz) (p. 364) Drugs that affect the functioning of the immune system.

proton pump inhibitor (PPI) (PRŌ-tŏn PŬMP ĭn-HĬB-ĭ-tŭr) (p. 363) A drug that blocks acid secretion in the stomach.

REVIEW OF RELATED PHYSIOLOGY AND PATHOPHYSIOLOGY

The upper GI system is responsible for taking in and moving food into the stomach. Digestion begins in the mouth, where chewing changes the food to a fine texture; saliva moistens it and begins the conversion of starch into simple sugars. The food is then swallowed, passing through the pharynx and down the esophagus to the stomach (Animation 20.1). Specialized cells in the stomach (*gastric* *glands*) secrete digestive enzymes and gastric juices, which act on the partially digested food. The stomach also physically churns and mixes the food. Stomach secretions include the enzyme pepsin, which acts on proteins; hydrochloric acid, needed for the action of pepsin; and the enzyme, gastric lipase, which begins the breakdown of fats. These acid substances that digest food also have the potential to damage or break down normal GI tissues.

The stomach secretes thick gel-like mucus to coat and protect it from contact with stomach acids. In most people, acid production is balanced by mucus secretion, and ulcers do not form. Whenever acid production exceeds mucus production, the risk for ulcers and tissue damage increases. Health problems, genetic and lifestyle influences, and certain drugs can decrease mucus production or increase acid secretion and upset the protective balance. The intestinal tract, unlike the stomach, does not secrete large amounts of the protective mucus. Instead, it relies on buffers such as bicarbonate from the pancreas to neutralize stomach acids before they reach the intestines.

The small intestine is made up of three segments, the duodenum, jejunum, and ileum (Animation 20.2). It breaks down food using enzymes and bile. The small intestine does most of the work of digestion and is where most nutrients are absorbed. Peristalsis moves food through, mixing with the digestive secretions from the pancreas and bile. The duodenum is largely responsible for the continuing breakdown process, with the jejunum and ileum mainly responsible for the absorption of nutrients into the bloodstream.

The large intestine (colon) is a 5- to 7-foot-long muscular tube (Animation 20.3). It is responsible for processing waste. Stool is waste left over from the digestive process which passes through the colon by means of peristalsis, transitioning from a liquid state to a solid form. As stool passes through the colon, any remaining water is absorbed. The stool itself is mostly food debris and bacteria. When the descending colon becomes full of stool, it is emptied into the rectum for elimination. The rectum, an 8-inch chamber that connects the colon to the anus, receives stool from the colon and holds it until elimination occurs. The last part of the digestive tract is the anus, which consists of the pelvic floor muscles and two other muscles called anal sphincters (internal and external), which relax for the elimination of waste products.

Gastroesophageal reflux disease (GERD) and *peptic ulcer disease* (PUD) affect the upper gastrointestinal (GI) system (mouth, esophagus, stomach, and upper part of the small intestine [duodenum]). GERD occurs when stomach contents leak backward into the esophagus. PUD may occur in the esophagus, stomach, or upper part of the duodenum. *Inflammatory bowel disease* (IBD) affects the lower GI system (small intestine, colon, and rectum).

GASTROINTESTINAL ULCERS

GI ulcers are fairly common. About 10% of people in the United States develop an ulcer during their lifetime. A GI ulcer is an open sore found in the mucosal lining of the stomach or duodenum where hydrochloric acid and pepsin are located. These ulcers are also commonly referred to as *peptic ulcer disease (PUD)*. When a peptic ulcer occurs in the stomach, it is called a *gastric ulcer*, and when an ulcer is formed in the duodenum, it is called a *duodenal ulcer* (Figure 20.1).

An *esophageal ulcer* is a hole in the lining of the esophagus that has been damaged by the acidic digestive juices secreted by the stomach cells. Esophageal ulcers usually

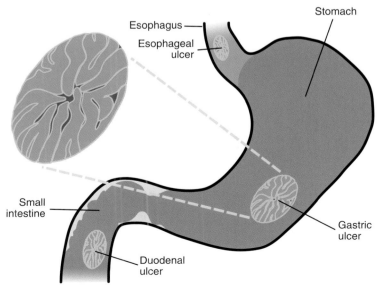

FIG. 20.1 Locations of gastric, duodenal, and esophageal ulcers.

Box 20.1	Factors in the Development of Peptic Ulcers

- Acid and pepsin
- Alcohol
- Caffeine
- *Helicobacter pylori* bacterial infection

- Nonsteroidal antiinflammatory drugs
- Smoking
- Stress

occur in the lower part of the esophagus near the stomach. This type of ulcer is often associated with chronic GERD when acidic stomach contents back up (reflux) into the esophagus.

In the past, the causes of peptic ulcers were believed to be excess acids and lifestyle factors such as stress and too many spicy foods. However, research has shown that 80% to 90% of gastric ulcers are caused by infection with the *Helicobacter pylori (H. pylori)* bacteria. *H. pylori* infection is present in 20% to 30% of people in the United States. Some people experience no signs or symptoms, whereas others develop ulcers. Today it is believed that lifestyle (e.g., stress and diet), along with excess acids and *H. pylori* infection, have roles in the development of ulcers; but *H. pylori* is the primary cause. Box 20.1 summarizes the factors that are suspected to have a role in the development of peptic ulcers.

Gastric mucosa resists damage, but when there is an increase in gastric acidity or a decrease in prostaglandins, which increase the production of bicarbonate and also produce the protective mucus, there is a danger of developing an ulcer (Figure 20.2). The mucosa breaks down, and an open sore or raw area develops in the stomach or upper part of the intestine (duodenum).

The most common symptom of a peptic ulcer is burning, gnawing pain caused by stomach acid coming into contact with the open wound (ulcer). The pain usually occurs somewhere between the navel (*umbilicus*) and the breastbone (*sternum*) and may last from a few minutes to many hours. It often occurs when the stomach is empty and can be relieved by eating foods that buffer stomach acids or taking a drug that reduces stomach acid such as an antacid. The pain may flare up at night or come and go for a few days to several weeks. Other symptoms of a gastric ulcer include vomiting blood (bright red or black), dark blood in the stool, nausea or vomiting, belching, unexplained weight loss, and chest pain.

Antibiotics are a very important part of the treatment plan for PUD. They are used to treat *H. pylori* in the GI tract, the major cause of GI ulcers. Commonly prescribed antibiotics include drugs such as clarithromycin (Biaxin), metronidazole (Flagyl), tetracycline (Sumycin), and amoxicillin (Amoxil). Treatment of ulcers involves not only drugs but also lifestyle changes. Recommended lifestyle changes include

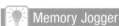

Memory Jogger

The primary cause of 80%–90% of GI ulcers is infection with the *H. pylori* bacteria.

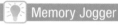

Memory Jogger

The most common symptom of a peptic ulcer is burning, gnawing pain that occurs between the umbilicus and sternum.

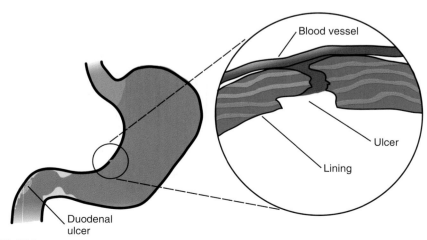

FIG. 20.2 Gastric ulcer pathophysiology: The mucosa breaks down and an open sore develops.

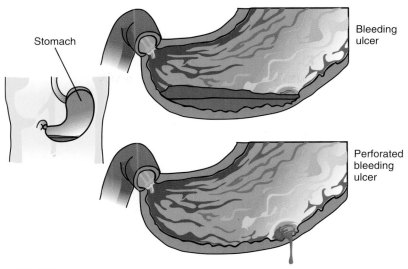

FIG. 20.3 A peptic ulcer may lead to bleeding, perforation, or other emergencies.

Box **20.2**	Signs That Indicate an Ulcer Is Getting Worse

- Blood in stools
- Continuing nausea or repeated vomiting
- Feeling cold or clammy
- Feeling weak or dizzy
- Losing weight
- Pain that doesn't go away after taking drugs
- Pain that radiates to the back
- Sudden severe pain
- Vomiting blood
- Vomiting food eaten hours or days ago

avoiding irritating foods, caffeine, and excessive alcohol. Smoking cessation is highly recommended because smoking slows ulcer healing and is related to the return of ulcers. Smoking increases acid secretion; reduces prostaglandin, mucus, and bicarbonate production; and decreases mucosal blood flow. Patients with a gastric ulcer are instructed to avoid excess stress and nonsteroidal antiinflammatory drugs (NSAIDs). NSAIDs are associated with the development of gastric upset and ulcers because they inhibit prostaglandins. As many as 15% of patients on long-term NSAID treatment may develop ulcers of the stomach or duodenum.

Although most ulcers heal within a few weeks with drug treatment, some serious complications may occur. When an ulcer damages GI tissues, blood vessels may also be damaged, resulting in a bleeding ulcer (Figure 20.3). Sometimes an ulcer causes a hole in the wall of the stomach or duodenum, allowing partially digested food and bacteria to enter the sterile abdominal cavity (*peritoneum*) and causing an inflammation and infection of the abdominal cavity (*peritonitis*). Signs that tell you an ulcer is getting worse are listed in Box 20.2.

GASTROESOPHAGEAL REFLUX DISEASE

Most people suffer from occasional heartburn, but when heartburn occurs daily, exposure of the mucosa of the esophagus to stomach acids can cause irritation and inflammation. *Gastroesophageal reflux disease* (GERD) is a condition in which the liquid contents of the stomach back up (*regurgitate* or *reflux*) into the esophagus. At the lower end of the esophagus where it connects to the stomach is a strong muscle ring called the *lower esophageal sphincter* (LES). The LES stays tightly shut except when food or liquids pass into the stomach. When closed it prevents stomach contents from backing up into the esophagus. Reflux or *regurgitation* happens when the LES

 Did You Know?

No special diet is recommended for the prevention or treatment of ulcers. A bland diet has not been shown to be effective.

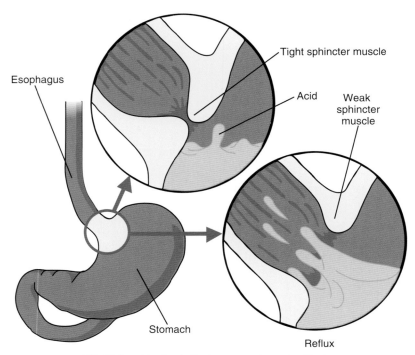

FIG. 20.4 Acid reflux in the lower esophageal sphincter.

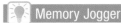

Memory Jogger

The cause of GERD is an LES that is not working correctly and allows acidic stomach contents to back up (reflux) and damage the esophagus.

Memory Jogger

The most common symptom of GERD is dyspepsia (heartburn).

is not working correctly (Figure 20.4). The LES may relax during periods of the day or night, or it may become too weak and constantly allow stomach contents to flow upward into the esophagus. When the LES is very weak and GERD is severe, a patient may need surgery to strengthen the LES.

Most people experience reflux occasionally; a person with GERD has reflux more often, and the stomach contents stay in the esophagus for longer periods of time. The regurgitated stomach contents contain stomach acids and pepsin and may also contain bile. These substances can injure the esophagus, causing inflammation and tissue damage, including ulcers. Risk factors for developing GERD are listed in Box 20.3.

The most common symptom of GERD is *dyspepsia* (heartburn). Other common symptoms include sour or bitter taste; bitter stomach fluid going into the mouth, especially during sleep; hoarseness; *water brash* (regurgitation of watery acid from the stomach); a repeated need to clear the throat; difficulty swallowing food or liquid; wheezing or coughing at night; and worsening of symptoms after eating or when bending over or lying down.

GERD is a chronic condition and treatment is lifelong. Treatment of GERD is divided into five stages (Box 20.4) and involves not only drugs but also lifestyle changes (Table 20.1) such as smoking cessation (because nicotine weakens the LES),

---

Box 20.3 **Risk Factors for Gastroesophageal Reflux Disease**

- Being overweight
- Being pregnant
- Certain diseases (e.g., diabetes, asthma, peptic ulcers)
- Certain drugs (e.g., nonsteroidal antiinflammatory drugs)
- Drinking alcohol and caffeinated beverages
- Eating foods with high acid content (e.g., tomatoes, orange juice)
- Eating fatty and spicy foods
- Lying down too soon after meals
- Smoking

Box 20.4   Stages of Treatment for Gastroesophageal Reflux Disease

Stage I: Lifestyle modifications
Stage II: As-needed drug therapy
- Antacid and/or antacid-containing alginic acid
- Over-the-counter histamine H_2 blocker

Stage III: Scheduled pharmacologic therapy
- Histamine H_2 blocker for 8–12 weeks
- For persistent symptoms: high-dose H_2 blocker or proton pump inhibitor for additional 8–12 weeks
- Proton pump inhibitors as first choice for documented erosive esophagitis

Stage IV: Maintenance therapy
- For patients with symptoms of relapse or complicated disease
- Lowest effective dosage of histamine H_2 blocker or proton pump inhibitor

Stage V: Surgery
- For patients with severe symptoms, erosive esophagitis, or disease complications
- Fundoplication procedure to strengthen lower esophageal sphincter

Table 20.1   Lifestyle Changes for Treatment of Gastroesophageal Reflux Disease

LIFESTYLE CHANGE	RATIONALE
Avoid eating within 3 hours of bedtime	Decreases risk of nighttime reflux
Stop smoking	Nicotine weakens the LES
Avoid alcohol (especially red wine), caffeine, chocolate, citrus fruits and juices, fatty foods, milk, peppermint, pepper seasoning, spearmint, and tomato products	These foods cause increased reflux
Decrease portions at mealtimes	Decreases reflux
Avoid tight-fitting clothes and bending after meals	Decreases reflux
Elevate the head of the bed or mattress 6–10 inches	Helps keep acid in stomach by gravity while sleeping
Lose weight if overweight	Relieves pressure on the stomach and LES

LES, Lower esophageal sphincter.

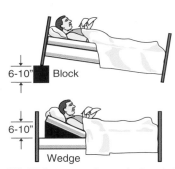

FIG. 20.5 How to elevate the head of the bed.

decreased dietary fat intake, weight reduction, and avoidance of large meals as well as foods that cause regurgitation. A patient with GERD is instructed to elevate the head of the bed at least 6 to 10 inches using blocks under the top bed legs or a pillow wedge (Figure 20.5). After meals, the patient with GERD should remain upright for 3 hours. Patients should also avoid foods that cause increased reflux such as chocolate, peppermint, alcohol, and caffeinated drinks.

Chewing gum after meals may be a useful treatment for GERD because it increases the production of saliva, which contains bicarbonate, and increases the rate of swallowing. The bicarbonate in saliva neutralizes acid in the esophagus and decreases the irritation of refluxed stomach contents.

Complications of GERD occur when the disease is severe or long-lasting. The constant irritation of the esophagus by stomach contents can lead to inflammation, ulcers, and bleeding. Bleeding can cause anemia. Over time, scarring of the esophagus can cause it to narrow, making swallowing difficult. Narrowing of the esophagus is called an *esophageal stricture*. Chronic GERD can cause changes in the cells of the esophagus, leading to precancerous cells and cancer. This condition is called *Barrett esophagus* and occurs in about 10% to 20% of patients with GERD. Barrett esophagus increases the risk of developing esophageal cancer.

⭐ Critical Point for Safety

Patients with GERD should avoid chocolate, peppermint, alcohol, nicotine, and caffeinated drinks because they lower the pressure of the LES and promote reflux.

QSEN: Safety

Did You Know?

Chewing gum after meals may prevent irritation of the esophagus associated with GERD.

INFLAMMATORY BOWEL DISEASES

Inflammatory bowel diseases (IBD) include Crohn disease (CD) and ulcerative colitis (UC). They are disorders that involve chronic inflammation of the gastrointestinal (GI) tract. According to the Centers for Disease Control and Prevention (CDC), there are around 3 million people in the United States with IBD. Crohn disease can affect any part of the GI tract but most commonly occurs in the final section of the small intestine and the colon. Ulcerative colitis causes inflammation in the large intestine (colon) (Figure 20.6). Table 20.2 provides a comparison of CD and UC.

Although the exact cause of IBD is unknown, it is a result of a defective immune system. The immune system incorrectly responds to environmental triggers causing inflammation of the GI tract. IBD likely has a genetic component so anyone with a family history of CD or UC is more likely to develop the condition. Common symptoms of IBD include persistent diarrhea, abdominal pain, rectal bleeding, bloody stools, weight loss, and fatigue.

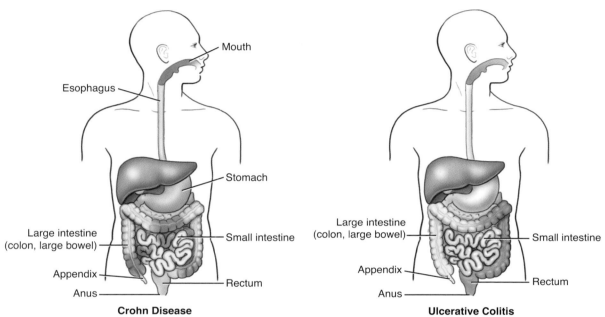

FIG. 20.6 Comparison of locations of Crohn disease and ulcerative colitis. (From Sorrentino, S.A., & Remmert, L. N. [2021]. *Mosby's textbook for nursing assistants* [10th ed.]. St. Louis: Elsevier.)

Table 20.2	Comparison between Crohn Disease and Ulcerative Colitis
CROHN DISEASE	**ULCERATIVE COLITIS**
Can affect any part of the gastrointestinal (GI) tract; most often occurs in the terminal portion of the small intestine and large intestine (colon)	Occurs in the large intestine (colon) and the rectum
Damaged areas appear in patches that are next to healthy tissue	Damaged areas are continuous (not patchy); usually starting at the rectum and spreading into the colon
Inflammation can reach through multiple layers of the walls of the GI tract	Inflammation is present only in the innermost layer of the colon
5–6 soft loose stools per day not bloody	10–20 liquid, bloody stools per day
Complications include fistulas and nutritional deficiencies	Complications include hemorrhage and nutritional deficiencies
Diagnosed by endoscopy	Diagnosed by colonoscopy

GENERAL ISSUES FOR DRUGS FOR PUD, GERD, AND IBD

There are several classes of drugs used to treat PUD, GERD, and IBD that have both different and common actions and effects. Responsibilities for these common actions and effects are listed in the following paragraphs. Specific responsibilities are listed with the discussion of each individual class of drugs.

⊛ PRIORITY ACTIONS TO TAKE *BEFORE* GIVING DRUGS FOR PUD, GERD, OR IBD

Be sure to obtain a complete list of drugs currently being used by the patient, including over-the-counter and herbal drugs. Not only can some drugs increase the risk for PUD or GERD, but the drugs used to treat these problems may interfere with the absorption of other drugs.

Obtain a baseline set of vital signs, including body temperature, and obtain a baseline weight. Ask patients about weight loss and fatigue, normal bowel habits, the appearance of stools, bleeding, vomiting, and reflux (location, duration, character, and factors that cause it to occur).

Listen to the abdomen with your stethoscope for bowel sounds, check for distention, and ask about abdominal pain. Instruct the patient to report any episodes of heartburn or reflux, as well as abdominal discomfort or bloody stools.

⊛ PRIORITY ACTIONS TO TAKE *AFTER* GIVING DRUGS FOR PUD, GERD, OR IBD

Be sure to recheck vital signs at least every 8 hours and weigh patients every morning. Also assess for abnormal heart rhythms (too fast, too slow, or irregular). Keep track of bowel movement frequency, consistency, and appearance. Recheck the abdomen for active bowel sounds and distention every shift. Remind the patient about the potential for altered bowel functions, including constipation and diarrhea. Ask patients about bowel movements every day. Record any episodes of reflux, heartburn, indigestion, abdominal discomfort, diarrhea, or bloody stools. Report abnormalities to the prescriber.

⊛ TEACHING PRIORITIES FOR PATIENTS TAKING DRUGS FOR PUD, GERD, OR IBD

- Take the drug exactly as prescribed for the period of time prescribed, even when you are feeling better.
- Take a missed dose as soon as possible but **never** take a double dose.
- Notify your prescriber for difficulty swallowing; persistent abdominal pain; vomiting blood (bright red or coffee grounds–appearing emesis); or black, tarry stools.
- Weigh yourself every morning at the same time, and report continued weight loss to your prescriber.
- Increasing your intake of fluid and fiber-containing foods, as well as exercising can help prevent constipation.
- Avoid alcohol, aspirin-containing products, NSAIDs, and foods that cause increased GI irritation because all of these substances increase the risk for ulcer development.

 Critical Point for Safety

Teach patients with PUD or GERD to avoid substances that cause increased GI irritation, such as alcohol, NSAIDs, and aspirin.

QSEN: Safety

TYPES OF DRUGS FOR PUD AND GERD

Antiulcer drugs are used to treat ulcers of the stomach and duodenum. **Histamine H_2 blockers** decrease the secretion of gastric acid, and **proton pump inhibitors (PPIs)** block the secretion of gastric acid. **Cytoprotective drugs** such as sucralfate (Carafate) are used to form a thick coating that covers an ulcer to protect the open sore from further damage and allows healing to occur. Antibiotics are used to treat *H. pylori* infections that are the major cause of ulcers.

Several groups of drugs are used to treat GERD. Drugs used to treat PUD such as histamine H_2 blockers and PPIs are also used to treat GERD. **Antacids** can neutralize stomach acid and decrease the ability of acid to irritate and inflame the esophagus. Metoclopramide (Reglan), a *promotility drug*, increases LES tone and helps to empty the stomach. *Antibiotics* are used to treat *H. pylori* infections, which cause GI ulcers.

Drugs used to treat IBD include aminosalicylates, corticosteroids, immunomodulators, and biologics. **Aminosalicylates** are compounds that contain 5-aminosalicylic acid (5-ASA) and reduce inflammation in the lining of the intestine. **Corticosteroids** lower the activity of the immune system and limit the inflammation in the digestive tract. They are used as short-term treatments for Crohn disease and for ulcerative colitis flares (worsening of the disease) because they reduce inflammation quickly, sometimes within a few days to a few months. The first two **immunomodulators** to be used widely for IBD were azathioprine (Imuran) and 6-mercaptopurine (6- MP, Purinethol), drugs that are chemically very similar. The purpose of these drugs is to maintain remission of Crohn disease and ulcerative colitis. **Biologics** are treatments for people with moderate to severe Crohn disease or ulcerative colitis. They are often prescribed as an option when other drugs such as immunosuppressants (e.g., azathioprine, mercaptopurine, methotrexate) or steroids have not been effective, or side effects have been hard to manage.

HISTAMINE H_2 BLOCKERS

How Histamine H_2 Blockers Work

Histamine H_2 blockers (antagonists) cause decreased stimulation of H_2 receptors in gastric cells that secrete hydrochloric acid *(parietal cells)*, leading to a decrease in gastric acid secretion. When histamine binds to receptors in the stomach lining, acid pumps are activated, releasing acid into the stomach. H_2 blockers prevent histamine from stimulating the pumps in the stomach that produce hydrochloric acid.

Histamine H_2 blockers are used to heal ulcers or relieve the symptoms and pain that occur with GERD. These drugs are available over-the-counter and by prescription. Over-the-counter H_2 blockers are lower dose and are useful for the prevention and relief of mild heartburn, indigestion, or sour stomach. Prescription-strength H_2 blockers come in higher doses and are used for moderate-to-severe forms of GERD.

Common names and doses of drugs for histamine H_2 blockers are listed in the following table. Due to possible cancer risk, all forms of ranitidine were recalled by the US Food and Drug Administration (FDA) in 2020, including over-the-counter Zantac. Ranitidine (Zantac) was found to contain N-nitrosodimethylamine, or NDMA, a known human carcinogen (cancer-causing substance). Nizatidine (Axid) has also been discontinued in the United States because of NDMA. Two versions of a new Zantac drug without ranitidine were made available over-the-counter for the US market in June 2021. These products include famotidine 10 mg as an original strength version and famotidine 20 mg as a maximum strength version. Be sure to consult a reliable drug resource for information on specific histamine H2 blockers.

Adult Dosages for Commonly Prescribed Histamine H_2 Blockers

Drug Category	Drug Name	Usual Maintenance Dose
Histamine H_2 Blockers	cimetidine (Tagamet)	800 mg orally twice daily or 400 mg orally four times per day for 12 weeks IV/IM: 300 mg every 6 hr for PUD *Special Considerations:* **Over-the-counter, 200 mg orally 30 min before food or beverages that are known to cause symptoms**
	famotidine (Pepcid)	20 mg orally twice daily for up to 6 weeks for GERD 20 mg orally once daily at bedtime for PUD IV: 20 mg every 6 hr when oral therapy is not feasible *Special Considerations:* **10 mg orally; take 15 min to 1 hr prior to eating a meal that is expected to cause symptoms**

Adult Dosages for Commonly Prescribed Histamine H₂ Blockers—cont'd

Drug Category	Drug Name	Usual Maintenance Dose
	ranitidine (Zantac)	OTC: 75–150 mg orally once or twice daily *Special Considerations:* **For prophylaxis, take before eating. Should not be taken for more than 2 weeks without consulting a health care provider**

GERD, Gastroesophageal reflux disease; *IM*, intramuscular; *IV*, intravenous; *PUD*, peptic ulcer disease.

Intended Responses of Histamine H₂ Blockers
- Secretion of gastric acid is decreased.
- Symptoms of GERD are decreased.
- Ulcers are healed and prevented.

Common Side Effects of Histamine H₂ Blockers
Side effects of these drugs are uncommon. However, the most common side effect of histamine H₂ blockers is confusion. Other common side effects include dizziness, drowsiness, headaches, altered sense of taste, constipation, diarrhea, nausea, impotence and decreased sperm count, anemia, neutropenia (decreased number of neutrophil white blood cells), and thrombocytopenia (low platelet count).

Possible Adverse Effects of Histamine H₂ Blockers
Adverse life-threatening effects of H₂ blockers include abnormal heart rhythms (dysrhythmias), seizures, decreased white blood cell count (*agranulocytosis*), and anemia caused by deficient red blood cell production by the bone marrow (*aplastic anemia*).

⭐ Priority Actions to Take *Before* Giving Histamine H₂ Blockers
In addition to the general responsibilities related to drugs for PUD and GERD (p. 363), check the patient's baseline level of consciousness because drowsiness and confusion are common side effects of these drugs. Use this information to determine patient responses to the drug. Also assess for current discomfort level with signs and symptoms, and ask about foods that may precipitate discomfort.

If prescribed more than once a day, give the drug with meals to prolong its therapeutic effects. If the patient is prescribed to take a histamine H₂ blocker once a day, give it at bedtime to prolong its effects when there is no food in the stomach, and reflux may be worse.

If the patient is to receive an intravenous (IV) drug, be sure to check the IV site at least every 2 to 4 hours for patency and signs of infection.

⭐ Priority Actions to Take *After* Giving Histamine H₂ Blockers
In addition to the general responsibilities related to drugs for PUD and GERD (p. 363), for inpatients, ensure that the call light is within easy reach and remind patients to call for help when getting out of bed because these drugs may cause dizziness or drowsiness. Ask patients about improvement and relief from PUD or GERD symptoms.

Watch for other side effects, including nausea or vomiting. Notify the prescriber for any signs of an allergic reaction (e.g., fever, sore throat, rashes); confusion; black, tarry stools; dizziness; or drowsiness.

⭐ Teaching Priorities for Patients Taking Histamine H₂ Blockers
In addition to the general precautions related to drugs for PUD and GERD (p. 363), include these teaching points and precautions:
- If you have been taking over-the-counter histamine H₂ blockers for more than 2 weeks see your prescriber if symptoms have not improved, because these drugs are to be used only for short-term treatment of GERD and ulcers. Also, signs and symptoms of GERD and PUD are similar to those of stomach cancer, which must be ruled out.

 Critical Point for Safety

Watch for confusion, the most common side effect, when giving histamine H₂ blockers, and report changes to the prescriber.

QSEN: Safety

Common Side Effects
Histamine H₂ Blockers

Confusion

Dizziness

Drowsiness

Headache

Taste changes

Nausea/ Vomiting, Diarrhea, Constipation

⭐ **Critical Point for Safety**

Teach patients to notify their prescriber if they have been taking over-the-counter H₂ blockers for more than 2 weeks and are still experiencing reflux.

QSEN: Safety

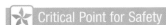

- Avoid smoking because it interferes with the action of histamine H_2 blockers. Discuss smoking cessation with your provider.
- Because these drugs may cause dizziness or drowsiness, avoid driving, operating dangerous machines, or engaging in any other activities that require alertness until you know how the drug affects you.
- Avoid irritating foods, alcohol, and aspirin because they are irritating to your GI system.
- Take the prescribed drug exactly as directed by your prescriber. Do **not** take a double dose.
- Report bruising, fatigue, diarrhea, black or tarry stools, sore throat, or rash to your prescriber because they may indicate worsening of the illness or an allergic reaction to the drug.

Life Span Considerations for Histamine H_2 Blockers

Considerations for pregnancy and lactation. Histamine H_2 blockers have a low likelihood of increasing the risk for birth defects or fetal harm. However, they have not been studied in pregnant women. A woman should always tell her health care provider if she is pregnant or planning to become pregnant. Pregnant women frequently experience heartburn. They should not take any drugs without consulting their health care provider. Instead, they should try nonpharmacologic and lifestyle changes. These drugs pass into breast milk and may cause undesired side effects in the breastfeeding infant. They should be avoided while breastfeeding.

Considerations for older adults. Older adults are more likely to experience confusion and dizziness because of increased sensitivity to the side effects of histamine H_2 blockers compared with younger adults. Teach family members to watch for changes in cognition or increased confusion. Teach older adults to take special precautions to avoid falls. Instruct them to change positions slowly and to use handrails when going up or down stairs. Suggest that older adults avoid driving or using heavy machinery until they know how the drug affects them.

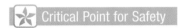

PROTON PUMP INHIBITORS

How Proton Pump Inhibitors Work

Normally, the stomach produces acid to help break down food in the process of digestion. When the acid irritates the mucosal lining of the stomach or duodenum, ulceration or bleeding can occur. **Proton pump inhibitors** (PPIs) work by completely blocking the production of stomach acid. These drugs block the action of "pumps" located in acid-secreting cells, which totally blocks stomach acid secretion.

PPIs are the most prescribed and powerful drugs used for treating PUD or GERD and should be used for only limited periods of time. They are used when H_2 blockers are not effective. Often PPIs are used in combination with antibiotics to treat *H. pylori* infections in the stomach.

Some are available over the counter; others require a prescription. Common names and doses of drugs for PPIs are listed in the following table. Be sure to consult a reliable drug resource for information on specific PPIs.

Adult Dosages for Commonly Prescribed Proton Pump Inhibitors

Drug Category	Drug Name	Usual Maintenance Dose
Proton Pump Inhibitors	dexlansoprazole (Dexilant, Kapidex)	30–60 mg orally once daily for 4 weeks
	esomeprazole magnesium (Nexium)	20 mg orally once daily every morning given 1 hr before the first meal of the day for 4 weeks ***Special Considerations:*** **If symptoms persist, may be given for an additional 4 weeks**

Adult Dosages for Commonly Prescribed Proton Pump Inhibitors—cont'd

Drug Category	Drug Name	Usual Maintenance Dose
	lansoprazole (Prevacid)	15 mg orally once daily for up to 14 days ***Special Considerations:* Full relief may take 1–4 days**
	omeprazole (Prilosec, Zegerid)	20 mg orally once daily with a full glass of water 30 min before breakfast for 14 days ***Special Considerations:* Full relief may take 1–4 days**
	pantoprazole (Protonix)	20–40 mg orally once daily for up to 14 days. IV: 40 mg once daily for 7–10 days ***Special Considerations:* Full relief may take 1–4 days**
	rabeprazole (Aciphex)	20 mg orally once daily for up to 14 days ***Special Considerations:* Full relief may take 1–4 days**

IV, Intravenous.

Intended Responses of Proton Pump Inhibitors
- Gastric acid secretion is decreased.
- Acid reflux is decreased.
- Ulcers are healed.

Common Side Effects of Proton Pump Inhibitors
Side effects rarely occur with PPIs. The most common side effects are diarrhea, constipation, belching and gas, abdominal pain, and headaches. Some patients report generally feeling ill while taking these drugs.

Lansoprazole (Prevacid), omeprazole (Prilosec), and rabeprazole (Aciphex) also may cause dizziness. In addition, rabeprazole may cause increased sun sensitivity (photosensitivity).

Long-term use of PPIs may lead to stomach infections because these drugs inhibit the production of stomach acids that help to kill bacteria. This may also lead to anemia because the loss of stomach acid reduces the digestion of protein essential for making new cells.

Possible Adverse Effects of Proton Pump Inhibitors
Allergic reactions are rare and include itching, dizziness, swollen ankles, muscle and joint pain, blurred vision, depression, and dry mouth. Some PPIs may cause serious skin reactions such as Stevens-Johnson syndrome or toxic epidermal necrolysis. Angioedema may also occur.

⊛ Priority Actions to Take *Before* Giving Proton Pump Inhibitors
In addition to the general responsibilities related to drugs for PUD and GERD (p. 363), give these drugs before meals, preferably in the morning. PPIs can be given with antacids.

Assess patients for bowel sounds and abdominal pain. Ask patients about any liver problems and check the result of any laboratory liver function tests.

If the patient is to be given an IV drug, be sure to check the IV site for patency and signs of infection or infiltration.

⊛ Priority Actions to Take *After* Giving Proton Pump Inhibitors
In addition to the general responsibilities related to drugs for PUD and GERD (p. 363), report any black, tarry stools to the prescriber immediately. These are indicators of upper GI bleeding, which can lead to severe hemorrhage.

 Do Not Confuse

rabeprazole *with* **aripiprazole**

An order for rabeprazole may be confused with aripiprazole. Rabeprazole is a PPI used to block gastric secretions, whereas aripiprazole is an antipsychotic drug used for schizophrenia and acute bipolar episodes.

QSEN: Safety

 Do Not Confuse

Prilosec *with* **Prinivil**

An order for Prilosec may be confused with Prinivil. Prilosec is a PPI used to block stomach acid secretion, whereas Prinivil is an angiotensin-converting enzyme inhibitor used to treat high blood pressure.

QSEN: Safety

Common Side Effects
Proton Pump Inhibitors

Diarrhea, Constipation, Gas, Abdominal pain   Headache

 Drug Alert

Administration Alert

For best effects, PPIs should be given before meals, preferably in the morning, because they suppress acid better when taken before a meal.

QSEN: Safety

 Critical Point for Safety

Black, tarry stools are never normal; they indicate bleeding and should be reported to the prescriber immediately.

QSEN: Safety

If lansoprazole, rabeprazole, or omeprazole is prescribed, teach the patient to call for help when getting out of bed because these drugs may cause dizziness. Be sure that the call light is within easy reach.

Ask patients about the relief of symptoms. Reassess for bowel sounds and abdominal distention.

★ Teaching Priorities for Patients Taking Proton Pump Inhibitors

In addition to the general precautions related to drugs for PUD and GERD (p. 363), include these teaching points and precautions:

- Take the drug exactly as prescribed and take it for the full time period, even if you are feeling better.
- Remember that these drugs do not cure the ulcer; they just change the GI environment so that healing is more likely to occur. Stopping the drug too soon can allow a partially healed ulcer to reopen.
- Report any black, tarry stools; diarrhea; abdominal pain; or persistent headaches to your prescriber immediately, because these are signs of bleeding and possible low blood volume (hypovolemia).
- If you are prescribed lansoprazole, omeprazole, or rabeprazole, avoid driving or engaging in other activities that require increased alertness because these drugs may cause dizziness.
- If you are prescribed rabeprazole, use sunscreen and wear protective clothing when going outdoors because this drug causes photosensitivity (increased sensitivity of the skin to light and other sources of ultraviolet rays).
- If you are diabetic, check your glucose more often because hypoglycemia (low blood sugar) can occur.
- Avoid alcohol, salicylates, and NSAIDs because they can cause GI irritation.

Life Span Considerations for Proton Pump Inhibitors

Considerations for pregnancy and lactation. Omeprazole, pantoprazole, and rabeprazole have a moderate likelihood of increasing the risk for birth defects or fetal harm. They are not safe for use during pregnancy because they may cause harm to the unborn child. The other PPI drugs have a low likelihood of increasing the risk for birth defects or fetal harm. They are considered safe for use during pregnancy, but the benefits must outweigh the risks. PPIs are not recommended for use during breastfeeding. A woman taking a PPI should tell her health care provider if she is pregnant or planning to become pregnant.

Considerations for older adults. There is an increased risk for side effects in older adults. PPIs have been associated with an increased risk for hip fractures because of decreased calcium absorption. Some studies have shown that short-term use of PPIs decreases the absorption of vitamin B_{12}. Older adults should have more frequent checkups to determine the effectiveness of the drug. In addition, the drug should be stopped in older adults when ulcers or inflammation have healed completely.

ANTACIDS

How Antacids Work

Many antacids are available over-the-counter without a prescription. **Antacids** are drugs that neutralize acids in the stomach. They are given by mouth to neutralize stomach acids and relieve heartburn and indigestion. Neutralizing stomach acids decreases the irritation and inflammation of the GI mucosa, especially the esophagus. Most antacids use salts of calcium, aluminum, or magnesium to neutralize the acid.

Common names and doses of a few antacids are listed in the following table. Be sure to consult a reliable drug resource for information on any specific antacid.

Adult Dosages for Commonly Prescribed Antacids

Drug Category	Drug Name	Usual Maintenance Dose
Antacids	aluminum hydroxide (AlternaGEL, Amphojel)	80–140 mEq (40–60 mL) orally given every 3–6 hr, or 1 and 3 hr after meals and at bedtime *Special Considerations:* **The recommended OTC dose is 600 mg orally given 5–6 times per day, after meals and at bedtime**
	calcium carbonate (Rolaids, TUMS)	Regular strength chewable tablets, 2–4 tablets orally as needed. Max: 12 tablets per day Ultra-strength chewable tablets, 2–3 tablets orally as needed. Max: 7 tablets per day *Special Considerations:* **Calcium carbonate can cause gastric hypersecretion and is *not* the preferred antacid for the adjunctive treatment of peptic ulcer disease**
	magnesium hydroxide/ aluminum hydroxide/ simethicone (Maalox, Milk of Magnesia, Mylanta)	400–1200 mg (5–15 mL of original strength suspension) as a single dose orally up to 4 times daily after meals and at bedtime. Max 60 mL/day

Intended Responses of Antacids

- Gastric acids are neutralized.
- There is relief from heartburn and indigestion.
- Symptoms of GERD are decreased.
- Ulcers are healing, and pain from ulcers is decreased.

Common Side Effects of Antacids

Side effects of antacids are very rare when they are taken as directed. They are more likely to occur if the drug is taken in large doses or over a long period of time or if the patient has kidney disease. The most common side effect of antacids containing calcium or aluminum salts is constipation. The most common side effect of antacids containing magnesium salts is diarrhea. Table 20.3 summarizes the side effects of antacids on the basis of their primary ingredients.

Common Side Effects

Antacids

Diarrhea, Constipation, Loss of appetite

Weakness, Fatigue

Table **20.3**	Common Side Effects of Antacids
TYPE OF ANTACID	**SIDE EFFECTS**
Aluminum containing	Bone pain, constipation, discomfort, loss of appetite, mood changes, muscle weakness, swelling of wrists or ankles, weight loss
Calcium containing	Constipation, decreased respiratory rate, difficult and frequent urination, fatigue, loss of appetite, mood changes, muscle pain, nausea and vomiting, nervousness, restlessness, twitching, unpleasant taste
Magnesium containing	Difficult or painful urination, dizziness, fatigue, irregular heart rhythm, light-headedness, loss of appetite, mood changes, muscle weakness, weight loss
Sodium bicarbonate containing	Decreased respiratory rate, fatigue, frequent urination, headache, loss of appetite, mood changes, muscle pain, nausea or vomiting, nervousness, restlessness, swelling of feet and lower legs, twitching

Possible Adverse Effects of Antacids

Adverse effects have not been reported when these drugs are taken appropriately. If not taken as directed they may cause bowel obstruction or fecal impaction.

⊛ Priority Actions to Take *Before* Giving Antacids

In addition to the general responsibilities related to drugs for PUD and GERD (p. 363), ensure that antacids are given 1 hour after or 2 hours before any other drug therapy. Antacids interfere with the absorption of other drugs and should not be taken at the same time.

Check calcium and magnesium laboratory values. Ask patients if they are experiencing constipation. Ask patients about pain including location, intensity, duration, and factors that cause or bring relief.

⊛ Priority Actions to Take *After* Giving Antacids

In addition to the general responsibilities related to drugs for PUD and GERD (p. 363), ask patients about symptom relief. Check patients daily for bowel movements. Report constipation or diarrhea to the prescriber.

⊛ Teaching Priorities for Patients Taking Antacids

In addition to the general precautions related to drugs for PUD and GERD (p. 363), include these teaching points and precautions:

- Contact your prescriber if you have been taking an antacid for more than 2 weeks and have not obtained relief because excessive use of antacids may cause or worsen kidney problems. Using calcium-based antacids too much may lead to the formation of kidney stones.
- Do not take an aluminum hydroxide or calcium antacid within 1 to 2 hours of other drugs without consulting your prescriber because these drugs affect the absorption of other drugs.
- If you have heart failure do **not** take sodium-containing antacids (e.g., Alka-Seltzer, Bromo-Seltzer) because they increase sodium and water retention. This problem causes an increase in the workload of the heart and can worsen heart failure.
- If you are taking an aluminum hydroxide or a calcium carbonate antacid you may experience the side effect of constipation.
- If you are taking a magnesium-containing antacid you may experience the side effect of diarrhea.
- Avoid taking antacids if you experience any signs of appendicitis or inflamed bowels such as cramping, pain, and soreness in the lower abdomen; bloating; and nausea and vomiting.
- If you are prescribed a liquid antacid always shake the bottle well before measuring your dose.

Life Span Considerations for Antacids

Pediatric considerations. Antacids should not be given to young children unless directed by the prescriber. Excessive amounts of antacids can change the pH of the blood and cause alkalosis.

Considerations for pregnancy and lactation. Magnesium hydroxide antacids have a low likelihood of increasing the risk for birth defects or fetal harm and are generally considered safe for use during pregnancy. Calcium carbonate and aluminum hydroxide antacids have a moderate likelihood of increasing the risk for birth defects or fetal harm. Long-term use of antacids may have negative effects on the fetus, and sodium-containing antacids should not be taken by women who tend to retain body water. Many antacids pass into breast milk, but they have not been reported to cause problems with breastfeeding babies.

Considerations for older adults. Older adults should not take aluminum-containing antacids if they have bone problems or Alzheimer disease because these drugs may cause these conditions to worsen.

Critical Point for Safety

Be sure to ask patients about antacid use because these drugs are readily available over the counter and can interfere with the absorption of other drugs.

QSEN: Safety

Critical Point for Safety

Teach patients to contact their prescriber if they have been taking an antacid for more than 2 weeks and continue to experience signs of reflux or an ulcer.

QSEN: Safety

Critical Point for Safety

Patients should not take an aluminum hydroxide or a calcium carbonate antacid within 1–2 hours of taking other drugs because they interfere with drug absorption in the GI tract.

QSEN: Safety

Critical Point for Safety

Patients with heart failure should **not** take sodium-containing antacids because they can cause salt and water retention and increase the workload of the heart.

QSEN: Safety

Critical Point for Safety

Older adults with bone problems or Alzheimer disease should not take aluminum-containing antacids because those drugs may cause these problems to worsen.

QSEN: Safety

CYTOPROTECTIVE DRUGS

How Cytoprotective Drugs Work

Cytoprotective (GI coating) drugs decrease acid damage to the stomach by coating the mucosal lining of the stomach and reducing the risk of developing an ulcer. Some cytoprotective drugs such as bismuth subsalicylate (Pepto-Bismol) are available over the counter.

Most of these drugs work by coating some part of the GI mucosa and reducing its exposure to stomach acids. Sucralfate (Carafate) is prescribed to protect open-sore areas in the GI tract and allow ulcers to heal. Sucralfate reacts with stomach acids to form a thick coating that covers the surface of an ulcer. This protects the open area from further damage. It also stops the effects of pepsin (a digestive enzyme that breaks down protein). Interestingly, this drug does not coat the normal stomach mucosa. Bismuth subsalicylate also coats the stomach and intestine protecting the mucosa. In addition, this drug inhibits the activity of *H. pylori* bacteria, helping to decrease GI infections.

The common doses of cytoprotective drugs are listed in the following table. Be sure to consult a reliable drug resource for more information about any specific cytoprotective drug.

Did You Know?

Sucralfate (Carafate) forms a protective coating over an ulcer but does not coat normal stomach mucosa.

Adult Dosages for Commonly Prescribed Cytoprotective Drugs

Drug Category	Drug Name	Usual Maintenance Dose
Cytoprotective	bismuth subsalicylate (Pepto-Bismol)	1050 mg (30 mL) orally every hour, as needed. Do not exceed 4 doses/day
	sucralfate (Carafate)	1 g orally four times per day on an empty stomach. Give before meals and at bedtime for 4–8 weeks depending on ulcer healing

Intended Responses of Cytoprotective Drugs

- Ulcers are protected to prevent further tissue damage.
- Ulcers are healed.

Common Side Effects of Cytoprotective Drugs

Side effects are rare with cytoprotective drugs. The most common side effect of sucralfate is constipation. Other side effects include dizziness; drowsiness; diarrhea; dry mouth; rashes; and gastric discomfort such as flatulence (gas), indigestion, and nausea.

Common Side Effects
Cytoprotective Drugs

Diarrhea, Constipation, Abdominal discomfort

Dizziness

Drowsiness

Dry mouth

Possible Adverse Effects of Cytoprotective Drugs

No life-threatening adverse effects have been documented with sucralfate. Bismuth subsalicylate (Pepto-Bismol) has caused changes in behavior with nausea and vomiting, as well as ringing in the ears.

✪ Priority Actions to Take *Before* Giving Cytoprotective Drugs

Be sure to review the general responsibilities related to drugs for PUD and GERD (p. 363) and assess abdominal discomfort before giving these drugs. Ask patients about previous ringing in the ears.

✪ Priority Actions to Take *After* Giving Cytoprotective Drugs

Be sure to review the general nursing responsibilities related to drugs for PUD and GERD (p. 363) after giving cytoprotective drugs. Ask patients about relief from GI pain and discomfort. Check for ringing in the ears. Monitor for behavioral changes as well as side effects.

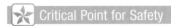

⊛ Teaching Priorities for Patients Taking Cytoprotective Drugs

In addition to the general precautions related to drugs for PUD and GERD (p. 363), include these teaching points and precautions:

* Take the drug exactly as directed by your prescriber for the full period of time (usually 4 to 8 weeks), even when feeling better.
* Increasing your fluid intake, dietary fiber (e.g., extra fruits, vegetables, and bran), and exercise help to prevent constipation, abdominal pain, and gas.
* Avoid taking antacids within 30 minutes of using these drugs because antacids will interfere with their action.

Life Span Considerations for Cytoprotective Drugs

Considerations for pregnancy and lactation. Sucralfate has a low likelihood of increasing the risk for birth defects or fetal harm and appears to be safe to use during pregnancy. However, extensive studies on pregnant women have not been conducted. A woman of childbearing years should be sure to tell her prescriber if she is breastfeeding an infant because it is not known whether sucralfate passes into breast milk. Teach patients who continue to breastfeed while taking these drugs to follow the tips in Box 1.1 in Chapter 1 to reduce infant exposure to the drugs.

PROMOTILITY DRUGS

How Promotility Drugs Work

When used to treat GERD, promotility drugs increase LES tone and the speed of emptying food out of the stomach. Metoclopramide (Reglan) increases stomach and small intestine contractions (peristalsis), helping to move food through the GI system. When food moves more quickly into the intestinal system, it is less likely to back up into the esophagus. Promotility drugs are **not** used to manage gastric or duodenal ulcers.

Metoclopramide is the promotility drug prescribed for treatment of GERD. It is usually given 30 minutes before meals and may be prescribed for 4 to 12 weeks. The common dosages for this drug are listed in the following table. For additional information on metoclopramide, see Chapter 19 and consult a reliable drug resource.

Adult Dosages for Commonly Prescribed Promotility Drugs

Drug Category	Drug Name	Usual Maintenance Dose
Promotility Drugs	metoclopramide (Reglan)	10–15 mg orally up to 4 times per day, 30 min before meals and at bedtime 10 mg IV or IM up to 4 times per day, 30 min before meals and at bedtime

OTHER DRUGS USED TO TREAT ULCERS

Antibiotics for *H. pylori* Infection

Antibiotics are essential to the treatment plan for PUD and are used to treat *H. pylori* infections of the GI tract. Common drugs and doses used to treat *H. pylori* infections are listed in the following table. See Chapter 6 for additional information on antibacterial drugs, Chapter 8 for information on antifungal drugs (metronidazole), and consult a reliable drug resource for additional information on any specific antibiotic drug for *H. pylori* infection.

Adult Dosages for Commonly Prescribed Promotility Drugs

Drug Category	Drug Name	Usual Maintenance Dose
Antibiotics	amoxicillin (Amoxil, Trimox)	1000 mg orally twice daily *Special Considerations:* **Usually given with another antibiotic and a proton pump inhibitor**

Adult Dosages for Commonly Prescribed Promotility Drugs—cont'd

Drug Category	Drug Name	Usual Maintenance Dose
	clarithromycin (Biaxin)	500 mg orally 3 times daily in combination with omeprazole for 14 days ***Special Considerations:* Usually given with a proton pump inhibitor**
	metronidazole (Flagyl)	500 mg orally 3 times daily in combination with clarithromycin and a proton pump inhibitor for 14 days as a first-line treatment option
	tetracycline (Sumycin, Tetracap)	500 mg orally 4 times daily in combination with bismuth subsalicylate, metronidazole, and a proton pump inhibitor for 10–14 days as a first-line treatment option

DRUGS FOR INFLAMMATORY BOWEL DISEASE

AMINOSALICYLATES

How Aminosalicylates Work

Aminosalicylates are a group of drugs that can help to control the symptoms of some inflammatory bowel diseases, including ulcerative colitis and Crohn disease. These drugs may also maintain remission for these conditions by preventing leucocyte (white blood cell) recruitment into the bowel wall. Aminosalicylates work by limiting the inflammation in the lining of the gastrointestinal tract. They may be prescribed as pills, enemas, or suppositories inserted through the rectum. The form prescribed depends on several factors, including where in the digestive tract the inflammation is located. Be sure to consult a reliable drug resource for more information about any specific aminosalicylate drug.

Adult Doses of Aminosalicylates for Management of Moderate to Severe UC and CD

Drug Category	Drug Name	Usual Maintenance Dose
Aminosalicylates	balsalazide (Colazol, Giazo)	2250 mg (3 × 750 mg capsules) orally 3 times per day (total daily dose of 6.75 g/day) for up to 8 weeks. May require 12 weeks treatment
	mesalamine 5-ASA (Apriso, Asacol, Canasa, Delzicol)	1600 mg orally 3 times daily for 6 weeks 1000 mg Per Rectum enema once daily at bedtime for 3–6 weeks For remission maintenance: 1500 mg orally once daily in the morning with or without meals
	olsalazine (Dipentum)	500 mg orally twice daily (Max: 1 g/day) for maintenance of remission of UC
	sulfasalazine (Azulfidine, Sulfazine)	500 mg orally every 6–8 hr for UC 3–6 g/day orally, given in divided doses for CD

Intended Responses of Aminosalicylates

- Decreased inflammation
- Induce and maintain remission in UC
- Improvement of symptoms
- Absence of pain and bleeding
- Decrease in number of diarrhea episodes

⇄ Do Not Confuse

metronidazole *with* **metformin**

An order for metronidazole may be confused with metformin. Metronidazole is an antifungal antibiotic, whereas metformin is an antidiabetic drug used for the management of type 2 diabetes.

QSEN: Safety

⇄ Do Not Confuse

olsalazine *with* **olanzapine**

An order for olsalazine may be confused with olanzapine. Olsalazine is an aminosalicylate used for treatment of ulcerative colitis and Crohn disease. Olanzapine is an antipsychotic drug used to treat schizophrenia acute manic episodes of bipolar disorder and acute agitation.

QSEN: Safety

⇄ Do Not Confuse

sulfasalazine *with* **sulfasoxazole**

An order for sulfasalazine may be confused with sulfasoxazole. Sulfasalazine is an aminosalicylate used for treatment of ulcerative colitis and Crohn disease. Sulfasoxazole is a sulfonamide antibiotic used to treat or prevent many different types of infections caused by bacteria, such as bladder infections, ear infections, or meningitis.

QSEN: Safety

Common Side Effects
Aminosalicylate Drugs

Headache   Nausea/Vomiting,
Abdominal
discomfort,
Diarrhea

Rash

 Critical Point for Safety

Sulfasalazine has a sulfa component. Be sure to ask patients about allergies to sulfa drugs, because this drug should not be given to a patient with sulfa drug allergies.

QSEN: Safety

 Critical Point for Safety

Give oral doses of aminosalicylates with a full glass of water to prevent crystals from forming in a patient's urine.

QSEN: Safety

Critical Point for Safety

After giving an aminosalicylate drug be sure to monitor for signs of allergic reactions including asthma-like symptoms, such as wheezing and trouble breathing; headaches, nasal congestion; changes in skin color; itching, skin rash, or hives; swelling of the hands, feet, and face; stomach pain or upset; and eczema. Report these to the prescriber immediately.

QSEN: Safety

 Drug Alert

Administration Alert

Before giving the enema form of mesalamine, shake the liquid well and instruct patients to hold the liquid in their colon for at least 20–40 min.

QSEN: Safety

Common Side Effects of Aminosalicylates

Common side effects of aminosalicylates include headache, nausea, abdominal pain and cramping, loss of appetite, vomiting, rash, and fever. These drugs may also cause diarrhea. Sulfasalazine can cause sun sensitivity.

Possible Adverse Effects of Aminosalicylates

Possible adverse effects of aminosalicylates include kidney injury. Patients with kidney problems should *not* take these drugs.

Sulfasalazine can cause a decrease in sperm production and function in male patients; however, sperm count becomes normal after the drug is discontinued. There is a sulfa component to this drug and it is *not* given to patients with sulfa allergies.

Pancreatitis is a rare adverse effect when mesalamine is prescribed. Diarrhea is a common adverse effect of olsalazine, and other possible effects include hair loss, pancreatitis, and pericarditis.

⭐ Priority Actions to Take *Before* Giving Aminosalicylates

In addition to the general actions to take before giving drugs for PUD, GERD, and IBD (p. 363), ask patients about kidney problems and ensure that ordered kidney functions laboratory tests are completed. Report any abnormal values to the prescriber. Ask patients about allergies to salicylate or sulfonamide drugs.

Assess patient stools for consistency, frequency, color, and presence of blood or mucous. Ask patients about abdominal pain or cramping.

Give patients a full glass of water to drink with each oral dose to prevent crystals from forming in the urine.

Explain the route of the prescribed drug to the patient (e.g., oral, or rectal enema). Instruct patients to hold the enema liquid in the colon for 20 to 40 minutes.

⭐ Priority Actions to Take *After* Giving Aminosalicylates

In addition to the general actions to take after giving drugs for PUD, GERD, and IBD (p. 363), continue to monitor patients' stools and ask about abdominal discomfort. Ask patients about worsening or improvement of symptoms. Continue to monitor renal function tests because renal toxicity may occur.

Monitor patients for allergic reactions to sulfonamide drugs (e.g., skin rash, hives, itchy eyes or skin, breathing problems, face swelling) or salicylates (e.g., asthma-like symptoms, such as wheezing and trouble breathing; headaches, nasal congestion; changes in skin color; itching, skin rash, or hives; swelling of the hands, feet, and face; stomach pain or upset; and eczema). Immediately notify the prescriber of allergic reactions because the drug will need to be discontinued.

⭐ Teaching Priorities for Patients Taking Aminosalicylates

In addition to teaching patients the general precautions related to drugs for PUD, GERD, and IBD (p. 363), include these teaching points and precautions:

- Take your medication exactly as instructed by your prescriber. Continue to take your prescribed drug even if you are feeling better.
- Take oral drugs with a full glass of water.
- If you are a male patient, you sperm count may be decreased while taking this drug; however, it will return to normal after you finish taking it.
- If you are prescribed the enema form of mesalamine, shake the liquid well and hold it in your colon for at least 20 to 40 minutes.
- If you are prescribed sulfasalazine, wear protective clothing and use sunscreen to prevent sunburn due to sun sensitivity.
- Notify your prescriber of abdominal discomfort, diarrhea with blood, headache, fever, rash, bruising, or chest pain because these may indicate an allergic reaction and the drug may need to be discontinued.
- Avoid driving or operating heavy or dangerous equipment until you know how the drug will affect you because dizziness may occur.

Life Span Considerations for Aminosalicylates

Considerations for pregnancy and lactation. Women who plan to become pregnant while taking sulfasalazine should take a dose of folate 2 mg orally daily. These drugs are considered safe to use during pregnancy and breastfeeding.

CORTICOSTEROIDS

How Corticosteroids Work

Corticosteroids are drugs similar to natural cortisol that prevent or limit inflammation by slowing or stopping inflammatory mediator production. Corticosteroids work like natural cortisol and are the most powerful agents to slow or stop production of most inflammatory mediators. When they enter inflammatory cells, corticosteroids bind to control points of protein synthesis in the cell and prevent the conversion of substances into active mediators that cause inflammation. Thus, they suppress both inflammatory responses and immune responses. They are used for short-term treatment of IBD. See Chapter 10 for additional information on corticosteroids. Be sure to consult a reliable drug resource for more information about any specific corticosteroid drug.

Adult Doses of Corticosteroids for Management of Moderate to Severe UC and CD

Drug Category	Drug Name	Usual Maintenance Dose
Oral Drugs	rednisone (Deltasone)	40–60 mg orally daily for 1–2 weeks, then taper daily dose by 5 mg weekly until at 20 mg orally once daily, and then continue with 2.5–5 mg decrements weekly ***Special Considerations:*** **Tapering this drug should generally not exceed 3 months**
	budesonide (Entocor)	9 mg orally once daily in the morning for up to 8 weeks. May taper to 6 mg orally once daily for 2 weeks prior to treatment cessation to minimize the risk of adrenal insufficiency
	hydrocortisone (Cortef, Solu-Cortef)	20 to 240 mg per day orally 2–4 divided doses
Rectal Foams	budesonide (Uceris)	2 mg (1 metered dose) rectally twice daily (in the morning and evening) for 2 weeks, then 2 mg (1 metered dose) rectally once daily (in the evening) for 4 weeks ***Special Considerations:*** **Evening doses are applied immediately prior to bedtime**
	hydrocortisone (Cortef, Solu-Cortef)	One applicatorful (90 mg of hydrocortisone acetate) rectally once daily or twice per day for 2–3 weeks, and every second day thereafter
Suppositories	hydrocortisone (Cortef, Solu-Cortef)	Insert 1 suppository rectally 2–3 times per day, for 2 weeks
Enemas	hydrocortisone (Cortef, Solu-Cortef)	100 mg rectally, as a retention enema, nightly for 21 nights or until clinical and proctological remission are achieved ***Special Considerations:*** **Clinical symptoms usually subside promptly within 3–5 days**

Intended Responses of Corticosteroids
- Decreased inflammation
- Improvement of symptoms

Common Side Effects of Corticosteroids
Common side effects of corticosteroids include increased risk for infections, especially candida (yeast/thrush) infections, dry mouth, and bad taste.

 Do Not Confuse

prednisone *with* **prednisolone**

An order for prednisone may be confused with prednisolone. Both drugs are immediate-acting corticosteroids used to decrease inflammation, and prednisolone is also used for immunosuppression. Double check the patient prescription to make sure the correct drug is given.

QSEN: Safety

Common Side Effects

Corticosteroids

Dry mouth,
Taste
changes

Possible Adverse Effects of Corticosteroids

Patients who are prescribed a systemic corticosteroid for more than a month experience some adverse effects, depending on the daily dose and how long they have been on the drug. The most common are infections, hypertension, diabetes, osteoporosis, avascular necrosis, myopathy, cataracts, and glaucoma. Other systemic effects may include hyperglycemia, increased appetite and weight gain, increased facial hair, mood swings, and bruising (see Chapter 10).

Long-term use of rectal suppositories can cause weakening of the anorectal muscles, also called steroid myopathy.

⭐ Priority Actions to Take *Before* Giving Corticosteroids

In addition to the general actions to take before giving drugs for PUD, GERD, and IBD (p. 363), inspect the patient's mouth and throat to assess whether an infection or thrush is present. Thrush appears as white or cream-colored patches of a cottage cheese–like coating on the mucous membranes, the roof of the mouth, and tongue. Check for any signs or symptoms of other infections.

Assess skin condition, especially the perianal area for excoriation, irritation, or ulceration related to stools. Document the patient's stools (e.g., color, consistency, number, frequency, presence of blood or mucous). Collect any required stool samples for laboratory analysis. Assess for bowel sounds and abdominal distention as well as bleeding.

Check baseline blood pressure, heart rate, and weight because prednisone can cause increased blood pressure, tachycardia, and fluid retention. Monitor intake and output. Assess for edema.

Also check baseline glucose because prednisone can cause hyperglycemia, and potassium because hypokalemia can occur.

Teach patients about the form of corticosteroids prescribed for them (e.g., oral, suppository, enema, or rectal foam).

⭐ Priority Actions to Take *After* Giving Corticosteroids

In addition to the general actions to take after giving drugs for PUD, GERD, and IBD (p. 363), continue to monitor for any signs or symptoms of infection, as well as frequency and nature of stools and skin problems. Notify the prescriber of any signs of infection. Assess for any signs or symptoms of adverse systemic effects of these drugs. Ask patients about improvement or worsening of symptoms of UC or CD.

Assist the patient to brush his or her teeth or to rinse with water or mouthwash to remove the drug from the oral cavity. This practice helps reduce the bad taste and mouth dryness, as well as decrease the risk for thrush and other oral infections.

Continue to monitor blood pressure, heart rate and rhythm, intake and output, and assess for increasing edema. Check glucose and potassium levels as well as daily weights. Notify the prescriber for any abnormalities.

⭐ Teaching Priorities for Patients Taking Corticosteroids

In addition to teaching patients the general precautions related to drugs for PUD, GERD, and IBD (p. 363), include these teaching points and precautions:

- Take the drug exactly as directed by your prescriber (e.g., oral, or rectal).
- Do **not** suddenly stop taking your prescribed corticosteroid drug because of the potential for adrenal insufficiency. Your adrenal glands require some time to begin producing cortisol again.
- Notify your prescriber of any signs or symptoms of infections (e.g., fever, sore throat, or sore mouth).
- Brush your teeth or rinse with water or mouthwash to remove the drug from your oral cavity because this will help with dry mouth and unpleasant taste, as well as prevention of thrush infection.
- Remember that these drugs are used for short-term control of IBD symptoms because long-term use increases the risk for systemic adverse effects (e.g., increased appetite, weight gain, changes in mood, muscle weakness, blurred vision, increased growth of body hair, easy bruising, and decreased resistance to infection).

- Rectal forms of these drugs are used to treat localized inflammation of the anus and rectum because they decrease the risk of systemic effects.
- Keep a record of the nature of your stools, noting any changes in frequency, consistency, color, or presence of blood. Notify your prescriber of blood in your stool.
- Notify your prescriber of any worsening or improvement in your symptoms.
- Consult your prescriber before taking any over-the-counter or herbal preparations.

Life Span Considerations for Corticosteroids

Considerations for pregnancy and lactation. Corticosteroids may increase the maternal risk of hypertension, edema, gestational diabetes, osteoporosis, premature rupture of membranes, and small-for-gestational-age babies. No adverse effects have been reported in breastfed infants with maternal use of any corticosteroid during breastfeeding. With high maternal doses, avoiding breastfeeding for 4 hours after a dose should markedly decrease the dose received by the infant.

IMMUNOMODULATORS

How Immunomodulators Work

Immunomodulators are substances that modify the immune system's response to a threat. Immunomodulators modulate and potentiate the immune system, by keeping it highly prepared for any threat. Immunomodulators work by suppressing the overly active immune response that occurs in IBD. 6-Mercaptopurine (6-MP) and azathioprine (Imuran) are closely related drugs as azathioprine is converted into 6MP in the body. Azathioprine and 6-Mercaptopurine, which are both chemically quite similar, are taken orally on a daily basis. Because these drugs can take 3 to 6 months to show improvement in symptoms, steroids are often prescribed at the same time to produce a more rapid response.

These drugs may also be prescribed with biologics to help prevent antibody formation which can lead to loss of response to biologics. Be sure to consult a reliable drug resource for more information about any specific biologic drug.

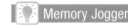
Memory Jogger

Immunomodulators may take 3–6 months to show improvement. Steroids can be prescribed to produce a more rapid response and improvement of symptoms.

Adult Doses of Immunomodulators for Management of Moderate to Severe UC and CD

Drug Category	Drug Name	Usual Maintenance Dose
Immunomodulators	azathioprine (Imuran)	For CD: 1.5–2.5 mg/kg/day orally, titrated to 25–50 mg orally once daily For UC: 2 to 2.5 mg/kg/day orally is the usual initial and maximal target (goal) dose range recommended as one option for maintenance treatment
	6-mercaptopurine (6-MP, Purinethol)	For CD: 0.75–1.5 mg/kg/day orally is the usual maximal dose range; doses are usually titrated to target from 25 or 50 mg orally once daily For UC: 1.5 mg/kg/day orally is the usual initial and maximal target (goal) dose range
	cyclosporine (Sandimmune)	2.5–15 mg/kg/day orally for Crohn disease (CD) 2 mg/kg IV is the targeted cyclosporine dose for rescue treatment of acute severe ulcerative colitis (UC)
	methotrexate (Rheumatrex)	12.5–15 mg orally once weekly as adjunctive therapy for reducing immunogenicity against biologic therapy 25 mg subcutaneous once weekly for treatment of active disease with dose-reduction to 15 mg subcutaneous once weekly for maintenance of remission of CD
	tacrolimus (Progral)	0.025 mg/kg orally twice daily initially, with dose titration to an optimal target tacrolimus serum trough level of 10–15 ng/mL, given for 2 weeks for UC

Intended Responses of Immunomodulators
- Decreased inflammatory response
- Immunosuppression
- Decreased need for long-term steroids
- Decrease episodes of flares

Common Side Effects of Immunomodulators
Increased risk for infections may occur with all immunomodulators. Common side effects of these drugs are listed by drug in the following table.

Drugs	Common Side Effects
Azathioprine & 6-mercaptopurine (6-MP)	Headache, nausea, vomiting, diarrhea, malaise, sores in the mouth, rash, fever, joint pain, alopecia, arthralgia, muscle wasting
Cyclosporine & Tacrolimus	Increased risk for infection; sleep problems; headache; tremors; candida infection; rash; hyperkalemia, hypomagnesemia, hyperlipidemia, hyperuricemia; tingling in fingers and feet; increased facial hair
Methotrexate	Flu-like symptoms (nausea, vomiting, headache, fatigue, diarrhea); severe mouth sores (candida); low white blood cell count; dizziness *Special Considerations:* **Some side effects of methotrexate can be prevented by the use of extra folic acid**

Headache Fatigue

Nausea/ Vomiting

Common Side Effects
Immunomodulators

Possible Adverse Effects of Immunomodulators
Azathioprine and 6-MP can cause pancreatitis, and bone marrow suppression as well as increased risk for serious bleeding. Return to normal production of blood cell production may take several weeks after these drugs are discontinued. Other risks with these drugs are increased risk for development of non-Hodgkin lymphoma, hepatotoxicity, and pancreatitis.

Cyclosporine may cause seizures, encephalopathy, hepatotoxicity, pancreatitis, nephrotoxicity, and increased risk of lymphoma.

Tacrolimus may cause seizures, hypertension, prolonged QT segment (may cause life-threatening dysrhythmias), GI bleeding, renal failure, anemia, lung problems, and anaphylaxis.

Methotrexate can cause scarring of the liver and lung inflammation. Liver scarring can be more severe with diabetes, obesity, and increased alcohol consumption. Other risks include renal failure, tumor lysis syndrome, leukopenia, thrombocytopenia, and anemia.

⭐ Priority Actions to Take *Before* Giving Immunomodulators
In addition to the general actions to take before giving drugs for PUD, GERD, and IBD (p. 363), check blood laboratory results (e.g., complete blood count, lipid profile, liver and kidney function tests). Ask patients about liver or kidney problems and if they have received influenza and vaccines for other transmissible infections such as pneumonia. Also, ask if they have received the shingles vaccine.

Assess for any signs of liver toxicity such as dark urine, jaundice, itching, and light-colored stools. Get a baseline weight and vital signs. Be sure to ask about alcohol consumption.

⭐ Priority Actions to Take *After* Giving Immunomodulators
In addition to the general actions to take after giving drugs for PUD, GERD, and IBD (p. 363), continue to monitor vital signs and laboratory test results. Weigh patients daily and monitor urine output. Assess urine for any changes in appearance. Report changes to the prescriber.

Monitor for any signs of infection or bleeding and notify the prescriber for signs of both these complications.

Assess for any vision or central nervous system changes (e.g., dizziness, confusion) and report these to the prescriber.

⊛ Teaching Priorities for Patients Taking Immunomodulators

In addition to teaching patients the general precautions related to drugs for PUD, GERD, and IBD (p. 363), include these teaching points and precautions:

- Take your prescribed drug exactly as directed by your prescriber. Remember that it may take 3 to 6 months to experience improvement in symptoms while taking these drugs.
- Avoid crowds or people with known infections to reduce your risk of infection.
- Notify your prescriber for any signs or symptoms of infection, changes in urine or decreased urine output, and signs of liver toxicity (e.g., dark urine, jaundice, itching, and light-colored stools).
- Report any mouth inflammation, bleeding, or white spots to your prescriber.
- Notify your prescriber of any changes in your level of consciousness, confusion, or dizziness.
- Avoid the use of regular razors because it increases the risk of bleeding.
- Wear protective clothing and sunscreen to protect from ultraviolet sun exposure.
- With methotrexate you may need a wig or hairpiece due to alopecia (hair loss).
- Avoid live forms of vaccines.
- Avoid consumption of alcohol and grapefruit juice.
- Visit your dentist regularly for dental care and to prevent mouth infections. Use a soft toothbrush to prevent bleeding of the gums.
- Consume 10 to 12 glasses of fluid each day.
- Some drugs (e.g., Azathioprine) cause GI symptoms, and taking them with food can decrease the discomfort.
- Weigh yourself every day and keep track of your weight.
- Use contraceptive measures during and for up to 12 weeks after treatment to avoid pregnancy.
- Keep all follow-up appointments to monitor progress and laboratory studies.

Critical Point for Safety

Monitor patients for signs of liver toxicity such as dark urine, jaundice, itching, and light-colored stools. Report these changes immediately to the prescriber.

QSEN: Safety

Life Span Considerations for Immunomodulators

Considerations for pregnancy and lactation. Women who are pregnant or plan to become pregnant should consult their prescribers before taking methotrexate and azathioprine. These drugs should be avoided by pregnant women. Both men and women should avoid methotrexate for several months before conception because it can lead to pregnancy loss or birth defects. Breastfeeding is avoided with tacrolimus.

Considerations for older adults. Older IBD patients are at higher risk of adverse events and less treatment responsiveness compared with younger patients.

BIOLOGICS

How Biologics Work

Biologics are a class of complex antiinflammatory drugs derived from living sources that target specific inflammatory cells, components, or products to modify chronic disorders associated with inflammation and tissue damage. They are made from biological instead of chemical processes and are often prescribed when other treatments such as aminosalicylates or immunomodulators do not work for ulcerative colitis (UC) or Crohn disease (CD). Thus, these drugs are not considered first-line treatments. Biologic drugs are given either by subcutaneous or intravenous routes. They do not work for everyone, and in some cases, they stop working overtime. The cost of using these drugs is very high, as much as $20,000 per year.

Gastrointestinal inflammation with UC and CD occurs with over-activity of the immune system. Biologics block some parts of this over-activity, decrease the inflammation, and help to improve symptoms. Some of these drugs are called anti-TNF

Critical Point for Safety

Biologics are given by subcutaneous or intravenous routes. Be sure to use appropriate injection techniques and monitor sites for injection reactions.

QSEN: Safety

drugs (e.g., infliximab, adalimumab, golimumab), which work to block a protein (tumor necrosis factor alpha) that promotes the inflammation process in the intestines. Another group of these drugs called integrin receptor antagonists (e.g., vedolizumab) stop integrins (molecules in the immune system) from attaching to cells in the lining of the intestines. Infliximab also helps heal and lower the number of intestinal fistulas associated with CD. Common names and doses of biologic drugs for UC and CD are listed in the following table. See Chapter 11 for additional information on biologics. Be sure to consult a reliable drug resource for more information about any specific biologic drug.

Adult Doses of Biologics for Management of Moderate to Severe UC and CD

Drug Category	Drug Name	Usual Maintenance Dose
Anti-TNF Drugs	adalimumab (Humira)	For CD and UC: 160 mg subcutaneously (given in 1 day or split over 2 consecutive days), then 80 mg subcutaneously 2 weeks later (day 15). On day 29, begin a maintenance dose of 40 mg subcutaneously every other week
	certolizumag (Cimzia)	For CD: 400 mg subcutaneously, given as two 200-mg subcutaneous injections, at weeks 0, 2, and 4 as monotherapy or concomitantly with non-biologic disease-modifying antirheumatic drugs (DMARDs). If clinical response occurs, administer 400 mg subcutaneously every 4 weeks as maintenance therapy
	golimumab (Simponi)	For UC: 200 mg subcutaneously on week 0, followed by 100 mg subcutaneously at week 2 for induction. For maintenance, give 100 mg subcutaneously every 4 weeks starting at week 6
	infliximab (Remicade)	For CD & UC: 5 mg/kg IV infusion at weeks 0, 2, and 6 as induction therapy. Thereafter, a maintenance regimen of 5 mg/kg IV infusion every 8 weeks
Integrin Receptor Antagonists	natalizumab (Tysabri)	For CD: 300 mg IV infusion given over 1 hr every 4 weeks
	ustekinumab (Stelera)	For CD & UC: First dose intravenous infusion is weight-based: *more than 85 kg*: 520 mg IV infusion as a single dose; *56 kg to 85 kg:* 390 mg IV infusion as a single dose; *55 kg or less:* 260 mg IV infusion as a single dose; then subcutaneous injection of 90 mg subcutaneously starting 8 weeks after initial intravenous induction dose, followed by 90 mg subcutaneously every 8 weeks thereafter
	vedolizumab (Entyvio)	For CD & UC: 300 mg IV infusion administered over 30 min at weeks 0, 2, and 6 as induction therapy. Thereafter, a maintenance regimen of 300 mg IV infusion is given every 8 weeks ** *Special Considerations:* Full response is usually observed by 6 weeks; patients who do not respond by week 14 are unlikely to respond with continued treatment and consideration should be given to discontinuing therapy in these patients**

Common Side Effects

Biologics

Injection site reaction

Headache

Nausea

Sore throat

Cough

Intended Responses of Biologics
- Improving GI symptoms with CD and UC
- Inducing and maintaining remission
- Preventing flares
- Decreasing need for hospitalization and surgery

Common Side Effects of Biologics
Common side effects of biologics include injection site reactions (e.g., redness, itching, rash, swelling, and pain), headaches, fever, chills, nausea, cough, feeling achy, and sore throat.

Possible Adverse Effects of Biologics

Possible adverse effects of biologics include increased risk for infection because of their effects on the immune system. Patients with previous infections such as tuberculosis or hepatitis B may experience reactivation of these conditions when they start on biologic therapy. Some biologics (e.g., infliximab) increase the risk of lymphoma (a type of blood cancer). Rarely, these drugs can cause liver problems (e.g., vedolizumab), joint pain (e.g., certolizumab), or nervous system problems (e.g., ustekinumab).

Priority Actions to Take *Before* Giving Biologics

In addition to the general actions to take before giving drugs for PUD, GERD, and IBD (p. 363), ask patients about prior infections such as tuberculosis and hepatitis B. Patients must be tested for tuberculosis a week before the first dose of a biologic is given, and the drug is **not** given the drug if the tuberculosis test is positive. Because of the effects of biologics on the immune system, ask if patients have been vaccinated for influenza and pneumonia.

Most biologics are given by subcutaneous injection, although some are given as an IV infusion. Allow the drug or prefilled syringe to come to room temperature before injecting (about 30 minutes after removing from refrigeration) and inspect the liquid. Do not use it if the drug is cloudy, discolored, or contains large particles. For subcutaneous injections select an appropriate site such as the upper arm, thigh, or abdomen (except for a 2-inch area surrounding the umbilicus), and be sure the skin is intact. After cleansing the area, pinch up the skin, insert the needle at a 90-degree angle, and inject it subcutaneously. Do **not** aspirate before injecting the drug. If a patient will be giving his or her own subcutaneous shots at home, teach them the correct technique and ask them to demonstrate how to give the shot (see Box 2.3 in Chapter 2 for steps for teaching a patient to self-inject a subcutaneous drug). Intravenous infusions are usually given in a physician's office or outpatient setting of a hospital. Depending on the drug, the infusion time may be between 30 minutes and 4 hours. Have emergency equipment for anaphylaxis available in the room where the patient is located because the risk for allergic reactions is relatively high. As a result of this risk, only a licensed health care professional should give the injection and a physician must be in the facility.

Priority Actions to Take *After* Giving Biologics

In addition to the general actions to take after giving drugs for PUD, GERD, and IBD (p. 363), monitor for any signs or symptoms of infection, as well as reactivation of tuberculosis or hepatitis B. Do **not** massage the site after injection. Ensure that the patient remains in the facility under observation for 30 to 60 minutes. Assess oxygenation and blood pressure every 5 to 10 minutes.

Teaching Priorities for Patients Taking Biologics

In addition to teaching patients the general precautions related to drugs for PUD, GERD, and IBD (p. 363), include these teaching points and precautions:

- Watch for the signs and symptoms of an allergic response because these may occur even several hours after the injection.
- Report allergic reactions immediately. Call 911 or go to the nearest emergency department if any symptoms of an allergic reaction occur.
- Notify your prescriber of any signs or symptoms of infection (e.g., fever, fatigue, cough, flu-like symptoms) immediately.
- Be sure to get vaccinated for influenza and pneumonia.
- If you or a family member will be doing self-administration of the drug, use the appropriate techniques taught for performing the actual injection, including how to select a site and the technique for giving the injection with a prefilled syringe or dosing pen (Box 2.3 in Chapter 2).
- Check with your health insurance if the cost of biologics is covered or if financial assistance is available to help cover the costs.

Critical Point for Safety

Monitor biologic drug injection sites for reactions (e.g., redness, itching, rash, swelling, and pain) because these drugs are given by injection (subcutaneous or intravenous) and these are common side effects of biologic drugs.

QSEN: Safety

Critical Point for Safety

Monitor patients with previous infections such as tuberculosis or hepatitis B carefully because they may experience reactivation of these conditions when started on biologic therapy.

QSEN: Safety

- Consult with your prescriber before taking any over-the-counter drugs, herbal supplements, or natural remedies.
- Avoid crowds and people who are ill.
- Notify your prescriber of any prior or new health problems. Also, inform your prescriber if your symptoms get worse.
- Be sure to keep all follow-up appointments with your prescriber including receiving laboratory testing, as well as subcutaneous injections or intravenous doses of biologic drugs.

Life Span Considerations for Biologics
Pediatric considerations. Biologics appear to be safe in both adults and children. However, the long-term safety in children and teens is unknown.

Considerations for pregnancy and lactation. Biologics do not increase the risk for miscarriages or congenital malformations and appear reasonably safe if used during the first half of pregnancy. There appears to be a low level of risk of using biologics during lactation. However, pharmaceutical manufacturers generally state that women should not breastfeed while using these drugs.

Considerations for older adults. Older adults have an increased risk for the development of malignancy and infection.

Get Ready for the NCLEX® Examination!

Key Points

- The most common cause of PUD is infection with the *H. pylori* bacteria.
- Antibiotics are essential to the treatment plan for PUD because of *H. pylori* infections.
- Complications of ulcers include bleeding, perforation, and gastric obstruction.
- GERD may damage the lining of the esophagus, causing inflammation.
- The cause of GERD is a lower esophageal sphincter that is not working correctly and allows stomach contents to back up (reflux) into the esophagus.
- Complications of GERD include ulcers; bleeding; strictures; and Barrett esophagus, a precancerous condition that may lead to the development of esophageal cancer.
- Patients with GERD should avoid chocolate, peppermint, alcohol, nicotine, and caffeinated drinks because they lower the pressure of the LES and promote reflux.
- Teach patients with PUD or GERD to avoid substances that cause increased GI irritation, such as alcohol, NSAIDs, and aspirin.
- Histamine H_2 blockers are available in lower doses over the counter for mild heartburn and indigestion. They are also available in higher doses by prescription for moderate-to-severe forms of GERD.
- Watch for confusion, the most common side effect, when giving histamine H_2 blockers.
- Smoking interferes with the action of histamine H_2 blockers.
- Teach patients to notify their prescriber if they have been taking over-the-counter H_2 blockers for more than 2 weeks and are still experiencing reflux.
- Patients taking histamine H_2 blockers should not smoke because smoking interferes with the action of these drugs.

- Monitor older adults closely because they are more likely to experience confusion and dizziness as side effects of histamine H_2 blockers.
- Black, tarry stools indicate bleeding and should always be reported to the prescriber.
- For best effects PPIs should be given before meals, preferably in the morning.
- Teach patients to take proton pump inhibitors for the full period of time recommended by the prescriber, even if they are feeling better.
- Teach older adults who have been prescribed PPIs to take a daily multivitamin because PPIs decrease the absorption of vitamin B_{12} and calcium.
- Be sure to ask patients about antacid use because these drugs are readily available over the counter.
- Teach patients to contact their prescriber if they have been taking an antacid for more than 2 weeks and continue to experience signs of reflux or an ulcer.
- Aluminum hydroxide antacids decrease the absorption of other drugs when taken within 1 to 2 hours.
- Patients with heart failure should not take sodium-containing antacids because they can cause salt and water retention and increase the workload of the heart.
- Older adults with bone problems or Alzheimer's disease should not take aluminum-containing antacids because those drugs may cause these problems to worsen.
- Teach patients taking cytoprotective drugs to prevent constipation by increasing intake of fluids and fiber-containing foods and exercising.
- Children should not be given bismuth subsalicylate (Pepto-Bismol) because it contains aspirin and may cause Reye syndrome.
- Sulfasalazine has a sulfa component. Be sure to ask patients about allergies to sulfa drugs, because this drug should not be given to a patient with sulfa drug allergies.

- When a patient is prescribed corticosteroids for IBD, inspect the patient's mouth and throat to assess whether an infection or thrush is present. Thrush appears as white or cream-colored patches of a cottage cheese–like coating on the mucous membranes, the roof of the mouth, and tongue.
- Because immunomodulators may take 3 to 6 months to show improvement, steroids may be prescribed to produce a more rapid response and improvement of symptoms.
- Monitor patients with previous infections such as tuberculosis or hepatitis B carefully because they may experience reactivation of these conditions when they start on biologic therapy.

Additional Learning Resources

Be sure to visit your Evolve website (http://evolve.elsevier.com/Workman/pharmacology/) for additional online resources.

SG Go to your Study Guide for additional learning activities to help you master this chapter content.

Review Questions

See *Answers to In-Text Review Questions* in the back of the book for answers to these questions.

1. The patient asks a nurse why does the backward flow of stomach contents into the esophagus cause tissue damage? What is the nurse's **best** response?

   A. "Because there are no digestive processes occurring in the esophagus."
   B. "The esophagus does not have any thick gel-like mucus to protect it from acid."
   C. "The esophagus secretes only bicarbonate, which is not strong enough to neutralize stomach acids."
   D. "The esophagus cannot expand with extra volume and the excessive stretching damages the muscle layer."

2. A patient with a history of GI ulcers reports feeling new onset burning, gnawing stomach pain. What is the nurse's **best** action?

   A. Assessing the patient's abdomen for the presence of active bowel sounds
   B. Administering the prescribed as-needed dose of liquid antacid
   C. Offering the patient food to buffer excess stomach acid
   D. Notifying the prescriber immediately

3. A patient who is prescribed sucralfate asks how this drug will help treat his gastric ulcer. What is the nurse's **best** response?

   A. "Sucralfate decreases secretion of gastric acids to help your ulcer heal."
   B. "Sucralfate completely blocks the secretion of gastric acids so your ulcer can heal."
   C. "Sucralfate treats the infection with *H. pylori* that is the major cause of gastric ulcers."
   D. "Sucralfate forms a thick coating to cover the ulcer, to protect from further damage and allow healing."

4. The patient with GERD asks the nurse how do histamine (H₂) blockers help heal gastric ulcers? What is the nurse's **best** response?

   A. "These drugs promote cell division."
   B. "Histamine H₂ blockers neutralize acids that are present in the stomach."
   C. "They decrease the amount of acid secreted by stomach cells."
   D. "They increase the rate that stomach contents move into the intestinal tract."

5. The nurse is teaching an older adult patient who has been prescribed famotidine, and his or her family about the drug. Which common side effect will the nurse instruct the patient's family to watch for and report to the prescriber?

   A. Confusion
   B. Anxiety
   C. Depression
   D. Psychosis

6. A patient who has been taking famotidine for the last month has all of the following blood laboratory results. Which result does the nurse report to the prescriber as soon as possible?

   A. International normalized ratio (INR) of 0.9
   B. Red blood cell count of 2 million/mm³
   C. White blood cell count of 8000/mm³
   D. Platelet count of 150,000/mm³

7. What should the nurse teach a patient about smoking and peptic ulcer disease? **Select all that apply.**

   A. Smoking increases acid secretion.
   B. Smoking is not related to ulcer formation.
   C. Smoking slows ulcer healing.
   D. Smoking is related to the reoccurrence of ulcers.
   E. Smoking decreases stomach mucus production.
   F. Smoking stimulates scar tissue formation in the stomach.

8. For which risk factors does the nurse screen when providing care for a patient who is developing GERD? **Select all that apply.**

   A. Being underweight
   B. Being pregnant
   C. Taking NSAID drugs
   D. Eating foods high in alkaline content
   E. Drinking caffeinated beverages
   F. Eating spicy foods
   G. Drinking 2 L of water daily

9. Why is the nurse concerned for older patients who are prescribed proton pump inhibitors and are at greater risk for drug-induced hip fracture?

   A. Induced drowsiness increases the risk for falling.
   B. Inhibited calcium absorption makes bones more fragile.
   C. Excessive potassium loss reduces muscle strength and balance.
   D. Anemia and fatigue prevent participation in exercise and reduce muscle weakness.

10. A patient with indigestion is prescribed aluminum hydroxide. To prevent the most common side effect of this drug, what precaution will the nurse teach this patient?

    A. "Take this drug 30 minutes before each meal."
    B. "Do not drink fluids for at least 30 minutes after taking this drug."
    C. "Be sure to consume a diet with lots of vegetables and other foods with fiber."
    D. "Report any episodes of diarrhea immediately to your prescriber."

11. Which assessments indicate to the nurse that a patient receiving an immunomodulator drug has liver toxicity?

    A. Darkened urine and light-colored stools
    B. Runny nose and blood-shot eyes
    C. Itching and hyperactive bowel sounds
    D. Swollen hands and decreased blood pressure

12. Which question is most important for the nurse ask a patient when a biologic drug is prescribed for inflammatory bowel disease?

    A. "Do you have any allergies to iodine or shellfish?"
    B. "Have you ever tested positive for tuberculosis or hepatitis?"
    C. "Does your health history include migraine headaches?"
    D. "Have you ever been prescribed corticosteroid drugs?"

Clinical Judgment

1. Which foods, activities, and drugs are **most important** for the nurse to teach the patient with peptic ulcer disease (PUD) to avoid? **Select all that apply.**

    A. Alcohol
    B. Stress
    C. Dairy products
    D. Exercising
    E. Smoking
    F. Spicy food
    G. Acetaminophen
    H. Nonsteroidal antiinflammatory drugs (NSAIDs)
    I. Carbonated beverages
    J. Caffeine

2. The nurse has taught a 57-year-old patient with peptic ulcer disease (PUD), who is prescribed rabeprazole, about proton pump inhibitor therapy. The patient is to take rabeprazole 20 mg orally for 6 weeks. Which patient statements indicate that the patient understands what the nurse has taught and which statements indicate that the patient needs more teaching? **Use an X to indicate which patient statements about issues related to this therapy are either Understood or Requires Further Teaching.**

PATIENT STATEMENT	UNDERSTOOD TEACHING	REQUIRES FURTHER TEACHING
"After I've been taking the rabeprazole for a couple of weeks my ulcer will be cured and I can stop taking it."		
"I will be sure to report any black and tarry looking bowel movements as well as diarrhea to my doctor."		
"I will be sure to take some time to sit in the sun whenever I can."		
"I will be careful not to drive until I know how this drug affects me because it can cause dizziness."		
"My doctor prescribed the rabeprazole because it will decrease the acid in my stomach so my ulcer can heal."		
"Once my prescription runs out, I will buy rabeprazole over-the-counter and take it so my ulcer doesn't come back."		

Drug Therapy for Diabetes

21

Learning Objectives

The content presented in this chapter should help you to:

1. Understand the physiology of normal blood glucose control (regulation) and the pathophysiology of diabetes mellitus.
2. Explain the names, actions, usual adult dosages, possible side effects, and adverse effects of antidiabetic drugs.
3. Describe priority actions to take before and after giving antidiabetic drugs.
4. Prioritize essential information to teach patients taking antidiabetic drugs.
5. Explain the names, actions, usual dosages, possible side effects, and adverse effects of insulin therapy.
6. Describe priority actions to take before and after giving insulin.
7. Prioritize essential information to teach patients taking insulin therapy.
8. Describe appropriate life span considerations for insulin therapy and for antidiabetic drugs.

Key Terms

alpha-glucosidase inhibitors (ĂL-fă-glū-KŌ-sĭ-dās ĭn-HĬB-ĭ-tŭrz) (p. 395) A class of noninsulin antidiabetic drugs that work by slowing the digestion of dietary starches and other complex carbohydrates by inhibiting an enzyme that breaks them down into glucose.

amylin analogs (ĂM-ĭ-lĭn Ă-nă-lŏgs) (p. 397) A class of noninsulin antidiabetic drugs that are chemically similar to natural amylin, which delays gastric emptying and lowers after-meal blood glucose levels

antidiabetic drugs (nŏn-Ĭn-sŭl-ĭn ăn-tĭ-dī-ă-BĔT-ĭk DRŬGZ) (p. 390) Oral and injectable drugs not related to insulin that use many actions to assist in lowering blood glucose levels.

diabetes mellitus (dī-ĕ-BĒ-tĕs MĔL-lĭ-tŭs) (p. 388) A metabolic disease that results from either the loss of the ability to make insulin or the loss of receptor sensitivity to the presence of insulin.

DPP-4 inhibitors (ĭn-HĬB-ĭ-tŭrz) (p. 396) A class of noninsulin antidiabetic drugs that works by inhibiting the enzyme DPP-IV, which normally breaks down and inactivates the incretin hormones, especially GLP-1. The result is an increase in the activity of normal incretin hormones.

glucagon (GLŪ-kă-gŏn) (p. 388) The hormone released by alpha cells of the pancreas and a synthetic drug that prevents hypoglycemia by breaking down glycogen from the liver into glucose.

glucose (GLŪ-kōs) (p. 386) The most common simple carbohydrate and the main fuel for the human body. Once inside cells, glucose is used to make the chemical energy substance adenosine triphosphate (ATP).

hyperglycemia (hī-pŭr-glī-SĒ-mē-ă) (p. 386) A blood glucose level above normal (higher than 110 mg/dL when fasting).

hypoglycemia (hī-pō-glī-SĒ-mē-ă) (p. 387) A blood glucose level below normal (lower than 70 mg/dL).

insulin (ĬN-sŭl-ĭn) (p. 386) The hormone produced by the beta cells of the pancreas that prevents blood glucose levels from becoming too high.

insulin sensitizers (ĬN-sŭl-ĭn SĔN-sĭ-tī-zŭrz) (p. 394) A class of noninsulin antidiabetic drugs known as sensitizers that increases the sensitivity of the insulin receptor to the binding of naturally secreted insulin, which improves the movement of glucose from the blood into the cells of the pancreas.

insulin stimulators (ĬN-sŭl-ĭn STĬM-yū-lā-tŭrz) (p. 392) A class of noninsulin antidiabetic drugs that works by stimulating the beta cells of the pancreas to release preformed insulin.

sodium-glucose cotransporter 2 (SGLT2) inhibitors (sō-de-um GLŪ-kōs kō-TRĂNS-pŏrt-ŭr ĭn-HĬB-ĭ-tŭrz) (p. 398) The newest class of noninsulin antidiabetic drugs that lower blood glucose levels by preventing kidney reabsorption of glucose that was filtered from the blood into the urine.

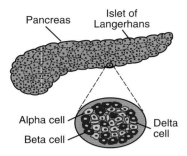

FIG. 21.1 Close-up view of the pancreas showing the islets of Langerhans that contain the glucagon-secreting alpha cells and the insulin-secreting beta cells.

Memory Jogger

Body cells need glucose and oxygen to make enough adenosine triphosphate (ATP) to perform all bodily functions.

Memory Jogger

The trigger for insulin synthesis and secretion is hyperglycemia, and its action is to restore normal blood glucose levels by allowing blood glucose to move into cells. Insulin *lowers* blood glucose levels.

RELATED PHYSIOLOGY AND PATHOPHYSIOLOGY OF ENDOCRINE PANCREATIC FUNCTION

ENDOCRINE PANCREAS PHYSIOLOGY

The pancreas is a digestive organ that has small islands of endocrine tissue within it, known as the islets of Langerhans. The digestive functions of the pancreas occur in the exocrine portions of the pancreas. Some of these functions include making and releasing digestive enzymes and producing bicarbonate. The endocrine pancreas regulates blood glucose levels by the secretion of two classic hormones, insulin and glucagon, from different cells within the islets of Langerhans (Figure 21.1). The beta cells produce and secrete insulin, which is the hormone that prevents blood glucose levels from becoming too high. The alpha cells produce and secrete glucagon, which is the hormone that prevents blood glucose levels from becoming too low. Together, these two hormones regulate glucose and ensure that the right amount is always present to provide enough energy for proper body *metabolism* (the energy use by each cell and amount of work performed within the body).

Glucose is the most common simple carbohydrate and the main source of fuel for the human body. Inside cells, it is used to form *adenosine triphosphate (ATP)*, which is the main chemical energy substance that drives most of the cellular reactions of the body. The body makes its own ATP, mostly from glucose when adequate oxygen also is present. ATP is the "fuel" that makes the body's "engine" run. For example, ATP provides the energy for skeletal muscle contraction for movement and maintenance of body temperature, heart muscle contraction for blood circulation, neuron excitation for thinking, and gastrointestinal work for food digestion. So for normal body function, people need a constant supply of glucose in the blood ready to enter cells and make sufficient amounts of ATP. However, too much glucose causes many problems.

An appropriate balance of insulin and glucagon, along with food intake, ensures that we always have the right amount of glucose in the blood. When a person has a blood glucose level within the normal range (between 70 and 110 mg/dL), he or she has *euglycemia* or is in a euglycemic state. Table 21.1 lists the laboratory values that indicate euglycemic glucose control.

Insulin

Insulin, often called the "hormone of plenty," prevents blood glucose levels from becoming too high (hyperglycemia). It is synthesized and released into the blood whenever blood glucose levels start to rise above normal levels. So, the trigger for insulin secretion is hyperglycemia, and insulin's action restores normal blood glucose levels by moving blood glucose into cells. Insulin binds to insulin receptors on the membranes of many cells (Animation 21.1). The result of having insulin bound to its receptors is that the cell membrane becomes more open (*permeable*) to glucose, allowing the blood glucose to enter the cell (Figure 21.2). As excess glucose leaves the blood and enters the cells, the blood glucose level returns to normal.

Table **21.1**	Laboratory Indicators of Adequate Blood Glucose Control
TEST	**VALUE**
Fasting blood glucose level	70–110 mg/dL
Hemoglobin A1c (A1C)	4%–6%
Spot blood glucose level[a]	Less than 150 mg/dL
Blood ketone body level	Negative
Urine glucose level	Negative
Urine ketone body level	Negative

[a]Random, not fasting.

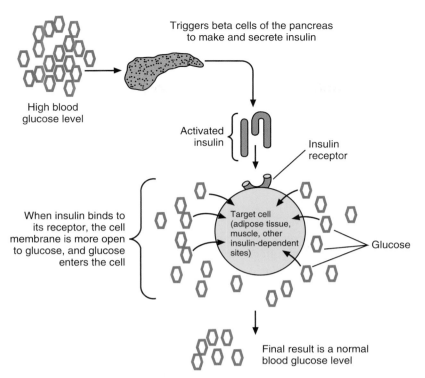

FIG. 21.2 Action of insulin.

Insulin is called the hormone of plenty because in a healthy person eating well makes blood levels of carbohydrates, proteins, and fats rise. When you have more than enough glucose to meet your energy needs, insulin allows the extra glucose to be converted to glycogen.

Glycogen is a starchy storage form of extra glucose. Molecules of glucose are linked together to form the trunk and branches of glycogen "trees" (Figure 21.3). In addition to glucose regulation, insulin also helps control protein and fat metabolism. Box 21.1 lists the effects of insulin.

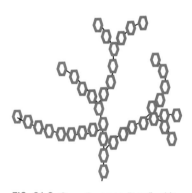

FIG. 21.3 One glycogen "tree" with 40 molecules of glucose stored in it.

Glucagon

If insulin were the only hormone controlling blood glucose levels, the body would be at risk for having blood glucose levels below normal (**hypoglycemia**). Low blood glucose levels reduce body metabolism because not enough glucose enters cells to make adequate amounts of ATP. If hypoglycemia is severe enough, all body metabolism is reduced (especially in the brain) and death can occur quickly. So balancing blood glucose levels to avoid hypoglycemia involves the action of the hormone glucagon.

⭐ Critical Point for Safety

When blood glucose levels are below 40 mg/dL, brain function decreases. When it falls below 25 mg/dL, death can occur within minutes. Hypoglycemia can lead to death much more quickly than hyperglycemia and requires rapid intervention.

QSEN: Safety

Box 21.1 Effects of Insulin

- Prevents blood glucose levels from rising too high
- Prevents muscle breakdown
- Stores fats inside fat cells
- Builds glycogen (stored form of glucose) in the liver and muscle
- Improves protein digestion and use in the body
- Increases the amount of energy produced in the cells
- Induces cell division for growth and wound healing
- Maintains blood levels of cholesterol and other fats within normal limits

Memory Jogger

The trigger for glucagon secretion is hypoglycemia, and its action is to restore the blood glucose level back up to normal. *Glucagon works in opposition to insulin.* Insulin causes blood glucose levels to decrease, preventing hyperglycemia. Glucagon causes blood glucose levels to rise, preventing hypoglycemia.

Glucagon is released by the alpha cells of the pancreas to prevent hypoglycemia by breaking down glycogen into glucose. It is released whenever blood glucose starts to fall below normal levels. The trigger for glucagon secretion is hypoglycemia, and its action is to raise the blood glucose level back up to normal. Glucagon starts actions that remove glucose from glycogen trees and allow the released free glucose to enter the blood (Figure 21.4). This action brings the blood glucose level back to normal (euglycemia). Because of glucagon, a person can go 10 to 12 hours without eating and not become so hypoglycemic that cells die.

The balance between insulin action and glucagon action keeps blood glucose levels in the normal range. Although the cell types for insulin and glucagon secretion are both in the pancreas, problems occur much more often with the cells that secrete insulin.

Insulin Enhancers

The beta cells of the pancreas also co-secrete two additional proteins along with insulin that increases insulin's effectiveness, the *incretin hormones* (especially *glucagon-like peptide 1 [GLP-1]*) and *amylin*. Like insulin, these substances are secreted when food is present in the stomach and blood glucose levels begin to rise. GLP-1 increases the rate of insulin secretion and slows the rate of stomach (gastric) emptying. This action allows glucose to enter the blood more slowly so that insulin secretion matches this rate to maintain euglycemia, and hyperglycemia does not occur. Amylin similarly helps prevent hyperglycemia by delaying gastric emptying and also by triggering a sense of satiety in the brain. *Satiety* sensation helps a person feel "full" or satisfied when eating and leads to the behavior of decreased food intake (less food intake; less hyperglycemia). Without these insulin enhancers, much more insulin would be needed to prevent hyperglycemia, and the balance of glucose uptake versus glucose storage would be more difficult to maintain.

PATHOPHYSIOLOGY OF THE ENDOCRINE PANCREAS: DIABETES MELLITUS

Diabetes mellitus (DM) is a common and complex metabolic disease that results from either the loss of the ability to make insulin or reduced receptor sensitivity to the

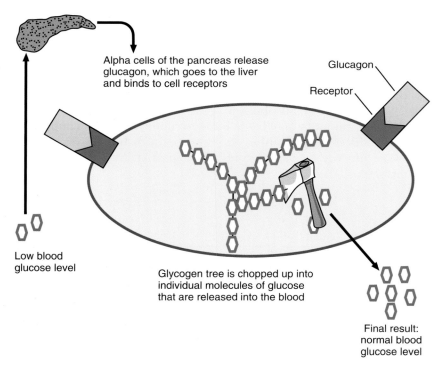

FIG. 21.4 Action of glucagon.

presence of insulin. The first result of either of these problems is hyperglycemia. There are a variety of types of DM but the two most common forms are type 1 (T1DM) and type 2 (T2DM). They differ in cause, usual age of onset, degree of insulin secretion remaining, and how they are treated. The two types have many of the same symptoms, and the long-term complications are the same. However, the drugs used to treat these disorders differ because people who have T1DM do not make any insulin and those with T2DM do continue to make some insulin but it is less effective at the cellular level.

About 35 million people in the United States have DM. More than 90% of those with the disease have T2DM and less than 10% have T1DM. Because people who have T2DM do produce insulin to some degree, symptoms are more subtle and the person may have the disorder for years before it is diagnosed. Often by the time it is diagnosed, some pathologic changes and organ damage have already occurred.

Type 1 Diabetes (T1DM)

Type 1 diabetes (T1DM) results when the beta cells of the pancreas no longer make and secrete any insulin. Usually, the beta cells have been destroyed, most often as part of an autoimmune response to a viral infection. In addition to loss of insulin production, beta cell production of incretins and amylin is also lost. Without insulin, the patient's blood glucose level becomes very high, but glucose cannot enter many cells. As a result, the body switches from using glucose to make ATP to using fat to make ATP. Overall, the body has less ATP available. Because insulin is no longer produced, patients who have T1DM must use insulin daily for the rest of their lives or receive a pancreas transplant.

Although T1DM can occur at any age, it most commonly begins in children and young adults. The first symptoms are caused by hyperglycemia. These include excessive hunger and eating (*polyphagia*), thirst, drinking more fluids than usual throughout the day (*polydipsia*), urinating more (*polyuria*), weight loss, and fatigue. The fasting blood glucose level is way above 110 mg/dL, and often glucose is present in the urine.

If T1DM is not treated with insulin, hyperglycemia worsens, and the body uses more fat for fuel. When fat is used to make ATP, a by-product is the formation of *ketoacids*. If these ketoacids form faster than they are eliminated, the patient develops *diabetic ketoacidosis (DKA)*, a serious complication that can result in coma and death.

Type 2 Diabetes (T2DM)

The cause of T2DM appears to be genetic, although not everyone with the known gene variations develops the disease. The biggest nongenetic risk factors for developing the disease are obesity and a sedentary lifestyle. With T2DM the person still has beta cells that make some insulin; however, the insulin receptors are not very sensitive to insulin. As a result, insulin does not bind as tightly to its receptors as it should, and less glucose moves from the blood into the cells. So, hyperglycemia is present with T2DM.

Long-Term Complications of Diabetes

Insulin is important for all types of metabolism, not just for glucose control. Without adequate amounts of insulin, the person with either type of diabetes has major changes in blood vessels that lead to organ damage, serious health problems, and early death. Box 21.2 lists many of the serious complications of untreated or poorly controlled diabetes. The long-term complications of the disease are the same for both T1DM and T2DM.

DRUG THERAPY FOR DIABETES

Drug therapy for diabetes reduces the risks for many long-term complications and extends life. Patients who are able to control blood glucose levels with a combination of drug therapy, diet, and regular exercise also live longer, healthier lives.

Memory Jogger

Diabetes is very common and type 2 DM is the most common type. Many people who have T2DM are unaware that they have this serious disorder until complications and organ damage are present.

Memory Jogger

Patients who have T1DM do not make their own insulin and must use insulin as a drug from other sources for glucose regulation.

Memory Jogger

Symptoms of untreated diabetes include excessive hunger, thirst, polydipsia, polyuria, weight loss, and fatigue.

Memory Jogger

Patients with T2DM make some of their own insulin, but the insulin receptors are resistant to binding with the insulin. This problem is most common among people who are overweight and sedentary. The incidence of T2DM has greatly increased in the past two decades as the incidence of obesity has risen, even among children.

Memory Jogger

Complications from untreated or poorly controlled diabetes include blindness; kidney failure; foot and leg amputations; hypertension; and increased risk for infection, heart attacks, and strokes.

Memory Jogger

The goal of drug therapy for T2DM is to keep blood glucose levels within target ranges and have reduced blood fat levels along with a close to normal body weight. *Causing hypoglycemia is to be avoided.*

Box 21.2   Complications of Poorly Controlled Diabetes

- Blindness
- Early death
- Erectile dysfunction
- High blood cholesterol levels
- High blood triglyceride levels
- Hypertension
- Increased risk for heart attack
- Increased risk for infection

- Increased risk for stroke
- Loss of touch sensation (peripheral neuropathy)
- Kidney failure
- Poor wound healing (especially on the feet and legs, leading to amputation)

The drug types used to manage diabetes are *insulin* and noninsulin *antidiabetic drugs.* **Antidiabetic drugs** include oral agents and some injectable drugs that increase the amounts of the natural insulin enhancers, incretins and amylin, which work with insulin. All patients with T1DM must receive *insulin* therapy as hormone replacement for the rest of their lives. For the patient who has T2DM and still makes some insulin, *antidiabetic drugs* help maintain normal blood glucose levels in a variety of ways. Because T2DM is most common and many more people use antidiabetic drug therapy, these drugs will be discussed first.

ANTIDIABETIC DRUG THERAPY

Antidiabetic drugs for T2DM used to be called hypoglycemic agents. However, because the goal of therapy is to help the person become euglycemic rather than hypoglycemic, the correct term is antidiabetic drug. Noninsulin **antidiabetic drugs** are oral and injectable drugs that use many actions to assist in lowering blood glucose levels. Because they work in different ways to control blood glucose levels, two or more drugs may be used together for best control. Some patients with T2DM also require insulin as temporary therapy during other illnesses or when the disease progresses to the point that therapy with diet, exercise, and antidiabetic drugs alone is insufficient to keep blood glucose levels within target ranges.

Antidiabetic agents for T2DM are classified by their actions to reduce blood glucose levels. The eight major classes of antidiabetic drugs are insulin "stimulators," biguanides, insulin sensitizers, alpha-glucosidase inhibitors, incretin mimetics (GLP-1 agonists), dipeptidyl peptidase-4 (DPP-4) inhibitors, amylin analogs, and sodium-glucose cotransporter 2 (SGLT2) inhibitors. The mechanism of action for each class of drugs is different and some classes contain more than one drug group. Which drug or drugs are used depends on how much beta-cell function is left, patient responses, and the patient's overall health. Often, more than one drug (from different classes) is used to reach the best blood glucose control. In this chapter, the drug dosages listed are for each drug prescribed alone. When drugs are used in combination, the dosages of one or more of the drugs in the combination are reduced.

General Issues for All Antidiabetic Drugs

Each class of antidiabetic drug has both unique and common actions and effects. Responsibilities for these common actions and effects are listed in the following paragraphs. Specific mechanisms of action, dosages, side effects and adverse effects, and responsibilities are listed with each individual class. Most drugs are started at a lower dosage and gradually increased to a level that is most effective for an individual patient.

Intended responses of antidiabetic drug therapy

- Laboratory values of blood glucose control are maintained within the patient's target ranges.
- Blood lipid levels are controlled.
- Progression of disease is slowed.
- Associated long-term organ damage is avoided.
- Patient's weight is normal or near-normal for height.

Memory Jogger

The eight classes of antidiabetic drugs are:
- Insulin stimulators
- Biguanides
- Insulin sensitizers
- Alpha-glucosidase inhibitors
- GLP-1 agonists
- DPP-4 inhibitors
- Amylin analogs
- SGLT2 inhibitors

Common side effects of antidiabetic drug therapy. The most common general side effects of antidiabetic drugs are nausea, vomiting, diarrhea, and rash. For injectable agents, the most common side effect is injection site reactions.

Possible adverse effects of antidiabetic drug therapy. *Hypoglycemia* is a constant possibility with antidiabetic drug therapy. Some drugs directly reduce blood drug levels and can lead to hypoglycemia. Other drugs prevent hyperglycemia but when taken along with an agent that directly lowers blood glucose levels, can potentiate a hypoglycemia episode. As stated earlier, hypoglycemia can quickly become worse, leading to shock and death. It must be avoided to prevent harm.

⭐ ***Priority actions to take*** *before* ***and*** *after* ***giving antidiabetic drugs***
Patients and their families are responsible for T2DM management at home using antidiabetic drug therapy. The most important nursing function is to provide extensive and appropriate teaching to patients and families so that they can self-manage these drugs safely. Dosing schedules can be complicated, with some drugs taken once daily, others multiple times of day, and still others on a weekly, rather than on a daily basis. Timing of dosages in coordination with meals is critically important for prevention of hypoglycemia, as well as for best overall glucose control. For injectable drugs given subcutaneously, use the teaching guide in Box 2.3 in Chapter 2 to help patients and families perform this technique correctly and safely. It is also critical to teach patients and families how to avoid, recognize, and manage episodes of hypoglycemia.

⭐ ***Teaching priorities for patients taking antidiabetic drugs***
Teach patients taking any antidiabetic drug regimen these general care issues and precautions:
- The best diabetes control occurs when your drug therapy is part of an overall lifestyle change that includes dietary modification and some level of regular exercise.
- Take your drug exactly as prescribed with regard to meals because not eating a meal with or shortly after taking these drugs can lead to dangerously low blood glucose levels.
- Keep a glucose source such as hard candies, glucose tablets or gel, sugar cubes, graham crackers, or saltine crackers with you at all times to take if you have symptoms of low blood glucose levels. These symptoms include hunger, headache, tremors, sweating, increased irritability, and an inability to concentrate or focus that can worsen to confusion.
- If you treat yourself for hypoglycemia, recheck your blood glucose level 15 minutes after eating the glucose source to determine whether more glucose is needed.
- Avoid drinking alcohol because it is likely to induce hypoglycemia. If alcohol is used, limit yourself to one serving and drink it either with food or right after you eat a meal.
- Always check your blood glucose level before performing an exercise session and avoid taking your drugs right before exercising. If your blood glucose level is below 80, do not exercise without eating first.
- If your drug is to be taken by subcutaneous injection, use the techniques taught to you to maintain sterility, ensure a correct dose, and prevent injection site reactions or complications.
- If you are ill and unable to eat or drink, **do not** take your regularly scheduled antidiabetic drugs without contacting your prescriber. Your prescriber will tell

Box 21.3	Signs and Symptoms of Hypoglycemia

- Anxiety, confusion, loss of consciousness
- Cool, clammy skin
- Headache
- Hunger
- Increased sweating
- Rapid, pounding heart rate
- Shakiness, tremors

Common Side Effects

Antidiabetic Drug Therapy

GI problems   Rash   Injection site reaction

⭐ **Critical Point for Safety**

The most frequent adverse effect of antidiabetic drug therapy is severe hypoglycemia, which can rapidly lead to shock and death. Symptoms include hunger, headache, tremors, sweating, and confusion. Teach patients and families how to avoid situations leading to hypoglycemia and steps to take to correct it.

QSEN: Safety

 Drug Alert

Teaching Alert

Teach patients taking antidiabetic drugs to avoid drinking alcohol because it is likely to induce hypoglycemia. If alcohol is used, it should be limited to one serving and taken either with food or right after a meal is completed.

QSEN: Safety

you whether the dose should be skipped or decreased and whether you need to go to a hospital.

- Wear a medical alert bracelet or carry a wallet card with you at all times that states you have diabetes and which drugs you take.
- Most of the antidiabetic drugs interact with hundreds of other drugs. Do not take other prescribed or over-the-counter drugs and supplements unless approved by your prescriber.

Life span considerations for antidiabetic drugs

Pediatric considerations. Although type 2 diabetes is becoming increasingly common among children starting around age 10 years as a result of the rising obesity problem, few antidiabetic drugs have been approved for use in children. Currently, the two drug classes that are approved for use in children are the biguanides and meglitinide analogs. Dosages for a child are based on how he or she responds to the drug rather than by size and weight.

Considerations for pregnancy and lactation. Diabetes is often more difficult to control during this physically stressful time. In addition, some patients who do not have diabetes may have problems with high blood glucose levels only during pregnancy. Insulin is the drug of choice for treating hyperglycemia during pregnancy. The antidiabetic drugs are not approved for use during pregnancy and breastfeeding.

Insulin Stimulators

Antidiabetic drug groups that are insulin stimulators are the second-generation sulfonylureas (*glimepiride, glipizide, glyburide*) and the meglitinide analogs (*nateglinide, repaglinide*). The table below lists the names and adult dosages of the most common drugs in this class for initial and progressive therapy. Dosage increases are individualized based on patient responses.

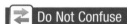
Critical Point for Safety

The only drug approved to manage diabetes during pregnancy is insulin. Breastfeeding when taking other antidiabetic drugs is not recommended because some do enter the breast milk and it is not known what effect they may have on the nursing infant.

QSEN: Safety

Do Not Confuse

glipizide *with* glyburide

An order for glipizide can be confused with glyburide. Although both drugs are oral antidiabetic drugs from the second-generation sulfonylurea class, the dosages are very different.

QSEN: Safety

Common Adult Dosages for Insulin Stimulator Antidiabetic Drugs

Drug Groups	Drug Names	Usual Maintenance Dosages
Sulfonylureas	glimepiride ❶ (Amaryl)	1–4 mg orally once daily with breakfast or first meal of the day
	glipzide ❶ (Glucatrol, Glucatrol XL)	10–15 mg orally daily 30 min before breakfast or first meal of the day
	glyburide ❶ (Diabeta, Glycron, Glynase, Micronase)	2.5–10 mg orally daily with breakfast or first meal of the day. Max: 20 mg daily
Meglitinide Analogs	nateglinide ❶ (Starlix)	120 mg orally 30 min before each meal of the day
	repaglinide ❶ (Prandin)	0.5–4 mg orally 30 min before each meal of the day (not to exceed 4 doses)

❶ High-alert drug.

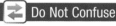
Do Not Confuse

Micronase *with* Microzide

An order for Micronase can be confused with Microzide. Micronase is an oral antidiabetic drug, whereas Microzide is a diuretic.

QSEN: Safety

How insulin stimulators work. Insulin stimulators work directly on the beta cells of the pancreas to release preformed insulin. The increased insulin then lowers blood glucose levels. These drugs require that significant numbers of healthy beta cells be present for this mechanism of action.

Additional side effects and possible adverse effects of insulin stimulators. In addition to the general common side effects and adverse effects of antidiabetic drugs, *sulfonylureas* also may cause increased sun sensitivity (photosensitivity), blurred vision, fluid retention, and anemia. *Meglitinides* also may cause dizziness, back pain, upper respiratory infections, and flu-like achiness.

⊛ *Teaching priorities for patients taking insulin stimulators*

In addition to the general teaching priorities on pp. 391–392, include these precautions and care issues for patients taking an insulin stimulator:

- Be sure to tell your prescriber if you have an allergy to sulfonamide antibiotics because it is likely that you will also have an allergy to the sulfonylureas and should not take these drugs.
- If you take a sulfonylurea (glimepiride, glipizide, or glyburide), avoid direct sunlight, use sunscreen, and wear protective clothing (including a hat) whenever you are outside because these drugs increase sun sensitivity and can cause a severe sunburn, even if you have darker skin.
- If you take either nateglinide or repaglinide and eat more than three meals in a day, also take the drug with each of the extra meals. If you miss a meal, skip that meal's drug dose to prevent hypoglycemia.

Biguanides: Metformin

Currently, metformin (*Fortamet, Glucophage, Glucophage XR, Riomet*) is the only drug in the biguanide class. Although an older drug, it is still in common use today because it has several mechanisms of action for effective blood glucose control. The usual dosage for the immediate-release formulation is 500 to 850 mg orally twice daily with meals. The extended-release dosage is 500 to 2000 mg orally once daily with the evening meal. All formulations of metformin are considered high-alert drugs.

How metformin works. One way metformin prevents hyperglycemia is by inhibiting liver conversion of glycogen into glucose and its release into the blood. This drug also slows intestinal absorption of glucose, which allows the patient's own insulin production to better match any increase in blood glucose level. Metformin also increases the sensitivity of insulin receptors so that more of the patient's own insulin binds effectively.

Additional side effects and possible adverse effects of metformin. In addition to the general common side effects and adverse effects of antidiabetic drugs, metformin can cause bloating, flatulence, indigestion, abdominal pain, and headache. A severe adverse effect of metformin is *lactic acidosis,* which is the buildup of lactic acid in tissues when not enough oxygen is present to allow metabolism to occur normally. Signs and symptoms of lactic acidosis are muscle aches, fatigue, drowsiness, abdominal pain, hypotension, and a slow, irregular heartbeat. Drinking alcohol, having liver disease, being dehydrated, or having kidney problems increases the risk for lactic acidosis.

Tests that involve the use of radio-opaque dye (such as urograms, angiograms, and other scans) can lead to kidney failure with metformin, usually within 48 hours. A patient who takes metformin may take the dose before receiving the dye but should not resume the drug again until 48 hours after testing with dye or surgery with anesthesia, or until good urine output has been reestablished.

Metformin must be used with caution in adults older than age 65. The older adult is more likely to have heart failure, poor circulation, kidney disease, or liver disease. All of these problems greatly increase the risk for the complication of lactic acidosis. If the drug is prescribed for an older adult, more careful monitoring of kidney and heart function is needed. Metformin is not recommended for patients older than age 80.

⊛ *Teaching priorities for patients taking metformin*

In addition to the general teaching priorities on pp. 391–392, include these precautions and care issues for patients taking metformin:

- Do not crush or chew the extended release (XR) metformin tablets because crushing the tablet destroys its time-release properties and may allow too much drug to enter your bloodstream at one time.

 Drug Alert

Teaching Alert

Meglitinide drug doses are matched to meals. If a meal is missed, that drug dose must also be missed to prevent hypoglycemia.

QSEN: Safety

 Memory Jogger

All formulations of metformin are considered high-alert drugs.

 Critical Point for Safety

Metformin can cause lactic acidosis. Do not give this drug within 48 hours to anyone who has had testing with radio-opaque dye unless adequate kidney function has been determined.

QSEN: Safety

- Take the drug with food.
- Many people experience gastrointestinal discomfort when first starting metformin. Often, these problems go away over time.
- Drink plenty of water (day and night) to avoid dehydration and a complication called lactic acidosis. This problem is more likely to occur when alcohol is used.
- Check with your prescriber 2 days before having any imaging procedure involving the use of dye. Depending on the dye, you may need to stop taking the drug before the procedure and not start taking it again for 48 hours or until your kidney function returns to normal after the procedure to prevent kidney problems.
- If you become pregnant, contact your prescriber immediately because metformin is not recommended during pregnancy.

Insulin Sensitizers: Thiazolidinediones

Insulin sensitizers are the thiazolidinediones or "glitizones" and "TZDs" that increase the sensitivity of the insulin receptor for insulin binding. The table below lists the names and adult dosages of the most common drugs in this class for initial and progressive therapy.

Adult Dosages for Insulin Sensitizers: Thiazolidinediones

Drug Names	Usual Maintenance Dosages
pioglitazone ❶ (Actos)	15–45 mg orally once daily
rosiglitizone ❶ (Avandia)	2–4 mg orally twice daily or 4–8 mg once daily

❶ High-alert drug.

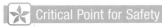
Do Not Confuse

Actos *with* Actonel

An order for Actos can be confused with Actonel. Actos is an oral antidiabetic drug from the thiazolidinedione class, whereas Actonel is a drug that prevents calcium loss from bones.

QSEN: Safety

How insulin sensitizers work. Insulin sensitizers do not act directly on the beta cells of the pancreas. Instead, they lower blood glucose levels by increasing the sensitivity of the insulin receptor to the binding of naturally secreted insulin, which improves the movement of glucose from the blood into the cells. These drugs also decrease liver conversion of glycogen into glucose. As a result, these drugs lower blood glucose levels to normal without causing hypoglycemia.

Additional side effects and possible adverse effects of insulin sensitizers. In addition to the general common side effects and adverse effects of antidiabetic drugs, TZDs may cause upper respiratory infections, headaches, muscle aches, fluid retention, weight gain, and anemia. These drugs, especially *rosiglitazone* (Avandia), may lead to heart failure as a result of water retention. In addition, rosiglitazone has a black box warning indicating that it should not be prescribed for anyone who has moderate to severe heart failure or who is at risk for heart failure. The edema associated with these drugs can cause macular edema in the eye and interfere with vision. The TZDs can cause liver impairment, leading to jaundice, higher-than-normal liver enzymes, and difficulty digesting fatty meals. In addition, cholesterol levels often increase during TZD therapy.

Critical Point for Safety

Do **not** give the thiazolidinediones to a patient with severe heart failure. Assess patients with mild heart failure frequently for indications of worsening heart failure such as rapid weight gain, hypotension, and difficulty breathing.

QSEN: Safety

⊛ ***Teaching priorities for patients taking insulin sensitizers***

In addition to the general teaching priorities on pp. 391–392, include these precautions and care issues for patients taking an insulin sensitizer:

- Check yourself daily for yellowing of your skin, the roof of your mouth, or whites of your eyes, which may indicate a liver problem. Also check for lack of appetite, dark urine, or pale stools. Notify your prescriber if you notice any of these symptoms.
- These drugs can cause or worsen heart failure. Weigh yourself daily. If your weight increases by more than 3 lb in 1 week, it may be an indication of heart failure. Also check your ankles for swelling daily, which is another indication of heart failure. If you have increasing difficulty breathing, weight gain, or ankle swelling, notify your prescriber immediately.
- Report persistent vision changes to your prescriber because these drugs can cause edema in the eye.

• Keep all appointments for laboratory work to check your liver function and cholesterol levels. This drug class often causes an increase in blood cholesterol levels.

Alpha-Glucosidase Inhibitors

Alpha-glucosidase inhibitors are a unique type of oral antidiabetic drug. The table below lists the names and adult dosages of the most common drugs in this class.

Usual Adult Dosages of Common Alpha-Glucosidase Inhibitors

Drug Names	Usual Maintenance Dosages
acarbose (Precos)	Initially: 25 mg orally 3 times daily with the first bite of a meal After 4 weeks: 50–100 mg orally 3 times daily with the first bite of a meal
miglitol (Glyset)	Initially: 25 mg orally 3 times daily with the first bite of a meal After 4 weeks: 50 mg orally 3 times daily with the first bite of a meal

How alpha-glucosidase inhibitors work. Alpha-glucosidase inhibitors are oral antidiabetic drugs that work by slowing the digestion of dietary starches and other complex carbohydrates by inhibiting an enzyme in the intestinal tract that breaks them down into glucose. The result of this action is that blood glucose does not rise as far or as fast after a meal. Drugs from this class do not cause hypoglycemia when taken as the only therapy for diabetes. These are the only antidiabetic drugs that are not considered "high-alert."

Additional side effects and possible adverse effects of alpha-glucosidase inhibitors. Although all oral antidiabetic drugs are associated with some gastrointestinal side effects, alpha-glucosidase inhibitors always cause these side effects because the intestinal tract is the site of their actions. These drugs are not to be used by anyone who is malnourished or has difficulty digesting or absorbing food, such as patients with ulcerative colitis or Crohn disease. The alpha-glucosidase inhibitors may induce liver impairment.

 Critical Point for Safety

The alpha-glucosidase inhibitors interfere with carbohydrate and glucose nutrient absorption. This class of drugs is contraindicated in patients who are already malnourished or have difficulty digesting or absorbing food, such as those with ulcerative colitis or Crohn disease. In such patients, excessive weight loss and iron deficiency anemia are more likely.

QSEN: Safety

⊛ ***Teaching priorities for patients taking alpha-glucosidase inhibitors***
In addition to the general teaching priorities on p. 391–392, include these precautions and care issues for patients taking an alpha-glucosidase inhibitor:

• This drug works by preventing the breakdown of starches to form glucose in your intestinal tract and are only effective with a meal. **If you do not eat a meal, do not take the drug.**
• Keep the individual tablets in their wrapped packages to prevent deterioration from exposure to moisture.
• Assess yourself weekly and report any skin yellowing, pain over the liver area, or darkening of the urine to your prescriber immediately because these drugs can reduce liver function.
• Gastrointestinal problems are very common because these drugs greatly increase gas formation. This problem is expected and does not represent a bad reaction to the drug.
• If you are ill with vomiting or diarrhea, stop taking the drug until you are able to eat normally again.
• Because these drugs interfere with intestinal absorption, it is best to take any other prescribed drugs either 2 hours before or 2 hours after taking this antidiabetic drug.

Incretin Mimetics: GLP-1 Agonists

The **GLP-1 agonists** are incretin mimetic drugs taken by subcutaneous (SC) injection that enhance insulin action. At present, these drugs are only approved for use with patients who have T2DM. The table below lists the names and adult dosages of the most common drugs in this class.

Adult Dosages of Common GLP-1 Agonists

Drug Names	Usual Maintenance Dosages
dulaglutide ❶ (TRULICITY)	Initially: 0.75 mg SC **weekly** Maintenance: 1.5–4.5 mg SC **weekly**
exenatide ❶ (Byetta)	5–10 mcg SC twice daily 30 min before morning and evening meals
exenatide XR ❶ (Bydureon, Bydureon BCise)	2 mg SC once **weekly**
liraglutide (Saxenda, Victoza)	Initially: 0.6 mg SC once daily for 1 week Maintenance: 1.2–1.8 mg SC once daily
lixisenatide ❶ (ADLYXIN)	Initially: 10 mcg SC once daily for 14 days Maintenance: 20 mcg SC once daily
semaglutide ❶ (OZEMPIC, Rybelsus, Wegovy)	Initially: 0.25 mg SC once **weekly** Maintenance: 0.25–1 mg SC once **weekly**

❶ High-alert drug; *SC*, subcutaneously.

How GLP-1 agonists work. GLP1 agonists work by acting like natural "gut" hormones (incretins) that are secreted with meals at the same time insulin is secreted and help lower blood glucose levels in several ways. They inhibit glucagon secretion thus reducing liver production of glucose and they delay gastric emptying. This slows the rate of glucose absorption into the blood and makes the person feel full. The actions of these drugs rely on pancreatic insulin production.

Additional side effects and possible adverse effects of GLP-1 agonists. In addition to the general common side effects and adverse effects of antidiabetic drugs, GLP-1 agonists are associated with an increased risk for pancreatitis with symptoms of persistent abdominal pain and nausea. These drugs are associated with an increased risk for certain types of thyroid cancer. They have a black box warning indicating the GLP-1 agonists are not to be used by anyone who has or has had thyroid cancer, or who has a close family member who has had thyroid cancer.

⊛ ***Teaching priorities for patients taking GLP-1 agonists***
In addition to the general teaching priorities on pp. 391–392, include these precautions and care issues for patients taking GLP-1 agonists:
- If you are prescribed to take dulaglutide, exenatide XL, or semaglutide, remember that these drugs are taken only once **weekly**, not daily. Taking one of these drugs more often than once per week can lead to a dangerous overdose.
- These drugs come in prefilled pens that contain a month's supply. Store the pens in the refrigerator and never freeze them. Warm temperatures, freezing temperatures, and exposure to light can make all these drugs lose their effectiveness.
- If you are performing self-injection of this drug, follow package directions for activating the pen and use the directions taught to you for subcutaneous injections (Box 2.3 in Chapter 2).
- Check your injection sites daily for indications of infection such as warmth, redness at or around the injection site, swelling, pain, skin that is firm to the touch, or foul-smelling drainage.
- If you notice a swelling at the front of your neck, notify your prescriber immediately because drugs from this class have an increased risk for thyroid cancer.
- If you develop persistent pain above or around your stomach and have nausea and vomiting, notify your prescriber because these are symptoms of pancreatitis, an adverse effect of this drug.

⬟ Critical Point for Safety

Some GLP-1 drugs are taken daily and others are taken **weekly**. Many patients are unfamiliar with drugs taken only once weekly. Teach patients who are prescribed to take a drug weekly **never** to take it daily. This would result in a severe overdose.

QSEN: Safety

Dipeptidyl Peptidase-4 (DPP-4) Inhibitors
The DPP-4 inhibitors are oral antidiabetic drugs taken along with at least one other antidiabetic drug to control blood glucose levels. The table below lists the names and adult dosages of the most common drugs in this class.

Adult Dosages of Common DPP-4 Inhibitors

Drug Names	Usual Maintenance Dosages
alogliptin ❶ (Nesina)	25 mg orally once daily
linagliptin ❶ (Trajenta)	5 mg orally once daily
saxagliptin ❶ (Onglyza)	2.5–5 mg orally once daily
sitagliptin ❶ (Januvia)	100 mg orally once daily

❶ High-alert drug.

How DPP-4 inhibitors work. DPP-4 inhibitors work by inhibiting the enzyme DDP-4, which normally breaks down and inactivates the incretin hormones, especially GLP-1. By inhibiting this enzyme, DPP-4 inhibitor drugs slow the inactivation of the natural incretin hormones. Thus, it increases the active incretin hormone levels in the body, reducing both before- and after-meal blood glucose levels. These drugs work only when blood glucose is elevated.

Additional side effects and possible adverse effects of DPP-4 inhibitors. In addition to the general common side effects and adverse effects of antidiabetic drugs, DPP-4 inhibitors may cause abdominal pain, pancreatitis, and an increased incidence of respiratory infections. They also are associated with a higher incidence of serious allergic reactions, including anaphylaxis, angioedema, and Stevens-Johnson syndrome. Some people have developed severe joint pain (arthralgia) while taking drugs from this class that becomes so disabling the drug needs to be discontinued.

⊛ *Teaching priorities for patients taking DPP-4 inhibitors.* In addition to the general teaching priorities on pp. 391–392, include these precautions and care issues for patients taking DPP-4 inhibitors:
* Drugs in this class have a higher risk for allergic reactions. If you have a rash, itching, or hives, notify your prescriber immediately. If you have swelling of the face, lips, or tongue, or difficulty breathing, call 911 immediately.
* If you develop persistent pain above or around your stomach and have nausea and vomiting, notify your prescriber because these are symptoms of pancreatitis, a possible adverse effect of this drug.
* If you develop severe joint pain while taking this drug, contact your prescriber. Some people may need to stop this drug if the joint pain interferes with their daily activities.

Amylin Analogs

Amylin analogs are synthetic oral antidiabetic drugs similar to the naturally produced amylin, which is an insulin enhancer. Currently, the only drug in this class is *pramlintide* (Symlin). This drug works to reduce hyperglycemia in three ways: delaying gastric emptying to lower the rate of glucose entry into the blood after meals; suppressing the liver conversion of glycogen into glucose; triggering the sensation of satiety in the brain. Because amylin is normally co-secreted by pancreatic beta cells along with insulin, amylin is absent in people with type 1 diabetes and present in very low levels in people with type 2 diabetes.

Pramlintide is the only noninsulin antidiabetic drug approved for use in both T1DM and T2DM. For people with T1DM, initial dosages start at 15 mcg subcutaneously immediately before each major meal. The dose is gradually increased up to 60 mcg. For people with T2DM, initial dosages start at 60 mcg subcutaneously immediately before each major meal and are gradually increased to 120 mcg/dose. For most people taking this drug, over time lower dosages of insulin and other antidiabetic drugs are required to maintain good glucose control.

Additional side effects and possible adverse effects of amylin analogs. Because pramlintide delays gastric emptying, it can reduce or delay the rate of absorption for

 Critical Point for Safety

Pramlintide, an amylin analog, is the only noninsulin antidiabetic drug approved for use in patients with T1DM, as well as for T2DM. However, dosages used to manage the two types of diabetes are different.

QSEN: Safety

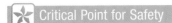

other drugs the patient takes, especially for those that have a desired rapid onset of action such as analgesics. The drug can cause significant nausea at the beginning of therapy that decreases over time. Pramlintide may cause pancreatitis. Because these injections are frequent (several times daily), fatty changes in the subcutaneous tissue are common. Lipodystrophy, in which the fatty tissue accumulates around an injection site, results in a lumpy skin appearance. Lipoatrophy, in which fatty tissue breaks down in an injection site area, results in a skin depression.

⭐ *Teaching priorities for patients taking amylin analogs.* In addition to the general teaching priorities on pp. 391–392, include these precautions and care issues for patients taking pramlintide:

- If you also inject insulin before meals, **do not** mix these two drugs in the same syringe, and be sure to use two completely different injection sites for each drug.
- Use the abdomen or the fronts and sides of the thighs as injection sites. **Do not** use the arms because drug absorption from the arms is variable and the drug may not be absorbed in time to work with the meal being eaten.
- Pramlintide comes in prefilled pens that do not contain a needle. These must be purchased separately. Store the pens in the refrigerator and never freeze them. Warm temperatures, freezing temperatures, and exposure to light can all make the drug lose its effectiveness.
- Follow package directions for activating the pen, cleaning the pen tip, and attaching the needle. Use the directions taught to you for subcutaneous injections.
- Check your injection sites daily for indications of infection such as warmth, redness at or around the injection site, swelling, pain, skin that is firm to the touch, or foul-smelling drainage.
- Because pramlintide makes insulin and all other antidiabetic drugs work better, you are at greater risk for developing low blood glucose levels. Check your blood glucose levels at least several times daily to identify and prevent your blood glucose level from becoming too low.
- Drugs in this class have a higher risk for allergic reactions. If you have a rash, itching, or hives, notify your prescriber immediately. If you have swelling of the face, lips, or tongue, or difficulty breathing, call 911 immediately.
- If you take prescribed drugs for other health problems, their absorption could be delayed if taken too close to the time pramlintide is injected. If possible, take other drugs at least an hour before or an hour after injecting pramlintide and eating a meal.
- If you develop persistent pain above or around your stomach and have nausea and vomiting, notify your prescriber because these are symptoms of pancreatitis, an adverse effect of this drug.

Sodium-Glucose Cotransporter 2 (SGLT2) Inhibitors

Sodium-glucose cotransporter 2 (SGLT2) inhibitors are a newer class of oral antidiabetic drugs that help remove glucose from the blood by preventing kidney reabsorption of filtered glucose. They are approved for use in patients with T2DM for blood glucose control. Additionally, SGLT2 inhibitors are approved for use to increase cardiac function in patients with heart failure and low ejection fractions. The table below lists the names and adult dosages of the most common drugs in this class.

Adult Dosages of Common Sodium-Glucose Cotransporter 2 (SGLT2) Inhibitors

Drug Name	Usual Maintenance Dosage
canagliflozin ❶ (Invokana)	100 mg orally daily before breakfast. Max dose: 300 mg
dapagliflozin ❶ (Farxiga)	5 mg orally once daily before breakfast. Max dose: 10 mg
empagliflozin ❶ (Jardiance)	10 mg orally once daily before breakfast. Max dose: 25 mg
ertugliflozin ❶ (Steglatro)	5 mg orally once daily in the morning.[a] Max dose: 15 mg

❶ High-alert drug; [a]can be taken with or without food.

How SGLT2 inhibitors work. Glucose from the blood is freely filtered in the glomerulus of the kidney. Much of it is reabsorbed back into the blood by specific transporters in the kidney tubules that also transport filtered sodium at the same time. For a healthy person with normal blood glucose levels, all filtered glucose is reabsorbed back into the blood and none is present in the urine. If glucose levels are high enough, the transporters cannot reabsorb it all and some glucose remains in the urine and is excreted. SGLT2 inhibitors lower blood glucose levels by preventing kidney reabsorption of filtered glucose back into the blood. As a result, most of the filtered glucose gets excreted in the urine and blood glucose levels are lower. By keeping more glucose in the urine, urine osmolarity is higher and a diuretic effect also occurs.

Additional side effects and possible adverse effects of SGLT2 inhibitors. In addition to the general common side effects and adverse effects of antidiabetic drugs, SGLT2 inhibitors are associated with an increased risk for pancreatitis. They also can increase urine output to the extent that dehydration and electrolyte imbalances can occur, especially of sodium and potassium. The fluid volume lost from the blood causes hypotension, dizziness, and an increased risk for falls. Because these drugs increase the amount of glucose in the urine, serious urinary tract infections including cystitis and pyelonephritis have occurred, along with an increased risk for vaginal infections. In addition, infections of the skin of the perineum have occurred, including a rare complication in which the perineal skin developed a life-threatening condition, called necrotizing fasciitis (tissue necrosis). This problem is also known as Fournier gangrene, and drugs in this class have a black box warning for it.

⊛ *Teaching priorities for patients taking SGLT2 inhibitors.* In addition to the general teaching priorities on pp. 391–392, include these precautions and care issues for patients taking SGLT2 inhibitors:

- Get up slowly from a lying or sitting position because this drug can lower your blood pressure and make you feel dizzy and unsteady on your feet. Use handrails when going up and down steps to prevent falls.
- Drink plenty of water and other fluids to prevent dehydration because this drug increases your urine output. Symptoms of dehydration include lightheadedness, dry mouth and mucous membranes, and dizziness on standing.
- If you develop pain and burning during urination, notify your prescriber immediately because urinary tract infections are more common and can be more serious when taking this drug.
- If the skin around your genitals becomes sore, swollen, reddened, or irritated, contact your prescriber to have him or her examine the area because some very serious skin infections have occurred among people taking this drug.
- If you develop persistent pain above or around your stomach and have nausea and vomiting, notify your prescriber because these are symptoms of pancreatitis, an adverse effect of this drug.

Combination Antidiabetic Drug Therapy

Often T2DM is best controlled using more than one antidiabetic drug. To simplify drug therapy, some oral drugs have been combined. The patient may not understand that a single tablet contains more than one drug. Be sure to teach the patient about the side effects, adverse effects, and issues that should be reported to their prescriber for both drugs contained in a combination tablet.

The table below lists examples of the most common current combination drug therapy for oral antidiabetic drugs that are still available in the United States. Consult a reliable drug reference for specific information about dosages and scheduling of these drugs and for the less common combination agents.

 Critical Point for Safety

Teach patients prescribed any combination oral antidiabetic drug that the single tablet does contain more than one drug and that the precautions and care issues needed include all the ones for each individual drug within the tablet.

QSEN: Safety

Common Oral Combination Antidiabetic Drugs for Type 2 Diabetes

Drug Name	Drugs Contained Within the Combination
Duetact	pioglitazone; glimepiride
Glyxambi	empagliflozin; linagliptin
Janumet	sitagliptin; metformin
Jentadueto	linagliptin; metformin
Kazano	alogliptin; metformin
Kombiglyze XR	metformin; sitagliptin
Segluromet	ertugliflozin; metformin
Steguljan	ertugliflozin; sitagliptin
Synjardy	empagliflozin; metformin
Trijardy XR	empagliflozin; linagliptin; extended-release metformin
Xigduo XR	dapagliflozin; metformin

Memory Jogger

Because insulin is destroyed by stomach acids and intestinal enzymes, it cannot be used as an oral drug. Most commonly it is injected subcutaneously, although inhaled formulations are now available.

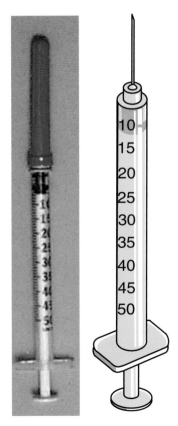

FIG. 21.5 50-unit (U-50) insulin syringes. (From Lilley, L., Harrington, S., & Snyder, J. [2007]. *Pharmacology and the nursing process* [5th ed.]. St. Louis: Mosby.)

INSULIN DRUG THERAPY

Insulin must be used as drug therapy for people with T1DM because they do not produce their own insulin. The goals of insulin therapy for T1DM are to maintain blood glucose levels within the normal range, avoid ketoacidosis, and prevent or delay the blood vessel changes that lead to organ damage. In addition, insulin may be an "add-on" drug for people with T2DM whose target blood glucose levels cannot be maintained with diet, exercise, and antidiabetic drug therapy. Insulin is a small protein that is destroyed by stomach acids and intestinal enzymes. As a result, it is most commonly taken parenterally. Recently, some forms of commercially available insulin are being atomized into a spray and inhaled through the nose.

Types of Insulin

Although some insulin is obtained from animal sources, today most of it is synthetic human insulin produced by recombinant DNA technology. Regardless of insulin type, it is a high-alert drug, meaning that it can cause serious harm if the wrong dose is given, if a dose is given to a patient for whom it was not prescribed, or if a dose is not given to a patient for whom it was prescribed.

For most patients with diabetes, insulin is injected subcutaneously using a special syringe with a short, thin needle (Figure 21.5). Special internal and external insulin pumps also can be used to deliver insulin either continuously as needed or hourly. Although both of these methods have advantages over regular injections, they are expensive and have some complications. Thus, most patients with T1DM use either standard insulin syringes or prefilled automatic syringes or pens to inject insulin from once to as many as 8 or 10 times each day.

Many types of insulin are available as therapy for T1DM, although all insulin works in the same way at the cellular level. Insulin types vary by how fast they work, how long the effects last (duration), and whether they are synthetic or come from animal sources. Table 21.2 lists the most common types of insulin for general injection and their features. Be sure to consult a reliable drug reference for more information about other specific insulin formulations.

How insulin drug therapy works. Just like the insulin the body makes, insulin injected into the body binds to insulin receptors on the membranes of many cells. The result of having the injected insulin bound to its receptor is that the cell membrane becomes more open to glucose, allowing glucose to leave the blood and enter cells (see Fig. 21.2). As glucose from the blood enters the cells, the blood glucose level is reduced to normal (euglycemia). If too much insulin is injected or

Table 21.2	Types and Durations of Insulin			
PREPARATION	**TRADE NAME**	**ONSET (hr)**	**PEAK (hr)**	**DURATION (hr)**
Rapid-Acting Insulin				
Insulin aspart	Fiasp, NovoLog	0.25	1–3	3–5
Insulin glulisine	Apidra, SoloStar,	0.3	0.5–1.5	3–4
Insulin lispro injection	Admelog, Humalog	0.25	0.5–1.5	5
Insulin human inhalation	Afrezza	0.25	0.1–1.5	3–4
Short-Acting Insulin				
Regular human insulin injection	Humulin R,	0.5	2–4	5–7
	Novolin R	0.5	2.5–5	8
	ReliOn R	0.5	2.5–5	8
Intermediate-Acting Insulin				
Isophane insulin NPH injection	Humulin N	1.5	4–12	10–16 or longer
	Iletin II NPH			
	Novolin N			
70% human insulin isophane suspension/30% human regular insulin injection	Humulin 70/30	0.5	6–10	10–16
	Novolin 70/30	0.5	6–10	10–16
50% human insulin isophane suspension/50% human insulin injection	Humulin 50/50	0.5	3–5	10–16 or longer
70% insulin aspart protamine suspension/30% insulin aspart injection	NovoLog Mix 70/30	0.25	1–4	18–24
75% insulin lispro protamine suspension/25% insulin lispro injection	Humalog Mix 75/25	0.25–5	2–3	12–24
	Humalog KwikPen Mix 75/25			
50% insulin lispro protamine suspension/50% insulin lispro injection	Humalog mix 50/50	0.25–5	2–3	12–24
	Humalog KwikPen Mix 50/50			
Long-Acting Insulin				
Insulin degludec	Treseba	1	12	42
Insulin detemir injection	Levemir	1	None	5.7–24
Insulin glargine injection	Basaglar, Lantus, Semglee, Toujeo	2	None	24
Insulin degludec/Insulin aspart	RYZODEG	0.25–0.75	2–4	24–30

if the patient's blood glucose level is not high enough when it is given, hypoglycemia can occur.

Intended responses of insulin drug therapy
- Blood glucose levels are in the normal range.
- There is no glucose or acetone in the urine.
- Blood lipid levels are at or close to the normal range.
- Long-term complications of diabetes are delayed

Common side effects of insulin drug therapy. Insulin as a drug has few side effects. Side effects are usually related to having repeated subcutaneous injections at one site or body area. These problems include injection site infections and changes in the skin and subcutaneous tissue at injection sites.

Possible adverse effects of insulin drug therapy. The main adverse effect of insulin is the lowering of blood glucose levels below normal (hypoglycemia). This action, sometimes called insulin shock, is dangerous because brain cells are very sensitive to low blood glucose levels and the patient can become nonresponsive very quickly. If the problem is not corrected quickly, the patient can die. The signs and symptoms of hypoglycemia are listed in Box 21.3.

Critical Point for Safety

Hypoglycemia is *always* a potential adverse effect of insulin therapy. Patients must learn to balance their carbohydrate intake with the timing of peak action for whatever insulin types they take to help prevent hypoglycemia.

QSEN: Safety

Insulin regimens. The goal of insulin therapy for patients with T1DM is to keep blood glucose levels within the normal range at all times. Better overall blood glucose control occurs with multiple injections of insulin each day.

An *insulin regimen* or program is the insulin injection schedule used to prevent hyperglycemia. The most effective regimens are those that provide insulin in a pattern that closely resembles the way insulin normally is released from the healthy pancreas. The normal pancreas releases a constant (basal) amount of insulin that keeps blood glucose levels normal between meals by balancing liver glucose production with whole-body glucose use. The normal pancreas is also stimulated by eating food to produce additional insulin to prevent blood glucose levels from rising too high after meals.

The total amount of insulin needed and how often it is needed for blood glucose control varies from patient to patient. Usually, the patient injects long-acting insulin at the beginning of the day for a basal dose. Shorter-acting insulin is taken before meals and snacks. The amount of insulin needed and injected is based on blood glucose levels. The patient checks his or her blood glucose level 2 to 12 times each day based on the specific insulin regimen, activity level, age, total amount of calories needed in a day, and how his or her blood glucose level responds to the insulin.

Some patients who have T1DM inject insulin as a combination of more than one insulin type administered just once daily. However, control of blood glucose is managed better when insulin injections of smaller dosages are used more frequently. Regardless of the type of regimen, whenever short-acting insulin is given before a meal, the meal should be eaten within 15 minutes after receiving the injection to avoid hypoglycemia.

The most recommended insulin regimen for best control is the intensified regimen. These regimens include a basal dose of intermediate- or long-acting insulin and multiple-bolus doses of short- or rapid-acting insulin designed to bring the next blood glucose value into the target range. Insulin dosage is based on the patient's blood glucose patterns. Usually, the patient must check the blood glucose levels at least eight times per day. Blood glucose testing 1 to 2 hours after meals and within 10 minutes before the next meal helps to determine how effective the bolus dose is.

⭐ *Priority actions to take **before** and **after** giving insulin.* Insulin drug errors are common and have serious consequences, including death. The many different types of insulin increase the risk for errors. It is important not to interchange insulin types and to ensure that the dose prescribed is the one given.

Test the patient's blood glucose level before giving insulin and make sure that the patient can and will eat within 15 minutes of the insulin injection to prevent hypoglycemia. It is best to ensure that the meal is actually on the unit before giving the insulin.

Check the order carefully for the exact type and amount of insulin to be injected. Do not interchange insulin types. Insulin preparations are available in U-50, U-100, and U-500 concentrations. The most commonly used preparation is U-100 insulin (100 units per mL). When doses are less than 50 units, they are usually administered with a U-50 syringe (50 units per 0.5 mL). This drug is available in a concentration of 50 units on a 0.5-mL volume. U-100 insulin provides 100 units of insulin in 1 mL of the drug. To give the correct amount of insulin, the syringe must be calibrated in the same units as the drug.

Check the insulin vial for color and clarity. Some insulin is supposed to be clear and colorless. This includes rapid-acting insulin, short-acting insulin, insulin glargine (Lantus), and insulin detemir (Levemir). If particles are present or if the liquid is cloudy, discard the insulin and open a new vial. All other insulin types have a cloudy appearance after they have been gently rotated.

Gently roll the insulin vial (or pen, cartridge, syringe, or other prefilled injection device) between your hands to mix and warm the insulin. Do not shake the vial because bubbles will form and the dose may not be accurate.

Drug Alert

Action/Interaction Alert

Whenever insulin is given before a meal, it is critical that the patient eats a meal of sufficient calories within 15 min of the insulin injection to prevent hypoglycemia.

QSEN: Safety

Critical Point for Safety

Insulin is a high-alert drug with serious consequences when dosages injected are not correct. Insulin types are not interchangeable. Double check the order and your calculation with another licensed health care professional to ensure that you are giving the prescribed dose.

QSEN: Safety

Drug Alert

Administration Alert

Always use an insulin syringe that is calibrated and marked in the same unit concentration as the insulin you are giving. **Never** use any syringe other than an insulin syringe to give insulin.

QSEN: Safety

Critical Point for Safety

Do not shake an insulin container before drawing up the drug because bubbles will form and the dose may not be accurate.

QSEN: Safety

Needles on insulin syringes are small gauge (28-gauge, 29-gauge, and 30-gauge) and vary in length from 4 to 12.7 mm. Use shorter needles for thinner patients and longer needles for patients who have more subcutaneous tissue. Check and recheck that the amount and type of insulin you have drawn up into the syringe is the amount ordered.

Usually, the abdomen is the preferred site for insulin injection (except for a 2-inch circle around the umbilicus). Other acceptable sites include the fronts and sides of the thighs. The upper arms are no longer recommended sites because the absorption of insulin after injection varies at this site and can make the peak action of insulin less predictable.

Cleanse the site with an alcohol swab, and grasp a fold of skin in your nondominant hand. Insert the needle at a 90-degree angle (a 45-degree angle if the patient is very thin), and inject the insulin without pulling back on the plunger. (It is not necessary to check for a blood return, and pulling tissue back into the needle can cause bruising and other tissue damage.)

After the injection is complete, withdraw the needle rapidly while supporting the skin. Do **not** massage the site because doing so can change the rate at which insulin is absorbed from the tissues.

Assess the patient hourly for signs and symptoms of hypoglycemia. These include confusion, cool and clammy skin, tremors, headache, hunger, and sweating (see Box 21.3). Keep a simple sugar (such as orange juice and sugar packets) on the unit. Ensure that the patient's meals or between-meal snacks are on time and that he or she eats them.

Assess the patient's response to insulin. Check blood glucose levels as often as ordered and whenever you suspect the patient may be hypoglycemic or hyperglycemic. Document the results.

⭐ *Teaching priorities for patients self-injecting insulin.* Most patients are frightened or overwhelmed at first by the whole process of drawing up and injecting the correct amount of insulin without contaminating the drug or the needle. A team approach to patient education, including a diabetes educator, can be very helpful. Usually teaching a patient how to self-inject insulin takes more than one teaching session and requires that he or she is alert enough to learn, can see well enough to ensure safe drug administration, and has good use of the arms, hands, and fingers to be able to perform the physical actions involved.

Teach patients to use the steps outlined in Box 2.3 in Chapter 2 for self-injection of insulin from a vial. Box 21.4 lists teaching tips for patients prescribed to use pen-style prefilled syringes or injectors. To begin teaching, use normal saline solution and the same type of insulin syringe that the patient will use at home. Demonstrate how to correctly draw up insulin into the syringe and inject it. Have the patient, and whomever the patient designates as a helper, "teach back" the techniques to you, complete with explanations in his or her own words. Remind patients to always have a spare bottle of each type of insulin that they use. Using the manufacturer's recommendations, teach them about how to store insulin and any prefilled syringes, cartridges, or pens between uses.

Instruct patients to check the injection site daily for any signs or symptoms of infection (warmth, redness, firmness to the touch, presence of drainage, pain in and around the area). Stress the need to report the presence of any symptom indicating infection to the prescriber *immediately* because infections can progress and become worse rapidly in patients who have diabetes.

Ensure that patients know the signs and symptoms of hypoglycemia (see Box 21.3). Urge them not to skip or delay meals. Tell them to always carry a glucose or carbohydrate source that contains at least 15 g of carbohydrate in a pocket or purse and to eat it at the first sign of hypoglycemia.

Stress to patients who are using multiple insulin injections daily the importance of keeping to the schedule for insulin injections and meals. For patients using insulin on an intensified injection regimen, there is more flexibility in meal timing because the injections are timed to the meals and blood glucose levels.

 Drug Alert

Administration Alert

After inserting the needle, inject the insulin without aspirating for blood, and do *not* massage the site after removing the needle.

QSEN: Safety

 Drug Alert

Teaching Alert

Teach patients the importance of having at least one other family member, friend, companion, or neighbor also know how to inject insulin safely for those times when patients cannot perform this action for themselves.

QSEN: Safety

| Box 21.4 | **Patient Education Guide for Using Pen-Style Injection Devices** |

- Wash your hands.
- Check the drug label to be sure it is what was prescribed.
- Remove the cap.
- Look at the insulin to be sure it is evenly mixed if it contains NPH and that there is no clumping of particles.
- Wipe the tip of the pen where the needle will attach with an alcohol swab.
- Remove the protective pull tab from the needle and screw it onto the pen until snug.
- Remove both the plastic outer cap and inner needle cap.
- Look at the dose window and turn the dosage knob to the appropriate dose.
- Holding the pen with the needle pointing upward, press the button until at least a drop of insulin appears. This is the

- "cold shot," "air shot," or "safety shot." Repeat this step if needed until a drop appears.
- Dial the number of units needed.
- Cleanse the injection site.
- Hold the pen perpendicular to and against the intended injection site with your thumb on the dosing knob.
- Press the dosing knob slowly all the way to dispense the dose.
- Hold the pen in place for 6–10 seconds; then withdraw from the skin.
- Replace the outer needle cap; unscrew until the needle is removed and dispose of the needle in a hard plastic or metal container.
- Replace the cap on the insulin pen.

Life span considerations for insulin

Pediatric considerations. Many children have T1DM and require insulin injections and blood testing of glucose levels. A child may have daily differences in the amount or type of food eaten and the amount of exercise experienced. These differences can make having good control over blood glucose levels a real challenge.

Considerations for pregnancy and lactation. Insulin is the treatment of choice for diabetes during pregnancy. Insulin needs change during pregnancy and often increase during the last 6 months. Reassure patients who use additional insulin injections during pregnancy that the extra injections usually are not needed once the pregnancy is over.

Considerations for older adults. T1DM is managed with insulin, and insulin use in an older adult can pose some special problems. Many older adults with T1DM have some degree of reduced vision and a decreased sense of touch as a result of the disease. These problems increase the risk for errors in insulin dosing, injection, and self-monitoring of blood glucose levels. Older patients may benefit from the use of prefilled insulin syringes, cartridges, or pens. Urge older adults with vision problems to use magnifying glasses and good light when testing blood glucose levels or withdrawing insulin.

The risk for hypoglycemia is increased in older adults, especially if they also take beta-adrenergic blocking drugs, warfarin (Coumadin), or other drugs that increase the hypoglycemic response. The older adult may eat less than a younger adult and must understand how to match insulin dosage and scheduling with food intake.

Drug Alert

Interaction Alert

The risk for hypoglycemia with insulin is increased when patients also take *beta-adrenergic blocking drugs*, *warfarin* (Coumadin), or other drugs that increase the hypoglycemic response.

QSEN: Safety

Get Ready for the NCLEX® Examination!

Key Points

- Body cells use glucose and oxygen to make the chemical energy substance ATP to use as fuel for cellular work in the body.
- Hypoglycemia can lead to brain cell dysfunction and death.
- A patient with type 1 diabetes (T1DM) does not make insulin and must take insulin for the rest of his or her life.
- A patient with type 2 diabetes (T2DM) still makes some insulin. The insulin does not interact well with its receptor.
- Complications from untreated or poorly controlled diabetes include blindness; kidney failure; foot and leg amputations; hypertension; and increased risk for infection, heart attacks, and strokes.
- Because the different types of antidiabetic drugs work in different ways, a patient may be prescribed to take more than one type.
- Remind patients to limit alcohol intake and drink only with or shortly after a full meal to prevent hypoglycemia.

- The most frequent adverse effect of antidiabetic drug therapy is severe hypoglycemia, which can rapidly lead to coma and death. Symptoms include hunger, headache, tremors, sweating, and confusion.
- The only drug approved to manage diabetes during pregnancy is insulin. Breastfeeding when taking other antidiabetic drugs is not recommended because some do enter the breast milk and it is not known what effect they may have on the nursing infant.
- Antidiabetic drugs that, when used alone, can cause hypoglycemia are the sulfonylureas, meglitinides, GLP-1 agonists, amylin analogs, DPP-4 inhibitors, and the SGLT2 inhibitors.
- For antidiabetic drugs that should be taken right before a meal or a substantial snack (alpha-glucosidase inhibitors, meglitinide analogs, amylin analogs), if a meal is skipped, that drug dose must also be skipped.
- With the insulin sensitizers and the alpha-glucosidase inhibitors the risk for serious hypoglycemia occurs only when the

drugs are used in combination with drugs that do cause hypoglycemia.

- Patients who have an allergy to sulfonamide antibiotics are very likely to have an allergy to sulfonylureas and should not take these drugs.
- Metformin can cause lactic acidosis. Do not give this drug within 48 hours to anyone who has had testing with radio-opaque dye unless kidney function has returned to normal.
- Do not give the thiazolidinediones to a patient with severe heart failure. Assess patients with mild heart failure frequently for indications of worsening heart failure such as rapid weight gain, hypotension, and difficulty breathing.
- The alpha-glucosidase inhibitors interfere with carbohydrate and glucose nutrient absorption. This class of drugs is contraindicated in patients who are already malnourished or have difficulty digesting or absorbing food, such as ulcerative colitis or Crohn disease. In such patients, excessive weight loss and iron deficiency anemia are more likely.
- Alpha-glucosidase inhibitors must be taken with the first bite of a meal because their actions occur in the intestinal tract to reduce glucose uptake.
- Some GLP-1 drugs are taken daily and others are taken **weekly**. Many patients are unfamiliar with drugs taken only once weekly. Teach patients who are prescribed to take a drug weekly **never** to take it daily. This would result in a severe overdose.
- Pramlintide, an amylin analog, is the only noninsulin antidiabetic drug approved for use in patients with T1DM, as well as for T2DM. However, the dosages required for treatment of the two types of diabetes are different.
- Although pramlintide is often taken at the same time as insulin, it must **never** be mixed in the same syringe as insulin or injected into a site within 2 inches of an insulin injection.

- Because pramlintide delays gastric emptying, it can reduce or delay the rate of absorption for other drugs the patient takes, especially for those that have a desired rapid onset of action such as analgesics. Teach patients to take other prescribed drugs at least 1 hour before or 1 hour after taking pramlintide and eating a meal to ensure absorption.
- Teach patients prescribed any combination oral antidiabetic drug that the single tablet does contain more than one drug and that the precautions and care issues needed include all the ones for each individual drug within the tablet.
- Hypoglycemia is *always* a potential adverse effect of insulin therapy. Patients must learn to balance their carbohydrate intake with the timing of peak action for whatever insulin types they take to help prevent hypoglycemia.
- Check the order carefully for the exact type and amount of insulin to be injected. Do not interchange insulin types.
- Use an insulin syringe that is marked off in the same concentration units as the insulin concentration you are injecting.
- Rotate the area for insulin injection within one injection site.
- Administer insulin as a subcutaneous injection, not an intramuscular injection.
- Do not pull back on the plunger before injecting the insulin and do not rub or massage the injection site.
- Determine how well an older adult who is to self-inject insulin can see the markings on the syringe and reach the injection site.

Additional Learning Resources

Be sure to visit your Evolve website (http://evolve.elsevier.com/Workman/pharmacology/) for additional online resources.

SG Go to your Study Guide for additional learning activities to help you master this chapter content.

Review Questions

See *Answers to In-Text Review Questions* in the back of the book for answers to these questions.

1. **How does insulin lower blood glucose levels?**

   A. Enhancing the enzymes that break down glucose
   B. Enhancing kidney excretion of glucose in the urine
   C. Increasing cell membrane permeability to glucose
   D. Converting glycogen into glucose in the liver and brain

2. **Why can't a patient with type 1 diabetes use an oral antidiabetic drug for blood glucose control?**

   A. Their pancreatic beta cells no longer produce insulin.
   B. Their drug receptors are no longer sensitive to insulin.
   C. They are unable to digest and absorb the oral antidiabetic drugs.
   D. Antidiabetic drugs cause further damage to the exocrine pancreas.

3. **Which question is most important for the nurse to ask a patient newly prescribed glyburide?**

   A. "Do you have any drug allergies?"
   B. "How long have you had diabetes?"
   C. "Have you ever had thyroid cancer?"
   D. "Are you able to give yourself an injection?"

4. **A patient asks the nurse how metformin will help to reduce her blood glucose levels. What is the nurse's best response?**

   A. Directly forcing your beta cells to release more insulin
   B. Inhibiting the enzyme that breaks down insulin
   C. Preventing the breakdown of glycogen into glucose
   D. Increasing your need for glucose

5. **A patient is newly prescribed miglitol for type 2 diabetes. How will the nurse instruct the patient to take this drug for best effect?**

   A. "Take this drug with the first bite of every meal."
   B. "This drug is to be taken only once daily before breakfast."
   C. "Inject this drug at least 2 inches away from the site you injected insulin."
   D. "Dissolve the drug in water or juice and take it at bedtime to avoid nausea."

6. **For which patient will the nurse question a prescription for rosiglitazone?**

   A. 28-year-old man with type 2 diabetes
   B. 40-year-old woman with a history of thyroid cancer
   C. 55-year-old woman with moderate osteoporosis
   D. 64-year-old man with moderate heart failure

7. Which precaution is **most important** for the nurse to teach a patient prescribed semaglutide to prevent harm?

   A. Only take this drug once weekly.
   B. Report any vision changes immediately.
   C. Do not mix in the same syringe with insulin.
   D. This drug can only be given by a health care professional.

8. Which statement made by a patient who is learning to self-inject insulin indicates to the nurse that more instruction is needed about insulin injection sites?

   A. "I can reach my thigh best, so I will use different areas of the same thigh."
   B. "By rotating sites within one area, my chance of having skin changes is less."
   C. "The abdominal site is best for me to use because it is closest to the pancreas."
   D. "If I change my injection site from my thigh to my arm, the insulin absorption may be different."

9. How will the nurse modify insulin injection technique for a patient who is 5 feet 10 inches tall and weighs 106 lb (48.1 kg)

   A. Using a 6 mm needle and injecting at a 90-degree angle
   B. Using a 6 mm needle and injecting at a 45-degree angle
   C. Using a 12.7 mm needle and injecting at a 90-degree angle
   D. Using a 12.7 mm needle and injecting at a 45-degree angle

10. The nurse is preparing to give a patient a dose of NPH insulin from an open vial and notes that the solution is cloudy. What is the nurse's **best** action to prevent harm?

    A. Warming the vial in a bowl of warm water until it reaches normal body temperature
    B. Returning the vial to the pharmacy and opening a fresh vial of NPH insulin
    C. Rolling the vial between the hands until the insulin is clear
    D. Checking the expiration date and drawing up the dose

Clinical Judgment

1. With which classes or groups of drugs for diabetes, when given as a single agent, will the nurse monitor the patient most closely for development of serious hypoglycemia? **Select all that apply.**

   A. Alpha-glucosidase inhibitors
   B. Amylin analogs
   C. Biguanides
   D. DPP-4 inhibitors
   E. GLP-1 agonists
   F. Insulin
   G. Meglitinides
   H. SGLT2 inhibitors
   I. Sulfonylureas
   J. Thiazolidinediones

2. The patient is a 48-year-old man newly diagnosed with type 2 diabetes mellitus. One month ago he attended a diabetes education session with a diabetes educator to learn more about his management plan. The plan included dietary modification, increasing his weight-bearing exercise to at least 150 minutes weekly, and self-injecting regular-release exenatide twice daily. He has returned to the clinic for follow-up on his health and evaluation of the effectiveness of the management plan. The nurse is assessing him, answering his questions, and reinforcing the diabetes education presented a month ago. **For each patient assessment finding at this visit, use an X to indicate whether the educational intervention implemented by the diabetes education was Effective (helped to meet expected outcomes), Ineffective (did not help to meet expected outcomes), or Unrelated (not related to the expected outcomes).**

ASSESSMENT FINDINGS	EFFECTIVE	INEFFECTIVE	UNRELATED
Weighs 10 lb (4.5 kg) less than 1 month ago			
Fasting blood glucose 132 mg/dL			
Serum sodium level 139 mEq/L			
A1C = 5.9%			
Reports drinking one 12-ounce beer daily with supper			
Eats a full meal within 30 min of injecting exenatide			
Reports using sunscreen of SPF 40 or wearing a hat when outdoors			
Walks at a moderate pace for 2 miles 5 days each week			

Drug Therapy for Thyroid and Adrenal Gland Problems

22

Learning Objectives

The content presented in this chapter should help you to:

1. Explain the names, actions, usual adult dosages, possible side effects, and adverse effects of drugs for thyroid problems and for adrenal gland problems.
2. Describe priority actions to take before and after giving drugs for thyroid and adrenal gland problems.
3. Prioritize essential information to teach patients taking drugs for thyroid or adrenal gland problems.
4. Explain appropriate life span considerations of drugs for thyroid and adrenal gland problems.

Key Terms

aldosterone (ăl-DŎS-tĕ-rōn) (p. 413) A hormone secreted by the adrenal cortex that regulates sodium and water balance.

corticosteroids (kōr-tĭ-kō-STĚR-ōydz) (p. 413) Drugs similar to natural cortisol, a hormone secreted by the adrenal cortex that is essential for life.

thyroid hormone agonists (THĬ-rōyd HŎR-mōn Ă-gŏn-ĭsts) (p. 409) Drugs that mimic the effect of thyroid hormones, T_3 and T_4, helping to regulate metabolism.

The endocrine system consists of many different glands that secrete one or more hormones into the blood, which then circulates everywhere until it reaches its target tissue(s). A *target tissue* is a tissue or organ that is affected or controlled by the hormone. For example, the ovary is an endocrine gland that secretes estrogen. The main target tissues of estrogen are the uterine lining and certain breast cells. The endocrine system helps to regulate metabolism and all body functions. This chapter focuses on drug therapy for problems of the thyroid and adrenal endocrine glands. Hormones from these two glands are essential for life and affect all body cells.

REVIEW OF RELATED PHYSIOLOGY AND PATHOPHYSIOLOGY OF THYROID FUNCTION

The thyroid gland is located in the front of the neck just below the Adam's apple. It produces two thyroid hormones: thyroxine (T_4) and triiodothyronine (T_3). These two hormones are formed from the amino acid tyrosine and the mineral iodine. T_3 is the active thyroid hormone, and T_4 is converted to T_3.

When T_3 and T_4 leave the thyroid gland and enter other body cells, they bind to receptors inside the cell, and activate the genes for metabolism (Animation 22.1). *Metabolism* is the energy use of each cell and the amount of work performed in the body. Thyroid hormones increase the rate of metabolism in every cell they enter, speeding up the energy use and work output of each cell. Important functions controlled by thyroid hormones include:

- Assisting in brain development before birth and during early childhood
- Maintaining brain function throughout the life span
- Helping maintain the ability to think, remember, and learn
- Maintaining heart and skeletal muscle function
- Ensuring continued production of other hormones
- Maintaining effective respiratory function and cell uptake of oxygen

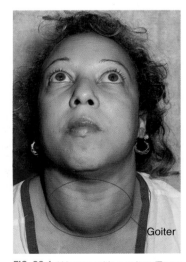

Goiter

FIG. 22.1 Woman with a goiter. (From Ignatavicius, D. D., & Workman, M. L. [2016]. *Medical-surgical nursing: Patient-centered collaborative care* [8th ed.]. Philadelphia: Saunders.)

 Memory Jogger

Thyroid hormones are essential for life because they regulate whole body metabolism.

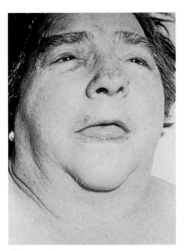

FIG. 22.2 Facial appearance of a woman with severe hypothyroidism. (From Ignatavicius, D. D., & Workman, M. L. [2016]. *Medical-surgical nursing: Patient-centered collaborative care* [8th ed.]. Philadelphia: Saunders.)

 Memory Jogger

A goiter can be present when the thyroid gland is overactive or underactive.

| Box 22.1 | Signs and Symptoms of Hypothyroidism |

ADULTS
- Constipation
- Decreased scalp hair, increased body hair
- Edema of the face, around the eyes, and on the shins
- Feels cold all the time
- Lacks energy, sleeps excessively
- Lower than normal body temperature
- Menstrual irregularities
- No interest in sex
- Slow heart rate
- Slow respiratory rate
- Speaks slowly
- Thickened, waxy-feeling skin
- Thick tongue
- Thinks slowly
- Weight gain

INFANTS AND CHILDREN
- Constipation
- Excess facial and body hair
- Reduced cognition
- Poor eater
- Protruding tongue
- Short stature
- Sleeps excessively

HYPOTHYROIDISM

Hypothyroidism is a condition of low thyroid function (underactive thyroid) causing low blood levels of thyroid hormones (THs) and slow metabolism. Thyroid cells may fail to produce enough thyroid hormones because they have been damaged and no longer function, or because the person's diet does not include enough iodine or tyrosine to make thyroid hormones.

When the production of T_3 and T_4 is too low or absent, the blood levels of the hormones decline, and the patient's entire body metabolism is slowed, sometimes to dangerously low levels. In an effort to increase thyroid hormone production, the thyroid gland cells can divide, making the whole thyroid gland larger and forming a goiter, which is a distinct swelling in the neck. *The presence of a goiter indicates that the patient has a thyroid problem but does not indicate whether the thyroid is underactive or overactive.* Figure 22.1 shows a patient with a goiter. Box 22.1 lists other common symptoms of hypothyroidism.

When left untreated, hypothyroidism can slow metabolism to such a low level that the heart stops functioning and death occurs. This severe type of hypothyroidism is called *myxedema* and is a medical emergency requiring immediate attention. Figure 22.2 shows a woman with severe hypothyroidism. Figure 22.3 shows an infant with hypothyroidism.

Thyroid Hormone Replacement (Agonist) Drugs

Keeping thyroid hormone function at the right level is essential for overall health. If the thyroid is not making these hormones at all or not making enough, replacement of thyroid hormones is needed to keep the metabolism of all cells, tissues, and organs functioning at the proper level. The goal of thyroid hormone agonist therapy is to ensure that the patient's whole-body metabolism is as close to normal as possible. The two most common drugs used for this purpose are levothyroxine and liothyronine. Of the two, levothyroxine is the one most recommended. For some patients, a combination of the two drugs is used.

Usual Adult Dosages for Thyroid Hormone Agonists

Drug Name	Usual Maintenance Dosage
levothyroxine (Estre, Levothroid, Synthroid, Unithroid)	Initial dosage of 1 mcg/kg orally once daily. Doses are slowly increased by 12.5–25 mcg increments every 4–6 weeks until desired response is evident
liothyronine (Cytomel, Triostat)	Initial dosage of 25 mcg orally once daily. Doses slowly increased by 25 mcg/day or less every 1–2 weeks. Typical maintenance dose: 25–75 mcg orally once daily
levothyroxine/liothyronine (Thyrolar)	Initial dosage of 1 tablet of (25 mcg T_4/6.25 mcg T_3) orally once daily. Doses increased slowly to a typical maintenance dose of 50–100 mcg T_4 with 12.5–25 mcg T_3 orally daily

How thyroid hormone agonists work. Thyroid hormone replacement drugs are thyroid hormone agonists, which mimic the effect of the thyroid hormones T_3 and T_4, helping to regulate metabolism. They work just like the patient's own thyroid hormones by entering the blood and going into all cells. Once inside the cells, the drug binds to receptors on the DNA and activates the genes for metabolism. Just like T_3 and T_4, these drugs increase the rate of metabolism in all cells they enter, speeding up the energy use and work output of each cell. When a person has an underactive thyroid gland causing hypothyroidism, he or she usually takes thyroid hormone agonists for the rest of his or her life.

Intended responses of thyroid hormone agonists
- Body temperature is normal.
- Level of activity is normal.
- Heart rate, blood pressure, and respiratory rate are normal for the patient's age and size.
- Body weight is maintained when the patient takes in the amount of calories needed for his or her age, size, and activity level.
- The patient is mentally alert; he or she is able to remember people, places, and events from the recent and distant past.
- Bowel movement pattern is normal for the patient's usual bowel habits.

Common side effects of thyroid hormone agonists. Thyroid hormone agonist drugs have few nonhormonal side effects. In general, the side effects are really those of an overdose of the drug, and the symptoms are those of hyperthyroidism.

Possible adverse effects of thyroid hormone agonists. The most serious adverse effect of thyroid hormone agonists is an increase in the activity of the cardiac and nervous systems. The increase in cardiac activity can overwork the heart and lead to anginal chest pain, a heart attack, and heart failure.

In the nervous system, the increased activity can lead to seizures. Seizures are rare but can occur in any patient taking high doses of thyroid hormone agonists. However, they are more likely to occur in the patient who already has a seizure disorder.

Thyroid hormone agonists enhance the action of drugs that reduce blood clotting (anticoagulants), especially warfarin (Coumadin). This action can lead to excessive bruising and bleeding.

⭐ ***Priority actions to take*** before ***giving thyroid hormone agonists.*** Before giving the first dose of a thyroid hormone agonist, assess the patient's blood pressure and heart rate and rhythm. The side effects and adverse effects of thyroid hormone agonists increase metabolic rate and cardiac activity.

Check the dose and the specific drug name carefully. Thyroid hormone agonists are **not** interchangeable because the strength of each drug varies.

Food and fiber impair the absorption of thyroid hormone agonists from the intestinal tract. Ensure that the drug is given 2 to 3 hours before a meal or fiber supplement or at least 3 hours after a meal or fiber supplement.

⭐ ***Priority actions to take*** after ***giving thyroid hormone agonists.*** Assess the patient's blood pressure and heart rate and rhythm to determine whether the drug is working and if there are side effects. Ask the patient whether he or she has any chest pain or discomfort. This symptom may be the first indication of an adverse cardiac effect.

If the patient also takes a drug that affects blood clotting, especially warfarin (Coumadin), assess at least once each shift for any sign of increased bleeding and review the international normalized ratio (INR) and blood counts (Table 1.6 in Chapter 1). Look for bleeding from the gums; unusual or excessive bruising anywhere on

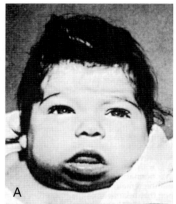

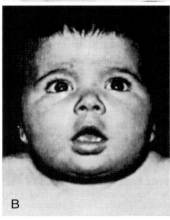

FIG. 22.3 Facial appearance of an infant with hypothyroidism before treatment (A) and after thyroid hormone replacement therapy (B). (From Behrman, R. E., Kliegman, R. M., & Jenson, H. B. [2004]. *Nelson textbook of pediatrics* [17th ed.]. Philadelphia: Saunders.)

Common Side Effects
Thyroid Hormone Agonists

Hypertension   Insomnia   Diarrhea

Tachycardia   Weight loss

⭐ Critical Point for Safety

Never substitute one type or brand of thyroid hormone replacement drug with another. Drug strengths vary (e.g., liothyronine is four times as potent as levothyroxine), and patient responses vary.

QSEN: Safety

Drug Alert

Interaction Alert

Thyroid hormone agonists increase the action of warfarin (Coumadin), increasing the risk for bleeding. Assess the patient for excessive bleeding. Review laboratory reports of blood counts and INR to determine the patient's risk (Table 1.6 in Chapter 1).

QSEN: Safety

Drug Alert

Teaching Alert

Teach patients to take thyroid drugs 2–3 hours before or at least 3 hours after eating a meal or taking a fiber supplement to prevent interference with absorption.

QSEN: Safety

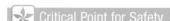 Critical Point for Safety

Remind pregnant women who have hypothyroidism to be sure to continue thyroid hormone agonist therapy. If they stop taking the drug, the pregnancy is at risk and the fetus may not develop properly.

QSEN: Safety

the skin; bleeding around intravenous (IV) sites or for more than 5 minutes after discontinuing an IV; and for the presence of blood in urine, stool, or vomitus.

⭐ *Teaching priorities for patients taking thyroid hormone agonists.* When a patient is diagnosed with hypothyroidism and is first prescribed a thyroid hormone replacement drug, the dose for the first several weeks is low. Usually, it is increased slowly every 2 to 3 weeks until the patient has normal blood levels of TH and signs of normal metabolism. The teaching priorities for patients taking thyroid hormone agonists include:

* Do not increase the dose beyond what is prescribed for you. Increasing the drug too quickly can lead to adverse effects such as heart attack or seizures.
* Check your pulse each morning before taking the drug and again each evening before going to bed. If the pulse rate becomes 20 beats higher than the normal rate for 1 week or if it becomes consistently irregular, notify your prescriber.
* Call 911 or go to the emergency department immediately if you have chest pain.
* Remember that you need to take the drug daily to maintain normal body function. If you are ill and cannot take the drug orally, contact your prescriber to get an injected dose of the drug.
* Do not stop the drug suddenly or change the dose (up or down) without contacting your prescriber.
* Take the drug 2 to 3 hours before a meal or before taking a fiber supplement or at least 3 hours after a meal or after taking the supplement because food or a fiber supplement reduces the absorption of the drug.
* If you also take warfarin (Coumadin), keep all follow-up appointments and appointments for blood-clotting tests because these drugs increase the effectiveness of warfarin. Also avoid situations that can lead to bleeding and other drugs (such as aspirin) that can make bleeding worse.

Life span considerations for thyroid hormone agonists

Pediatric considerations. Children may develop hypothyroidism or may have been born with the problem. They must take thyroid hormone replacement drugs for their entire life. During infancy and early childhood, when the patient is going through periods of rapid growth, he or she actually needs a higher drug amount per kilogram of body weight than an adult!

Considerations for pregnancy and lactation. Women with hypothyroidism usually have difficulty becoming pregnant. Once pregnant, however, thyroid hormone replacement drugs are safe to take during pregnancy. In fact, *for a pregnant woman who has hypothyroidism, not taking the drug can lead to problems with the pregnancy and the fetus.* Pregnant women often need a higher dose of the drug. Because thyroid hormone replacement drugs can enter breast milk and increase the infant's metabolism, the mother taking these drugs should not breastfeed.

Considerations for older adults. The metabolism of older adults is more sensitive to thyroid hormone replacement drugs, and they are more likely to have adverse cardiac and nervous system effects. For this reason, older adults who need these drugs are usually prescribed a lower dose than younger adults. In addition, older adults are more likely to have diabetes. Thyroid hormone replacement drugs change the effectiveness of insulin and other drugs for diabetes. Often drugs for diabetes need to be increased to prevent high blood sugar levels (*hyperglycemia*). Teach older adults with diabetes and hypothyroidism to check their blood glucose levels more frequently.

HYPERTHYROIDISM

Hyperthyroidism is an increase in thyroid gland activity, causing high blood levels of thyroid hormones (T_3 and T_4) and symptoms of increased metabolism. This health problem is also called an overactive thyroid. Thyroid cells may produce excessive thyroid hormones for several reasons, but the most common type of hyperthyroidism

Box 22.2	Signs and Symptoms of Hyperthyroidism

GENERAL SYMPTOMS
- Diarrhea
- Difficulty sleeping
- Feeling too warm most of the time
- Fine tremors of the hands
- Heartbeat irregularities
- High blood pressure
- Higher than normal body temperature
- Menstrual irregularities
- Rapid heart rate
- Sweating
- Thinning of scalp hair
- Weight loss

ADDITIONAL SYMPTOMS SPECIFIC TO GRAVES DISEASE ONLY
- Blurred vision
- Bulging or protruding eyes (exophthalmia)

is Graves disease. As a result of hyperthyroidism with excessive production of thyroid hormones, the patient's body metabolism is much faster or greater than normal. With some types of hyperthyroidism, such as Graves disease, the patient also has a goiter.

Another name for hyperthyroidism is *thyrotoxicosis,* because the side effects of excessive thyroid hormones can cause toxic side effects to some organs. Symptoms of hyperthyroidism from any cause are listed in Box 22.2. The excess thyroid hormones increase the metabolism of all cells above normal levels and make every organ work harder, especially the heart. Additional symptoms that occur only with hyperthyroidism caused by Graves disease include bulging or protruding eyes (*exophthalmos*) (Figure 22.4) and blurred vision.

When hyperthyroidism is severe, it is called *thyroid crisis* or *thyroid storm.* This condition is an extreme state of hyperthyroidism in which all symptoms are more severe and life threatening. The patient has a fever, dangerously high blood pressure, and a rapid, irregular heartbeat. Symptoms can develop quickly. If not treated, this problem can lead to seizures, heart failure, and death.

Most often, hyperthyroidism is a permanent health problem that is treated by destroying all or part of the thyroid gland by using radiation to destroy thyroid cells or by surgical removal (*thyroidectomy*). Drug therapy with antithyroid drugs to reduce thyroid production of hormones is often used before surgery. If the patient is too ill for surgery or radiation, antithyroid drugs may be used long-term in place of these treatments. Additional drugs, such as beta-blockers, may be used to help control the cardiac problems associated with the disorder, but these drugs do not change the hyperthyroidism.

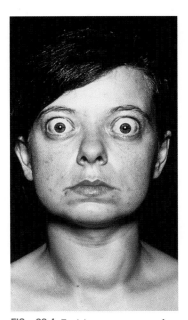

FIG. 22.4 Facial appearance of a woman with hyperthyroidism from Graves disease. Note the bulging eyes, goiter, and lack of body fat. (From Ignatavicius, D. D., & Workman, M. L. [2016]. *Medical-surgical nursing: Patient-centered collaborative care* [8th ed.]. Philadelphia: Saunders.)

Antithyroid Drugs

The main recommended antithyroid drug in the United States is methimazole. Another drug, propylthiouracil, is a second-line drug but rarely used because of severe toxicities. Although symptoms usually begin to improve within several weeks to months after starting antithyroid drugs, antithyroid drug therapy usually continues for at least a year.

Usual Adult Dosages for Antithyroid Drugs

Drug Name	Usual Maintenance Dosage
methimazole (Northyx, Tapazole)	Initially, 5–20 (depending on hyperthyroid severity) orally every 8 hr until symptoms controlled; then 2–5 mg orally every 8 hr
propylthiouracil (PTUl)	Initially, 100–200 mg orally every 8 hr. Maintenance doses: 30–50 mg orally every 8 hr

How antithyroid drugs work. Methimazole enters the thyroid gland and combines with the enzyme responsible for connecting iodine (iodide) with tyrosine to make

Do Not Confuse

methimazole *with* **metolazone**

An order for methimazole can be confused with metolazone. Methimazole is a thyroid-suppressing drug, whereas metolazone is a diuretic.

QSEN: Safety

 Do Not Confuse

propylthiouracil *with* **Purinethol**

An order for propylthiouracil can be confused with Purinethol. Propylthiouracil is a thyroid-suppressing drug, whereas Purinethol is a cancer chemotherapy drug.

QSEN: Safety

Common Side Effects

Antithyroid Drugs

Rash

Nausea

Headache

Muscle aches

active T_3 and T_4. This action keeps the enzyme so busy working on the drug that it does not have the opportunity to make active thyroid hormones. Methimazole does not affect the hormones already formed and stored in the thyroid gland, so it may take as long as 3 or 4 weeks for a person to use all of the existing thyroid hormones made and stored before the drug was started.

Intended responses of antithyroid drugs
- Body temperature is normal.
- Level of activity is normal.
- Heart rate, blood pressure, and respiratory rate are normal for the patient's age and size.
- Body weight is maintained when the patient takes in the amount of calories needed for his or her age, size, and activity level.
- Bowel movement pattern is normal for the patient's usual bowel habits.

Common side effects of antithyroid drugs. Antithyroid drugs have many minor side effects. These include rash, loss of taste sensation, headache, muscle and joint aches, itchiness, drowsiness, nausea, vomiting, lymph node enlargement, and swelling of the feet and ankles.

Possible adverse effects of antithyroid drugs. A major adverse effect of antithyroid drugs is bone marrow suppression, which reduces the production of blood cells. As a result, the patient is less resistant to infection and more likely to be anemic.

Both drugs, especially propylthiouracil, can be *hepatotoxic* (liver toxic). The severe hepatoxicity is the main reason why propylthiouracil is rarely prescribed. Less often, these drugs can also damage the kidneys.

Antithyroid drugs enhance the action of drugs that reduce blood clotting (anticoagulants), especially warfarin (Coumadin). This action increases the risk for excessive bruising and bleeding.

Antithyroid drugs have the potential to reduce thyroid function below normal, to the hypothyroid state. If this condition persists, the patient may need to take thyroid agonists.

⭐ **Priority actions to take before and after giving antithyroid drugs.** Ask female patients who are within child-bearing age whether they are pregnant, planning to become pregnant, or are breastfeeding. Antithyroid drugs can cause harm to the fetus and can cause hypothyroidism in a breastfed infant.

Check the patient's liver function tests before giving these drugs because of the risk for liver toxicity. If a patient already has a liver problem, the effects of the drugs on the liver are worse and occur at lower doses.

Assess patients who also take a drug that affects blood clotting, especially warfarin (Coumadin), at least once each shift for any sign of increased bleeding. Look for bleeding from the gums; unusual or excessive bruising anywhere on the skin; bleeding around IV sites or for more than 5 minutes after discontinuing an IV; and the presence of blood in urine, stool, or vomit.

Assess the patient daily for yellowing of the skin or sclera (jaundice), which is a symptom of liver problems.

Review the patient's white blood cell count (WBC) because bone marrow suppression is possible with reduced WBC counts. Low WBC counts increase the risk for infection.

⭐ **Teaching priorities for patients taking antithyroid drugs.** The effects of hyperthyroidism are severe and potentially dangerous. Close adherence to drug therapy as well as monitoring for complications are essential. Teach patients the following care issues and precautions:
- If you are also taking warfarin (Coumadin), keep all follow-up appointments and appointments for blood-clotting tests because these drugs increase the

effectiveness of warfarin. Also, avoid situations that can lead to bleeding and other drugs, such as aspirin, that can make bleeding worse.

- Avoid crowds and people who are ill because the drug reduces your production of white blood cells and increases your risk for infection.
- Check the color of the roof of your mouth and the whites of your eyes every day for the presence of a yellow tinge. If this is present, report this change to your prescriber as soon as possible.

Life span considerations for antithyroid drugs

Considerations for pregnancy and lactation. Antithyroid drugs have a high likelihood of increasing the risk for birth defects or fetal damage and can cause miscarriages. These drugs should not be given during pregnancy unless the disorder is severe and the benefits of treatment are thought to outweigh the risks in a life-threatening situation or when other treatments are not available. Women taking an antithyroid drug should not breastfeed because the drug could cause hypothyroidism in the infant.

Considerations for older adults. Older adults taking thyroid-suppressing drugs are more likely to have an adverse effect, and adverse effects are more likely to be severe. The older patient's resistance to infection is already lower than that of a younger adult because of age-related changes that occur in the immune system. Decreased bone marrow activity makes this problem worse. Many older adults also take warfarin (Coumadin). The effects of warfarin are increased when the patient also takes a thyroid-suppressing drug.

REVIEW OF RELATED PHYSIOLOGY AND PATHOPHYSIOLOGY OF ADRENAL GLAND FUNCTION

ADRENAL INSUFFICIENCY

The adrenal glands are small, triangular-shaped endocrine glands that sit on top of the kidneys (Figure 22.5). These two glands have two layers: the thick outermost layer, known as the cortex; and the inner layer, known as the medulla (Figure 22.6). The cortex secretes two main types of steroid hormones, cortisol and aldosterone. Cortisol, a glucocorticoid, is essential for life and functions to regulate:

- The body's response to stress
- Carbohydrate, protein, and fat metabolism
- Emotional stability
- Immune function
- Sodium and water balance
- Normal excitability of heart muscle cells

Aldosterone is a mineral corticoid hormone secreted by the adrenal cortex that regulates sodium and water balance.

Adrenal insufficiency, also called *Addison disease*, usually results in greatly reduced secretion of both cortisol and aldosterone. Common causes of adrenal insufficiency include autoimmune diseases attacking and destroying the adrenal glands, adrenalectomy, abdominal radiation therapy, and disorders of the anterior pituitary gland. Signs and symptoms of adrenal insufficiency include hypoglycemia, salt craving, muscle weakness, hypotension, fatigue, low serum sodium levels, and high serum potassium levels. Depending on the cause, some people also have darkening of the skin. Without supplementation or replacement of cortisol and aldosterone, the person with adrenal insufficiency would eventually die.

Adrenal Hormone Replacement Drugs

Cortisol and aldosterone deficiencies are corrected by replacement therapy. Therapy may be temporary or permanent depending on the specific cause of adrenal insufficiency. **Corticosteroids** (also called glucocorticoids) are drugs similar to natural cortisol. These drugs, especially prednisone, correct cortisol deficiency or absence. Chapter 10 discusses corticosteroid therapy in detail.

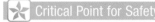

Critical Point for Safety

Antithyroid drugs are best avoided during pregnancy because they can cause birth defects and fetal harm. Determine whether a female patient of child-bearing age is pregnant. Instruct sexually active women to use two reliable methods of birth control while on antithyroid drug therapy. Breastfeeding is contraindicated during antithyroid drug therapy.

QSEN: Safety

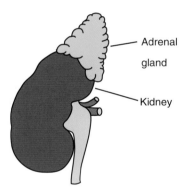

FIG. 22.5 Location of adrenal gland on top of kidney.

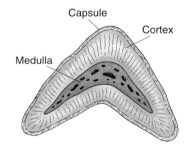

FIG. 22.6 Adrenal gland layers. (From Ignatavicius, D. D., & Workman, M. L. [2016]. *Medical-surgical nursing: Patient-centered collaborative care* [8th ed.]. Philadelphia: Saunders.)

Common Side Effects

Fludrocortisone

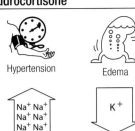

Hypertension   Edema

Hypernatremia   Hypokalemia

Aldosterone deficiency is partially helped by corticosteroid therapy, but more assistance is needed to regulate sodium and potassium balance. So, cortisol replacement is often supplemented with an additional mineralocorticoid hormone replacement, fludrocortisone (Florinef). This drug acts in a similar manner to aldosterone and results in greater reabsorption of sodium with increased excretion of potassium. These actions help correct or prevent hyponatremia, hyperkalemia, and hypotension. The usual adult dosage is 0.1 to 0.2 mg orally once daily.

Common side effects of fludrocortisone therapy. Side effects of fludrocortisone therapy are associated with the drug's action on fluid and electrolyte balance. Common problems include hypertension, edema formation, low blood potassium levels, and high blood sodium levels.

Possible adverse effects of fludrocortisone. The most common adverse effect of fludrocortisone is congestive heart failure (CHF). If CHF develops, the drug dose is either reduced or stopped.

⭐ ***Priority actions to take before and after giving fludrocortisone.*** Fluid and electrolyte balance, especially sodium and potassium balance, are profoundly affected by fludrocortisone therapy. The normal range for serum sodium is 135 to 145 mEq/L (mmol/L) and the normal range for serum potassium is 3.5 to 5.0 mEq/L (mmol/L). Adrenal insufficiency causes low sodium levels (*hyponatremia*) and high potassium levels (*hyperkalemia*). Fludrocortisone therapy can cause just the opposite: high sodium levels (*hypernatremia*) and low potassium levels (*hypokalemia*). Although rapid changes in either electrolyte can be dangerous, potassium imbalances are more likely to be life-threatening. A major nursing responsibility is monitoring serum sodium and potassium values. Review the electrolyte laboratory results as often as they are taken. Use these to determine therapy effectiveness and to identify possible complications early. Report abnormal electrolyte levels, especially hyperkalemia, to the prescriber immediately and assess the patient's respiratory (rate and depth) and cardiac status (blood pressure, heart rate, and rhythm).

⭐ ***Teaching priorities for patients taking fludrocortisone.*** Because fludrocortisone is typically used along with a corticosteroid, remind patients of the usual corticosteroid therapy precautions listed in Chapter 10. In addition, teach patients the following care issues and precautions:
- Take fludrocortisone at the same time daily with food to prevent gastrointestinal problems.
- Weigh yourself daily and keep a record of it because the drug can cause fluid retention with weight gain, edema, and heart failure.
- Report a weight gain of 2 lb in a day or 3 lb in a week to your prescriber immediately.
- Take your pulse at least twice each day. If the rate is persistently higher than 90 or lower than 60 and is irregular, notify your prescriber immediately.

ADRENAL GLAND HYPERFUNCTION

Unlike adrenal gland insufficiency, in which *all* adrenal hormones are deficient, with adrenal gland hyperfunction, most commonly either cortisol is excessively secreted (hypercortisolism or Cushing disease) or aldosterone is excessively secreted (hyperaldosteronism). Excessive secretion of both types of hormones at the same time is less common. Adrenal gland hyperfunction can result in a problem within the adrenal gland, often an adrenal gland tumor, or it can be a result of problems in the pituitary gland that overproduce hormones that stimulate the adrenal gland to produce adrenal hormones in excess.

When adrenal gland hyperfunction is caused by a problem in the adrenal gland, surgery is the most common treatment. If both adrenal glands are removed, the patient will have adrenal insufficiency and must take life-long replacement corticosteroids and fludrocortisone. Before surgery, and for patients who are not able to have surgery, drug therapy can help manage the problems caused by adrenal gland hyperfunction.

Drugs for Adrenal Gland Hyperfunction

A variety of drugs are used to suppress adrenal hormones in the person whose hyperfunction is related to the adrenal gland rather than the pituitary gland. Some drugs target and suppress cortisol production directly or indirectly when cortisol is oversecreted. Other drugs are aldosterone blocking drugs (mineralocorticoid receptor antagonists) that prevent or control excessive aldosterone production (*hyperaldosteronism*).

Adult Dosages of Common Drugs for Adrenal Gland Hyperfunction

Drug Class	Drug Name	Usual Maintenance Dosage
Direct Inhibitors of Cortisol Synthesis	metyrapone (Metopirone)	125–1500 mg orally every 6–8 hr
	mitotane (Lysodren)	0.5–2 g orally every 6–8 hr
	osilodrostat (ISTURISA)	Initial dose: 2 mg orally every 12 hr until cortisol levels decrease. Maintenance: 2–7 mg orally every 12 hr
Corticosteroid Receptor Antagonists	mifepristone (Korlym)	300 mg orally once daily; can be increased to 1200 mg orally daily
Mineralocorticoid Receptor Antagonists	spironolactone (Aldactone, CAROSPIR)	Initially: 100–400 mg orally daily. Maintenance doses are lower but vary

How adrenal suppressing drugs work. Adrenal gland synthesis of cortisol requires multiple steps and several different enzymes. Direct inhibitors of cortisol synthesis, *metyrapone* (Metopirone), *mitotane* (Lysodren), and *osilodrostat* (ISTURISA), each disrupt the cortisol synthesis pathway by inhibiting specific enzymes in the adrenal gland that convert precursor substances into cortisol. Inhibiting any of these enzymes reduces the amount of cortisol present. *Mifepristone* (Korlym) doesn't lower cortisol levels but instead blocks corticosteroid receptors to reduce the action of cortisol. It is approved for use only in people who have type 2 diabetes and hyperglycemia along with hypercortisolism.

Excessive secretion of aldosterone changes kidney function and causes increased excretion of potassium while increasing reabsorption of sodium and water. Drug therapy strictly for hyperaldosteronism requires mineralocorticoid receptor antagonists (aldosterone antagonists) that bind to and block aldosterone receptors in the kidney tubules.

An aldosterone antagonist is *spironolactone* (Aldactone). Although the drug does not decrease aldosterone levels, it reduces the effects of aldosterone and prevents potassium loss and excessive sodium and water reabsorption. It is also used for blood pressure control.

Intended responses of adrenal suppressing drugs
- Reduced blood levels of glucocorticoids (cortisol) and aldosterone
- Normal blood levels of sodium and potassium
- Normal blood levels of glucose
- Normal blood pressure

Common side effects of adrenal suppressing drugs. All drugs for suppression of cortisol production and use are likely to cause headache, nausea, vomiting, dizziness, hypertension, skin rashes, and dizziness. *Mitotane* can also cause bloody urine (hematuria). *Mifepristone* causes many side effects, including menstrual irregularities.

 Memory Jogger

Aldosterone is known as the "sodium and water" saving hormone.

Common Side Effects

Drugs for Cortisol Suppression

Headache   Nausea/ Vomiting   Dizziness

Hypertension   Rash

Common Side Effects
Aldosterone Antagonists

Na⁺ Na⁺
Na⁺ Na⁺
Na⁺ Na⁺
Hyperkalemia

Na⁺
Hyponatremia

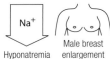
Male breast
enlargement

Acne

Hypotension

⭐ Critical Point for Safety

Acute adrenal insufficiency can result from adrenal suppressing drugs. Symptoms include hypoglycemia, salt craving, muscle weakness, hypotension, and fatigue. Levels of cortisol must be monitored regularly.

QSEN: Safety

In addition to the common side effects listed above, *spironolactone* can also cause hyperkalemia and increased sex hormone levels (especially testosterone), leading to acne, increased body hair (*hirsutism*), and breast enlargement in men (*gynecomastia*). The effect on sodium and water can cause hyponatremia and hypotension.

Possible adverse effects of adrenal suppressing drugs. All drugs for the suppression of cortisol production and use can cause acute adrenal insufficiency, which is a life-threatening complication. Symptoms of acute adrenal insufficiency include hypoglycemia, salt craving, muscle weakness, hypotension, and fatigue. The cortisol levels of patients taking these drugs must be monitored closely.

Because these drugs and the aldosterone antagonists affect fluid and electrolytes, which have profound effects on the electrical conduction system of the heart, many dysrhythmias are possible, usually as an indirect (secondary) response. *Osilodrostat* can prolong the QT interval.

Mifepristone is also a drug used to induce abortion and can cause pregnancy loss. *Aldosterone antagonists* cause amenorrhea and have been shown to cause infertility in laboratory animals.

Steroid hormones, including cortisol and aldosterone, are processed by the liver. Drugs that change the activity of these hormones can increase serum cholesterol levels and reduce liver function.

⭐ *Teaching priorities for patients taking adrenal suppressing drugs.* Conditions of adrenal gland hyperfunction are often chronic and managed on an outpatient basis. Teach patients taking adrenal suppressing drugs the following care issues and precautions:

- These drugs can over-suppress your adrenal gland, which can be dangerous. If you develop persistent symptoms of low blood glucose levels (hunger, headache, shakiness, dizziness, weakness), a sense that you need more salt (salt craving), and increased fatigue, notify your prescriber immediately.
- Because these drugs alter blood levels of sodium, potassium, and cortisol, keep all appointments for laboratory blood work.
- If these drugs cause you to have nausea, vomiting, and other gastrointestinal upsets, take them with food.
- Metyrapone must be taken with food.
- These drugs can cause drowsiness in some people. Do not drive or operate heavy machinery until you know how the drug affects you.
- Take your pulse at least twice daily. If the rate is persistently higher than 90 or lower than 60, or is irregular, notify your prescriber immediately.
- Notify your prescriber if you develop yellowing of your skin or eyes, darkening of your urine, or lighter stools. These symptoms are signs of liver problems, which may occur when taking a drug for adrenal gland problems.
- If you take mifepristone and are a woman of childbearing age who is sexually active, use two reliable forms of birth control while taking mifepristone.
- If you become pregnant while taking any drug for an adrenal gland problem, notify your prescriber immediately.

Life span considerations for adrenal suppressing drugs.

Considerations for pregnancy and lactation. *Mifepristone* is absolutely contraindicated during pregnancy because of the very high risk for pregnancy loss. None of the drugs used to suppress adrenal hormone production are approved for use in children or in women who are pregnant or breastfeeding. However, the risk of taking direct cortisol inhibitors or aldosterone antagonists while pregnant must be weighed against the seriousness of the adrenal hyperfunction. These drugs are not to be taken while breastfeeding because of the serious suppression of the infant's adrenal function.

Get Ready for the NCLEX® Examination!

Key Points

- Proper thyroid function is essential for life. Both an underactive thyroid gland (causing hypothyroidism) and an overactive thyroid gland (causing hyperthyroidism) must be treated.
- Thyroid problems are very common.
- Side effects and adverse effects of thyroid hormone agonists resemble hyperthyroidism.
- Infants and young children may need a higher dose (in terms of micrograms per kilogram of body weight) of thyroid hormone agonists than adults and older adults need.
- Thyroid crisis (or thyroid storm) is an emergency situation. The death rate for thyroid crisis is about 30%, even when the patient is treated correctly.
- Teach patients taking thyroid hormone agonists not to stop the drug suddenly or change the dose of the drug without consulting their prescriber.
- When thyroid hormone agonists are first started, the dose is low and is increased slowly until the patient gets to the dose that keeps metabolism at a normal level.
- Teach patients to take thyroid drugs 2 to 3 hours before or at least 3 hours after eating a meal or taking a fiber supplement to prevent interference with absorption.
- Thyroid hormone agonists increase a patient's blood sugar level; patients with diabetes may need higher doses of insulin or other antidiabetic drugs.
- Never substitute one type or brand of thyroid hormone replacement drug with another. Drug strengths vary (e.g., liothyronine is four times as potent as levothyroxine), and patient responses vary.
- Thyroid hormone agonists increase the action of warfarin (Coumadin), increasing the risk for bleeding. Assess the patient for excessive bleeding. Review laboratory reports of blood counts and INR to determine the patient's bleeding risk.
- Remind pregnant women who have hypothyroidism to be sure to continue thyroid hormone agonist therapy. If they stop taking the drug, the pregnancy is at risk and the fetus may not develop properly.
- The effects of antithyroid drugs may not be seen until 3 to 4 weeks after therapy has started because of the existing thyroid hormones stored in the gland.
- Antithyroid drugs are best avoided during pregnancy because they can cause birth defects and fetal harm. If breastfeeding occurs while taking antithyroid drugs, the infant can develop hypothyroidism.
- Adrenal cortex hormones (glucocorticoids and aldosterone) are essential for life.
- Glucocorticoid deficiency is corrected with cortisol hormone replacement therapy, and aldosterone deficiency is corrected with fludrocortisone, often along with glucocorticoid replacement.
- Assess patients being managed for adrenal gland problems frequently for cardiac indications of hyperkalemia and hypokalemia, which can be life-threatening. Symptoms of *hyperkalemia* include bradycardia; hypotension; and ECG changes of tall, peaked T waves, prolonged PR intervals, flat or absent P waves, and wide QRS complexes. Symptoms *of hypokalemia* include weak, thready, irregular pulse, and hypotension.
- Acute renal insufficiency can result from adrenal suppressing drugs. Symptoms include hypoglycemia, salt craving, muscle weakness, hypotension, and fatigue. Levels of cortisol must be monitored regularly.
- Drugs to suppress adrenal hormone production are not approved for use in children, pregnant women, or women who are breastfeeding.

Additional Learning Resources

⊕ Be sure to visit your Evolve website (http://evolve.elsevier.com/Workman/pharmacology/) for additional online resources.

SG Go to your Study Guide for additional learning activities to help you master this chapter content.

Review Questions

See *Answers to In-Text Review Questions* in the back of the book for answers to these questions.

1. **Why do thyroid problems (hypothyroidism and hyperthyroidism) cause such wide-spread symptoms?**

   A. The disorder is often present for weeks to months before diagnosis.
   B. The hormones produced by the thyroid are essential for life.
   C. Thyroid hormones affect the metabolism of all cells and organs.
   D. The goiter from hypothyroidism is malignant and interrupts lung and cardiac function.

2. **A patient with hypothyroidism as a result of an autoimmune (Hashimoto thyroiditis) disease asks how long thyroid replacement drugs will need to be taken. What is the nurse's best response?**

   A. "You will need to take the thyroid replacement drug until the goiter is completely gone."
   B. "You will need thyroid replacement drugs for the rest of your life because thyroid function will not return."
   C. "After the infection causing the problem is cured with antibiotics, you will no longer need to take the thyroid replacement drugs."
   D. "When your thyroid function studies indicate a normal blood level of thyroid hormones, you will be able to discontinue the drugs."

3. Which assessment is **most important** for the nurse to perform before giving a patient the first oral dose of a thyroid hormone agonist?

   A. Measuring heart rate and rhythm
   B. Checking core body temperature
   C. Asking about previous allergic drug reactions
   D. Listening to bowel sounds in all four abdominal quadrants

4. Which precaution is **most important** for the nurse to teach a patient starting thyroid hormone agonist therapy (HRT) to **prevent harm**?

   A. "Take the drug at the same time every day."
   B. "Avoid caffeinated beverages and foods."
   C. "Get plenty of sleep and take one nap daily."
   D. "Take the drug exactly as prescribed."

5. A patient who has hyperthyroidism is prescribed to take methimazole. Which coexisting health problem or therapy alerts the nurse to a potential problem or interaction?

   A. Chronic hepatitis B
   B. Open-angle glaucoma
   C. Type 2 diabetes mellitus
   D. Pacemaker for heart failure

6. Which report from a patient who has hypothyroidism and is taking levothyroxine indicates to the nurse that more teaching is necessary?

   A. "I take the drug at the same time every day."
   B. "I always drink a full glass of water when I take the pill."
   C. "Even though the pill is small, I mix it with pudding to make is easier to swallow."
   D. "Most often, I take the drug as early in the morning as possible to prevent it from keeping me awake at night."

7. A patient who has been taking methimazole for 1 week reports to the nurse that she has not noticed a change in any of her symptoms. What is the nurse's **best** action?

   A. Documenting the report as the only action
   B. Reassuring the patient that this is a normal response
   C. Notifying the prescriber and asking about increasing the dosage
   D. Asking the patient whether she has been faithful about taking the drug as prescribed.

8. A patient who has been taking fludrocortisone for the past month now has all of the following new onset problems. Which problem is **most important** for the nurse to notify the prescriber about immediately?

   A. 5 lb weight loss
   B. Increased flatulence
   C. Continuous shortness of breath
   D. Edema of both feet at the end of the day

9. Which electrolyte laboratory values indicate to the nurse monitoring a patient with adrenal insufficiency undergoing IV therapy with hydrocortisol that the patient is responding positively to this drug therapy?

   A. Serum sodium 147 mEq/L (mmol/L); serum potassium 7.1 mEq/L (mmol/L)
   B. Serum sodium 137 mEq/L (mmol/L); serum potassium 4.9 mEq/L (mmol/L)
   C. Serum sodium 127 mEq/L (mmol/L); serum potassium 2.8 mEq/L (mmol/L)
   D. Serum sodium 119 mEq/L ((mmol/L); serum potassium 6.2 mEq/L (mmol/L)

10. In reviewing the electrolytes of a patient taking a drug to suppress adrenal gland function, the nurse notes the serum potassium level has increased from 4.6 mEq/L (mmol/L) to 6.1 mEq/L (mmol/L). Which assessment is **most important** for the nurse to perform first?

    A. Deep tendon reflexes
    B. Oxygen saturation
    C. Pulse rate and rhythm
    D. Respiratory rate and depth

Clinical Judgment

1. Which precautions are **most important** for the nurse to teach for preventing harm to a patient who remains at continuing risk for adrenal hypofunction and is taking a corticosteroid and fludrocortisone? **Select all that apply.**

   A. Avoid crowds and people who are ill.
   B. Check your heart rate for irregular or skipped beats twice daily.
   C. Do not choose low-sodium versions of prepared foods.
   D. Get up slowly from sitting or lying positions.
   E. Keep a source of glucose, such as candy, with you at all times.
   F. Never skip your hormone replacement drugs.
   G. Always take these drugs with food.

2. The patient is a 22-year-old student who was just diagnosed with hypothyroidism after gaining 40 lb in 5 months, constantly feeling cold, and sleeping 12 hours daily. She is a little concerned that her recent mental slowness may be permanent. She is prescribed to start taking levothyroxine today. The nurse is developing a teaching plan with take-home instructions/precautions about this drug. **Use an X to indicate which instructions are Most Relevant, Not Relevant, or Potentially Harmful at this time for this patient with regard to levothyroxine therapy.**

INSTRUCTION/PRECAUTION	MOST RELEVANT	NOT RELEVANT	POTENTIALLY HARMFUL
Without a family history of hypothyroidism, your disease is probably milder and you may be able to stop the therapy once the symptoms have gone away.			
Drink a full glass of water with each day's dose and increase your overall daily water intake.			
If you forget a day's dose, be sure to take a double dose the next day.			
Try to take the drug at the same time every day so that you do not forget to take it.			
You do not need to change your usual food choices but be sure to take this drug at least 2–3 hours before or 3 hours after eating a meal or taking a fiber supplement.			
As your metabolism increases, you should recover your usual mental alertness and cognition.			
If you have any chest pain, call 911 or go to the nearest emergency department immediately.			
Do not increase or decrease the dose of the drug unless your prescriber tells you to do so.			
Keep the tablets in the container that came from the pharmacy rather than using a daily pill organizer.			

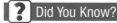

23 | Drug Therapy for Seizures

http://evolve.elsevier.com/Workman/pharmacology/

Learning Objectives

The content presented in this chapter should help you to:

1. Describe how different classes of drugs are used to treat seizures.
2. Discuss the common names, actions, usual adult dosages, possible side effects, and adverse effects of drugs for seizures.
3. Discuss the priority actions to take *before* and *after* giving commonly prescribed drugs for seizures.
4. Prioritize essential information to teach patients and their families and caregivers about commonly prescribed drugs for seizures.
5. Explain appropriate life span considerations of drugs for seizures.

Key Terms

broad-spectrum antiepileptic drugs (AEDs) (BRŌD SPĔK-trŭm ăn-tī-ĕp-ĭl-LĔP-tĭk DRŪGZ) (p. 431) Broad-spectrum AED may be the best choice of treatment when a patient has more than one type of seizure. These drugs are designed to treat or prevent seizures in more than one part of the brain. Broad-spectrum AEDs are effective in the treatment of a wide variety of seizures (e.g., partial plus absence or myoclonic seizures).

first-line drugs for seizures (p. 425) The exact action of first-line drugs for partial or generalized seizures is not known, but these drugs cause a decrease in the voltage, frequency, and spread of electrical impulses within the motor cortex of the brain, which leads to decreased seizure activity.

narrow-spectrum antiepileptic drugs (AEDs) (NĂR-rō SPĔK-trŭm ăn-tī-ĕp-ĭl-LĔP-tĭk DRŪGZ) (p. 426) Narrow-spectrum AEDs are designed for specific types of seizures. These drugs are often used to treat or prevent seizures that occur in a specific part of the brain on a regular basis. Narrow-spectrum AEDs primarily are for the treatment of focal or partial seizures.

second-line drugs for seizures (p. 436) Alternative drugs used for the treatment of seizures and are often used along with another seizure drug.

status epilepticus (STĂT-ŭs ĕp-ĭl-LĔP-tĭ-kŭs) (p. 424) A prolonged seizure (usually defined as lasting longer than 30 minutes) or a series of repeated seizures; a continuous state of seizure activity that may occur in almost any seizure type.

RELATED PHYSIOLOGY AND PATHOPHYSIOLOGY OF SEIZURES

When the brain is working normally, electrical impulses are orderly and organized. These impulses help the brain communicate with the spinal cord, nerves, muscles, and other parts of the brain. When electrical impulses are not orderly and organized, a *seizure* with abnormal impulses results (Figure 23.1). Often seizures occur when nerve cells fire in a more rapid and less controlled manner (Figure 23.2). These abnormal neuron firings can affect movement, senses, concentration, communication, and level of consciousness. After a seizure, most people experience confusion for a period of time.

A single seizure is fairly common and not a chronic problem. About 3.4 million (3 million adults, 470,000 children) people in the United States who have had a single seizure will (~60%) never experience another one. A person with repeated seizures has a *seizure disorder*, sometimes called *epilepsy*. Although seizures may begin at any age, most begin during early childhood or late adulthood. Seizures are frightening and can range from minor to life threatening.

> **? Did You Know?**
>
> Although 10% of Americans experience a seizure at some time during their lives, about 60% of them never experience another seizure.

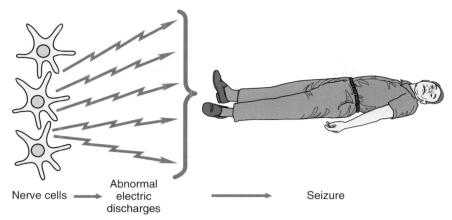

FIG. 23.1 The cause of seizures.

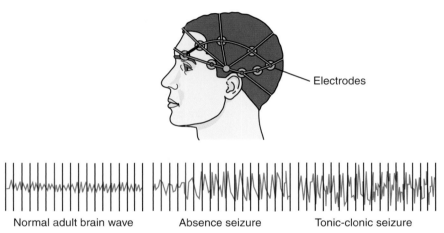

FIG. 23.2 Brain activity during a seizure.

CAUSES OF SEIZURES

Although certain factors are known to cause seizures (Table 23.1), for many people the cause is unknown. Several risk factors increase the possibility of seizures (Box 23.1). For adults, the most common causes include head injury, stroke, and tumor. Certain drugs may lead to seizures (Box 23.2). For children, the most common causes include fever, head injury, central nervous system infection, hypoxia, and electrolyte imbalances.

Stimuli that cause irritation to the brain such as injury, drugs, lack of sleep, infections, and low levels of oxygen may cause a seizure in anyone. However, when a person has a seizure disorder, seizures are more likely to occur during periods of increased emotional or physical stress. Risk factors associated with worsening of a well-controlled seizure disorder include pregnancy and lack of sleep (Box 23.3).

TYPES OF SEIZURES

Signs and symptoms of a seizure may vary widely, ranging from staring off into space to loss of consciousness and violent jerky movements. The type of seizure experienced depends on the part of the brain that is affected, the cause of the seizure, and the person's response. Some people experience an *aura*, a strange sensation (e.g., smell, visual, sound, or taste) that occurs before each seizure. Commonly a seizure

 Did You Know?

The cause of most seizures is unknown.

 Drug Alert

Monitoring Alert

A person who has a seizure disorder is more likely to have a seizure during times of increased emotional or physical stress.

QSEN: Safety

Table 23.1   Common Causes of Seizures

CAUSE	CHARACTERISTICS
Brain injury	Any age—mostly young adults
	Damage to brain membranes
	Seizures begin within 2 years of injury
Degenerative disorders (e.g., dementias)	Mostly affect older adults
Developmental/genetic	Condition present at birth
	Injury near birth; hypoxia at birth
	Seizures begin during infancy or early childhood
Disorders affecting blood vessels (e.g., stroke, transient ischemic attacks)	Most common cause of seizures after age 60
Idiopathic (no known cause)	Usually begin between ages 5 and 20
	Can occur at any age
	No other neurologic abnormalities present
	Family history of seizures present
Infections (e.g., meningitis, encephalitis, brain abscess, immune disorders)	Affect any age
	Reversible cause of seizures
	May be caused by acute severe infection in any part of the body
	Sometimes related to chronic infections
Metabolic abnormalities	Affect any age
	Diabetic complications
	Electrolyte abnormalities
	Kidney failure
	Nutritional deficiencies
	Phenylketonuria—causes seizures during infancy
	Metabolic diseases
	Use of cocaine, amphetamines, alcohol, other illicit drugs
	Alcohol or drug withdrawal
Tumors	Affect any age—most likely after age 30
	Partial (focal) seizures more common
	May progress to generalized seizures

Box 23.1   Risk Factors for Seizures

- Abnormal blood vessels in the brain
- Alcohol misuse/withdrawal
- Autoimmune disorders (e.g., Multiple Sclerosis, Systemic Lupus Eyrthematosus)
- Brain infections
- Drugs (see Box 23.2)
- Drug withdrawal
- Emotional stress
- Family history
- High fevers
- Head injury with bleeding

- Lack of sleep
- Hormone changes
- Hyperventilation
- Hyponatremia (low sodium)
- Lack of food
- Metabolic disorders
- Sensory stimuli (for example, flashing lights)
- Sleep deprivation
- Brain tumors
- COVID-19 infection

Box **23.2**   **Common Seizure-Causing Drugs**

- Antidepressants
- Bupropion alcohol
- Cocaine and other street drugs
- Excessive doses of antiseizure drugs
- Oral contraceptives
- Phenothiazines
- Theophylline

Box **23.3**   **Risk Factors for Worsening of Seizures with a Well-Controlled Seizure Disorder**

- Illness
- Lack of sleep
- Pregnancy
- Prescribed drugs (see Box 23.2)
- Skipping doses of antiseizure drugs
- Use of alcohol or street drugs

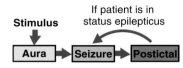

FIG. 23.3 Typical seizure. During status epilepticus the patient experiences a state of continuous seizure.

consists of an aura followed by the seizure and then a *postictal phase* usually characterized by confusion, lethargy, and decreased responsiveness (Figure 23.3). Most seizures are brief, lasting a few seconds to a few minutes.

General Onset Seizures

General onset seizures affect most or all areas of the brain. There are six types of generalized seizures (Table 23.2).

Generalized tonic-clonic seizures (also known as grand mal seizures) last 2 to 5 minutes, with stiffening or rigidity of the arm and leg muscles and immediate loss of consciousness. Spasm of the respiratory muscles can cause forced exhalation, sounding like a scream, called the *epileptic cry*.

Clonic seizures are characterized by muscle contraction and relaxation. Patients may bite their tongues or become incontinent.

Tonic seizures include a sudden increase in muscle tone; loss of consciousness; and autonomic signs such as rapid heart rate, sweating, pupil dilation, flushing, and loss of bowel function and bladder control for 30 seconds to several minutes. After the seizure, patients are often tired, confused, or lethargic for an hour or more.

Absence seizures (also known as *petit mal* seizures) are more common in children and tend to occur in families. They are brief (lasting no more than 20 seconds) and cause symptoms that indicate a lapse in awareness such as blank staring (a child may appear to be daydreaming). After the seizure, the child returns to normal immediately.

Myoclonic seizures cause brief jerking or stiffening of the extremities that lasts a few seconds. It may involve one or more extremities, and the jerking contractions may be asymmetric (stronger on one side of the body) or symmetric (the same on both sides of the body).

Atonic seizures, also called drop seizures, cause the loss of motor control for a few seconds, which can cause a patient to suddenly collapse, fall down, or drop their head. This type of seizure is followed by postictal (after the seizure) confusion.

 Memory Jogger

Before a seizure, a strange sensation called an *aura* may occur. After a seizure, a period of confusion, lethargy, and decreased responsiveness (*postictal phase*) usually occurs.

Seizures are categorized as general onset seizures, focal onset seizures, and seizures of unknown onset. In addition, a condition known as status epilepticus can occur, which is life-threatening.

 Memory Jogger

The two major groups of seizures are general onset and focal seizures.

 Memory Jogger

The six types of general onset seizures are generalized tonic-clonic, tonic, clonic, absence, myoclonic, and atonic.

Table **23.2**	**Types of Generalized Seizures**
TYPE	**SYMPTOMS**
Tonic-clonic (grand mal)	Convulsions, muscle rigidity, unconsciousness
Tonic	Muscle stiffness, rigidity
Atonic	Loss of muscle tone
Absence (petit mal)	Brief loss of consciousness
Myoclonic	Sporadic (isolated) jerking movements
Clonic	Repetitive jerking movements

Table **23.3**	Types of Focal Seizures
TYPE	**SYMPTOMS**
Simple partial motor	Head-turning, jerking, muscle rigidity, spasms
Simple partial sensory	Unusual sensations affecting either vision, hearing, smell, taste, or touch
Simple partial psychologic	Memory or emotional disturbance
Complex	Automatisms (for example, chewing, fidgeting, lip smacking, walking and other repetitive involuntary but coordinated movements)
Partial with secondary generalization	Symptoms that are initially associated with a preservation of consciousness, which then evolves into a loss of consciousness and convulsions

Focal Onset Seizures

Previously called partial seizures, focal onset seizures begin in one area of the brain. The two major types are simple and complex (Table 23.3). With a *simple focal onset seizure,* the patient remains conscious. Before the seizure, a patient may report an aura. During the seizure, the patient remains conscious. One-sided movement of an extremity, unusual sensations, or autonomic changes (e.g., heart rate, flushing, epigastric discomfort) may occur. *Complex focal onset seizures* cause patients to lose consciousness for 1 to 3 minutes. During this type of seizure, patients may have automatisms (automatic, unconscious actions) such as lip smacking, patting, or picking at clothes. Often, they experience amnesia during the period after a seizure. A *partial seizure with secondary generalization* begins with symptoms that are associated with preserving consciousness, followed by evolution to loss of consciousness and convulsions (sudden, violent, irregular movement of a limb or of the body).

Status Epilepticus

Status epilepticus is a life-threatening, prolonged seizure (usually defined as lasting longer than 30 minutes) or a series of repeated seizures without a recovery phase (postictal period), that may occur with almost any type of seizure. The risk for status epilepticus increases when a seizure is prolonged or when a series of seizures occur. Rapid recognition and treatment of this disorder are essential to prevent brain damage. Actions for treating this life-threatening condition include protecting the airway, providing oxygen, establishing intravenous (IV) access to give 5 to 10 mg of diazepam (Valium) by slow IV injection, and determining and treating the cause.

NONDRUG FOCUS OF SEIZURE MANAGEMENT

Controlling and preventing seizure activity are important for many reasons. During a seizure, the patient may have no control over motor activities, which can lead to accidents when the person is driving a car or handling heavy and dangerous equipment. Falls are common during seizures. So, the patient having a seizure is at risk for trauma and loss of motor control and could endanger self and others. In addition, confusion and incontinence (common during or after a seizure) reduce a person's productivity and are embarrassing.

Although antiseizure drugs are a major part of treating and controlling seizures, other important components include precautions such as keeping the airway open, placing a saline lock to give IV drugs, removing harmful objects, raising bedside rails, and keeping the bed at its lowest position. Padded side rails are useful as a safety measure to prevent injuries during seizure activity. The actions taken during a seizure should be correct for the type of seizure. For example, for a simple focal seizure, watch the patient and document the time the seizure occurred and how long it lasted. For a general onset seizure, cushion the head, loosen any clothing around

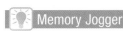

Memory Jogger

The two main types of focal onset seizures are simple and complex.

Drug Alert

Action/Intervention Alert

Without rapid recognition and treatment, status epilepticus can result in brain damage, coma, and death.

QSEN: Safety

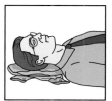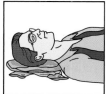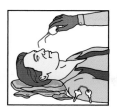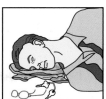

| Help the person to the floor and cushion the head | Loosen any clothing around the neck | Remove any sharp objects | Turn the person on one side |

FIG. 23.4 What to do if you witness a generalized or complex partial seizure.

the neck, remove anything that could cause injury to the patient, and turn him or her to one side to prevent aspiration and let secretions drain (Figure 23.4).

TYPES OF ANTIEPILEPTIC DRUGS (AEDs)

Antiepileptic drugs (AEDs) are a major part of the management and control of seizures. The goal of seizure drug therapy is the control and elimination of seizures. The choice of drugs prescribed is based on the type of seizure. These drugs are started one at a time. If a prescribed drug (**first-line drug**) does not work, either the dose may be increased or another drug may be tried (**second-line drug**). Sometimes it takes more than one drug to control a patient's seizure disorder. The use of these first-line narrow- and broad-spectrum drugs involves a balance between keeping a therapeutic level of the drug in the blood and avoiding serious side effects. Drugs for seizures include broad- and narrow-spectrum medications. All AEDs must be taken on time to maintain the blood level and control seizures.

GENERAL ISSUES RELATED TO AEDs

Antiseizure drugs include narrow- and broad-spectrum drugs. Responsibilities for common actions and effects are listed in the following paragraphs. Specific responsibilities are listed in the discussions of each group of antiepileptic drugs (AEDs).

⬤ Priority Actions to Take *Before* Giving Any AED

Always get a complete list of drugs that the patient is taking, including over-the-counter and herbal preparations. Some AEDs, especially phenytoin, interact with many other drugs. For example, the effects of anticoagulants may be increased, putting the patient at greater risk for bleeding.

Assess baseline vital signs, level of consciousness, and gait. Ask a patient to describe the nature of his or her seizures. Find out whether an aura occurs before each seizure. If an aura occurs, ask the patient to describe it. Instruct patients to notify the health care providers if they sense that a seizure may occur. Document patient responses.

To reduce the risk of injury during a seizure, be sure the patient's bed is in the lowest position and that the side rails are raised and padded. Ensure that the call light is within easy reach.

Ask female patients of childbearing age if they are pregnant, planning to become pregnant, or breastfeeding because some AEDs can cause fetal damage.

⬤ Priority Actions to Take *After* Giving Any AED

Reassess the patient's level of consciousness. Assess his or her vital signs. Because these drugs can cause dizziness or drowsiness, remind the patient to call for help when getting out of bed and make sure that the call light is within easy reach.

 Memory Jogger

Drugs for seizures include broad- and narrow-spectrum medications, and sometimes more than one drug is needed to control seizures.

 Drug Alert

Administration Alert

All AEDs must be taken on time to maintain the blood level and control seizures.

QSEN: Safety

 Drug Alert

Action/Intervention Alert

Drugs for focal and generalized seizures can increase the effects of anticoagulant drugs. Watch for abnormal bleeding.

QSEN: Safety

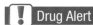

Action/Intervention Alert

Because drugs for focal and generalized seizures can cause dizziness and drowsiness, a patient should not get out of bed without assistance until the effects of the drug are known.

QSEN: Safety

Action/Intervention Alert

Patients taking drugs to prevent generalized or focal seizures should not drink alcohol because it can increase the side effects of dizziness or drowsiness and may trigger a seizure in some people.

QSEN: Safety

Drug Alert

Teaching Alert

While prescribed and taking any AED, patients should be taught to avoid grapefruit and grapefruit juice because they may increase the effects of these drugs.

QSEN: Safety

Monitor the patient for seizure activity and be prepared to manage a seizure if one occurs (for example, protect the airway and protect the patient from injury; see Figure 23.4).

✪ Teaching Priorities for Patients Taking Any AED

- Keep follow-up appointments with your prescriber to monitor control of the seizures and for periodic laboratory tests to monitor blood levels of these drugs.
- Take the drug exactly as prescribed and do not suddenly stop taking any AED because this may lead to seizures.
- Take a missed dose as soon as possible but do **not** take a double dose.
- Report symptoms of side effects and adverse effects immediately to your prescriber.
- Ask your prescriber before taking any over-the-counter drugs, including herbal supplements.
- Because these drugs can cause dizziness or drowsiness, avoid driving, operating dangerous machinery, or doing anything that requires mental alertness until you know how the drug affects you.
- Get out of bed or a chair slowly to avoid accidental falls.
- Avoid alcohol while taking these drugs because it can cause increased drowsiness or dizziness and, in some people, can trigger a seizure.
- Obtain and wear a medical alert bracelet and carry an identification card with you that states your diagnosis, prescribed drugs, and prescriber's name.
- Take your AEDs with food if gastrointestinal (GI) symptoms occur and drink plenty of water.
- While taking any antiepileptic drug, avoid grapefruit and grapefruit juice because these may increase the action of the drug and can lead to more side effects or adverse effects.
- If you are to have surgery of any kind, including dental surgery, be sure to tell your surgeon or dentist about the use of these drugs because of the increased risk for bleeding.

NARROW-SPECTRUM ANTIEPILEPTIC DRUGS (AEDs)

How Narrow-Spectrum AEDs Work

Narrow-spectrum AEDs are prescribed for specific types of seizures. They are used to treat or prevent seizures that occur regularly in a specific part of the brain (e.g., focal seizures). The exact action of some AEDs is not known, but in general, they act on the brain and nervous system. The use of these drugs causes a decrease in the voltage, frequency, and spread of electrical impulses within the motor cortex of the brain, which leads to decreased seizure activity.

Narrow-Spectrum AEDs and Their Actions

Drug	Action
carbamazepine	Decreases impulse transmission by affecting sodium channels in neurons
eslicarbazepine	Blocks sodium channels to slow the nerve firing sequence in seizures
ethosuximide	Increases the seizure threshold making it more difficult for the brain to start a seizure; causes CNS depression
gabapentin	Decreases abnormal excitement in the brain
lacosamide	Selectively enhances slow inactivation of sodium channels
oxcarbazepine	Blocks voltage-sensitive sodium channels
phenobarbital	Controls the abnormal electrical activity in the brain that occurs during a seizure
phenytoin	Decreases abnormal electrical activity in the brain
pregabalin	Reduces the synaptic release of several neurotransmitters
tiagabine	Binds to recognition sites associated with the GABA uptake carrier
vigabatrin	Inhibits the GABA-degrading enzyme, GABA transaminase

Generic names, brand names, uses, and common adult dosages of narrow-spectrum AEDs are listed in the following table. The Food and Drug Administration (FDA) has approved the following narrow-spectrum AEDs for treatment of seizures and epilepsy. Be sure to consult a reliable drug resource for specific information about any narrow-spectrum AEDs.

 Memory Jogger

Gabapentin (Neurontin) is also often used to control pain from chronic neuropathy and fibromyalgia.

Dosages and Uses for Common Narrow-Spectrum Antiepileptic Drugs (AEDs)

Drug	Uses	Dosage
carbamazepine (Carbatrol, Tegretol)	Generalized tonic/clonic seizures Refractory epilepsy Mixed seizures	Tablets and extended release: 200 mg orally twice daily; increase in weekly increments of 200 mg/day, as needed, up to 1600 mg orally per day given in 3 or 4 divided doses. There is no conversion from immediate to extended-release formulations Oral suspension: 100 mg orally 4 times daily. Increase in weekly increments of 200 mg/day, as needed, up to 1600 mg orally per day given in 3 or 4 divided doses
eslicarbazepine (Aptiom)	Focal seizures	400 mg orally once daily. Treatment may be initiated at 800 mg orally once daily if the need for seizure reduction outweighs an increased risk of adverse reactions. Monotherapy: 800 mg orally once daily Add-on therapy: 1600 mg orally once daily
ethosuximide (Zarontin)	Absence seizures	250 mg orally twice daily; usual dose is 20 mg/kg/day in 2 divided doses. Max: 1.5 g/day in divided doses
everolimus (Afinitor, Zortress)	Focal seizures caused by tuberous sclerosis	5 mg/m^2/dose orally once daily, then titrate dose to achieve a target trough concentration of 5–15 ng/mL. Adjust dose at 1- to 2-week intervals based on trough concentrations
gabapentin (Neurontin)	Focal seizures	300 mg orally 3 times per day. May increase using 300, 400, 600, or 800 mg dosage forms orally given 3 times per day *Special Considerations:* **Do not give doses less frequently than every 12 hours**
lacosamide (Vimpat)	Focal seizures Tonic/clonic seizures	100 mg orally twice daily initially; may increase by 100 mg/day at weekly intervals. Recommended maintenance dose is 150 to 200 mg orally twice daily. 100 mg IV twice daily initially; may increase by 100 mg/day at weekly intervals. Recommended maintenance dose is 150 to 200 mg PO twice daily. When discontinuing therapy, withdraw gradually over at least 1 week
oxcarbazepine (Oxtellar XR Trileptal)	Generalized tonic/clonic seizures Focal seizures	300 mg orally twice daily, initially. Titrate by 300 mg/day every third day to a dose of 1200 mg/day XR 600 mg/day PO once daily, initially. Titrate by 600 mg/day every week to a dose of 1200 to 2400 mg/day
phenobarbital	Some focal and generalized seizures Refractory epilepsy	1–3 mg/kg/day orally or IV/IM in 1–2 divided doses. Gradually titrate dosage based on patient response and serum concentrations
phenytoin (Dilantin, Phenytek)	Some focal and generalized seizures Refractory epilepsy	**Oral loading dose**: 15–20 mg/kg orally for non-emergent loading doses in a patient not currently on phenytoin; the loading dose should be divided and administered in no more than 400 mg/dose every 2–3 hr. 300 mg daily (extended release) or 100 mg 3 times daily (immediate release). Maintenance dose: 4 to 7 mg/kg/day orally; slow release (SR) can be given as 1 dose/day; tablets, oral suspension, prompt release given as 2–3 divided doses **IV dose**: 10–20 mg/kg (Max. 1000 mg) at a rate not to exceed 50 mg/min **Status epilepticus**: 15–20 mg/kg/dose IV administered at a rate not to exceed 50 mg/min
pregabalin (Lyrica)	Add-on treatment for focal seizures	150 mg/day orally divided into 2 or 3 doses, initially. May increase dose weekly based on efficacy and tolerability. Max: 600 mg/day
tiagabine (Gabitril)	Add-on treatment for focal seizures	4 mg/day orally for 1 week. Titrate weekly by 4–8 mg, not to exceed 56 mg/day in 2–4 divided doses
vigabatrin (Sabril)	Add-on treatment for focal impaired awareness seizures	500 mg orally twice daily initially. Titrate in 500 mg/day increments at weekly intervals based on patient response. Recommended dose: 1500 mg orally twice daily

Common Side Effects

Narrow-Spectrum AEDs

Ataxia,   Hypotension   Drowsiness
Dizziness

Headache   Nausea/
                 Vomiting

Intended Responses of Narrow-Spectrum AEDs

* Seizures are controlled and prevented.
* Abnormal electrical impulses are decreased.

Common Side Effects of Narrow-Spectrum AEDs

Common side effects of drugs for narrow-spectrum AEDs include ataxia (loss of coordination, clumsiness), dizziness, light-headedness, and drowsiness. *Phenytoin* often causes GI symptoms such as indigestion, nausea, and vomiting. *Phenytoin* also may cause double vision (diplopia), rapid involuntary movement of the eyes (nystagmus), hypotension, excessive growth of gum tissue (gingival hyperplasia), excessive growth of hair in areas not normally hairy (hypertrichosis), and rashes.

Common Side Effects of Narrow-Spectrum AEDs

Drug	Side Effects
carbamazepine	Drowsiness, dizziness, headaches and feeling or being sick
eslicarbazepine	Dizziness, difficulty with balance, rapid and repeated eye movements that are uncontrolled, excessive tiredness, sleepiness, weakness, forgetfulness or memory loss, difficulty concentrating
ethosuximide	Cramps, hiccups, increased hair growth on the face, nausea or vomiting, nearsightedness, pain or discomfort (in the chest, upper stomach, or throat), unusual drowsiness, dullness, tiredness, weakness, or feeling of sluggishness, weight loss
gabapentin	Drowsiness, tiredness or weakness, dizziness, headache, uncontrollable shaking of a part of your body, double or blurred vision, unsteadiness, anxiety
lacosamide	Nausea, vomiting, diarrhea, blurred or double vision, uncontrollable eye movements, dizziness, headache, drowsiness
oxcarbazepine	Dizziness, drowsiness, tiredness, nausea/vomiting, stomach/abdominal pain, headache, trouble sleeping, or constipation
phenobarbital	Drowsiness, headache, dizziness, excitement or increased activity (especially in children), nausea, vomiting
phenytoin	Headaches, feeling drowsy, sleepy or dizzy; feeling nervous, unsteady or shaky; feeling or being sick (nausea or vomiting), constipation, sore or swollen gums, mild skin rash
pregabalin	Dizziness, drowsiness, swelling in hands and feet, trouble concentrating, increased appetite, weight gain
tiagabine	Dizziness or lightheadedness, drowsiness, lack of energy or weakness; wobbliness, unsteadiness, or incoordination causing difficulty walking; depression, hostility or anger, irritability, confusion
vigabatrin	Problems walking or feeling uncoordinated, dizziness, shaking (tremors), joint pain, memory problems and not thinking clearly, eye problems (blurry vision, double vision, and eye movements that you cannot control)

Side effects for which the patient should be instructed to call the prescriber immediately include difficulty coordinating movements; skin rashes; easy bruising; tiny, purple-colored skin spots (petechiae, an indication of bleeding beneath the skin); bloody nose; or any unusual bleeding. These side effects likely indicate allergic and adverse reactions to these drugs.

Possible Adverse Effects of Narrow-Spectrum AEDs

Allergic reactions are an adverse effect of most narrow-spectrum AEDs. Adverse effects of both *carbamazepine* and *phenytoin* include neutropenia (a decrease in the number of white blood cells [WBCs] with sore throat, fever, and chills), and aplastic anemia (anemia caused by too few red blood cells [RBCs] produced by the bone marrow). A patient who develops neutropenia is at risk for life-threatening infections, whereas a patient with aplastic anemia does not have enough RBCs to carry oxygen to the tissues and cells.

Carbamazepine can also cause thrombocytopenia (low platelet count), increasing a patient's risk for severe bleeding. *Phenytoin* can lead to Stevens-Johnson syndrome (see Chapter 1), a serious and life-threatening body-wide (systemic) allergic reaction with a rash involving burnlike sores on the skin and mucous membranes. This syndrome usually indicates a serious allergic reaction to a drug.

The adverse events of *eslicarbazepine* are dizziness, somnolence, nausea, headache, diplopia, vomiting, fatigue, vertigo, ataxia, blurred vision, and tremor. *Ethosuximide* may cause serious allergic reactions affecting multiple body organs (e.g., liver or kidney). *Gabapentin* can cause life-threatening breathing problems, as well as thoughts about suicide or behavior changes.

The most serious adverse effect reported with *lacosamide* is cardiac conduction disturbances (e.g., sinus node dysfunction). Adverse effects of *oxcarbazepine* are related to the central nervous system and digestive system, including fatigue, drowsiness, diplopia, dizziness, nausea and vomiting. Long-term use of *oxcarbazepine* may also cause hyponatremia (low sodium).

When *gabapentin* is prescribed for a patient who is taking morphine, increased blood levels of gabapentin can occur, possibly leading to toxicity. A lower dose of gabapentin, morphine, or both may be required to avoid side effects.

Several life-threatening adverse effects are associated with *phenobarbital*, including closure of the larynx, which blocks the passage of air to the lungs (laryngospasm); circulatory collapse (shock); and decreased number of WBCs (neutropenia). Additional adverse effects include respiratory depression when high doses are prescribed, CNS depression, coma, and death. Swelling similar to that seen in urticaria (hives) can occur beneath the skin instead of on the surface. Other adverse effects include deep swelling around the eyes and lips and sometimes of the hands and feet (angioedema; see Chapter 1) and hypersensitive reaction to the administration of a foreign serum (serum sickness), which is characterized by fever, swelling, skin rash, and enlargement of the lymph nodes. Phenobarbital is one of the first AEDs and is not used as commonly now because of its many adverse effects.

⊛ Priority Actions to Take *Before* Giving Narrow-Spectrum AEDs

In addition to the general responsibilities related to AEDs (p. 425), if the patient is to receive an IV drug such as *phenytoin*, make sure to check the IV site for patency and solution compatibility. Use normal saline because this drug precipitates (forms solid particles) due to chemical incompatibility with dextrose solutions.

Be sure to schedule at least 2 hours between gabapentin and antacid drugs.

Ask older adults about the presence of liver or kidney problems.

If the patient is to receive any IV drug form (e.g., *phenobarbital, phenytoin)*, be sure to check that the IV site is patent and the IV solution is compatible with the drug.

⊛ Priority Actions to Take *After* Giving Narrow-Spectrum AEDs

In addition to the general responsibilities related to AEDs (p. 425), assess the patient's gait. Remind him or her about the importance of frequent and careful mouth care.

Be sure to ask the patient about nausea and vomiting. If GI symptoms develop, give these drugs with food or a snack. Remind the patient to drink plenty of water because these drugs dry the mouth and increase urine excretion.

Watch for side effects such as abnormal bleeding and report these to the prescriber especially if the patient is receiving anticoagulant therapy.

⊛ Teaching Priorities for Patients Taking Narrow-Spectrum AEDs

In addition to the general precautions related to AEDs (p. 426), include these teaching points and precautions:

- You may need to have occasional laboratory tests done to check blood levels of these drugs or to check for liver damage.
- If you are a female patient of childbearing age, birth control pills may not work effectively while taking these drugs. To prevent pregnancy, you may need to use another form of contraception.

 Drug Alert

Interaction Alert

When a patient takes morphine at the same time as *gabapentin* (Neurontin), the blood level of gabapentin is increased and could become toxic.

QSEN: Safety

 Drug Alert

Administration Alert

Do **not** use dextrose solutions with IV phenytoin because it causes precipitation as a result of chemical incompatibility.

QSEN: Safety

 Drug Alert

Teaching Alert

Drugs for generalized and focal seizures interfere with the effects of birth control pills. Women may need to use another form of contraception to avoid becoming pregnant.

QSEN: Safety

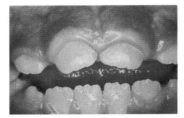

FIG. 23.5 Developmental gingival enlargement (overgrowth).

- Carbamazepine (Tegretol) can make your skin more sensitive to sunlight. Be sure to wear protective clothing and sunscreen, and avoid the use of sun lamps or tanning beds.
- Phenytoin (Dilantin) can cause extra growth of gum tissues. Be sure to visit your dentist regularly and brush and floss your teeth carefully.
- Take phenytoin at least 2 to 3 hours before or after using antacids because antacids decrease absorption of phenytoin.
- If you have diabetes and are prescribed gabapentin, this drug may affect a dipstick test for protein in the urine *(proteinuria)*.
- You should take gabapentin (Neurontin) at least 2 hours after an antacid because antacids can decrease absorption of this drug.
- If you are prescribed phenobarbital, take it only for the period of time it is prescribed, because it may become habit forming.
- Phenobarbital interferes with the actions of birth control pills. If you are a woman taking this drug you should use another form of contraception to prevent pregnancy. Be sure to notify your prescriber immediately if you are pregnant, breastfeeding, or planning to become pregnant.
- If you are prescribed phenobarbital, avoid alcohol because it adds to the drowsiness that this drug may cause.
- Avoid suddenly stopping drugs for seizures because the frequency of seizures may increase or change.

Life Span Considerations for Narrow-Spectrum AEDs

Pediatric considerations. *Carbamazepine* is preferred over *phenobarbital* for children because it has fewer adverse effects on behavior and alertness. *Phenytoin* must be used carefully for children because of extra growth of gums while taking the drug. Children are more likely to have behavioral changes while taking *carbamazepine*. Adolescents often require increased dosages of antiseizure drugs because of growth and hormone changes. Adolescents are at risk to stop taking this drug to avoid changes to the skin and gums and to fit in more closely with their peers (Figure 23.5). *Gabapentin* may cause fever, hyperactivity, and hostile or aggressive behavior in children because they are much more sensitive to the effects of this drug and are at increased risk of side effects.

Considerations for pregnancy and lactation. Several narrow-spectrum AEDs (e.g., carbamazepine and phenytoin) have a high likelihood of increasing the risk for birth defects or fetal damage and may be used during pregnancy only if the potential benefits outweigh the risks to the fetus. A seizure during pregnancy can result in oxygen loss to the fetus or physical injury to the mother or fetus if a fall occurs. Some infants have been born with low birth weight, small head sizes, skull or facial defects, underdeveloped fingernails, and delayed growth when mothers took large doses of these drugs during pregnancy. Carbamazepine passes into breast milk. Recent research indicates that most AEDs are considered safe or moderately safe during breastfeeding and most mothers with epilepsy are encouraged to breastfeed.

Taking *phenytoin* during pregnancy increases the risk of children born with cleft palate. Fetal hydantoin syndrome is a rare disorder that is caused by exposure of a fetus to phenytoin. The symptoms of this disorder may include abnormalities of the skull and facial features, growth deficiencies, underdeveloped nails of the fingers and toes, and/or mild developmental delays.

Considerations for older adults. Older adults are more sensitive to the effects of these drugs and may experience confusion, restlessness, nervousness, and abnormal heart rhythms. Older adults may also experience chest pain. Monitor heart rate and rhythm more frequently. Teach older adults to check their pulse at least once daily and to report abnormal or irregular beats to the prescriber. Stress the importance of calling 911 or getting to the nearest emergency department if chest pain occurs, especially if it is accompanied by shortness of breath.

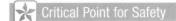

Gabapentin is more slowly eliminated from an older adult's body. Because of this, older adults may need to be started on a lower drug dose.

BROAD-SPECTRUM ANTIEPILEPTIC DRUGS (AEDs)

Broad-spectrum AEDs are the best choice of treatment when a patient has more than one type of seizure. They are designed to treat or prevent seizures in more than one part of the brain. Broad-spectrum AEDs are effective in the treatment of a wide variety of seizures.

How Broad-Spectrum AEDs Work

AEDs may have multiple mechanisms of action to block seizures. While they are called "antiepileptic," AEDs do **not** cure epilepsy. They suppress seizures as long as the drugs are in the body. These drugs decrease the likeliness of the brain having seizures by altering and reducing the excessive electrical activity (excitability) of the neurons that normally cause a seizure. Broad-spectrum anti-epileptic drugs are the best and most logical choice at the start of the treatment for seizures.

Broad-Spectrum AEDs and Their Actions

Drug	Action
acetazolamide	Inhibit the enzyme carbonic anhydrase
brivaracetam	Exact action is unknown
cannabidiol	Inhibition of intracellular calcium release decreases excitatory currents and seizure activity
cenobamate	Partly described, the drug acts on voltage-gated sodium channels through a pronounced action on persistent rather than transient currents
clobazam	Not fully understood, thought to involve potentiation of GABAergic neurotransmission resulting from binding at a benzodiazepine site at the GABA(A) receptor
clonazepam	Enhances the activity of the inhibitory neurotransmitter gamma-aminobutyric acid (GABA) in the central nervous system
clorazepate	Enhances the activity of the inhibitory neurotransmitter gamma-aminobutyric acid (GABA) in the central nervous system
diazepam	Enhances the inhibitory action of GABA, decreases inhibition in neuronal networks and affects calcium ion transport
divalproex	Increases the concentration of gamma-aminobutyric acid (GABA) in the brain
ethosuximide	Inhibits NADPH-linked aldehyde reductase necessary for the formation of gamma-hydroxybutyrate
felbamate	Dual actions on excitatory (NMDA) and inhibitory (GABA) brain mechanisms
fenfluramine	Causes the release of serotonin by disrupting vesicular storage of the neurotransmitter, and reversing serotonin transporter function
lamotrigine	Blocks sodium channels, stabilizing the electrical activity of the brain
levetiracetam	Modulation of synaptic neurotransmitter release through binding to the synaptic vesicle protein SV2A in the brain
lorazepam	Binds to a type of GABA receptor, called GABAA, and activates it in a similar way to GABA, to reduce the uncontrolled firing of neurons that causes seizures
methsuxamide	Elevates the seizure threshold and reduces the frequency of attacks through depression of nerve transmission in the cortex
perampanel	Excitatory neurotransmitter; exact antiepileptic mechanism in humans is unknown
primidone	Alters sodium and calcium channel transport, reducing the frequency of nerve firing
rufinamide	Exact mechanism is unknown, but thought to be modulation of activity in sodium channels
stiripentol	Inhibition of GABA reuptake from the synaptic cleft
topiramate	Helps prevent brain cells from working as fast as a seizure requires them to; thus, seizures can be stopped when they are just beginning
valproic acid	Increases availability of the neurotransmitter gamma-aminobutyric acid (GABA)
zonisamide	Decreases abnormal electrical activity in the brain

Generic names, brand names, uses, and common adult dosages of broad-spectrum AEDs are listed in the following table. The FDA has approved these broad-spectrum AEDs for the treatment of seizures or epilepsy. Be sure to consult a reliable drug resource for specific information about these broad-spectrum AEDs.

Dosages and Uses for Common Broad-Spectrum Antiepileptic Drugs (AEDs)

Drug	Uses	Dosage
acetazolamide (Diamox)	Adjunctive agent for refractory epilepsy	8–30 mg/kg/day orally, given in up to 4 divided doses. Usual maintenance dosage is 375–1000 mg/day
brivaracetam (Briviact)	Focal seizures	50 mg orally twice daily IV 50 mg twice daily Adjust dosage to 25 to 100 mg orally or IV twice daily based on clinical response and tolerability
cannabidiol (Epidiolex)	Seizures caused by tuberous sclerosis, [a]Dravet syndrome, [b]Lennox-Gastaut syndrome	2.5 mg/kg/dose orally twice daily; increase in weekly increments of 2.5 mg/kg/dose twice daily as tolerated to the recommended maintenance dosage of 5 mg/kg/dose orally twice daily Max: 10 mg/kg/dose orally twice daily
cenobamate (Xcopri)	Focal aware or simple partial seizures	12.5 mg orally once daily for weeks 1 and 2, then 25 mg once daily for weeks 3 and 4, then 50 mg once daily for weeks 5 and 6, then 100 mg once daily for weeks 7 and 8, then 150 mg once daily for weeks 9 and 10, then 200 mg orally once daily
clobazam (Onfi, Sympazan)	Seizures caused by Lennox-Gastaut syndrome	Lennox-Gastaut syndrome: 5 mg orally twice daily initially. Titrate to 10 mg twice daily on Day 7, then 20 mg twice daily on Day 14. Dravet syndrome: 0.2–0.3 mg/kg/day PO divided twice daily initially; increase to a target dose of 0.5–1 mg/kg/day over 2–3 weeks. Max: 2 mg/kg/day
clonazepam (Klonopin)	Myoclonic, absence, and atonic seizures	1.5 mg/day orally, divided into 3 equal doses. This dosage may be increased by 0.5–1 mg every 3 days until seizures are controlled. Usual maintenance dose range is 2 to 8 mg/day. Max: 20 mg/day
clorazepate (Tranxene)	Add-on treatment for focal seizures	7.5 mg orally 2–3 times per day. Increase by no more than 7.5 mg per week. Max: 90 mg/day orally, given in 2–3 divided doses
diazepam (Valium)	Clusters of seizures and prolonged seizures	2–10 mg orally 2–4 times daily 5 to 10 mg IV every 10 to 15 minutes as needed up to a maximum of 30 mg **Status epilepticus**: 0.15–0.2 mg/kg/dose (Max: 10 mg/dose) IV; may repeat once in 5 min if needed. Max: 30 mg
ethosuximide (Zarontin)	Absence seizures	500 mg orally daily, increase by 250 mg every 4–7 days. Max 1.5 g/day
felbamate (Felbatol)	Treatment of all types of seizures that do not respond to other treatments	1200 mg/day orally in 3–4 divided doses. Increase dose in 600 mg increments every 2 weeks to 2400 mg/day orally
fenfluramine (Fintepla)	Seizures caused by Dravet syndrome or Lennox-Gastaut syndrome	0.1 mg/kg/dose orally twice daily, initially. May increase dose to 0.2 mg/kg/dose twice daily after 1 week and further increase dose to 0.35 mg/kg/dose twice daily after another week. Max: 26 mg/day
lamotrigine (Lamictal)	Focal, generalized tonic-clonic, and generalized seizures caused by Lennon-Gastaut syndrome	**With valproic acid:** *Adults:* 25 mg orally every day during weeks 1–2; increase to 100–200 mg/day slowly over several weeks; maximum dosage 200 mg/day **When used with other seizure drugs:** *Adults:* 50–500 mg orally daily in 2 divided doses; usual maintenance dose is 300 to 500 mg/day orally given in 2 divided doses
levetiracetam (Keppra)	Focal, generalized tonic-clonic, and myoclonic seizures	500 mg orally twice daily. Increase dose every 2 weeks by 500 mg/dose (e.g., 1000 mg/day) increments to a maximum recommended dosage of 1500 mg orally twice daily. Max: 3000 mg/day

Dosages and Uses for Common Broad-Spectrum Antiepileptic Drugs (AEDs)—cont'd

Drug	Uses	Dosage
lorazepam (Ativan)	All types of seizures; alcohol-related seizures, status epilepticus	**Acute alcohol-related seizure prophylaxis**: single dose of lorazepam 2 mg IV given within 6 hr of a witnessed ethanol-related seizure **Status epilepticus**: 4 mg IV given slowly at a rate of 2 mg/min. A second 4 mg dose may be given in 10–15 min if needed.
methsuxamide (Celontin)	Absence seizures, refractory epilepsy	300 mg orally daily for 1 week; increase, if necessary, at weekly intervals for 3 weeks by 300 mg increments, up to a maximum of 1.2 g/day orally given in 3–4 divided doses
perampanel (Fycompa)	Focal, generalized seizures; refractory epilepsy	2 mg orally once daily at bedtime initially; titrate by 2 mg/day increments at weekly intervals; recommended maintenance dosage is 8–12 mg/day. Max: 12 mg/day
primidone (Mysoline)	Focal, generalized tonic-clonic seizures	125–250 mg/day orally at bedtime; increase by 125–250 mg/day every 3–7 days Usual dose is 750–1500 mg/day in 3–4 divided doses. Max: 2 g/day
rufinamide (Banzel, Inovelon)	Add-on for seizures caused by Lennon-Gastaut syndrome, Refractory partial seizures	**Lennox-Gastaut syndrome**: 400–800 mg/day orally in 2 equally divided doses. Max: 3200 mg/day given in 2 equally divided doses **Refractory partial seizures**: 3200 mg/day orally given in 2 divided doses
stiripentol (Diacomit)	Seizures caused by Dravet syndrome	Dravet syndrome: 50 mg/kg/day orally administered in 2 or 3 divided doses. Max: 3000 mg/day
topiramate (Topamax)	All types of seizures	50 mg/day orally administered in 2 divided doses. Increase daily dose by 50 mg once per week during weeks 2, 3, and 4. Increase the daily dose by 100 mg once per week during weeks 5 and 6. Recommended final dose, 400 mg per day orally in 2 divided doses. Max: 400 mg/day
valproic acid (Depakene, Depakote)	Monotherapy or adjunctive therapy for simple or complex absence seizures	1015 mg/kg/day orally for partial seizures and 15 mg/kg/day orally for absence seizures. Give in divided doses if the total daily dose exceeds 250 mg. Max: 60 mg/kg/day
zonisamide (Zonegran)	Add-on for focal seizures	100 mg orally once daily. After 2 weeks, the dose may be increased to 200 mg once daily for at least 2 weeks; dose can then be increased to 300 mg once daily and 400 mg once daily, with the dose stable for at least 2 weeks to achieve steady state at each dose. Max: 600 mg/day

[a]Dravet syndrome, previously called **severe myoclonic epilepsy of infancy** (SMEI), is an epilepsy syndrome that begins in infancy or early childhood and includes symptoms ranging from mild to severe.

[b]Lennox-Gastaut syndrome (LGS) is **a type of epilepsy** where patients experience many different types of seizures.

Intended Responses of Broad-Spectrum AEDs
- Seizures are controlled and prevented.
- Abnormal electrical impulses are decreased.
- Resistance of CNS to abnormal stimuli is increased.

Side Effects of Broad-Spectrum AEDs
Common side effects of these drugs include the GI symptoms of nausea, vomiting, and indigestion. They also may cause loss of appetite (anorexia) and weight loss.

Common Side Effects of Broad-Spectrum AEDs

Drug	Side Effects
acetazolamide	Dizziness, lightheadedness, increased urination, blurred vision, dry mouth, drowsiness, loss of appetite, nausea, vomiting, diarrhea, or changes in taste
brivaracetam	Constipation, nausea, vomiting, extreme tiredness or lack of energy, mood problems
cannabidiol	Dry mouth, diarrhea, reduced appetite, drowsiness and fatigue

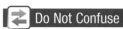 Do Not Confuse

Lamictal *with* **Lamisil**

An order for Lamictal may be confused with Lamisil. Lamictal is an antiseizure drug, whereas Lamisil is an antifungal, anti-infective drug.

QSEN: Safety

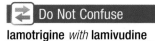 Do Not Confuse

lamotrigine *with* **lamivudine**

An order for lamotrigine may be confused with lamivudine. Lamotrigine is an antiseizure drug, whereas lamivudine is an anti-infective, antiretroviral drug used to treat human immune deficiency virus.

QSEN: Safety

Continued

Common Side Effects of Broad-Spectrum AEDs—cont'd

Drug	Side Effects
cenobamate	Blurred vision, double vision, or other changes in vision. It may also cause some people to become dizzy, drowsy, clumsy, or feel tired.
clobazam	Confusion, worsening of depression, hallucinations, suicidal thoughts, and unusual excitement, nervousness, or irritability
clonazepam	Drowsiness, dizziness, weakness, unsteadiness, depression, loss of orientation, headache, sleep disturbances, problems with thinking
clorazepate	Drowsiness, dizziness, tiredness, headache, nervousness, confusion, dry mouth
diazepam	Drowsiness, muscle weakness, fatigue, loss of control of body movements (ataxia)
divalproex	Diarrhea, dizziness, drowsiness, hair loss, blurred/double vision, change in menstrual periods, ringing in the ears, shakiness (tremor), unsteadiness
ethosuximide	Cramps, hiccups, increased hair growth, nausea or vomiting, near-sightedness; pain or discomfort in the chest, upper stomach, or throat; unusual drowsiness, dullness, tiredness, weakness, or feeling of sluggishness, weight loss
felbamate	Dizziness, drowsiness, sleep problems, weight loss, nausea, vomiting, double vision, taste changes
fenluramine	Chest pain, pounding heartbeats or fluttering in your chest; shortness of breath; unusual tiredness or weakness, feeling like you might pass out.
lamotrigine	Skin rashes and headaches, ataxia, insomnia, nausea
levetiracetam	Headaches, drowsiness, blocked nose, itchy throat
lorazepam	Drowsiness, dizziness, tiredness, muscle weakness, headache, blurred vision, sleep problems, loss or balance or coordination, forgetfulness, difficulty concentrating, nausea, vomiting, constipation, changes in appetite, rashes
methsuxamide	Drowsiness, dizziness, loss of muscle coordination, decreased appetite, headache, hiccups, nausea, vomiting, stomach cramps
perampanel	Dizziness, drowsiness, constipation, nausea, vomiting, headache, tiredness, weight gain
primidone	Dizziness, drowsiness, excitation, tiredness, headache, loss of appetite, nausea, or vomiting
rufinamide	Dizziness, drowsiness, fatigue, headache, nausea, and vomiting
stiripentol	Somnolence, decreased appetite, agitation, ataxia, weight decreased, hypotonia, nausea, tremor, dysarthria, and insomnia
topiramate	Dizziness, drowsiness, tiredness, speech and memory problems, vision problems, weight loss, taste changes, nausea, decreased appetite
valproic acid	Diarrhea, dizziness, drowsiness, hair loss, blurred/double vision, change in menstrual periods, ringing in the ears, shakiness (tremor), unsteadiness, taste changes
zonisamide	Dizziness, drowsiness, problems with memory or concentration, feeling agitated or irritable, loss of coordination, trouble walking, loss of appetite.

Common Side Effects

Broad-Spectrum AEDs

Ataxia,   Drowsiness   Headache
Dizziness

Nausea/Vomiting,   Weight loss
Loss of appetite

Other side effects of these drugs include mental confusion, drowsiness, dizziness, headaches, constipation, depression, and nervousness.

Patients taking these drugs should notify their prescriber immediately about symptoms of allergic reaction such as rashes, fever, and sore throat. The prescriber should also be notified immediately about signs of bleeding such as easy bruising, petechiae, bloody nose, or any unusual bleeding.

Possible Adverse Effects of Broad-Spectrum AEDs

Adverse effects of *ethosuximide* (Zarontin) include a decrease in the number of WBCs *(neutropenia)*; reduction in the number of erythrocytes, all types of WBCs, and blood platelets in the circulating blood (pancytopenia); and anemia caused by deficient RBC production in the bone marrow (aplastic anemia).

Valproic acid can lead to damage or destruction in the liver (hepatotoxicity), inflammation of the pancreas (pancreatitis), and bone marrow depression. Bone marrow depression can result in reduced production of RBCs, which causes anemia; reduced WBCs, which can result in infection; and reduced platelets, which can result in bleeding. Valproic acid may cause prolonged bleeding time.

Primidone decreases the effects of anticoagulant drugs, so higher doses of an anticoagulant may be needed to achieve therapeutic effects.

Clonazepam is a benzodiazepine CNS drug with the life-threatening adverse reaction of respiratory depression. *Lamotrigine* can lead to Stevens-Johnson syndrome, a serious and life-threatening body-wide (systemic) allergic reaction with a rash involving the skin and mucous membranes (see Chapter 1). It can also lead to toxic epidermal necrolysis, a life-threatening skin disorder characterized by blistering and peeling of the top layer of skin. Sudden withdrawal of *pregabalin* can increase the frequency of seizure activity. This drug should be gradually withdrawn over a week.

✪ Priority Actions to Take *Before* Giving *Broad*-Spectrum AEDs

In addition to the general responsibilities related to antiseizure drugs (p. 425), review the patient's baseline coagulation laboratory, liver function, and blood count test results. Obtain a baseline weight for the patient. Assess level of consciousness, energy level, and vision to provide a baseline for assessment before giving these drugs.

✪ Priority Actions to Take *After* Giving Broad-Spectrum AEDs

In addition to the general responsibilities related to antiseizure drugs (p. 425), check the patient's weight every day. If the patient develops GI distress, give these drugs with food.

Be sure to assess for and ask about side effects and watch for adverse effects of these drugs. Notify the prescriber if side effects or adverse effects occur. If the patient develops a rash, hold the drug and notify the prescriber immediately. To minimize the risk of severe rashes, the dose of *lamotrigine* (Lamictal) can be increased very slowly over 6 to 7 weeks. If the patient is taking lamotrigine, skin rash can be the first sign of Stevens-Johnson syndrome (see Chapter 1) or toxic epidermal necrolysis.

✪ Teaching Priorities for Patients Taking Broad-Spectrum AEDs

In addition to the general precautions related to AEDs (p. 426), include these teaching points and precautions:
- Take your prescribed drug(s) exactly as directed and take missed doses as soon as possible but **not** to take double doses.
- Do **not** stop taking these drugs suddenly because seizures may occur.
- If you are scheduled for surgery, including dental surgery, notify your surgeon or dentist about the use of these drugs.
- If you are prescribed ethosuximide (Zarontin) protect your eyes by wearing dark glasses because this drug can make your eyes more sensitive to light.
- Valproic acid (Depakote, Depacon) can lead to blood problems that can cause slowed healing and increased risk for infection. Notify your prescriber immediately if you notice symptoms of infection (e.g., fever, redness, chills, coughing, fatigue, headache, muscle aches).
- Notify your prescriber immediately about any signs of allergic reactions to these drugs, including skin rashes, fever, flu-like symptoms, and swollen glands.
- Notify your prescriber immediately if seizure activity increases or changes.

Action/Intervention Alert

Give drugs for seizures with food if GI symptoms such as nausea, vomiting, and stomach upset develop.

QSEN: Safety

Action/Intervention Alert

If a patient develops a rash, do not give the drug and notify the prescriber immediately because this may indicate an allergic reaction.

QSEN: Safety

Teaching Alert

Teach patients to **never** suddenly stop taking AEDs because this may cause seizures to occur.

QSEN: Safety

Teaching Alert

Teach patients taking *ethosuximide* (Zarontin) to wear dark glasses when going out into bright light.

QSEN: Safety

Action/Intervention Alert

Monitor a patient who is taking *valproic acid* (Depakote) closely for wound healing and signs of infection.

QSEN: Safety

Teaching Alert

Teach patients to notify their prescriber immediately if seizure activity increases or changes in any way.

QSEN: Safety

- If you are prescribed clonazepam, take it only for the period it is prescribed because it may become habit forming.
- Primidone (Mysoline) interferes with the actions of birth control pills. If you are a woman taking this drug, you should use another form of contraception to prevent pregnancy. Notify your prescriber immediately if you become pregnant, are breastfeeding, or are planning to become pregnant.
- If you are prescribed primidone or lamotrigine, avoid alcohol because it adds to the drowsiness that these drugs may cause.
- If you are prescribed lamotrigine, be sure to use sunscreen and wear protective clothes to prevent photosensitivity reactions (even if you have dark skin).
- If you smoke while taking clonazepam (Klonopin) be aware that cigarette smoking may decrease the effectiveness of this drug and a higher dose of the drug may be needed for it to be effective.
- Avoid suddenly stopping all drugs for seizures because the frequency of seizures may increase or change.

Life Span Considerations for Broad-Spectrum AEDs

Pediatric considerations. Children younger than 2 years of age are at increased risk for liver damage that may lead to death with valproic acid. Growing children who take drugs for seizures often need dose increases as they grow. Adolescence is a physically and emotionally stressful time with an increased risk for seizure occurrences. Children have a higher incidence of rashes with lamotrigine.

Considerations for pregnancy and lactation. Valproic acid has a high likelihood of increasing the risk for birth defects or fetal damage. During pregnancy it has been associated with developmental defects, low IQ, birth defects, congenital anomalies, and damage to the infant's liver. This drug also passes into breast milk and should not be used while a mother is breastfeeding. Women are more likely to experience dizziness when taking lamotrigine. Primidone may cause increased birth defects, and there have been reports of newborns with bleeding problems. Lamotrigine limits the body's production of folic acid. Folic acid deficiency during pregnancy is associated with a variety of birth defects. To prevent deficiency during pregnancy, a woman taking lamotrigine should take folic acid supplements throughout the pregnancy. With clonazepam, and primidone, animal studies have shown that newborns have lower weight and have a lower survival rate. These drugs pass into breast milk and should not be taken by a woman who is breastfeeding because they may cause unwanted side effects in infants.

Considerations for older adults. Valproic acid should be used cautiously in older adults because they may be more sensitive to its side effects such as sleepiness and dizziness. Teach older adults to take special precautions to avoid falls. Instruct them to change positions slowly and to use handrails when going up or down stairs. Suggest that older adults avoid driving or using dangerous machines until they know how the drugs will affect them.

Older adults are also more sensitive to these drugs and more likely to develop side effects. They may develop unusual restlessness or excitement with *primidone*. *Lamotrigine* is more slowly eliminated from an older adult's body. Because of this, older adults may need to be started on a lower drug dose.

SECOND-LINE (ALTERNATIVE) DRUGS FOR SEIZURES

Second-line drugs for seizures are drugs for the treatment of seizures often prescribed with another seizure drug or when an AED does not work. Included in this group are *phenobarbital* and *primidone* (Mysoline), which increase the body's threshold against seizure activity by blocking or slowing the spread of abnormal impulses. A big disadvantage of *phenobarbital* is that it can lead to physical dependence. *Primidone* is

Drug Alert

Teaching Alert

Teach patients **not** to smoke while taking *clonazepam* (Klonopin) because smoking decreases the effective of this drug and a higher dosage may be prescribed for it to be effective.

QSEN: Safety

Drug Alert

Teaching Alert

During pregnancy a woman prescribed lamotrigine will need to take folic acid supplements to prevent birth defects.

QSEN: Safety

Drug Alert

Action/Intervention Alert

Children and older adults are more sensitive to the effects of antiseizure drugs (AEDs) and are more likely to develop side effects. Monitor these patients carefully.

QSEN: Safety

turned into phenobarbital by the body and acts in the same way as phenobarbital. *Gabapentin* (Neurontin) and *lamotrigine* (Lamictal) stabilize the membranes of neurons to decrease seizure activity. The action of *clonazepam* (Klonopin) is not well understood but may be related to inhibition (slowing or stopping) of transmission of abnormal impulses. *Pregabalin* (Lyrica) is used to decrease the frequency of partial seizures.

Second-line drugs for seizures are often prescribed with other seizure medications, causing an increased risk for side effects. When more than one AEDs are prescribed together, lower doses may be needed. For more information on any of these drugs, please see the previous sections on narrow-spectrum and wide-spectrum drugs for seizures for more information on these drugs.

Get Ready for the NCLEX® Examination!

Key Points

- Although 10% of Americans experience a single seizure at some time during their lives, the majority never experience another seizure.
- Abnormal electrical impulses in the brain cause seizures to occur.
- The cause of many abnormal electrical impulses in the brain leading to seizures is not known.
- The most common ages for onset of seizures are early childhood and late adulthood.
- A person who has seizures is more likely to have a seizure during times of increased emotional or physical stress.
- A typical seizure consists of an aura, the seizure, and a postictal period.
- Status epilepticus is a prolonged seizure or a series of repeated seizures without enough time for recovery between seizures that can lead to brain damage, coma, and death.
- The exact action of most antiseizure drugs is not known, but these drugs decrease the voltage, frequency, and spread of abnormal electrical impulses in the brain.
- Drugs for seizures include broad- and narrow-spectrum medications, and sometimes more than one drug is needed to control seizures.
- Drugs for focal and generalized seizures can increase the effects of anticoagulant drugs. Assess patients for abnormal bleeding.
- Because drugs for focal and generalized seizures can cause dizziness and drowsiness, a patient should not get out of bed without assistance until the effects of the drug are known.
- Patients taking drugs to prevent generalized or focal seizures should not drink alcohol because it can increase the side effects of dizziness or drowsiness.
- While prescribed and taking any antiseizure drug, patients should be taught to avoid grapefruit and grapefruit juice because they may increase the effects of these drugs.
- Many drugs for seizures interfere with the effects of birth control pills, and women should be taught to use an alternative form of contraception to prevent pregnancy.
- Antacids decrease the absorption of antiseizure drugs and should be given at least 2 to 3 hours before or after taking these drugs.

- Patients should be instructed to notify their prescriber immediately if seizure activity increases or changes in any way.
- Patients who suddenly stop taking antiseizure drugs are at high risk for having a seizure.
- Report signs of allergic reaction or abnormal bleeding immediately to the prescriber.
- Give drugs for seizures with food if GI symptoms such as nausea, vomiting, and stomach upset develop.
- *Narrow-spectrum AEDs* are prescribed for specific types of seizures while *broad-spectrum AEDs* are effective in the treatment of a wide variety of seizures.
- Teach patients taking drugs for generalized and focal seizures to notify their prescriber immediately for signs of allergic or adverse reactions.
- When a patient takes morphine at the same time as *gabapentin* (Neurontin), the blood level of gabapentin is increased and could become toxic.
- Do **not** use dextrose solutions with IV *phenytoin* because it causes precipitation as a result of chemical incompatibility.
- Patients taking *phenytoin* (Dilantin) should see their dentist regularly because of extra growth of the gums that occurs while taking this drug.
- Assess older adults who have been narrow-spectrum AEDs for focal or generalized seizures for abnormal heart rhythms and chest pain. Report these occurrences immediately to the prescriber.
- Teach patients not to smoke while taking *clonazepam* (Klonopin) because smoking decreases the effective of this drug and a higher dosage may be prescribed for it to be effective.
- Children and older adults are more sensitive to the effects of antiseizure drugs (AEDs) and are more likely to develop side effects. Monitor these patients carefully.

Additional Learning Resources

Be sure to visit your Evolve website (http://evolve.elsevier.com/Workman/pharmacology/) for additional online resources.

SG Go to your Study Guide for additional learning activities to help you master this chapter content.

Review Questions

See *Answers to In-Text Review Questions* in the back of the book for answers to these questions.

1. A patient with a seizure disorder tells the nurse about training to participate in a marathon run. What is the **most important** information for the nurse to teach the patient at this time?

   A. "Your seizure medications prohibit training for this stressful event."
   B. "During times of increased physical stress, you are more likely to have a seizure."
   C. "Be sure to watch your diet because during training you will need more calories."
   D. "Start your exercise program slowly and gradually build up your strength."

2. A patient with a seizure disorder asks the nurse why she always sees bright spots before experiencing a seizure. What is the nurse's **best** response?

   A. "Some people experience a strange sensation called an aura before each seizure."
   B. "This is an unusual occurrence. I will notify your prescriber right away."
   C. "Bright spots before a seizure could indicate pressure in your brain from a tumor."
   D. "After the seizure do you feel confused, lethargic, and unable to respond to people?"

3. Which sign or symptom does the nurse expect to find when assessing a patient who is having an absence seizure?

   A. Rigidity of arm and leg muscles
   B. Automatisms such as lip smacking
   C. Blank staring as if daydreaming
   D. One-sided movement of an extremity

4. A patient who has been prescribed phenytoin reports gum swelling around the teeth. What is the nurse's **best** action?

   A. Tell the patient to document this unexpected change by taking a photograph.
   B. Instruct the patient to stop the drug and notify the prescriber immediately.
   C. Reassure the patient that this is a common and expected side effect.
   D. Remind the patient to brush teeth gently and avoid flossing.

5. A patient who has been taking carbamazepine for 2 months has all of the following blood laboratory results. Which result does the nurse report to the prescriber **immediately**?

   A. White blood cell (WBC) count 2200/mm³
   B. Platelet count 300,000/mm³
   C. Potassium 3.6 mEq/L
   D. Sodium 132 mEq/L

6. A female patient with a seizure disorder who is taking birth control pills is prescribed valproic acid. What information is **most important** for the nurse to include in this patient's teaching plan?

   A. "Do not drive a car until you know how this drug will affect you."
   B. "Be sure to change positions slowly when getting out of bed."

   C. "Avoid consumption of grapefruit or grapefruit juice."
   D. "Plan to use another form of contraception."

7. A patient who has been prescribed ethosuximide twice daily (every 12 hr) for absence seizures reports that the morning dose was missed 10 hr ago. What is the nurse's **best** advice?

   A. "Skip today's second dose as well as the dose you already missed."
   B. "Take the missed dose now and the regularly scheduled dose in 2 hours."
   C. "Take the missed dose and the regularly scheduled second dose immediately."
   D. "Take the regularly scheduled second dose now and forget about the morning dose."

8. A patient who has been prescribed ethosuximide tells the nurse about experiencing an upset stomach after each dose of the drug. What is the nurse's **best** action?

   A. Administering a dose of an antinausea drug
   B. Instructing the patient to take the drug with a full glass of water
   C. Giving the drug with meals or a snack
   D. Elevating the head of the bed to avoid aspiration

9. A patient is prescribed lamotrigine for seizure control. The drug received from the pharmacy is Lamisil. What is the nurse's **best** action?

   A. Administering the drug as prescribed
   B. Holding the dose and calling the pharmacy immediately
   C. Asking the patient whether he or she recognizes the tablet
   D. Notifying the prescriber that the usual brand of lamotrigine is not available

10. A patient who is prescribed gabapentin is also taking morphine sulfate for severe pain. What dosage adjustment will the nurse expect?

    A. Decreased dosage of gabapentin
    B. Increased dosage of gabapentin
    C. Decreased dosage of morphine
    D. Increased dosage of morphine

11. How will the nurse document the seizure activity for a patient who experiences a sudden loss of muscle tone for a few seconds followed by confusion?

    A. Partial seizures
    B. Atonic seizures
    C. Myoclonic seizures
    D. Tonic-clonic seizures

12. A patient is prescribed valproic acid 340 mg intravenously. The available drug solution is 500 mg in 5 mL. How many milliliters will the nurse give for this dose?

    A. 1.4 mL
    B. 2.4 mL
    C. 3.4 mL
    D. 4.4 mL

Clinical Judgment

1. Which factors are common causes of seizures in adults? **Select all that apply.**

   A. Emotional stress
   B. Liver failure
   C. Heart dysrhythmias
   D. Tumors
   E. Lack of sleep
   F. Asthma
   G. Sun exposure
   H. Physical stress
   I. Head injury
   J. Stroke

2. The nurse is providing a teaching session in the community for several women of child-bearing age who are diagnosed with a seizure disorder and prescribed antiepileptic drugs (AEDs). Which teaching points are appropriate for the teaching session, not appropriate for the teaching session, or may cause harm? **Place an X in the columns to indicate which teaching points Should Be Included, which Should Not Be Included, and which May Cause Harm If Included.**

TEACHING POINT	SHOULD BE INCLUDED	SHOULD NOT BE INCLUDED	MAY CAUSE HARM IF INCLUDED
Valproic acid has a high likelihood of increasing the risk for birth defects or fetal damage.			
Breastfeeding while taking AEDs is safe and recommended.			
A woman taking lamotrigine should take folic acid supplements throughout the pregnancy.			
If you are taking phenobarbital, you can use birth control pills to prevent pregnancy.			
Primidone had been reported to cause bleeding problems in newborn infants.			
Fetal hydantoin syndrome is a rare disorder that is caused by exposure of a fetus to gabapentin.			
If you are prescribed primidone or lamotrigine, you may consume only 1–2 alcoholic drinks per day.			
Valproic acid during pregnancy has been associated with developmental defects, low IQ, birth defects, congenital anomalies, and damage to the infant's liver.			

24 Drug Therapy for Alzheimer's and Parkinson's Diseases

Learning Objectives

The content presented in this chapter should help you to:

1. Describe how different classes of drugs are used to treat Alzheimer's disease and Parkinson's disease.
2. Describe the names, actions, usual adult dosages, possible side effects, and adverse effects of drugs for Alzheimer's disease.
3. Discuss the priority actions to take *before* and *after* giving commonly prescribed drugs for Alzheimer's disease.
4. Prioritize essential information to teach patients and their families and caregivers about commonly prescribed drugs for Alzheimer's disease.

5. Describe the names, actions, usual adult dosages, possible side effects, and adverse effects of drugs for Parkinson's disease.
6. Discuss the priority actions to take *before* and *after* giving commonly prescribed drugs for Parkinson's disease.
7. Prioritize essential information to teach patients and their families and caregivers about commonly prescribed drugs for Parkinson's disease.
8. Explain life span considerations for drugs for Alzheimer's and Parkinson's disease.

Key Terms

anticholinergic drugs (ăn-tĭ-kō-lĭn-ĔRJ-ĭk DRŬGZ) (p. 448) (See Chapter 19.)

catechol-*O*-methyltransferase (COMT) inhibitors (KĂ-tĕ-kŏl Ō MĔ-thŭl-TRĂNS-fŭr-ās ĭn-HĬB-ĭ-tŏrz) (p. 448) A group of drugs used to treat Parkinson's disease that allow a larger amount of levodopa to reach the brain, which raises dopamine levels in the brain and reduces symptoms.

cholinesterase/acetylcholinesterase inhibitors (KŌ-lĭn-ĔS-tĕr-ās/ăs-ĕ-tĭl-KŌ-lĭn-ĔS-tĕr-ās ĭn-HĬB-ĭ-tŏrz) (p. 443) A group of drugs used to treat Alzheimer's disease that reduce the activity of the enzyme acetylcholinesterase which breaks down

acetylcholine in the synapses of neurons to keep levels of acetylcholine higher and slow the progress of the disease.

dopaminergic/dopamine agonists (DŌ-pă-mĭ-nĕr-jĭk/DŌ-pă-mēn ĂG-ŏ-nĭsts) (p. 448) A group of drugs used to treat Parkinson's disease that increase the amount of dopamine activity in the brain, thus reducing tremor and muscle rigidity, and improving movement.

monoamine oxidase B (MAO-B) inhibitors (MŎ-nō-ă-mēn ŎK-sĭ-dās ĭn-HĬB-ĭ-tŏrz) (p. 448) A group of drugs used to treat Parkinson's disease that inhibit the enzyme that breaks down dopamine in the brain.

OVERVIEW

Alzheimer's disease and *Parkinson's disease* are both progressive neurologic disorders that occur more commonly in older adults. Parkinson's disease is a neurodegenerative disease with slow and progressive degeneration of the nervous system. Alzheimer's disease is the most common form of dementia. Both illnesses involve interrupted transmission of nerve impulses. Transmission of these impulses is normally helped by the presence of *neurotransmitters* (e.g., dopamine, acetylcholine), which are chemicals that transmit messages from one nerve cell *(neuron)* to another (see Figure 25.3 in Chapter 25).

ALZHEIMER'S DISEASE

Alzheimer's disease (AD) is a progressive and incurable condition that destroys brain cells, with gradual loss of intellectual abilities such as memory and extreme changes in personality and behavior. It is the most feared and most common form of dementia. *Dementia* is a brain disorder that seriously affects a person's ability to perform activities of daily living (ADLs), including loss of intellectual functions (e.g., thinking, remembering, and reasoning). It is estimated in 2021 that 6.2 million Americans age 65 and older are living with Alzheimer's dementia in the United States (2021 Alzheimer's disease facts and figures), and it affects about 50 million people worldwide. Dementia is currently the seventh leading cause of death among all diseases and one of the major causes of disability and dependency among older people globally. It involves physical, psychological, social, and economic impacts on people living with dementia and on their care providers, families, and society.

REVIEW OF RELATED PHYSIOLOGY AND PATHOPHYSIOLOGY FOR ALZHEIMER'S DISEASE

Pathophysiological changes with Alzheimer's disease are twofold (Animation 24.1). First is the presence of large amounts of the protein beta-amyloid (Abeta), which clumps together and forms plaques between cells in the brain. Second, other proteins twist and form tangles within the cell bodies of the neurons. (The nerve axons and dendrites are **not** tangled.) As a result, neurons die in the areas of the brain that are important to memory and other essential mental abilities (Figure 24.1). Connections between nerve cells are also disrupted. Levels of chemicals (e.g., acetylcholine) in the brain that carry messages between nerve cells are lower.

No single cause has been established for Alzheimer's disease. Instead, a combination of factors has been proposed. Age is the greatest risk factor. Genetics also plays a role in the development of this condition. Mutations in the *APOEe4* gene and several other genes are associated with an increased risk for AD. People with Down syndrome, a common disorder involving an extra chromosome number 21 (trisomy 21), have an increased risk for Alzheimer's disease by age 50 to 60 years. A person who has a severe head injury or whiplash injury may also be at increased risk of developing dementia. People who smoke or have high blood pressure or high cholesterol levels also seem to have a higher risk for Alzheimer's disease.

Alzheimer's disease symptoms begin very slowly. In the early stage, the first symptom may be mild forgetfulness, which can be confused with age-related memory changes. Table 24.1 provides a list of symptoms that occur during

 Did You Know?

Alzheimer's disease is more common in older adults but can affect people as young as age 30.

 Memory Jogger

With Alzheimer's disease, neurons die in the areas of the brain that are essential for memory and important mental abilities such as language.

? Did You Know?

A person with Down syndrome who lives to the age of 50–60 years is at increased risk for developing Alzheimer's disease.

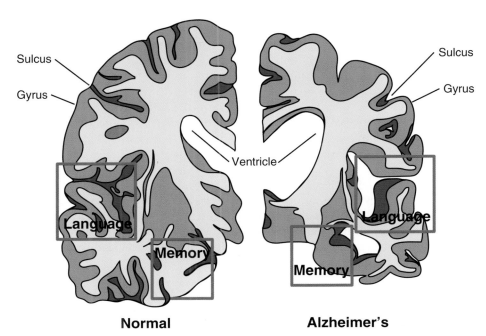

FIG. 24.1 Cross sections of a normal brain and a brain affected by Alzheimer's disease. Neurons die in areas of the brain important to memory and language.

Table **24.1**	Symptoms of Alzheimer's Disease
STAGE	**SYMPTOMS**
Early	Forgetfulness • Difficulty recalling events and activities • Difficulty remembering names of familiar people and things • Inability to solve simple mathematics problems
Middle	Beginning to have difficulty speaking, understanding, reading, and writing Failure to recognize familiar people and places Forgetting how to perform simple tasks such as brushing teeth and combing hair Inability to think clearly
Late	Aggressiveness Anxiety Need for total care Wandering away from home

different stages of the disease. As the disease progresses, symptoms are more noticeable, and family members seek medical help. In the late stages of the disease, the patient will need total care to prevent complications of immobility, aspiration, urinary tract infections, pneumonia, and pressure ulcers, which commonly lead to death in these patients.

There is no test for diagnosing Alzheimer's disease. The only absolute way to confirm that a patient has this illness is to see the plaques and tangles in the brain tissue, which can be done only by autopsy after the patient dies. Diagnosis is made by excluding other possible causes (for example, thyroid problems, drug reactions, depression, brain tumors, and blood vessel diseases). Brief cognitive assessment tools (e.g., mini-mental state exam, Montreal cognitive assessment) can aid in the early identification of early and mild dementia. On the basis of symptom assessment, health history, tests of memory and problem solving, and brain scan, a diagnosis of probable Alzheimer's disease can be made. Supporting tests for diagnosis include cerebrospinal fluid analysis and amyloid positron-emission tomography (PET) imaging.

There is no cure for Alzheimer's disease. Early diagnosis is important because it helps patients and families plan for the future, makes it possible for the patient with dementia to benefit from drugs that can slow the progression of the disease, and helps the patient and family to identify sources of advice and support. No treatment can stop the progression of Alzheimer's disease. Drug therapy may help prevent symptoms from becoming worse for a limited time and allow the patient to continue performing some daily activities for a longer period. Drugs may also be prescribed to help control behavioral symptoms such as sleeplessness, agitation, wandering, anxiety, and depression.

? Did You Know?

The only way to absolutely diagnose Alzheimer's disease is to look for plaques and tangles in brain tissue by autopsy after the patient's death.

Memory Jogger

Drugs prescribed for Alzheimer's disease and Parkinson's disease can help control the symptoms but **cannot** cure the disease.

TYPES OF DRUGS FOR ALZHEIMER'S DISEASE

No drug has been developed that protects neurons from the changes that occur with Alzheimer's disease. Drug treatments have been developed that may change the disease progression, or may temporarily slow the progression of symptoms in some patients. These drugs are categorized into biologic agents and classic agents.

Biologic Agents for Alzheimer's Disease (AD)

How biologic agents for AD work. Aducanumab (Aduhelm) is a biologic therapy agent consisting of an amyloid beta-directed monoclonal antibody approved by the U.S. Food and Drug Administration (FDA) for treatment of Alzheimer's disease in June 2021. While research continues, this is the first drug to focus on the underlying biology of the disease. It is the first treatment that may prevent beta-amyloid from clumping into plaques or remove beta-amyloid plaques that have formed to help the body clear the beta-amyloid from the brain. These actions are likely to decrease both cognitive and functional decline in Alzheimer's patients. However, there is no evidence that aducanumab can restore lost memories or cognitive function. Supporting the need for early diagnosis of Alzheimer's disease, aducanumab is prescribed for patients with mild cognitive impairment (MCI) or the mild dementia stage of the illness. This drug is given intravenously in an acute care setting, or an infusion therapy center.

Adult Dosages for Commonly Prescribed Amyloid Beta-Directed Monoclonal Antibodies

Drug Name	Usual Maintenance Dose
aducanumab (Aduhelm)	IV infusions given over 45–60 min every 4 weeks (at least 21 days apart) Infusions 1–2: 1 mg/kg IV every 4 weeks Infusions 3–4: 3 mg/kg IV every 4 weeks Infusions 5–6: 6 mg/kg IV every 4 weeks Infusion 7 and beyond: 10 mg/kg IV every 4 weeks

Intended responses of biologic agents for AD
- Prevention of beta-amyloid clumping into plaques
- Removal of beta-amyloid plaques
- Decrease in cognitive and functional decline

Common side effects of biologic agents for AD. The most common side effects include amyloid-related imaging abnormalities (ARIAs) such as headache, dizziness, nausea, confusion, and vision changes. These symptoms are usually due to a temporary swelling in areas of the brain and resolve over time.

Possible adverse effects of biologic agents for AD. A potentially serious side effect is an allergic reaction. Some patients develop small amounts of bleeding in or on the surface of the brain with swelling which may lead to ARIA symptoms, or may not cause symptoms. Increased risk for falls occurs with this drug.

Classic Drugs for Alzheimer's Disease (AD)
How classic drugs for AD work. Cholinesterase/acetylcholinesterase inhibitors reduce the activity of the enzyme acetylcholinesterase that breaks down acetylcholine in the synapses of neurons. This action keeps levels of acetylcholine higher. These drugs are used for early to moderate stages of Alzheimer's disease and their effects are temporary. The three drugs in this category, donepezil (Aricept), rivastigmine (Exelon), and galantamine (Reminyl), are the main drugs used for Alzheimer's treatment.

Glutamate regulators block the amino acid glutamate at *N*-methyl-D-aspartate receptors in the brain, preventing overstimulation (overstimulation of these receptors damages neurons and appears to be one cause of Alzheimer's disease). The only current drug in this class is *memantine* (Namenda). It can be effective in helping modify dementia (temporarily) in some patients with moderate-to-severe Alzheimer's disease.

Orexin receptor antagonists are thought to inhibit the activity of orexin, a neurotransmitter involved in the sleep-wake cycle. The only current drug in this class is *suvorexant* (Belsomra). It is used to treat insomnia that occurs with dementia and is prescribed for mild to moderate Alzheimer's disease.

Generic names, trade names, and common adult dosages of these drugs are listed in the following table. Be sure to consult a reliable drug resource for specific information about any other less common drugs used for Alzheimer's disease.

Common Side Effects
Biologic Agents

Headache   Nausea   Dizziness

Confusion   Vision changes

Adult Dosages for Commonly Prescribed Classic Drugs for Alzheimer's Disease

Drug Category	Drug Name	Usual Maintenance Dose
Cholinesterase Inhibitors	donepezil (Aricept)	5 mg orally at bedtime; increase to 10 mg after 4–6 weeks Transdermal dosage: apply 1 patch (delivers 5 mg/day of donepezil) topically to the back (avoiding the spine) once every 7 days **Approved for treatment of all stages of AD**
	galantamine (Razadyne, Reminyl)	4 mg orally twice daily with food, increase at 4-week intervals to 12 mg twice daily Extended-release: 8 mg once daily in the morning with food, increase at 4-week intervals to initial maintenance dose 16 mg/day. Max: 24 mg/day **For treatment of mild-to-moderate AD**
	rivastigmine (Exelon, Exelon Patch)	1.5 mg orally twice daily with food; after 4 weeks, may increase to 3 mg orally twice daily. Patch: apply 1 patch (4.6 mg) at a different body site once daily, may increase to a 9.5-mg patch. **For treatment of mild-to-moderate AD**
Glutamate Regulators	memantine (Namenda, Nameda XR)	5 mg orally daily; increase to 5 mg twice daily, then 5 mg in am and 10 mg in pm; maximum dosage 10 mg twice daily Extended Release: 7 mg orally once daily. Titrate in 7-mg increments at no sooner than 1 week intervals up to the recommended target dose of 28 mg once daily **For moderate-to-severe AD**
Orexin Receptor Antagonists	suvorexant (Belsomra)	10 mg orally taken no more than once per night and within 30 min of going to bed, with at least 7 hr remaining before the planned time of awakening for insomnia **For treatment of mild-to-moderate AD**

Do Not Confuse

Aricept *with* **Aciphex**

An order for Aricept may be confused with Aciphex. Aricept is an acetylcholinesterase inhibitor used for Alzheimer's disease, whereas Aciphex is a proton pump inhibitor used to treat gastroesophageal reflux disease (GERD) and gastric ulcers.

QSEN: Safety

Do Not Confuse

Reminyl *with* **Robinul**

An order for Reminyl may be confused with Robinul. Reminyl is an acetylcholinesterase inhibitor used for Alzheimer's disease, whereas Robinul is an anticholinergic agent that inhibits salivation and excessive respiratory secretions.

QSEN: Safety

Common Side Effects

Drugs for Alzheimer's Disease

Dizziness

Headache

Fatigue

Nausea/Vomiting, Diarrhea, Abdominal cramps

Intended responses of classic drugs for AD
- Dementia with Alzheimer's disease decreases temporarily.
- Degradation of acetylcholine is inhibited.
- Progression of Alzheimer's disease symptoms is slowed.
- Cognitive function in patients with Alzheimer's disease is improved.

Common side effects of classic drugs for AD. The most common side effects of cholinesterase/acetylcholinesterase inhibitors are nausea, vomiting, diarrhea, stomach cramps, headaches, dizziness, fatigue, weakness, insomnia, and loss of appetite *(anorexia).*

Side effects of suvorexant for insomnia include impaired alertness and motor coordination, worsening of depression, sleep behaviors (e.g., sleep-walking).

Possible adverse effects of classic drugs for AD. Adverse effects of cholinesterase/ acetylcholinesterase inhibitors include abnormal heart rhythms such as bradycardia and atrial fibrillation. Although uncommon, all of these drugs may cause gastrointestinal (GI) bleeding. Two additional uncommon but serious adverse effects include difficulty urinating and seizures. Adverse effects of memantine include shortness of breath and hallucinations. Risks associated with these drugs when a patient needs surgery with general anesthesia include awakening more slowly, respiratory depression, and an increased likelihood of experiencing confusion and delirium.

Symptoms of overdose with these drugs include upset stomach, vomiting, drooling, sweating, slow heartbeat (bradycardia), difficulty breathing, muscle weakness, and seizures. Report these effects to the prescriber immediately.

Suvorexant may cause impaired respiratory function.

✪ *Priority actions to take before giving classic drugs for AD.* Obtain a complete list of drugs currently being used by the patient, including over-the-counter and herbal products. Assess the patient for baseline cognitive function (e.g., memory, attention, reasoning, language, and ability to perform simple tasks).

Obtain a baseline weight. Assess baseline blood pressure and heart rate and rhythm. Ask about recent nausea, vomiting, loss of appetite, and weight loss. Have the patient or caregiver tell you about their usual urinary output pattern. Check the patient's hemoglobin and hematocrit levels.

Assess swallowing because patients may develop difficulty as the disease progresses and be at risk for aspiration. Drugs may need to be crushed or given in liquid form. Do *not* crush time-released pills or open time-released capsules.

Ask about a history of liver or kidney problems which may affect the metabolism of these drugs. Also ask about previous problems with GI bleeding or ulcers.

Before giving *suvorexant* for insomnia, ensure that the patient has at least 7 hours remaining before the planned time of awakening.

✪ *Priority actions to take after giving classic drugs for AD.* Reassess the patient's cognitive function often. Watch for changes in memory, attention, reasoning, language, and ability to perform simple tasks. Cognitive assessment is a long-term task because changes may take time to appear.

Recheck and monitor the patient's heart rate and rhythm, and blood pressure. Monitor intake and output and daily weights. Assess for signs of low hemoglobin or hematocrit. Continue to monitor the patient's swallowing ability. Watch him or her for potential seizure activity.

Because these drugs may cause dizziness and fatigue, instruct any in-patient to call for help when getting out of bed and ensure that the call light is within easy reach. Instruct patients at home to also call for help getting up. Suggest the use of a bell or other call device for help.

Ask the patient about nausea, vomiting, and GI discomfort. Check stools or emesis for signs of GI bleeding. Notify the prescriber if side effects occur.

After giving suvorexant for insomnia, monitor for changes in alertness or motor activity. Assess for worsening of depression or suicidal thoughts, as well as sleepwalking. Monitor respiratory status.

✪ *Teaching priorities for care providers and patients taking classic drugs for AD.* The patient with AD may be unable to self-administer prescribed drugs. For this reason, include the person providing home care for the patient in addition to the patient when giving instructions for precautions related to the drugs for AD management. Be sure to include any specific precautions related to proper storage.

- If you have difficulty swallowing tablets or capsules, they may be crushed or ordered in a liquid form.
- Do *not* crush extended-release drugs.
- Your prescribed drugs must be taken exactly as instructed by your prescriber.
- Be sure to keep follow-up appointments to monitor the progress of controlling the symptoms of the disease.
- Report side effects and signs of allergic or toxic reactions to your prescriber immediately.
- These drugs may cause dizziness, weakness, and fatigue. Be careful to get up slowly.
- To prevent injuries, use handrails when going up or down stairs, and when getting into or out of the bathtub or shower.
- Notify your prescriber of any signs of bleeding.

 Drug Alert

Administration Alert

Assess a patient's ability to swallow before giving drugs for Alzheimer's disease because he or she may be at risk for aspiration.

QSEN: Safety

 Drug Alert

Action/Intervention Alert

Because acetylcholinesterase inhibitors may cause GI bleeding, monitor the patient carefully for any signs of bleeding.

QSEN: Safety

 Drug Alert

Teaching Alert

Teach care providers to remind patients to use the bathroom every 2 hr to avoid incontinence episodes while taking drugs for Alzheimer's disease.

QSEN: Safety

Drug Alert

Administration Alert

Give *galantamine* (Reminyl, Razadyne) and *rivastigmine* (Exelon) twice a day with food to minimize the GI upset that is common with these drugs.

QSEN: Safety

- When suvorexant is taken for insomnia, it must be used only once per night, and taken within 30 minutes of going to bed, with at least 7 hours remaining before the planned time of your awakening.
- Take donepezil (Aricept) at bedtime and galantamine (Reminyl, Razadyne) and rivastigmine (Exelon) twice a day with food.
- Notify your prescriber about any changes in cognitive function.

Life span considerations for classic drugs for AD

Considerations for older adults. All of these drugs should be used cautiously in patients with histories of GI bleeding, liver disease, kidney disease, or heart disease. Rivastigmine should also be used cautiously for patients with asthma or chronic obstructive pulmonary disease (COPD). Older, frail women should not take more than 5 mg/day of donepezil because the drug has been associated with significant weight loss. This drug should be used with caution in any older adult with low body weight.

Because these drugs increase urination, the older adult, especially one who is confused, may have more episodes of incontinence. Remind family members to ensure that the older adult has the opportunity to use the bathroom every 2 hours while awake and at least once during the night.

PARKINSON'S DISEASE

REVIEW OF RELATED PHYSIOLOGY AND PATHOPHYSIOLOGY FOR PARKINSON'S DISEASE

Parkinson's disease (PD) is a slow, progressive, degenerative disease of the nervous system. In the United States, about 1 million people are affected by this disease. It affects 1 in 20 people older than 80 and commonly begins between the ages of 50 and 79.

Normally, when the brain initiates an impulse to move a muscle, the impulse passes through the basal ganglia. The function of the basal ganglia is to make muscle movements smooth and coordinate changes in posture. Basal ganglia release chemical messengers called *neurotransmitters* (for example, dopamine) that trigger the next nerve cell in the pathway to send an impulse. In Parkinson's disease nerve cells degenerate in a part of the basal ganglia called the *substantia nigra* (Figure 24.2). This

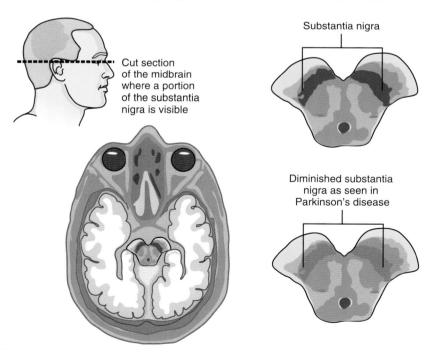

FIG. 24.2 In Parkinson's disease, nerve cells in the substantia nigra degenerate, and less dopamine is produced. This results in fewer connections between the nerve cells in the basal ganglia and in decreased smooth movements.

causes a decrease in the production of dopamine and in the number of connections between nerve cells in the basal ganglia. As a result, the basal ganglia are less able to produce smooth movements. These changes cause symptoms of increased tremor, lack of coordination, and slowed or reduced movements *(bradykinesia)*. Parkinson's disease begins subtly and progresses gradually. Symptoms appear when the amount of dopamine decreases in the brain.

The symptoms appear gradually and increase in severity as the disease progresses. Symptoms may be motor or nonmotor (Box 24.1). For many patients, the initial symptom is a coarse, rhythmic *tremor* of the hand while the hand is at rest, also called a *pill-rolling tremor.* As the disease progresses, muscles become rigid, movements become slow and difficult to initiate, and stiffness occurs. When the disease is advanced, the patient may suddenly stop walking, quicken his or her steps, or stumble-run to avoid falling. Posture becomes stooped, and balance becomes difficult to maintain.

The exact cause of Parkinson's disease is not known, but many factors may play a part. Age, especially age 50 and older, is a major risk factor. Genetic and environmental factors may cause the development of this condition. Two abnormal genes have been identified in people affected by Parkinson's disease before age 40. Environmental factors such as exposure to weak toxins or pesticides (e.g., Paraquat) over a long period of time are thought to lead to Parkinson's disease in genetically predisposed people. Several drugs have caused secondary Parkinson's disease (Table 24.2).

There is no specific test or marker for diagnosing Parkinson's disease. Diagnosis is based on symptoms. A diagnosis of Parkinson's disease is probable if drug therapy improves symptoms and other diseases have been ruled out. There is no cure for Parkinson's disease.

Memory Jogger

The **four major symptoms** of Parkinson's disease are:
- Tremor at rest
- Rigidity
- Bradykinesia (slow movements and difficulty starting to move)
- Abnormal gait

Box 24.1   Symptoms of Parkinson's Disease

MOTOR SYMPTOMS	NONMOTOR SYMPTOMS
• Bradykinesia	• Constipation
• Decreased arm swing when walking	• Decreased sense of smell
• Difficulty rising from a chair	• Depression
• Difficulty turning in bed	• Drooling
• Lack of facial expression	• Increased sweating
• Micrographia (small handwriting)	• Low voice volume
• Postural instability	• Male erectile dysfunction
• Rigidity and freezing in place	• Painful foot cramps
• Stooped, shuffling gait	• Sleep disturbance
• Tremor	• Urinary frequency and urgency

Table 24.2   Drugs That Cause Secondary Parkinson's Disease

CATEGORY	DRUG NAME
Antiemetics	prochlorperazine (Compazine)
Antihypertensives	reserpine (Serpasil)
Antipsychotics	chlorpromazine (Thorazine) fluphenazine (Prolixin) haloperidol (Haldol) mesoridazine (Serentil) perphenazine (Trilafon) risperidone (Risperdal) thioridazine (Mellaril) trifluoperazine (Stelazine)
Gastrointestinal motility drugs	metoclopramide (Reglan)
Illicit drugs	methcathinone—a psychoactive stimulant N-MPTP (1-methyl-4-phenyl-1,2,3,6-tetrahydropyridine)—a contaminant found in illicit drugs

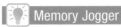
TYPES OF DRUGS FOR PARKINSON'S DISEASE

The four main types of drugs for treating Parkinson's disease are dopaminergic/dopamine agonists, COMT inhibitors, MAO-B inhibitors, and anticholinergics. Goals of drug therapy include minimizing disability, reducing possible side effects of drug therapy, and helping the patient maintain a high quality of life. Drug therapy may make movement easier and prolong normal function for several years.

How Drugs for Parkinson's Disease Work

No drugs have been developed that will cure or reverse the progression of Parkinson's disease. However, certain drugs can be used effectively to control the symptoms of the disease.

Drugs are prescribed to improve movement and enable patients to function effectively. The period of time that drugs for Parkinson's disease remain effective varies. For some patients, they may work for several years, whereas for others they may work for only a short period.

Dopaminergic/dopamine agonists increase the amount of dopamine activity in the brain, thereby reducing tremor and muscle rigidity and improving movement. Carbidopa prevents levodopa from being converted to dopamine before it reaches the brain. When carbidopa is added to levodopa, lower doses of levodopa can be used, leading to reduced side effects such as nausea and vomiting. Dopamine agonist drugs stimulate dopamine receptors to relieve symptoms and delay the onset of motor complications. The mechanism of action for the dopamine agonist rotigotine (Neupro) is unknown.

Catechol-*O*-methyltransferase (COMT) inhibitors allow a larger amount of levodopa to reach the brain, which raises dopamine levels in the brain. They help provide a more stable, constant supply of levodopa, which makes its beneficial effects last longer.

Monoamine oxidase B (MAO-B) inhibitors inhibit the enzyme that breaks down dopamine in the brain. As a result, more dopamine is available, and the progression of Parkinson's disease is slowed.

Anticholinergic drugs are effective against tremors and rigidity. These drugs block cholinergic nerve impulses that help control the muscles of the arms, legs, and body. They also restrict the action of acetylcholine, an important chemical messenger in the brain that helps regulate muscle movement, sweat gland function, and intestinal function.

Generic names, trade names, and dosages of the most commonly prescribed drugs are listed in the following table. Be sure to consult a reliable drug resource for specific information about less common drugs used to treat Parkinson's disease.

Adult Dosages for Commonly Prescribed Drugs for Parkinson's Disease

Drug Category	Drug Name	Usual Maintenance Dose
Dopaminergic/ Dopamine Agonists	apomorphine (Apokyn)	Subcutaneous: Initial dose is 0.1 mL (1 mg) subcutaneously. If a positive response is not obtained, give a 0.2 mL (2 mg) subcutaneous dose at least 30 min after the initial dose. Then, if no response, give 0.4 mL (4 mg) subcutaneously at least 30 min after the second dose
	bromocriptine (Cycloset, Parlodel)	1.25–2.5 mg orally twice daily with meals; increase at 2–7-day intervals by 2.5 mg/day to a maximum dosage 30 mg/day in divided doses; always give with meals. Usual dose range: 10 to 30 mg/day
	carbidopa/levodopa (Atamet, Duopa, Parcopa, Rytary, Sinemet, Sinemet CR)	25 mg carbidopa/100 mg levodopa orally 3 times daily. Extended-release: 50 mg carbidopa/200 mg levodopa twice daily

Adult Dosages for Commonly Prescribed Drugs for Parkinson's Disease—cont'd

Drug Category	Drug Name	Usual Maintenance Dose
	pramipexole (Mirapex, Mirapex ER)	0.125 mg orally 3 times daily initially; dosage range 1.5–4.5 mg/day in 3 divided doses Extended release: 0.375 mg orally once daily
	ropinirole (Requip, Requip XL)	0.25 mg orally 3 times daily for 1 week, then gradually increase at weekly intervals up to 24 mg/day in 3 divided doses of 8 mg Extended-release: 2 mg once daily, increase at 1–2-week intervals by 2 mg/day, maximum dosage 24 mg/day
COMT Inhibitors	entacapone (Comtan)	200 mg orally given with each dose of carbidopa/levodopa; maximum dosage 1600 mg/day (8 doses)
	tolcapone (Tasmar)	100 mg orally 3 times daily given with first dose given with dose of carbidopa/levodopa; max dose 600 mg/day
MAO-B Inhibitors	rasagiline (Azilect)	1 mg orally once daily; 0.5–1 mg once daily when combined with levodopa. Max: 1 mg/day orally due to the risk of hypertension
	selegiline (Carbex, Eldepryl, Zelapar)	5 mg orally twice daily with breakfast and lunch; oral dissolving tablet: 1.25 mg dissolved in mouth once daily (in the morning before breakfast) for 6 weeks, then may increase to 2.5 mg once daily
Anticholinergic Drugs	benztropine (Cogentin)	0.5–1 mg/day orally or intramuscularly (IM) at bedtime Dosage range: 0.5–6 mg/day in 1 or more divided doses
	trihexyphenidyl (Artane)	1 mg orally initially, then increase by 2 mg every 3–5 days until 6–10 mg/day orally is reached. Usually given 3 times a day with meals, or 4 times a day with meals and at bedtime
Dopamine Agonists	rotigotine (Neupro)	Initially, apply 1 patch (2 mg/24 hr) transdermally once daily. May increase patch dose by 2 mg/24 hr. Max: 6 mg/day

⇄ **Do Not Confuse**

Mirapex *with* **MiraLax**

An order for Mirapex can be confused with MiraLax. Mirapex is a dopamine agonist used to treat the symptoms of Parkinson's disease, whereas MiraLax is an osmotic laxative used to treat constipation.

QSEN: Safety

Intended Responses of Drugs for Parkinson's Disease
- Signs and symptoms of Parkinson's disease are decreased
- Tremor and rigidity of Parkinson's disease are relieved.

Common Side Effects of Drugs for Parkinson's Disease
The most common side effects of drugs to treat Parkinson's disease are dizziness, nausea, and hypotension. Common side effects of these drugs are summarized by drug or drug group in the following table.

Common Side Effects of Drugs for Parkinson's Disease

Drugs or Drug Groups	Side Effects
Anticholinergic Drugs	Blurred vision, constipation, dizziness, dry eyes, dry mouth, nervousness, sedation
carbidopa-levodopa (Sinemet)	Involuntary movements (dyskinesia), nausea and vomiting

Continued

Common Side Effects of Drugs for Parkinson's Disease—cont'd

Drugs or Drug Groups	Side Effects
COMT Inhibitors	Constipation, diarrhea, dyskinesia, dystonia (slow movement or extended spasm in a group of muscles), headache, sleep disorder
Dopamine Agonists	Amnesia, chest pain, constipation, dizziness, dry mouth, dyskinesia, dyspepsia, flushing, hallucinations, hypotension, nausea and vomiting, pallor, rhinorrhea (runny nose), somnolence, sweating, weakness, yawning
MAO-B Inhibitors	Confusion, dizziness, dry mouth, nausea, vivid dreams and hallucinations

Possible Adverse Effects of Drugs for Parkinson's Disease

Serious adverse effects of *carbidopa-levodopa* (Sinemet) include depression with suicidal tendencies, neutropenia (decreased number of white blood cells), and neuroleptic malignant syndrome (dysfunction of the autonomic nervous system, the branch of the nervous system responsible for regulating involuntary actions such as heart rate, blood pressure, digestion, and sweating; muscle tone; body temperature; and consciousness).

Apomorphine (Apokyn) can cause life-threatening central nervous system (CNS) depression, including respiratory depression, coma, and cardiac arrest.

Bromocriptine (Parlodel) may lead to shock or acute myocardial infarction. Pramipexole (Mirapex) can cause sleep attacks *(narcolepsy).*

COMT inhibitors can cause neuroleptic malignant syndrome or rhabdomyolysis, a serious and potentially fatal effect involving the destruction or degeneration of skeletal muscle. Signs and symptoms of this disorder include muscle aches; muscle weakness; and dark, cola-colored urine.

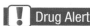 **Priority Actions to Take *Before* Giving Drugs for Parkinson's Disease**

Obtain a complete list of drugs currently being used by the patient, including over-the-counter and herbal products. Assess blood pressure, heart rate, and respiratory rate for a baseline. Assess baseline neurologic and mental status. Examine for baseline dyskinesia (impairment of voluntary motions), rigidity, tremors, and gait. Assess swallowing ability.

Ask women of childbearing age if they are pregnant or planning to become pregnant. Ask the patient about kidney or liver disease, which may affect the metabolism of these drugs.

Teach patients and their care providers that extended-release forms of these drugs must be swallowed whole and not chewed or split in half. Be sure to give *apomorphine* (Apokyn) subcutaneously and not intravenously.

Remove the old patch before applying a new *rotigotine* (Neupro) patch to a different area of clean, dry skin at the same time daily. Press firmly for 20 to 30 seconds, especially around the edges for good adherence. After removing the old patch, be sure to wash the site with soap and water to remove any adhesive or drug.

 Priority Actions to Take *After* Giving Drugs for Parkinson's Disease

Regularly reassess the patient's vital signs, including blood pressure, heart rate, and respiratory, rate every 4 to 8 hours. Because of side effects such as dizziness and hypotension, instruct the patient to call for help when getting out of bed and ensure that the call light is within easy reach. Tell the patient to change positions slowly when moving from lying down to sitting or standing.

Reassess the patient's mental status and watch for confusion or hallucinations. Watch the patient taking ropinirole (Requip) for episodes of falling asleep suddenly (narcolepsy). Report this immediately to the prescriber because the drug may need to be discontinued.

Table 24.3	Signs and Symptoms of Adverse Effects of Drugs Used to Treat Parkinson's Disease		
ADVERSE EFFECT	**SIGNS AND SYMPTOMS**	**ADVERSE EFFECT**	**SIGNS AND SYMPTOMS**
Neuroleptic malignant syndrome	Changes in cognition, including agitation, delirium, and coma High fever Muscle rigidity Muscle tremors Pharyngitis Unstable blood pressure	Rhabdomyolysis	Dark red or cola-colored urine Fatigue Generalized weakness Joint pain Muscle stiffness or aching Muscle tenderness Seizures Unintentional weight gain Weakness of the affected muscle(s)
Neutropenia	Anal ulcers Decreased immune response Fever Increased risk of bacterial infections Painful mouth ulcers Sore throat		

Ask the patient about side effects such as nausea and vomiting. Watch for side effects or adverse effects and report them immediately to the prescriber. Signs and symptoms of such adverse effects as neutropenia, neuroleptic malignant syndrome, and rhabdomyolysis are summarized in Table 24.3. Observe the patient for signs of drug allergic reactions such as rashes, hives, or changes in respiratory status.

After giving these drugs, be sure to monitor the patient's intake and output and assess for bladder distention because some drugs can cause urine retention. Monitor the patient for difficulty swallowing, which could increase the risk for aspiration.

Keep track of bowel movements and check bowel sounds because some drugs for Parkinson's disease can cause constipation or diarrhea.

Reassess dyskinesia, rigidity, tremors, and gait while the patient is taking drugs for Parkinson's disease.

Monitor skin condition for patients receiving the *rotigotine* (Neupro) patch. Be sure to rotate the site and do not apply to the same site more than once every 14 days. Always wash your hands after handling these patches.

⊛ Teaching Priorities for Care Providers and Patients Taking Drugs for Parkinson's Disease

- Include the person providing home care when teaching about these drugs.
- Instruct the home care provider(s) to report any changes in swallowing ability to the prescriber because of the increased risk of aspiration.
- Instruct home care providers and patients to take drugs for Parkinson's disease exactly as prescribed.
- It is essential to keep follow-up appointments to monitor the progress of treatment.
- Notify the prescriber if symptoms of Parkinson's disease (e.g., shaking, stiffness, and slow movement) become worse.
- Report any side effects immediately to your prescriber.
- Consult the prescriber or pharmacist before taking any over-the-counter or herbal products.
- Missed doses of drugs for Parkinson's disease should be taken as soon as possible. However, if it is almost time for the next dose, skip the missed dose to avoid taking a double dose of these drugs.
- Some drugs for Parkinson's disease are started at lower doses and gradually increased by the prescriber to best control the symptoms.
- These drugs can be used to control symptoms but do **not** cure the disease.

 Drug Alert

Action/Intervention Alert

To determine the effectiveness of drug therapy for Parkinson's disease, regularly reassess the patient for dyskinesia, rigidity, tremors, and gait.

QSEN: Safety

 Drug Alert

Teaching Alert

Patients and care providers are taught to notify their prescriber immediately if symptoms of Parkinson's disease such as shaking, stiffness, and slow movement become worse.

QSEN: Safety

- Avoid stopping these drugs suddenly because symptoms may become much worse.
- Be careful not to overdo physical activities but gradually increase activities to avoid falls and injuries.
- Always notify your surgeons or dentists when taking these drugs before having any surgical procedure.
- Drugs such as selegiline (Carbex) may cause photosensitivity. Wear protective clothing and sunscreen and avoid excessive sun exposure.
- Because of side effects such as dizziness and drowsiness, avoid driving, operating machines, or doing anything that requires increased alertness until you know how your drugs will affect you.
- Avoid alcohol or other CNS depressants because they can add to the drowsiness sometimes caused by drugs for Parkinson's disease.
- Change positions slowly because of the possible side effect of hypotension.
- Take drugs that cause GI upset with food or milk.
- If you are prescribed anticholinergic drugs, be sure to have regular eye examinations because these drugs can cause blurred vision.
- Dry mouth can be kept to a minimum by frequent mouth care, ice chips, or sugarless candy.
- If you are prescribed entacapone (Comtan) this drug may change your urine to a brownish-orange color. This is an expected side effect that is *not* harmful.
- If you are prescribed an MAO-B inhibitor such as selegiline (Carbex) or rasagiline (Azilect), avoid the foods listed in Box 24.2 while taking these drugs and for 2 weeks after stopping them.
- Avoid large amounts of chocolate, coffee, tea, or colas with caffeine. These foods contain tyramine, an amino acid that can cause a hypertensive crisis in patients receiving MAO inhibitor therapy.
- Anticholinergic drugs can cause decreased perspiration. If you are taking these drugs, be careful about overheating in hot weather.
- Taking the combination of *carbidopa-levodopa* (Sinemet) can cause the darkening of urine or perspiration.
- Report any changes in skin lesions immediately to the prescriber because carbidopa-levodopa can activate malignant melanoma. This drug may be contraindicated if you have a history of melanoma.
- If you are prescribed *apomorphine* (Apokyn) at home you will need special teaching about how to give the subcutaneous injections and how to care for the special dosing pen used to give this drug. Your home care provider will be included in this teaching because your muscle rigidity and tremors may make it difficult or impossible to self-inject.
- If you are prescribed the *rotigotine* (Neupro) patch system, you and your care provider will be taught how to correctly apply the patch, care of sites, rotation of sites, and washing hands after handling the patches.

 Drug Alert

Teaching Alert

While taking *selegiline* (Carbex) or *rasagiline* (Azilect), patients should avoid foods that contain tyramine (see Box 24.2).

QSEN: Safety

 Drug Alert

Teaching Alert

Teach patients taking anticholinergic drugs to remain indoors in an air-conditioned setting during hot weather.

QSEN: Safety

Drug Alert

Teaching Alert

Because *carbidopa-levodopa* may activate malignant melanoma, instruct patients to watch for and report any changes in skin lesions to their prescriber immediately.

QSEN: Safety

Box 24.2	Foods to Avoid When Taking MAO Inhibitors

• Aged cheeses	• Pickled herring
• Avocados	• Poultry
• Bananas	• Raisins
• Figs	• Red wine
• Beer	• Salami
• Broad beans	• Sauerkraut
• Dried sausage	• Sour cream
• Fish	• Soy sauce
• Liver	• Yeast extract
• Meats prepared with tenderizer	• Yogurt

Life Span Considerations for Drugs for Parkinson's Disease

Considerations for pregnancy and lactation. Although Parkinson's disease is very rare in women of childbearing age, bromocriptine (Parlodel) is usually not recommended during pregnancy or breastfeeding. It stops the production of breast milk. Most drugs for Parkinson's disease have a moderate likelihood of increasing the risk for birth defects or fetal harm. They have not been tested in pregnancy or breastfeeding and should not be used unless the benefits outweigh the risks.

Considerations for older adults. Older adults should be aware that they may experience confusion, hallucinations, and uncontrolled body movements because they are more sensitive to the effects of these drugs.

The older adult with Parkinson's disease is already unstable when walking and is at increased risk for falls. The drugs can cause a rapid decrease in blood pressure. Remind older adults to sit on the side of the bed for a few moments before attempting to stand and to change positions slowly. Instruct them to wear shoes, rather than slippers, for better stability and to use handrails when going up or down stairs. Assess the older adult's need for assistive devices, such as a cane or a walker for ambulating.

Drugs for Treatment of "Off" Times with Parkinson's Disease

Most drugs for the treatment of PD work on controlling the symptoms. "On" times are periods when commonly used drugs are working adequately and symptoms of the disease are controlled. "Off" times are periods when these drugs wear off and PD symptoms (e.g., tremor, rigidity, difficulty walking) reappear. These drugs for PD are used when needed for "Off" episodes in adults with Parkinson's treated with regular carbidopa/levodopa medicine. They do not replace regular carbidopa/levodopa medicine. Generic names, trade names, and dosages of these drugs are listed in the following table. Be sure to consult a reliable drug resource for specific information about less common drugs used to treat Parkinson's disease.

For the Treatment of "Off" Times in Parkinson's Disease as an Adjunct to Carbidopa/Levodopa

Drug	Dosage
apomorphine HCL (Kynmobi)	Initial dose: 2 mg (0.2 mL) subcutaneous; 10 mg sublingual as needed; not to exceed 5 doses/day **Carefully monitor blood pressure and heart rate**
istradefylline (Nourianz)	20 mg orally once daily. Adjust the dose based on efficacy response and tolerability. Max: 40 mg orally once daily
levodopa (Inbrija)	Inhale the contents of 2 capsules (42 mg per capsule for a total of 84 mg) via oral inhalation with the provided inhaler as needed for "off" symptoms up to 5 times daily **DO NOT swallow the capsules. Use inhaler provided by manufacturer.** Max: 420 mg/day via oral inhalation
opicapone (Ongentys)	50 mg orally once daily at bedtime, on an empty stomach
safinamide (Xadago)	Initial dose 50 mg orally once a day Maintenance dose: After 2 weeks, may increase dose to 100 mg orally once a day. Max: 100 mg/day

Drugs for Treatment of Hallucinations and Delusion with Parkinson's Disease

Pimavanserin (Nuplazid) is a newer drug for the treatment of hallucinations and delusions associated with PD. This drug is given as 1 capsule (34 mg) orally once a day. The capsule can be opened and mixed with a tablespoon (15 mL) of applesauce, yogurt, pudding, or a nutritional supplement. It has a **safety warning** because this drug can increase the risk of death in older patients with dementia-related psychosis.

Get Ready for the NCLEX® Examination!

Key Points

- Alzheimer's disease and Parkinson's disease are both progressive neurologic disorders that occur more often with aging.
- There is no cure for either Alzheimer's disease or Parkinson's disease. Treatment focuses on controlling symptoms.
- Drugs prescribed for Alzheimer's disease and Parkinson's disease can help control the symptoms but **cannot** cure the disease. Patient safety is a major concern for patients with Parkinson's disease and Alzheimer's disease.
- Alzheimer's disease is the most common form of dementia and affects a person's ability to perform activities of daily living.
- With Alzheimer's disease, neurons essential to memory and cognitive function die.
- Mild forgetfulness, the first symptom of Alzheimer's disease, can be confused with age-related memory changes.
- Because acetylcholinesterase inhibitors may cause GI bleeding, monitor the patient carefully for any signs of bleeding.
- Assess a patient's ability to swallow before giving drugs for Alzheimer's disease because he or she may be at risk for aspiration.
- Give *galantamine* (Reminyl, Razadyne) and *rivastigmine* (Exelon) twice a day with food to minimize the GI upset that is common with these drugs.
- With Parkinson's disease, there is a deficit of chemical messengers called *neurotransmitters* that facilitate transmission of brain impulses.
- The major symptoms of Parkinson's disease are tremor at rest, rigidity, bradykinesia, and abnormal gait. (Tremor is often the initial symptom.)
- Always ask patients taking COMT inhibitor drugs about muscle aches or weakness; these are symptoms of rhabdomyolysis, which is an adverse effect of these drugs.
- Be sure to give *apomorphine* subcutaneously and not intravenously because intravenous drugs are immediately absorbed and act very rapidly.
- Immediately report episodes of narcolepsy to the prescriber for a patient taking *ropinirole* (Requip).
- To determine the effectiveness of drug therapy for Parkinson's disease, regularly reassess the patient for dyskinesia, rigidity, tremors, and gait.
- Teach care providers and patients to report worsening of Parkinson's disease symptoms immediately to the prescriber.
- While taking *selegiline* (Carbex) or *rasagiline* (Azilect), patients should avoid foods that contain tyramine.
- Teach patients taking anticholinergic drugs to remain indoors in an air-conditioned setting during hot weather.
- Because *carbidopa-levodopa* may activate malignant melanoma, instruct patients to watch for and report any changes in skin lesions to their prescriber immediately.

Additional Learning Resources

🌐 Be sure to visit your Evolve website (http://evolve.elsevier.com/Workman/pharmacology/) for additional online resources.

SG Go to your Study Guide for additional learning activities to help you master this chapter content.

Review Questions

See *Answers to In-Text Review Questions* in the back of the book for answers to these questions.

1. **What is the common underlying pathophysiology of both Alzheimer's disease and Parkinson's disease?**

   A. Both are neurodegenerative diseases.
   B. Both are forms of dementia.
   C. Both involve interrupted transmission of nerve impulses.
   D. Both are primarily caused and directly related to environmental factors.

2. **Which symptom is often the earliest that the nurse will assess in a patient with Alzheimer's disease?**

   A. Difficulty solving simple math problems
   B. Problems performing simple tasks
   C. Mild forgetfulness
   D. Inability to read

3. **For which patient will the nurse assess **most** closely for symptoms of Alzheimer's disease?**

   A. 45-year-old with Down syndrome
   B. 50-year-old with a whiplash injury
   C. 60-year-old with hypertension
   D. 75-year-old with a smoking history

4. **Which teaching strategy by the nurse **best** supports safe medication administration for patients with Alzheimer's disease?**

   A. Include the patient's care provider when teaching about the patient's drugs.
   B. Provide written guidelines about each drug to the patient.
   C. Create a chart listing the drugs, dosages, and times they should be taken.
   D. Suggest that the patient set up the drugs each week in labeled boxes.

5. **A patient with Alzheimer's disease is prescribed rivastigmine. What action does the nurse take to **prevent** a common side effect?**

   A. Providing a full glass of water when the drug is taken.
   B. Giving the drug with meals twice a day.
   C. Assessing the patient's level of consciousness.
   D. Keeping an accurate record of all patient food intake.

6. **What is the **most important** precaution for the nurse to teach a patient who is prescribed transdermal rivastigmine?**

   A. Always remove old patches daily and apply the new patch to a different site.
   B. Report any difficulty starting the urinary stream to your prescriber immediately.

C. Place the patch on the neck or forehead so that the drug reaches the brain more quickly.

D. For best drug absorption, hold a warm wet washcloth over the patch for 5 minutes after applying it.

7. A patient with Parkinson's disease who has been prescribed entacapone tells the nurse about muscle aches, weakness, and having dark cola-colored urine. What is the nurse's **best** action?

A. Sending a urine specimen to the laboratory for urinalysis

B. Helping the patient back to bed and instructing him or her to rest

C. Telling the patient that these are expected side effects of the drug

D. Holding the drug and notifying the prescriber immediately

8. Which blood laboratory test result is most important for the nurse to check before administering the first prescribed dose of carbidopa-levodopa to a patient with Parkinson's disease?

A. International normalized ratio (INR)

B. Blood urea nitrogen (BUN) level

C. White blood cell (WBC) count

D. Lactate dehydrogenase (LDH)

9. For which adverse effect does the nurse monitor in a patient with Parkinson's disease after administering ropinirole?

A. Neuroleptic malignant syndrome

B. Depression with suicidal tendencies

C. Central nervous system depression

D. Narcolepsy or "sleep attacks"

10. A patient taking entacapone for Parkinson's disease informs the nurse that his urine is now brownish-orange in color. What is the nurse's **best** action?

A. Explaining that this is an expected side effect and is not harmful

B. Collecting a urine sample and sending it to the laboratory for urinalysis

C. Holding the drug and immediately notifying the prescriber.

D. Instructing the patient to increase his intake of fluids.

11. Which **major** symptoms of Parkinson's disease will the nurse expect to find on assessment when a patient is newly diagnosed? **Select all that apply.**

A. Bradycardia

B. Rigidity

C. Abnormal gait

D. Tremor at rest

E. Sleeplessness

F. Lack of facial expression

12. A patient with Parkinson's disease is prescribed tolcapone 200 mg three times a day. The drug is available in 100-mg tablets. How many tablets does the nurse give for each dose?

A. 1

B. 2

C. 3

D. 4

Clinical Judgment

1. A 68-year-old patient diagnosed with Parkinson's disease has been prescribed Rasagiline to help control symptoms including tremor, rigidity, and bradykinesia. The nurse is preparing a teaching plan for the patient and his care provider. Which foods must the nurse teach the patient and care provider to avoid? **Select all that apply**.

A. Spinach

B. Aged cheeses

C. Sour cream

D. Fresh apples

E. Soy sauce

F. Chicken breast

G. Liver

H. Yogurt

I. Grapes

J. Salami

2. A 73-year-old female patient with Parkinson's disease (PD) has been prescribed carbidopa/levodopa to control her symptoms. Over the past nine months, she has experienced increased episodes of symptom return after taking her medication. Additionally, the patient has begun experiencing hallucinations along with the usual PD symptoms. The health care provider prescribes istradefylline 20 mg orally, and pimavanserin 1 capsule (34 mg) orally. The nurse provides teaching to the patient's home care provider about these new drugs. **Place an X in the appropriate column to indicate which statements by the home care provider of the patient with PD indicate a Correct Understanding of this drug therapy and which statements indicate that More Instruction Is Needed.**

HOME CARE PROVIDER STATEMENT	CORRECT UNDERSTANDING	MORE INSTRUCTION NEEDED
"Now that the patient is taking istradefylline, she will no longer need to take her carbidopa/levodopa."		
"Istradefylline is given for 'off' times when the usual drugs wear off and PD symptoms reappear."		
"The istradefylline can be given up to 5 times a day to control PD symptoms."		
"Pimavanserin is a drug used for treatment of the patient's hallucinations."		
"When the patient has difficulty swallowing capsules, I can open the pimavanserin and mix it with a teaspoon of applesauce."		
"Because of her age, the patient has no additional risk while taking pimavanserin."		

Drug Therapy for Psychiatric Problems

Learning Objectives

The content presented in this chapter should help you to:

1. Describe the different classes of drugs used to treat depression, anxiety, and psychosis.
2. Discuss the common names, actions, usual adult dosages, possible side effects, and adverse effects of drugs for depression and anxiety.
3. Discuss the priority actions to take *before* and *after* giving commonly prescribed drugs for depression and anxiety.
4. Prioritize essential information to teach patients and their families and caregivers about commonly prescribed drugs for depression and anxiety.

5. Explain appropriate life span considerations for drugs for depression and anxiety.
6. Discuss common names, actions, usual adult dosages, possible side effects, and adverse effects of antipsychotic drugs.
7. Discuss the priority actions to take *before* and *after* giving commonly prescribed antipsychotic drugs.
8. Prioritize essential information to teach patients and their families and caregivers about commonly prescribed antipsychotic drugs.
9. Explain appropriate life span considerations for antipsychotic drugs.

Key Terms

antianxiety drug (ăn-tē-ăng-ZĪ-ĕ-tē DRŬG) (p. 469) A drug that eases anxiety; also known as an anxiolytic.

antidepressant drug (ăn-tē-dē-PRĔS-sĕnt DRŬG) (p. 460) A drug used to treat the symptoms of depression.

antipsychotic drug (ăn-tē-sī-KŎT-ĭk DRŬG) (p. 474) A drug used to treat psychosis; also called *major tranquilizers* and *neuroleptics*.

benzodiazepine (bĕn-zō-dī-ĂZ-ĕ-pēn) (p. 469) A type of drug commonly used to treat anxiety, produce sedation, or relax muscles.

norepinephrine and dopamine reuptake inhibitors (NDRIs) (nŏr-ĕp-ĭ-NĔF-rĭn DŌ-pĕ-mēn rē-ŬP-tāk ĭn-HĬB-ĭ-tŭrz) (p. 461) Antidepressant drugs that block the action of specific transporter proteins, increasing the amount of active

norepinephrine and dopamine neurotransmitters throughout the brain.

selective serotonin reuptake inhibitors (SSRIs) (sĕ-LĔK-tĭv sĕr-ō-TŌ-nĭn rē-ŬP-tāk ĭn-HĬB-ĭ-tŭrz) (p. 460) Antidepressant drugs that act by blocking the reuptake of serotonin, making more serotonin available to act on receptors in the brain.

serotonin and norepinephrine reuptake inhibitors (SNRIs) (sĕr-ō-TŌ-nĭn nŏr-ĕp-ĭ-NĔF-rĭn rē-ŬP-tāk ĭn-HĬB-ĭ-tŭrz) (p. 461) Antidepressants that block the uptake of serotonin and norepinephrine.

tricyclic antidepressants (TCAs) (trī-SĪK-lĭk ăn-tē-dē-PRĔS-sĕnts) (p. 460) Antidepressant drugs that act by blocking the reuptake of norepinephrine and serotonin and making more of these substances available to act on receptors in the brain.

OVERVIEW

Depression, anxiety, and psychosis are major psychiatric illnesses. As many as 30% of people in the United States report symptoms of depression, while only about 10% experience major depression. Anxiety affects as much as 18% of the population in the United States each year. The incidence of schizophrenia, a major psychotic disorder, is about 1% in the United States. The chronic nature of these illnesses presents many challenges for treatment.

Psychiatric disorders can include affective or emotional instability, behavioral problems, and cognitive dysfunction or impairment. Mental illness may be of biological (e.g., anatomic, chemical, or genetic) or psychological (e.g., emotional trauma or conflict) origin and may affect a person's ability to function in society and relationships. Treatment includes psychotherapy (sometimes called "Talk Therapy") and brain stimulation therapies (implantation of devices to send electrical signals to the brain). Drug therapy plays a major role in treating many mental disorders and conditions.

GENERAL ISSUES RELATED TO DRUG THERAPY FOR PSYCHIATRIC PROBLEMS

Drug therapy is extremely important in the management of many psychiatric problems. General responsibilities with drugs for depression, anxiety, and psychosis are discussed in the following paragraphs, followed by chapter sections related to specific categories of drugs for each type of illness. Be sure to use the principles listed in Chapter 2 when administering any drug for a psychiatric problem.

⊛ PRIORITY ACTIONS TO TAKE *BEFORE* GIVING ANY DRUG FOR PSYCHIATRIC PROBLEMS

Always obtain a complete list of the patient's current drugs, including over-the-counter and herbal preparations, because many adverse interactions are possible. Check vital signs, including blood pressure, heart rate, respiratory rate, and temperature to establish a baseline. Check and record the patient's weight because some drug doses are based on this and others may induce weight changes. Assess all patients for risk for falls and apply precautions if needed. If the drug is to be given intravenously, assess the IV site and ensure that it is patent. Ask women of childbearing age if they are pregnant or breastfeeding, or if they plan to become pregnant.

Assess each patient's mental status and ask about suicidal thoughts or plans. Notify the prescriber immediately if the patient has a suicide plan. Place patients on suicide precautions if needed.

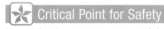

Critical Point for Safety

Immediately report any suicidal thoughts or suicide plans to the prescriber.

QSEN: Safety

⊛ PRIORITY ACTIONS TO TAKE *AFTER* GIVING ANY DRUG FOR PSYCHIATRIC PROBLEMS

Recheck the patient's blood pressure and heart rate and rhythm, and monitor for decreased blood pressure and abnormal heart rhythms. Because of the increased risk for dizziness, instruct patients to call for assistance when getting out of bed and ensure that the call light is within easy reach. Continue to monitor patients for dizziness, drowsiness, or light-headedness. Watch for side effects and adverse effects and report changes to the prescriber. Reassess a patient's mental status and continue to monitor for suicidal ideation or a suicide plan.

⊛ TEACHING PRIORITIES FOR PATIENTS TAKING ANY DRUG FOR PSYCHIATRIC PROBLEMS

For any patient who is prescribed any drug for a psychiatric problem, use these general teaching points:

- Take your prescribed drugs exactly as directed by your prescriber and pharmacist.
- Keep all follow-up appointments to monitor the progress of your treatment.
- Report any side effects to your prescriber immediately.
- If a drug dose is missed, take it as soon as possible unless it is almost time for the next dose. If it is almost time for the next dose do not take the missing dose but take your regularly scheduled dose. **Never** take a double dose of these drugs.
- Avoid driving, operating heavy or complicated equipment, or doing anything requiring alertness until the effects of your drug(s) are known, because of side effects such as drowsiness, dizziness, and impaired (blurred) vision.
- Change positions slowly because of the risk for hypotension and dizziness.
- Check your blood pressure and heart rate daily and notify your prescriber of high or low values.
- If you are a woman of child-bearing age, be sure to notify your prescriber if you are pregnant, plan to become pregnant, or are breastfeeding.
- Avoid alcohol while taking these drugs because alcohol may increase drowsiness and central nervous system (CNS) depression.
- Notify all health care providers about any psychiatric drugs you are taking before having any surgical procedures, including dental surgery, because many of these drugs work on the CNS, causing side effects such as hypotension, dizziness, and drowsiness.

Drug Alert

Interaction Alert

Patients taking an antidepressant that causes drowsiness should avoid alcohol because it can increase the drowsiness.

QSEN: Safety

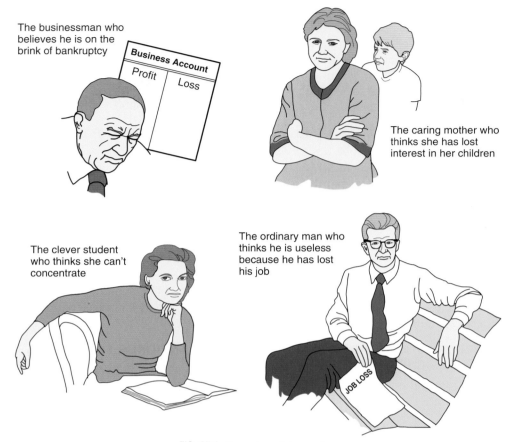

The businessman who believes he is on the brink of bankruptcy

The caring mother who thinks she has lost interest in her children

The clever student who thinks she can't concentrate

The ordinary man who thinks he is useless because he has lost his job

FIG. 25.1 Examples of depression.

- Obtain and wear a medical alert bracelet or carry an identification card stating your diagnosis and the name(s) of the drug(s) you are taking.

REVIEW OF RELATED PHYSIOLOGY AND PATHOPHYSIOLOGY OF DEPRESSION

Depression is an illness characterized by persistent feelings of sadness, despair, loss of energy, and difficulty dealing with normal daily life. It involves the body, mood, and thoughts. Depression affects how a person eats and sleeps, how a person feels about himself or herself and relates to others, as well as how he or she thinks about things. It interferes with the ability to function normally and causes pain and suffering for patients and their loved ones. Figure 25.1 gives some examples of depression.

The exact cause of depression is unknown, but theories include heredity, changes in neurotransmitter levels, altered neuroendocrine function, and psychosocial factors. Table 25.1 summarizes factors often associated with depression.

Research suggests that depression may be caused by an imbalance of brain chemicals called *neurotransmitters* (e.g., serotonin, dopamine, and norepinephrine) (Animation 25.1). Communication between neurons in the brain occurs by the movement of these chemicals across a small gap called the *synapse*. Neurotransmitters are small chemical hormones released from one neuron at the presynaptic nerve terminal that cross the synapse, where they may be accepted by the next neuron at a specialized site called a receptor (Figure 25.2). When neurotransmitter levels decrease or become imbalanced, the neurons are less able to communicate with each other, which may lead to depression and other mood changes.

Depression typically develops in the middle teens, 20s, or 30s, but it can occur at any age. Women are twice as likely as men to experience depression, and men are less likely than women to seek treatment. Because depression is often mistaken for a

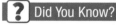 **Did You Know?**

Women are twice as likely as men to experience depression; men are less likely to seek treatment.

Table 25.1	Factors Associated with Depression
Factors	**Examples**
Physical factors	Extreme stress Trauma Environmental conditions
Chemicals	Dopamine Norepinephrine Serotonin
Heredity	First-degree relatives
Psychosocial factors	Abuse Separations of losses Introversion
Gender	Women twice as much as men Post-menopause Postpartum Thyroid dysfunction
Seasonal	Climates with long, severe winter
Physical illness	Thyroid disorders Adrenal disorders Brain tumors Stroke AIDS Parkinson disease Multiple sclerosis
Drugs	Corticosteroids Beta blockers Antipsychotics Reserpine Abuse of alcohol or amphetamines
Exposure to heavy metals	Lead Mercury

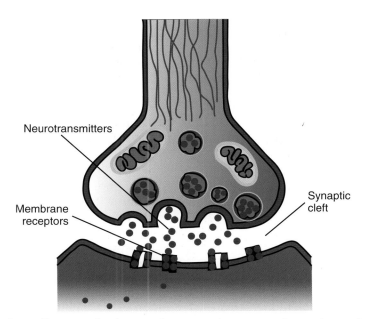

FIG. 25.2 Neurotransmitters carry signals across the synapse from a neuron to receptors on the next neuron.

normal part of aging, many older adults with depression may be undiagnosed or untreated. Children and adolescents with depression often pretend to be sick, refuse to go to school, get into trouble in school, have negative outlooks, and feel misunderstood. Many people with depression do not seek treatment because they do not recognize the condition as a treatable illness.

TYPES OF DEPRESSION

While it is normal to feel down occasionally, when a person is sad most of the time and it affects daily life, they may be experiencing clinical depression. There are several types of depression that may be caused by life events, or chemical changes in the brain. Table 25.2 lists types of depression, definitions, and signs and symptoms of each type.

Major depression is a disabling mental disorder marked by a persistent low mood, lack of pleasure in life, and increased risk of suicide. Diagnosis is based on the presence of five or more depression symptoms that last 2 weeks or more (Box 25.1). Major depression may occur just once or several times during a person's lifetime.

Bipolar disorder, formerly called "manic depression," is characterized by cycling moods from severe highs (*mania*) to severe lows (depression). Mood changes may be sudden and dramatic, or they may be gradual. During a low cycle, the person has symptoms of depression (see Box 25.1). During a high cycle, he or she may be overactive, overly talkative, and full of energy. Mania can affect thought processes, judgment, and social behavior. Box 25.2 summarizes symptoms of mania. Untreated mania may progress to psychosis.

Diagnosis of depression is based on identifying symptoms (see Box 25.1). A complete physical examination is important to rule out physical disorders such as thyroid disease, anemia, and viral infections. A detailed history by a qualified health care professional is important to discover specific factors in a patient's life that may contribute to depression.

The most common treatments for depression include counseling or psychotherapy and antidepressant drugs. Depression treatment is individualized, taking into account the severity and cause of the depression episode(s). Most patients with depression are treated as outpatients; however, when a person has suicidal thoughts (also called *suicidal ideation*), and particularly if the person has a suicide plan, hospitalization may be required. With treatment, symptoms can be well controlled. Figure 25.3 shows the cycle of depression, including how and when to intervene for effective treatment with medications and psychotherapy.

ANTIDEPRESSANTS

How Antidepressants Work

Antidepressant drugs are used to treat people with depression. Prescribing and using these prescription drugs can lead to the improvement of symptoms, particularly when patients also receive some form of psychotherapy or counseling.

The two most common groups of drugs used to treat depression are **selective serotonin reuptake inhibitors (SSRIs)** and **tricyclic antidepressants (TCAs)**. SSRIs have fewer side effects and are more commonly prescribed than TCAs. With most of these drugs, it can take as long as 8 weeks for symptoms of depression to improve. Often depression is chronic, and patients must continue to take antidepressants even when they have no symptoms to keep the depression from returning.

SSRIs work by increasing the amount of serotonin in the brain at any one time. Serotonin is one of the chemical messengers (neurotransmitters) that carry signals between brain nerve cells (neurons). SSRIs block the reabsorption (reuptake) of serotonin into neurons (Figure 25.4).

TCAs act on approximately five different neurotransmitter pathways to achieve their effects. They block the reuptake of serotonin and norepinephrine in presynaptic terminals, which leads to increased concentration of these neurotransmitters in the synaptic cleft. The effects of these drugs occur immediately, but the patient's symptoms often do not respond or improve for 2 to 8 weeks.

Memory Jogger

Bipolar disorder is characterized by cycling moods—from severe highs to severe lows.

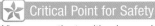

Critical Point for Safety

When a patient with depression has suicidal thoughts and a suicide plan, hospitalization may be required for the patient's safety.

QSEN: Safety

Memory Jogger

The two most common groups of drugs prescribed to treat depression are SSRIs and TCAs.

Table **25.2**   Types of Depression

Type of Depression	Definition	Signs and Symptoms
Major depression	Patient feels sad most of the time on most days of the week	• Loss of interest or pleasure in your activities • Weight loss or gain • Trouble getting to sleep or feeling sleepy during the day • Feeling restless and agitated, or else very sluggish and slowed down physically or mentally • Being tired and without energy • Feeling worthless or guilty • Trouble concentrating or making decisions • Thoughts of suicide
Persistent depressive disorder	Depression that lasts 2 years or longer	• Change in your appetite (not eating enough or overeating) • Sleeping too little or too much • Lack of energy, or fatigue • Low self-esteem • Trouble concentrating or making decisions • Feeling hopeless
Bipolar disorder	Sometimes called "manic depression"	• Mood episodes that range from extremes of high energy with an "up" mood to low "depressive" periods • In the low phase, patient has symptoms of major depression
Seasonal affective disorder	Period of depression associated with winter months and decreased sunlight	• Typically goes away during spring and summer • Light therapy can help with symptoms
Psychotic depression	Depression associated with psychotic symptoms	• Hallucinations • Delusions • Paranoia
Peripartum (postpartum) depression	Depression that occurs within weeks to months after childbirth	• Similar to major depression
Premenstrual dysphoric disorder (PMDD)	Depression and other symptoms at start of monthly menstruation	• Mood swings • Irritability • Anxiety • Trouble concentrating • Change in appetite or sleep habits • Feelings of being overwhelmed
Situational depression	Depressed mood when having trouble managing a stressful event in your life	• Occurs after a stressful event (e.g., death in your family, a divorce, or losing a job)
Atypical depression	A "specifier" that describes a pattern of depressive symptoms. A positive event can temporarily improve mood.	• Increased appetite • Sleeping more than usual • Feeling of heaviness in your arms and legs • Oversensitive to criticism

Box **25.1**   Symptoms of Depression

- Abrupt changes in eating habits
- Chronic fatigue; being slowed down
- Decreased ability to perform normal daily tasks
- Decreased appetite and/or weight loss or overeating and weight gain
- Difficulty concentrating, remembering, or making decisions
- Feelings of hopelessness or pessimism
- Inability to experience pleasure in hobbies and activities that were once enjoyed
- Insomnia, early morning awakening, or oversleeping
- Irritability
- Numb or empty feeling or absence of any feelings at all
- Persistent feeling of worthlessness, guilt, helplessness, or sadness
- Persistent physical symptoms that do not respond to treatment (e.g., headaches, digestive disorders, chronic pain)
- Recurrent thoughts of death or suicide
- Restlessness

Norepinephrine and dopamine reuptake inhibitors (NDRIs, e.g., *mirtazapine* [Remeron], *trazodone* [Desyrel]) correct the imbalance of the neurotransmitters dopamine and norepinephrine.

Serotonin and norepinephrine reuptake inhibitors (SNRIs, e.g., *desvenlafaxine* [Pristiq], *duloxetine* [Cymbalta]) block the uptake of serotonin and norepinephrine.

Box 25.2 **Symptoms of Mania**

- Abnormal or excessive elation
- Decreased need for sleep
- Grandiose notions
- Inappropriate social behavior
- Increased sexual desire
- Increased talking
- Markedly increased energy
- Poor judgment
- Racing thoughts
- Unusual irritability

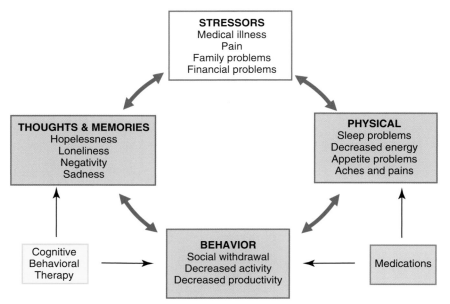

FIG. 25.3 The cycle of depression.

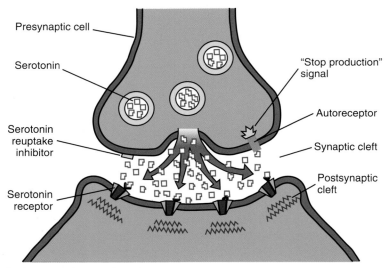

FIG. 25.4 Selective serotonin reuptake inhibitor drugs increase the amount of serotonin in the brain by blocking reuptake of neurotransmitters by neurons.

Bupropion (Wellbutrin) is an oral antidepressant drug from the aminoketone class. It is not a tricyclic antidepressant and is unrelated to other known antidepressants. The action of bupropion is not fully understood. It selectively inhibits the neuronal reuptake of dopamine. The onset of antidepressant effects takes 1 to 3 weeks, and the maximal effect may not be noted for 4 weeks. Its uses include attention-deficit hyperactivity disorder (ADHD), depression, diabetic neuropathy, neuropathic pain, postherpetic neuralgia, seasonal affective disorder (SAD), and tobacco cessation.

MAOIs (monoamine oxidase inhibitors) (e.g., phenelzine [Nardil], selegiline [Emsam]) are seldom used for the treatment of depression and are considered drugs of *last resort* for patients who have not responded to other drugs. This is because of their high potential for toxicity (including hypertensive crisis), dietary restrictions (avoidance of tyramine-containing foods), and many drug interactions. If a patient is prescribed an MAOI, consult a reliable drug source for information on the drug and its use for the treatment of depression.

Generic names, trade names, and adult dosages of common antidepressants are listed in the following table. Be sure to consult a reliable drug resource for specific information about less common drugs used to treat depression.

Dosages for Common Antidepressant Drugs

Drug Group	Drug	Usual Adult Dosage
SSRIs	citalopram (Celexa)	20 mg orally once daily. Titrate in increments of 20 mg at intervals of no less than 1 week based on response and tolerability. Max: 40 mg/day
	escitalopram (Lexapro)	10 mg orally once daily. May be increased to 20 mg once daily after a minimum of 1 week. Max: 20 mg/day
	fluoxetine (Prozac, Prozac Weekly, Sarafem, Selfemra)	20 mg/day orally initially. May increase dose after several weeks by 10–20 mg as needed and tolerated. A less frequent or lower dosage should be considered for geriatric adults. Max: 80 mg/day. Weekly maintenance for depression: 90 mg orally once weekly
	fluvoxamine (Luvox, Luvox CR)	50 mg orally once daily at bedtime. Increase at weekly intervals by 50 mg/day according to response and tolerability. Geriatric patients may require a reduced initial dose and slower titration. Average effective dose 100 mg/day. Max: 150 mg/day
	paroxetine (Paxil, Paxil CR, Brisdelle, Pexeva)	20 mg orally once daily usually in the morning. Increase in increments of 10 mg at a minimum of weekly intervals. Max: 50 mg/day. Debilitated or geriatric adults: 10 mg orally once daily initially, may increase if needed by 10 mg at a minimum of weekly intervals. Max: 40 mg/day. CR: 25 mg orally once daily initially, usually in the morning. May increase if needed in increments of 12.5 mg at a minimum of weekly intervals. Max: 62.5 mg/day
	sertraline (Zoloft)	50 mg orally once daily. A lower initial dose may be used (e.g., 25 mg orally once daily) to minimize adverse effects. May increase at intervals of not less than 1 week. Sertraline capsules may be initiated in patients who have taken 100–125 mg doses daily for at least 1 week. Max: 200 mg/day
TCAs	amitriptyline (Elavil, Tryptanol, Vanatrip)	Initially, 75 mg/day orally, given in divided doses, or 50–100 mg once daily at bedtime. Max (hospitalized patients): 300 mg/day. Usual maintenance dosage: 50–100 mg/day
	amoxapine (Amoxapine Tablets)	50 mg orally 2–3 times per day initially. May titrate to 100 mg 2–3 times per day by the end of the first week of treatment. Max (hospitalized): 600 mg/day in at least 2 divided doses

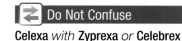

Do Not Confuse

Celexa *with* **Zyprexa** *or* **Celebrex**

An order for Celexa may be confused with Zyprexa or Celebrex. Celexa is an SSRI drug used to treat depression, whereas Zyprexa is an antipsychotic drug used to treat psychotic disorders. Celebrex is a nonsteroidal antiinflammatory drug (NSAID) used to treat osteoarthritis and rheumatoid arthritis.

QSEN: Safety

Continued

Dosages for Common Antidepressant Drugs—cont'd

Drug Group	Drug	Usual Adult Dosage
	clomipramine (Anafranil)	25 mg orally once daily, may gradually increase in the first 2 weeks to 100 mg/day. Max: 250 mg/day. After titration, the total daily dose may be given every night at bedtime to minimize daytime sedation
	desipramine (Norpramin)	50–75 mg/day orally initially, in single or divided doses. Titrate daily dose by 25–50 mg at weekly intervals. Usual adult dosage: 100–200 mg per day. Max: 300 mg/day
	doxepin (Prudoxin, Silenor, Sinequan, Zonalon)	75 mg/day orally as a single dose at bedtime or in 2–3 divided doses. May increase gradually depending on response and tolerability. Usual effective adult dose: 75–150 mg/day; 300 mg/day may be required in more severely ill patients
	imipramine (Tofranil, Tofranil PM)	75 mg/day orally; initial dosing at bedtime may help minimize daytime sedation. Hospitalized patient. Usual maintenance dose: 50-150 mg/day. Max: 300 mg/day
SNRIs	desvenlafaxine (Pristiq, Khedezla)	50 mg orally once daily, initially. Dose range: 50–400 mg/day. Max: 400 mg/day
	duloxetine (Cymbalta, Drizalma, Irenka)	20 mg orally twice daily or 60 mg/day as a single dose or in 2 divided doses initially. May give 30 mg/day for 1 week, then increase to 60 mg/day. Target maintenance dose is 60 mg/day; dividing the dose may increase tolerability. Max: 120 mg/day
	levomilnacipran (Fetzima)	20 mg/day orally for 2 days, then increase to 40 mg/day. Dose may be increased in increments of 40 mg at intervals of at least 2 days. Recommended dose range is 40–120 mg once daily, with or without food. Max: 120 mg once daily
	venlafaxine (Effexor, Effexor XR)	75 mg/day orally given in 2 or 3 divided doses, initially. May increase by 75 mg/day at intervals no less than every 4 days. Recommended outpatient max: 225 mg/day
NDRIs	mirtazapine (Remeron)	15 mg orally once daily at bedtime, initially. May titrate no sooner than every 1–2 weeks. Geriatric patients may need slower titration schedules. Effective dose range 15–45 mg/day. Max: 45 mg/day
	nefazodone (Serzone)	100 mg orally twice daily. May increase in increments of 100–200 mg/day at weekly intervals as tolerated and needed. Effective dose range 300–600 mg/day given in 2 divided doses
	trazodone (Desyrel, Oleptro)	150 mg/day orally in divided doses; may increase by 50 mg/day every 3–4 days as needed based on clinical response. Max: 400 mg/day for outpatients and 600 mg/day for inpatients
Aminoketones	bupropion (Wellbutrin, Wellbutrin SR, Wellbutrin XL, Zyban)	100 mg orally twice daily; titrate after no less than 3 days to 100 mg 3 times per day if needed; no single dose should exceed 150 mg. Antidepressant effects take 1–4 weeks

🔁 **Do Not Confuse**

trazodone *with* **tramadol**

An order for trazodone may be confused with tramadol. Trazodone is a combined reuptake inhibitor and receptor blocker used to treat depression, whereas tramadol is an opioid analgesic used to treat moderate to moderately severe pain.

QSEN: Safety

🔁 **Do Not Confuse**

Wellbutrin SR *with* **Wellbutrin XL**

An order for Wellbutrin SR can be confused with Wellbutrin XL. Both drugs are Aminoketones used to treat depression. However, Wellbutrin SR is a slow-release form of the drug given twice a day, whereas Wellbutrin XL is an extended-release form of the drug given once a day.

QSEN: Safety

Intended Responses of Antidepressants
- Depression is corrected.
- Symptoms of depressed mood are decreased.

Common Side Effects of Antidepressants
The most common side effects of drugs for depression are nausea and vomiting, weight gain, diarrhea, drowsiness (sleepiness), and sexual problems (e.g., decreased libido, impotence). Side effects occur more often in the first few days and often improve over time.

SSRI drugs have many side effects. The most common side effects include drowsiness, dizziness, fatigue, insomnia, GI upset (e.g., nausea, diarrhea, dyspepsia, and flatulence), and impotence with decreased interest in sexual activity. Other side effects include apathy, anxiety, nervousness, confusion, headache, weakness, abdominal pain, anorexia, dry mouth, increased saliva, increased sweating, weight gain, and tremors. Venlafaxine (Effexor) can cause increased blood pressure.

Common side effects of TCAs include lethargy, sedation, drowsiness, fatigue, blurred vision, dry eyes, dry mouth, hypotension, and constipation.

The most common side effects of SNRIs are nausea and dry mouth. NDRIs may also cause tachycardia, sore throat, tremors, GI and muscle pain, and tinnitus. Most side effects improve within a few weeks.

Common side effects of bupropion (Wellbutrin) include headache, weight loss, dry mouth, trouble sleeping (insomnia), nausea, dizziness, constipation, fast heartbeat, and sore throat. These usually improve over the first or second week after the drug is prescribed.

Possible Adverse Effects of Antidepressants
TCAs such as *amitriptyline* (Elavil), *desipramine* (Norpramin), *imipramine* (Tofranil), and *nortriptyline* (Aventyl) may cause serious adverse cardiac effects, including unstable ventricular dysrhythmias (abnormal heart rhythms) or asystole (absence of a heart rhythm).

Venlafaxine (Effexor), *duloxetine* (Cymbalta), and *bupropion* (Wellbutrin) may cause seizures. *Mirtazapine* (Remeron) can lead to neutropenia (decreased white blood cells [WBCs]), which increases the risk of infection. *Nefazodone* has been known to cause liver failure or liver toxicity.

Thoughts of suicide may increase in children, adolescents, and young adults when taking antidepressants; a warning appears on all labels for these drugs.

Signs of allergic reactions to antidepressants include chest pain, increased or irregular heart rhythm, shortness of breath, fever, hives, rash, itching, difficulty breathing or swallowing, swelling, decreased coordination, shaking hands (tremors), dizziness, light-headedness, and thoughts of hurting oneself.

Serotonin syndrome is a rare adverse effect that occurs when levels of serotonin are very high. Signs and symptoms of serotonin syndrome include anxiety, agitation, sweating, confusion, tremors, restlessness, lack of coordination, and rapid heart rate.

⊛ Priority Actions to Take *Before* Giving Antidepressants
In addition to the general responsibilities related to drugs for psychiatric problems (p. 457), ask whether the patient has a family history of depression. Ask about usual bowel patterns, fluid intake, and diet. Notify the prescriber if the patient is taking the herbal preparation St. John's wort (an herbal preparation used to treat depression). Ask patients prescribed a TCA drug about their smoking history.

Common Side Effects
Antidepressants

Dizziness

Hypotension

Drowsiness, Fatigue

Nausea/Vomiting, Diarrhea, Flatulence, Dyspepsia, Constipation

Impotence, Decreased libido

⚠ Drug Alert
Monitoring Alert

Assess patients taking antidepressant drugs for suicidal thoughts and report any positive findings immediately to the prescriber.

QSEN: Safety

Drug Alert

Interaction Alert

Be sure to ask a patient about the use of St. John's wort, an herbal product used to treat depression. It should not be taken with antidepressant drugs because it might increase the risk of the accumulation of high levels of serotonin in the patient's body.

QSEN: Safety

Drug Alert

Interaction Alert

Wellbutrin may be prescribed as Wellbutrin SR, the sustained-release form, which is administered in two doses at least 8 hr apart. Wellbutrin XL extended-release tablets should be taken once a day in the morning. Wellbutrin SR and XL tablets should be swallowed whole and never chewed, divided, or crushed.

QSEN: Safety

Drug Alert

Interaction Alert

Ask patients taking a TCA drug about smoking because smoking cigarettes may decrease the effectiveness of these drugs.

QSEN: Safety

Drug Alert

Teaching Alert

Be sure to teach patients who are taking an antidepressant that it may take 1–8 weeks before symptoms of depression improve.

QSEN: Safety

Critical Point for Safety

Instruct patients **not** to stop taking an antidepressant without first talking to their prescriber.

QSEN: Safety

Drug Alert

Action/Intervention Alert

Monitor children and adolescents carefully because antidepressant drugs may increase the risk of suicidal thoughts or actions.

QSEN: Safety

If a patient is taking a TCA, ask about smoking because smoking cigarettes may decrease the effectiveness of these drugs.

 Priority Actions to Take *After* Giving Antidepressants

In addition to the general responsibilities related to drugs for psychiatric problems (p. 457), reassess the patient's mental status to determine his or her response to drugs. Monitor the patient for drug side effects, adverse effects, or allergic reactions and report them to the prescriber. Recheck blood pressure and heart rate, and report any abnormalities. Assess for suicidal thoughts and report these to the prescriber immediately.

 Teaching Priorities for Patients Taking Antidepressants

In addition to the general responsibilities related to teaching patients about drugs for psychiatric problems (p. 457), include these teaching points and precautions:

- Your prescriber may start with a low drug dose and gradually increase it until therapeutic antidepressant effects are achieved.
- It may take 1 to 8 weeks before your symptoms of depression improve.
- Take your antidepressant drug even when you are feeling well.
- Antidepressants can control the symptoms of depression but will **not** cure depression.
- Antidepressants may need to be discontinued gradually to avoid adverse effects.
- If you are prescribed Wellbutrin, understand that it works by correcting the imbalance of the neurotransmitters dopamine and norepinephrine and that it may be prescribed as Wellbutrin SR (sustained-release form, which is taken in two doses at least 8 hours apart) or Wellbutrin XL (extended-release tablets that should be taken only once a day in the morning). Wellbutrin SR and XL tablets should be taken whole. Never chew, divide, or crush them.
- Frequent mouth rinses and good oral hygiene can minimize the effects of dry mouth.
- If you are prescribed an SSRI drug, take the dose once a day in the morning or evening.

Life Span Considerations for Antidepressants

Pediatric considerations. SSRIs, TCAs, and other antidepressant drugs should be used with caution in depressed children and adolescents because the risk for suicidal thoughts or actions may increase while taking these drugs. Fluoxetine (Prozac) may cause unusual excitement, restlessness, irritability, or trouble sleeping in children because they are more sensitive to the effects of this drug. Venlafaxine (Effexor) may slow growth and weight gain in children. A child's growth should be monitored carefully while taking this drug.

Considerations for pregnancy and lactation. SSRIs have a moderate likelihood of increasing the risk for birth defects or fetal harm when tested in animals. However, these drugs have not been tested during pregnancy. Paroxetine (Paxil) should be avoided in pregnancy. Some SSRIs pass through breast milk and may have unwanted effects such as drowsiness, decreased feeding, and weight loss in the breastfeeding infant. TCAs have a moderate to high likelihood of increasing the risk for birth defects or fetal harm.

Considerations for older adults. Older adults may require lower doses of SSRIs because of possible increased reaction to the effects and side effects of these drugs and slower metabolism of drugs such as escitalopram (Lexapro). Older patients with kidney disease or liver failure should be given lower doses of these drugs because they are metabolized by the liver and kidneys.

REVIEW OF RELATED PHYSIOLOGY AND PATHOPHYSIOLOGY OF ANXIETY

Anxiety is defined as a feeling of worry, nervousness, or unease, typically about an imminent event or something with an uncertain outcome. It includes feelings of

| Box 25.3 | **Symptoms of Anxiety** |

PANIC DISORDER
- Chest pain
- Chills or hot flashes
- Dizziness
- Feeling of being detached from the world (derealization)
- Fear of dying
- Nausea
- Numbness and tingling
- Palpitations
- Sense of choking
- Shortness of breath
- Sweating
- Trembling

GENERALIZED ANXIETY DISORDER
- Difficulty concentrating
- Easy fatigue
- Excessive, unrealistic worry
- Irritability
- Muscle tension
- Restlessness
- Sleep disturbance

PHOBIC DISORDER
- Intense, persistent, recurrent fear of certain objects (e.g., snakes, spiders, blood)
- Intense, persistent, recurrent fear of certain situations (e.g., heights, speaking in front of a group, public places)
- Panic attack possibly triggered by objects and situations

OBSESSIVE-COMPULSIVE DISORDER
- Obsessive thoughts such as:
  - Excessive focus on religious or moral ideas
  - Fear of being contaminated by germs or dirt or contaminating others
  - Fear of causing harm to yourself or others
  - Fear of losing or not having things you might need
  - Intrusive sexually explicit or violent thoughts and images
  - Order and symmetry—the idea that everything must line up "just right"
  - Superstitions—excessive attention to something considered lucky or unlucky
- Compulsive behaviors such as:
  - Accumulating "junk" such as old newspapers, magazines, empty food containers, or other things for which you do not have a use
  - Counting, tapping, repeating certain words, or doing other senseless things to reduce anxiety
  - Excessively double-checking things such as locks, appliances, and switches
  - Ordering or making groups of things even or arranging things "just so"
  - Praying excessively or engaging in rituals triggered by religious fear
  - Repeatedly checking in on loved ones to make sure they are safe
  - Spending a lot of time washing or cleaning

STRESS DISORDERS (POSTTRAUMATIC STRESS DISORDER)
- Avoiding activities, places, or people associated with the triggering event
- Being hypervigilant
- Difficulty concentrating
- Difficulty sleeping
- Feeling a general sense of doom and gloom along with decreased positive emotions and hopes for the future

apprehension, fear, or worry. It can occur without a cause and may not be based on a real-life situation. Symptoms of anxiety vary with the type of anxiety disorder (Box 25.3).

In the central nervous system (CNS), the important mediators of anxiety disorder symptoms are norepinephrine, serotonin, dopamine, and gamma-aminobutyric acid (GABA) (Animation 25.2). Other neurotransmitters and peptide (e.g., corticotropin-releasing factor) may also be involved. Peripherally, the autonomic nervous system, especially the sympathetic nervous system, mediates many of the symptoms.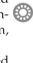

Anxiety that is perceived as out of proportion with what is normal or expected may escalate through a feedback circle (Figure 25.5). Physical symptoms may affect the heart (e.g., increased rate, pounding), lungs (e.g., increased rate and depth, shortness of breath), and nervous system (e.g., tremors, headaches). Emotional symptoms of anxiety include apprehension, dread, irritability, restlessness, and difficulty concentrating. Causes and factors associated with anxiety include mental conditions, physical conditions, the effects of drugs, or a combination of these causes. Box 25.4 summarizes the causes of the mental condition and the external factors associated with anxiety.

TYPES OF ANXIETY

Common anxiety disorders include panic disorder, generalized anxiety disorder, phobic disorder, obsessive-compulsive disorder, and posttraumatic stress disorder (PTSD).

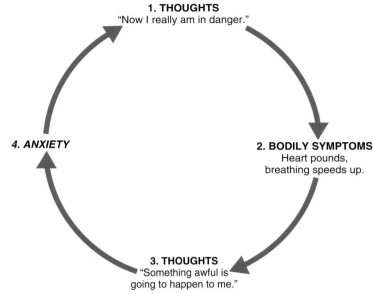

FIG. 25.5 The circle of anxiety.

Box 25.4	**Causes and External Factors Associated with Anxiety**

- Financial stress
- Lack of oxygen such as high-altitude sickness, emphysema, pulmonary embolus, and pneumonia (in older adults)
- Side effect of medication
- Stress at work
- Stress from a serious medical illness
- Stress from emotional trauma such as death of a loved one
- Stress from school
- Stress in personal relationships such as marriage
- Symptoms of a medical illness
- Use of illicit drugs such as cocaine

Panic disorders are separate and intense periods of fear or feelings of doom that develop over a short period of time, such as 10 minutes. A panic attack, the main symptom of panic disorder, is characterized by anxiety or terror and usually lasts between 15 and 30 minutes.

Generalized anxiety disorder (GAD) occurs when a person experiences excessive, almost daily anxiety and worry for more than 6 months. It affects about 3% of the population in the United States. Women are twice as likely as men to be affected. GAD most often begins during childhood or adolescence, but it may begin at any age.

Phobic disorders are intense, persistent, recurrent fears of certain objects (e.g., snakes) or situations (e.g., speaking in front of a group) that can cause a panic attack.

Obsessive-compulsive disorder (OCD) is characterized by obsessive thoughts and compulsive actions. The person with OCD becomes trapped in a pattern of repetitive thoughts and behaviors that do not make sense and are distressing but are very difficult to overcome. An example is a person who repeatedly washes his or her hands because of a fear of germs.

Posttraumatic stress disorder (PTSD) leads to anxiety and is caused by exposure to death or near-death experiences such as floods, fires, earthquakes, shootings, automobile accidents, or war. The traumatic experience recurs in thoughts and dreams.

Treatment of anxiety depends on the cause. Short-term anxiety attacks can be treated at home with interventions such as talking with a supportive person, meditating, taking a warm bath, resting in a dark room, or performing deep-breathing exercises. Strategies for coping with anxiety and stress include eating a well-balanced diet, getting enough sleep, exercising regularly, limiting caffeine and alcohol, avoiding nicotine and recreational drugs, using relaxation techniques, and balancing fun

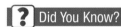

Did You Know?

Women are twice as likely as men to develop GAD.

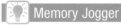

Memory Jogger

The common anxiety disorders include panic disorder, GAD, phobic disorder, OCD, and PTSD.

activities with responsibilities. Group therapy may be useful for anxieties such as fear of flying.

Physical conditions contributing to or causing anxiety may be treated with drugs or surgery. An example of a physical cause of anxiety is a tumor called a *pheochromocytoma,* which causes the adrenal glands to produce excessive amounts of adrenaline. Surgical removal of this tumor can resolve the symptoms of anxiety. Symptoms of hyperthyroidism include anxiety. Careful diagnosis is essential because many of the symptoms of hyperthyroidism are also found in anxiety disorder. Hyperthyroidism and anxiety are often confused. Medical or surgical treatment of hyperthyroidism can also resolve the anxiety. Counseling or psychotherapy may also be helpful. Antianxiety drugs are often prescribed to control the symptoms of anxiety.

ANTIANXIETY DRUGS

How Antianxiety Drugs Work

Mild anxiety is a common experience and usually requires no drug treatment. Moderate-to-severe anxiety is a symptom of psychiatric disorders such as phobia, panic disorder, OCD, and PTSD.

Chronic and severe anxiety are treated with **antianxiety drugs**, also called *anxiolytics* or *minor tranquilizers.* Most drugs used to treat anxiety also cause sedation or sleep and are likely to cause *dependence* (the psychologic craving for, or physiologic reliance on, a chemical substance) when taken for an extended period.

Benzodiazepines are CNS depressants that increase the inhibitory actions of gamma-aminobutyric acid (GABA) in the brain. GABA is a neurotransmitter that transmits messages from brain cell to brain cell. It sends a message to the brain neurons to slow down or stop firing. This quiets the brain and decreases anxiety. Diazepam (Valium) has a longer half-life, which makes it a less attractive choice than other benzodiazepine drugs. When treating anxiety disorders, benzodiazepines are generally used for temporary management of anxiety symptoms.

In the past, *benzodiazepines* were the most commonly prescribed drugs for treatment of anxiety. When taken as directed, these drugs allow many patients with anxiety to lead nearly normal lives. Other drug classes, such as SSRIs and buspirone, are now prescribed to treat anxiety more commonly than benzodiazepines because they have milder side effects and patients are less likely to become dependent on them. The major benefit of benzodiazepines is that they act within 30 minutes and may be given as needed, whereas it may take SSRIs 3 to 5 weeks to control anxiety. Benzodiazepines also decrease symptoms of alcohol withdrawal and prevent delirium tremens.

SSRIs relieve anxiety by affecting the action of the neurotransmitter serotonin in the brain. Serotonin stays in the synaptic gap longer, and the transmission of impulses is slowed. It is also theorized that these drugs may affect the limbic system, which is the part of the brain associated with emotions. They calm and relax people with anxiety; however, they may take several weeks to become effective.

Buspirone (BuSpar) binds the neuroreceptors for serotonin and dopamine in the brain and increases norepinephrine metabolism to relieve anxiety. Binding the neurotransmitters slows the transmission of impulses and quiets the brain to relieve anxiety.

Pregabalin is an antiseizure drug that, like benzodiazepines, increases the action of GABA, which is thought to be its mechanism for decreasing anxiety. *Hydroxyzine* is an antihistamine that causes sedation. It is used to treat insomnia that is caused by anxiety.

Generic names, trade names, and adult dosages of drugs for anxiety are listed in the following table. Be sure to consult a reliable drug resource for information about less common antianxiety drugs. For additional information on SSRI drugs prescribed for anxiety (e.g., citalopram, escitalopram, fluoxetine, fluvoxamine, paroxetine, sertraline), see the depression drugs section in this chapter (p. 463).

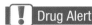 **Drug Alert**

Action/Intervention Alert

Monitor patients taking antianxiety drugs for signs of dependence because most of these drugs are likely to cause dependence when taken for a long time.

QSEN: Safety

 Drug Alert

Teaching Alert

Teach patients that it may take SSRI drugs 3 to 5 weeks to control anxiety.

QSEN: Safety

 Did You Know?

Beta blockers, which are usually prescribed for hypertension, are sometimes prescribed for patients facing anxiety-producing events such as performing on stage or making a speech.

Dosages for Common Antianxiety Drugs

Drug Group	Drug Name	Usual Adult Dosage
Benzodiazepines	alprazolam (Xanax, Niravam)	0.25–0.5 mg orally 3 times per day. Increase dose as tolerated at intervals of 3–4 days. Max 4 mg/day in divided doses
	clonazepam (Klonopin)	0.25 mg orally twice daily initially, increasing to the recommended dose of 1 mg/day after 3 days according to response and tolerability. Max 4 mg/day
	chlordiazepoxide (Librium)	5–10 mg orally 3–4 times per day for mild to moderate symptoms, or 20–25 mg 3–4 times per day for severe symptoms. Max: 100 mg/day
	clorazepate (Tranxene)	7.5–15 mg orally twice daily, or 15 mg once daily at bedtime. Usual maintenance dose is 15 mg twice daily. Max: 60 mg/day
	diazepam (Valium)	2–10 mg orally 2–4 times per day depending upon the severity of the symptoms. Max: 40 mg/day for ambulatory care 2–5 mg IM or IV. May repeat in 3–4 hr. For severe anxiety disorders and symptoms of anxiety, 5–10 mg IM or IV; repeat in 3 to 4 hours if necessary
	lorazepam (Ativan)	2–3 mg/day orally given in 2–3 divided doses. Usual dosage is 2–6 mg/day. Max: 10 mg/day *Special Considerations:* **When a higher dosage is needed, the evening dose should be increased before the daytime doses**
	oxazepam (Serax)	10–15 mg orally 3–4 times per day. For anxiety associated with depression, use 15–30 mg 3–4 times per day
Anxiolytics	buspirone (BuSpar)	7.5 mg orally twice daily initially, then increase as needed by 5 mg/day every 2–3 days. Usual maintenance dose: 15–30 mg/day administered in 2–3 divided doses. Max: 60 mg/day
Anticonvulsants	pregabalin (Lyrica)	75 mg orally twice daily, initially. May increase dose to 150 mg twice daily after 1 week based on efficacy and tolerability. Usual dose: 150 to 300 mg twice daily. Max: 300 mg PO twice daily
Antihistamines	hydroxyzine (Atarax, Hyzine, Rezine, Vistaril)	50–100 mg orally 4 times daily as needed. 50–100 mg IM initially; may repeat every 4–6 hr as needed
Beta Blockers	propranolol (Inderal)	10–80 mg orally, given 1 hr prior to the anxiety-producing event

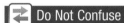 **Do Not Confuse**

Klonopin *with* **Clonidine**

An order for Klonopin may be confused with Clonidine. Klonopin (clonazepam) is a benzodiazepine drug used to treat anxiety and psychosis, whereas Clonidine is a central-acting adrenergic drug used to treat hypertension.

QSEN: Safety

 Do Not Confuse

buspirone *with* **bupropion**

An order for buspirone can be confused with bupropion. Buspirone is an antianxiety drug whereas bupropion is an antidepressant drug.

QSEN: Safety

Intended Responses of Antianxiety Drugs
- Anxiety is relieved without too much sedation.
- Symptoms of anxiety are decreased.
- Sense of well-being is improved.

Common Side Effects of Antianxiety Drugs

The most common side effects of benzodiazepines are related to their CNS effects. They include drowsiness, dizziness, light-headedness, fatigue, ataxia, and unsteadiness. Other side effects include sleepiness, depression, lethargy, apathy, memory impairment, disorientation, amnesia, delirium, headache, slurred speech, behavioral changes, euphoria, dysarthria, and inability to perform complex mental functions. Additional common side effects include nervousness, irritability, difficulty concentrating, a "glassy-eyed" appearance, changes in heart rate and blood pressure, changes in bowel function, and skin rashes. With *chlordiazepoxide* (Librium), there is pain at intramuscular sites after injection.

Common side effects of *buspirone* include dizziness and drowsiness. Others may include excitement, fatigue, headache, insomnia, nervousness, weakness, blurred vision, nasal congestion, sore throat, tinnitus, chest pain, palpitations, tachycardia, nausea, rash, myalgia, lack of coordination, numbness, paresthesia, clammy skin, and sweating.

Possible Adverse Effects of Antianxiety Drugs

Life-threatening adverse effects of *benzodiazepines* include seizures and coma. *Buspirone* can result in hallucinations and heart failure.

Suddenly stopping a *benzodiazepine* can cause a potentially life-threatening reaction of withdrawal symptoms, including nervousness, restlessness, tremulousness, weakness, and seizures. The patient may become dehydrated or delirious or may develop insomnia, confusion, and visual or auditory hallucinations.

Suicidal ideation (creating a plan to carry out suicide) may occur with patients taking *clonazepam* (Klonopin).

⭐ Priority Actions to Take *Before* Giving Antianxiety Drugs

In addition to the general responsibilities related to drugs for psychiatric problems (p. 457), check for a history of drug or substance dependencies. Assess patients for baseline levels of anxiety, symptoms, and stressors that lead to or cause anxiety. Check baseline vital signs and assess the patient's gait for steadiness. Ask about any suicidal thoughts or plans. Ask patients if they use herbal supplements because several are used to treat anxiety (e.g., St. John's wort, ginkgo biloba, valerian). Ask women of child-bearing age if they are pregnant, breastfeeding, or plan to become pregnant.

⭐ Priority Actions to Take *After* Giving Antianxiety Drugs

In addition to the general responsibilities related to drugs for psychiatric problems (p. 457), assess gait for steadiness. Continue to monitor the level of anxiety to assess the effectiveness of the drug. Assess for and continue to monitor the patient for suicidal ideation or suicidal plans. Recheck blood pressure and heart rate and report any abnormalities to the prescriber.

Because of the tendency to become dependent on *benzodiazepines*, give these drugs only as prescribed. While patients are taking these drugs, observe for signs of dependency and report them to the prescriber.

⭐ Teaching Priorities for Patients Taking Antianxiety Drugs

In addition to the general responsibilities related to teaching patients about drugs for psychiatric problems (p. 457), include these teaching points and precautions:

- Take these drugs, especially benzodiazepines, exactly as prescribed to decrease the chance of dependence.
- If you have suicidal thoughts, report this immediately to your prescriber.
- While taking antianxiety drugs, avoid drinking alcohol, taking sleeping pills, or taking prescription pain drugs at the same time because of the danger of more severe CNS depression.
- Your prescriber may want to taper you off of benzodiazepine drugs gradually because stopping them suddenly can cause withdrawal symptoms such as sweating, vomiting, muscle cramps, tremors, or seizures.
- Report any signs of dependence immediately to your prescriber.
- Do not take *benzodiazepines* with antacids because antacids decrease their absorption. Take these drugs 1 hour before or 2 hours after an antacid.
- If you are prescribed *alprazolam* (Xanax), *diazepam* (Valium), *midazolam* (Versed), *triazolam* (Halcion), or *buspirone* (BuSpar), avoid drinking grapefruit juice while taking these drugs because grapefruit juice slows their metabolism and causes increased blood concentration of these drugs, which can lead to overdose symptoms.

Common Side Effects
Antianxiety Drugs

Dizziness, Unsteadiness, Ataxia	Drowsiness, Fatigue
Headache	Impotence, Decreased libido

⭐ Critical Point for Safety

Patients should **not** stop taking benzodiazepine drugs suddenly because of the risk for life-threatening withdrawal symptoms, including nervousness, restlessness, tremulousness, weakness, and seizures.

QSEN: Safety

⚠ Drug Alert

Teaching Alert

Teach patients to avoid using alcohol, sleeping pills, or prescription pain drugs while taking antianxiety drugs.

QSEN: Safety

⚠ Drug Alert

Teaching Alert

Teach patients to take *benzodiazepines* exactly as prescribed to decrease the risk of developing dependence on these drugs.

QSEN: Safety

⚠ Drug Alert

Teaching Alert

Teach patients that the signs of dependence on benzodiazepines include:
- Strong desire or need to continue taking the drug
- Need to increase the dose to feel the effects of the drug
- Withdrawal effects after the drug is stopped (e.g., irritability, nervousness, trouble sleeping, abdominal cramps, trembling, or shaking)

QSEN: Safety

⚠ Drug Alert

Teaching Alert

Teach patients taking a benzodiazepine to take the drug 1 hr before or 2 hr after an antacid.

QSEN: Safety

Drug Alert

Teaching Alert

Teach patients who take alprazolam, diazepam, midazolam, triazolam, or buspirone to avoid drinking grapefruit juice.

QSEN: Safety

Critical Point for Safety

Benzodiazepines should not be used during pregnancy because the fetus can become dependent on these drugs and experience withdrawal symptoms after birth.

QSEN: Safety

Drug Alert

Teaching Alert

Teach family members to watch for and report changes in cognition or decreased mental alertness in older adults taking antianxiety drugs.

QSEN: Safety

Memory Jogger

Psychotic disorder symptoms include delusions, illusions, and hallucinations.

• Do not use over-the-counter herbal products or supplements unless approved by your prescriber. Always consult with your prescriber before taking any over-the-counter drugs.

Life Span Considerations for Antianxiety Drugs

Pediatric considerations. Children are more sensitive to the effects of benzodiazepines and more likely to experience side effects. Using clonazepam (Klonopin) during childhood may cause decreased mental and physical growth. Clonazepam should not be used in children younger than 18 years with panic disorders because safety and effectiveness have not been established.

Considerations for pregnancy and lactation. Benzodiazepines have a high likelihood of increasing the risk for birth defects or fetal harm and should not be used during pregnancy. Chlordiazepoxide (Librium) and diazepam have caused birth defects when used during the first trimester of pregnancy. The use of benzodiazepines during later pregnancy causes the fetus to become dependent on these drugs and can cause withdrawal symptoms after birth. These drugs should not be taken when a woman is breastfeeding because they can cause drowsiness, difficulty with feeding, and weight loss in the infant. Physical dependence and withdrawal symptoms may also occur in breastfed infants.

SSRI drugs should not be used during pregnancy because they have been linked to increased risk for premature births, stillbirths, birth defects, and miscarriage. *Hydroxyzine* is also avoided because it may cause birth defects.

Considerations for older adults. Older adults are more sensitive to the effects of benzodiazepines and are more at risk for side effects. Older adults should be monitored for respiratory depression. Benzodiazepines may cause daytime drowsiness, falls, and injuries. Teach older adults to change positions slowly and to use handrails when going up or down stairs. Instruct family members to assess older adults who are taking benzodiazepines for changes in cognition or reduced mental alertness. Low doses of benzodiazepines should be used with these patients because they are more sensitive to the effects and side effects of these drugs. Drowsiness may be much more intense in older adults. Instruct them not to drive or use dangerous equipment until they know how the drug will affect them. Chlordiazepoxide and clorazepate (Tranxene) are not recommended for older adults because they have a long half-life. Buspirone should be started at 5 mg twice a day for these patients.

REVIEW OF RELATED PHYSIOLOGY AND PATHOPHYSIOLOGY OF PSYCHOSIS

Psychosis is defined as a severe mental disorder in which thought and emotions are so impaired that contact is lost with external reality. It includes a loss of contact with reality, which may be brief or long term. Common symptoms of psychosis include *delusions* (false ideas about what is occurring or personal identity), *illusions* (mistaken perceptions), and *hallucinations* (seeing or hearing things that are not there). An example of a delusion is when a person exaggerates his or her sense of self-importance and is convinced that he or she has special powers, talents, or abilities. The person may believe that he or she is a famous movie star or a saint. An example of an illusion is when a person thinks that he or she hears voices in the wind. The most common type of hallucination is hearing imaginary voices (*auditory hallucination*) that give commands, make comments, or warn of impending danger. A visual hallucination occurs when a person sees something that is not there, such as a bright light, a shape, or a human figure. A person who is experiencing a psychotic episode may be unaware that anything is wrong and unable to ask for help. Other symptoms of psychosis are listed in Box 25.5.

Box 25.5 Symptoms of Psychosis

- Confusion
- Depression and sometimes suicidal thoughts
- Disorganized thoughts or speech
- Emotion exhibited in an abnormal manner
- Extreme excitement (mania)

- False beliefs (delusions)
- Loss of touch with reality
- Mistaken perceptions (illusions)
- Seeing, hearing, feeling, or perceiving things that are not there (hallucinations)
- Unfounded fears or suspicions

Box 25.6 Potential Causes of Psychosis

- Alcohol and other drugs
- Bipolar disorders (manic depression)
- Brain tumors
- Dementia (Alzheimer's and other degenerative brain disorders)

- Epilepsy
- Psychotic depression
- Schizophrenia
- Stroke

While the exact cause of psychotic disorders is not known, the pathophysiology of psychosis involves an interaction between extrinsic, drug-related, and intrinsic, disease-related components such as neurochemicals (e.g., dopamine, serotonin, acetylcholine) and structural abnormalities, visual processing deficits, sleep dysregulation, and genetics (schizophrenia tends to run in families). These disorders may develop because the brain overreacts to neurotransmitters (substances that carry messages between nerves) in the brain. It is believed that dopamine plays an important role in psychosis. Dopamine is a neurotransmitter, one of many chemicals that the brain uses to transmit information from brain cell to brain cell. Psychosis may be caused by a variety of medical or psychiatric problems. Box 25.6 lists potential causes of psychosis.

Treatment of psychosis can be complex and includes psychologic therapies such as counseling, guided discussion, and cognitive behavior therapy to help change or eliminate unwanted thoughts or beliefs. Antipsychotic drugs are important in the treatment of psychosis because they help to decrease auditory hallucinations and delusions and stabilize thinking and behavior. Hospital care may be needed to ensure patients safety because people with psychosis may harm themselves or others. Many symptoms of psychosis can be better controlled with long-term treatment.

TYPES OF PSYCHOSIS

The most common psychotic disorder is *schizophrenia* (Animation 25.3). This illness causes behavior changes, delusions, and hallucinations that last longer than 6 months and affect social interaction, school, and work.

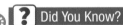 **?** Did You Know?

Schizophrenia is the most common type of psychotic disorder.

Schizoaffective disorder occurs when a person has symptoms of both schizophrenia and a mood disorder, such as depression or bipolar disorder. With *schizophreniform disorder* there are symptoms of schizophrenia, but the symptoms last for a shorter time: between 1 and 6 months. A *brief psychotic disorder* occurs when a person experiences a sudden, short period of psychotic behavior that is often in response to a very stressful event, such as a death in the family. Recovery is often quick, usually less than a month. With a *delusional disorder*, a person has a delusion (a false, fixed belief) involving a real-life situation that could be true but isn't, such as being followed, being plotted against, or having a disease. The delusion lasts for at least 1 month.

Psychoses may be *substance-induced* caused by the use of or withdrawal from drugs, such as hallucinogens and crack cocaine. These result in hallucinations, delusions, or confused speech. *Psychosis due to a medical condition* includes hallucinations, delusions, or other symptoms resulting from another illness that affects brain function, such as a head injury or tumor.

Memory Jogger

Antipsychotic drugs (major tranquilizers) are the drugs most commonly prescribed to treat psychosis. Most antipsychotic drugs work by causing CNS depression.

Critical Point for Safety

Antipsychotic drugs should never be used to restrain patients who wander, have insomnia, or are uncooperative.

QSEN: Safety

ANTIPSYCHOTIC DRUG THERAPIES

How Antipsychotic Drugs Work

Antipsychotic drugs, sometimes called *neuroleptics* or *major tranquilizers*, are prescribed to treat and control the symptoms of psychosis such as hallucinations, illusions, and delusions. These drugs produce a tranquilizing effect that helps to relax the CNS, allowing patients to function appropriately and effectively. They also control or reduce the symptoms of other psychiatric disorders that may lead to psychosis such as bipolar disorder. Antipsychotic drugs have a short-term sedative effect and a long-term effect of decreasing the risk of psychotic episodes. Most are available in oral forms (pills, capsules) and some are available in parenteral form (intravenous, intramuscular).

All antipsychotic drugs tend to block dopamine receptors in the dopamine pathways in the brain. The normal effect of releasing the neurotransmitter dopamine is decreased. The transmission of impulses is decreased, which in turn decreases the symptoms of hallucinations, illusions, and delusions.

Major tranquilizers are the most commonly prescribed drugs for psychosis. Another drug used to treat psychosis is *lithium carbonate* (Lithonate) used for mania.

Antipsychotic drugs are occasionally used to treat acute delirium. The danger of using these drugs includes prolonged or worsening agitation, especially when using older drugs such as *haloperidol* (Haldol). These drugs should no longer be prescribed for patients with dementia unless the patient is agitated, aggressive, or showing psychotic behavior that is distressing to patients or dangerous to others. Antipsychotic drugs should never be used at the whim of a caregiver for the sole purpose of sedation to restrain patients who wander, have insomnia, or do not cooperate.

Typical antipsychotic drugs (first generation [e.g., haloperidol, chlorpromazine]) are well known and continue to be useful in the treatment of severe psychoses especially when the newer drugs are not effective. The drawback of these drugs is the high risk of side effects or adverse effects. *Atypical antipsychotic drugs* (second generation [e.g., clozapine, olanzapine]) are less likely to result in side effects or adverse effects and unlikely to produce extrapyramidal effects such as tremors, paranoia, anxiety, and dystonia.

Generic names, trade names, and usual adult dosages of antipsychotic drugs are listed in the following table. Be sure to consult a reliable resource for additional information about any antipsychotic drug.

Dosages for Common Antipsychotic Drugs

Drug Group	Drug	Usual Adult Dosage
Typical Antipsychotic Drugs	chlorpromazine (Thorazine)	10 mg orally 3–4 times per day or 25 mg 2–3 times per day. Intramuscular: 25 mg
	fluphenazine (Prolixin)	2.5–10 mg/day orally, given in 2 or 3 divided doses (every 6 or 8 hr); may increase gradually as needed and tolerated. A therapeutic effect is achieved with less than 20 mg/day, given as divided doses every 6–8 hr. Usual max: 20 mg/day
	haloperidol (Haldol)	0.5–2 mg orally 2–3 times per day with moderate symptomatology or in debilitated patients. For severe, chronic, or refractory target symptoms, initiate with 3–5 mg given 2–3 times per day. Max: 100 mg/day
	loxapine (Loxitane)	10 mg orally twice daily. Titrate fairly rapidly during the first 7–10 days. For severe cases, initial dose of 50 mg/day may be necessary. Usual maintenance dose is 60–100 mg/day given as a single bedtime dose or divided doses twice daily. Max: 250 mg/day

Dosages for Common Antipsychotic Drugs—cont'd

Drug Group	Drug	Usual Adult Dosage
	molindone (Moban)	50–75 mg/day orally in 3 or 4 divided doses. May increase to 100 mg/day after 3 or 4 days depending on severity of symptoms. Max: 225 mg/day
	perphenazine (Trilafon)	4–8 mg orally 3 times per day. For hospitalized psychotic patients, 8–16 mg initially 2–4 times per day; avoid dosages greater than 64 mg/day **Special Considerations: After the dosage is stabilized, perphenazine may be given as a single bedtime dose or in 2 divided doses ($^1/_3$ in the morning and $^2/_3$ at bedtime) to improve compliance**
	thioridazine (Mellaril)	50–100 mg orally 3 times per day depending on the severity of symptoms. Titrate gradually to a total daily dose ranging from 200 to 800 mg/day based on response and tolerability. Max: 800 mg/day **Special Considerations: Used when patients fail to respond to other antipsychotic drugs**
	thiothixene (Navane)	2 mg orally 3 times daily or 5 mg twice daily. Single daily dose may be used. Usual optimal dosage is 20–30 mg/day given in divided doses. Doses up to 60 mg/day may be necessary for severe conditions
	trifluoperazine (Stelazine)	Initially 2–5 mg orally once or twice daily. Increase as needed. Usual dose range: 15–20 mg/day, but may require 40 mg/day or more
Atypical Antipsychotic Drugs	aripiprazole (Abilify)	10 mg–15 mg orally once daily. Max: 30 mg/day
	clozapine (Clozaril)	12.5 mg orally once or twice daily on the first day. After day 1, the dose may be titrated by 25–50 mg every day over 2 weeks, if well tolerated, to a dose of 300–450 mg/day, in divided doses. Max: 900 mg/day
	olanzapine (Zyprexa)	**Adults not at risk for hypotension:** 5–10 mg orally once daily initially, with a target dose of 10 mg/day within several days. Max: 20 mg/day **Adults at risk for hypotension:** 5 mg orally once daily; dose increases should be performed cautiously.
	quetiapine (Seroquel)	25 mg orally twice daily on day 1. Increase by 25–50 mg, on day 2 and day 3 to a target range of 300–400 mg/day in divided doses 2 or 3 times per day, by day 4. Further dosage adjustments in increments/decrements of 25–50 mg twice a day, at intervals of at least 2 days. Recommended maintenance dose range: 400–800 mg/day. Max: 800 mg/day
	risperidone (Risperdal)	2 mg/day orally given as a single dose or as 1 mg twice per day. Adjust dose at intervals of at least 24 hr and in increments of 1–2 mg/day. Effective range: 4–16 mg/day. Max: 16 mg/day

 Do Not Confuse

Clozaril *with* Colazal

An order for Clozaril may be confused with Colazal. Clozaril is an antipsychotic drug used to treat psychotic disorders, whereas Colazal is a GI antiinflammatory drug used to treat mild to moderate ulcerative colitis.

QSEN: Safety

 Do Not Confuse

Zyprexa *with* Celexa *or* Zyrtec

An order for Zyprexa may be confused with Celexa or Zyrtec. Zyprexa is used to treat psychotic disorders, whereas Celexa is an SSRI drug used to treat depression and Zyrtec is an antihistamine used to treat allergies.

QSEN: Safety

Continued

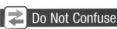
Do Not Confuse

chlorpromazine *with* **chlorpropamide**

An order for chlorpromazine may be confused with chlorpropamide. Chlorpromazine is an antipsychotic drug used to treat psychosis, whereas chlorpropamide is a sulfonylurea used to treat type 2 diabetes.

QSEN: Safety

Dosages for Common Antipsychotic Drugs—cont'd

Drug Group	Drug	Usual Adult Dosage
Other Drugs	ziprasidone (Geodon)	20 mg orally twice daily with food. Increase as needed at intervals of 2 days or more. Max: 80 mg twice per day
	lithium carbonate (Eskalith, Lithonate)	300–600 mg orally 3 times a day. Titrate dose by 300 mg every 3 days. Usual dosage range: 600 mg orally 2 or 3 times per day
	prochlorperazine (Compazine, Compro)	For schizophrenia: Outpatient: 5–10 mg orally 3–4 times per day Inpatient: 10 mg orally 3–4 times per day; 10–20 mg IM initially; may repeat every 1–4 hr as needed

Intended Responses of Antipsychotic Drugs
- Signs and symptoms of psychosis, including hallucinations, illusions, and delusions, are decreased.
- Behavior is improved (or there is less antisocial behavior).
- Schizophrenic behavior is decreased.
- Suicidal thoughts and behaviors are decreased.

Common Side Effects of Antipsychotic Drugs
Early in treatment, common side effects of antipsychotic drugs related to CNS depression may include sedation and drowsiness, dizziness when changing positions, lethargy, restlessness, insomnia, and GI upset (e.g., nausea, vomiting, and diarrhea). Other side effects include agitation, headache, hypotension, tachycardia, muscle spasms, tremor, weakness, dry mouth, dry eyes, blurred vision, weight gain, photosensitivity, and constipation.

Possible Adverse Effects of Antipsychotic Drugs
Several life-threatening adverse effects can occur with antipsychotic drugs. *Tardive dyskinesia* (Figure 25.6), a disorder characterized by involuntary movements (extrapyramidal symptoms) most often affecting the mouth, lips, and tongue and sometimes the trunk or other parts of the body such as arms and legs, can be caused by antipsychotics. However, this adverse effect is much more common with typical (first-generation) drugs. Several drugs sometimes cause seizures, including clozapine, haloperidol, olanzapine, quetiapine, and lithium.

Neuroleptic malignant syndrome is a rare, potentially life-threatening disorder involving dysfunction of the autonomic nervous system. The autonomic nervous system is the branch of the nervous system responsible for regulating such involuntary actions as heart rate, blood pressure, digestion, and sweating. Muscle tone becomes

Common Side Effects

Antipsychotic Drugs

Dizziness

Insomnia

Drowsiness/Sedation

GI upset, Nausea/Vomiting, Diarrhea

Hand tremors

Photosensitivity

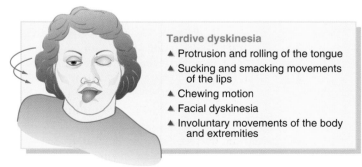

Tardive dyskinesia
- Protrusion and rolling of the tongue
- Sucking and smacking movements of the lips
- Chewing motion
- Facial dyskinesia
- Involuntary movements of the body and extremities

FIG. 25.6 Tardive dyskinesia symptoms. (Modified from McCuistion, L. E., Yeager, J. J., Winton, M. B., & DiMaggio, K. [2023]. *Pharmacology: A patient-centered nursing process approach* [11th ed.]. St. Louis: Elsevier.)

rigid with tremors, body temperature and respiratory rate are markedly elevated, heart rate is tachycardic, blood pressure may be elevated or decreased, and consciousness is also severely affected. All antipsychotic drugs can cause this syndrome.

Neutropenia (decreased white blood cells) can result from taking clozapine or prochlorperazine. Clozapine can also cause myocarditis (inflammation of the heart muscle).

Quetiapine (Seroquel) and risperidone (Risperdal) cause an increased risk of death in older adults with dementia.

Lithium toxicity (overdose) can occur if a patient receives too much of the drug. Symptoms of lithium toxicity include severe nausea and vomiting, severe hand tremors, confusion, and vision changes.

⭐ Priority Actions to Take *Before* Giving Antipsychotic Drugs
In addition to the general responsibilities related to drugs for psychiatric problems (p. 457), monitor fluid intake and urine output. Obtain a baseline weight.

Assess baseline level of psychosis. Check orientation, mood, and behavior. Be sure to observe that patients swallow these drugs. Ask about suicidal thoughts or plans.

Ask patients about smoking because smoking may decrease the effectiveness of olanzapine and clozapine.

⭐ Priority Actions to Take *After* Giving Antipsychotic Drugs
In addition to the general responsibilities related to drugs for psychiatric problems (p. 457), monitor intake and output and daily weight. Monitor bowel function. Report constipation to the prescriber and encourage the patient to drink extra fluids.

Reassess the patient's mental status, monitoring orientation, mood, and behavior for changes. Watch for sedation, side effects, and adverse effects. Continue to monitor for suicidal thoughts.

Give antipsychotic drugs with food if the patient develops GI upset symptoms.

⭐ Teaching Priorities for Patients Taking Antipsychotic Drugs
In addition to the general responsibilities related to drugs for psychiatric problems (p. 457), include these teaching points and precautions:
- Your prescriber may start with a low dose and gradually increase it to achieve therapeutic effects.
- Immediately report side effects and adverse effects of these drugs to your prescriber if any of these symptoms occur.
- Immediately report sore throat, unusual bleeding or bruising, rash, or tremors to your prescriber.
- Your prescriber may instruct you about the importance of psychotherapy and may recommend this along with the prescribed drugs to help keep your psychosis under control.
- Avoid alcohol and other CNS depressants while taking these drugs.
- Monitor your bowel function and increase activity, fluid intake, and fiber-containing foods to prevent constipation.
- Take your drugs at least 2 hours apart from antacids to prevent decreased absorption.
- Take your drugs with food if GI upset occurs.
- Some of these drugs may cause urine to be abnormally colored (e.g., prochlorperazine may turn urine pink or reddish-brown).
- Wear protective clothing, hats, and sunscreens when outdoors to protect against severe sunburn, which is a common side effect of these drugs.
- Use frequent mouth rinses and good oral care to help minimize the side effect of dry mouth.
- If you are prescribed quetiapine (Seroquel), avoid temperature extremes because this drug impairs body temperature regulation.
- If you are prescribed quetiapine (Seroquel) or olanzapine (Zyprexa), avoid grapefruit and grapefruit juice during therapy. Grapefruit can interfere with the

Action/Intervention Alert

Before giving an antipsychotic, be sure to ask the patient about suicidal thoughts and initiate suicide precautions if needed.

QSEN: Safety

Action/Intervention Alert

Encourage patients taking antipsychotic drugs to drink extra fluids to prevent constipation.

QSEN: Safety

Action/Intervention Alert

Discuss with patients the importance of psychotherapy in addition to antipsychotic drug therapy to help keep their psychosis under control.

QSEN: Safety

Teaching Alert

Tell patients taking prochlorperazine (Compazine, Compro) that it may turn their urine pink or reddish-brown.

QSEN: Safety

Critical Point for Safety

Instruct patients taking quetiapine (Seroquel) to avoid temperature extremes because this drug impairs body temperature regulation.

QSEN: Safety

Drug Alert

Teaching Alert

Instruct patients taking lithium carbonate to have a blood level drawn 4–7 days after beginning to take the drug, and once a month thereafter. Teach the symptoms of lithium toxicity (severe nausea and vomiting, severe hand tremors, confusion, and vision changes) and instruct that they notify the prescriber immediately if the lithium level is high (above 1.2 mEq/L) or these symptoms occur.

QSEN: Safety

Drug Alert

Teaching Alert

To prevent falls, teach older adults to change positions slowly while taking chlorpromazine (Thorazine) because it can cause a rapid drop in blood pressure.

QSEN: Safety

metabolism of the drug, causing increased blood levels and increased risk for side effects or adverse effects.

- If you are prescribed lithium, your blood serum lithium level should be checked between 4 and 7 days following initiation of the drug and then once a month. Blood levels of this drug can become too high. If severe nausea and vomiting, severe hand tremors, confusion, and vision changes develop, contact your prescriber immediately.

Life Span Considerations for Antipsychotic Drugs

Pediatric considerations. Side effects and adverse effects are more likely in children because they are more sensitive to the effects of these drugs.

Considerations for pregnancy and lactation. Drugs for psychosis have a moderate risk of the increased likelihood for birth defects or fetal harm and should be avoided during pregnancy. These drugs may cross the placenta and cause unwanted side effects such as involuntary movements in the newborn infant. These drugs should not be taken during breastfeeding. Lithium has a high risk of the increased likelihood for birth defects or fetal harm and should be avoided during pregnancy and breastfeeding.

Considerations for older adults. Side effects and adverse effects are more likely in older adults because they are more sensitive to the effects of these drugs. They should start with lower doses of all antipsychotic drugs. Older adults with renal insufficiency should also be started with lower doses.

Most antipsychotic drugs, especially *chlorpromazine* (Thorazine), can cause a rapid fall in blood pressure when changing from a sitting to a standing position (orthostatic hypotension). Teach older adults to change positions slowly and to sit on the edge of the bed for a few moments before standing. Remind them to always use handrails when going up or down stairs.

Lithium can cause excessive urination and quickly lead to dehydration, especially in older adults. Remind older adults to drink daily about the same amount of fluid they lose in urination. Also, remind them to notify the prescriber if they are too nauseated and cannot take in as much fluid as they should.

Get Ready for the NCLEX® Examination!

Key Points

- Psychiatric disorders can include affective or emotional instability, behavioral problems, and cognitive dysfunction or impairment.
- Mental illness can be caused by biologic or psychologic factors.
- Drug therapy is extremely important in the management of many psychiatric problems.
- Depression can be mistaken as part of the aging process, and many older adults go undiagnosed and untreated.
- Many people with depression do not seek treatment because they do not recognize that it is a treatable illness.
- Patients taking an antidepressant that causes drowsiness should avoid alcohol because it can increase the drowsiness.
- When a patient with depression has suicidal thoughts and a suicide plan, hospitalization may be required for the patient's safety.
- The two most common groups of drugs prescribed to treat depression are SSRIs and TCAs.

- Assess for and immediately report any suicidal thoughts or suicide plans to the prescriber.
- Be sure to ask a patient about the use of St. John's wort, an herbal product used to treat depression. It should not be taken with antidepressant drugs because it might increase the risk of the accumulation of high levels of serotonin in your body.
- Any SR or XL antipsychotic drugs should be swallowed whole and never chewed, divided, or crushed.
- Ask patients taking a TCA drug for depression about smoking because smoking cigarettes may decrease the effectiveness of these drugs.
- Teach patients who are taking any antidepressant that it may take 2 to 8 weeks before symptoms of depression improve.
- Instruct patients to **never** stop taking an antidepressant without first talking to their prescriber.
- Monitor children and adolescents carefully because antidepressant drugs may increase the risk of suicidal thoughts or actions.
- The common anxiety disorders include panic disorder, GAD, phobic disorder, OCD, and PTSD.

- Monitor patients taking antianxiety drugs for signs of dependence because many of these drugs, especially benzodiazepines, are likely to cause dependence when taken for a long time.
- Teach patients that it may take SSRI drugs 3 to 5 weeks to control anxiety.
- Physical reactions such as increased heart rate, sweating, trembling, fatigue, and weakness often occur with anxiety.
- Beta blockers, which are usually prescribed for hypertension, are sometimes prescribed for patients facing anxiety-producing events such as performing on stage or making a speech.
- Patients should **not** stop taking benzodiazepine drugs suddenly because of the risk for life-threatening withdrawal symptoms, including nervousness, restlessness, tremulousness, weakness, and seizures.
- Teach patients to avoid using alcohol, sleeping pills, or prescription pain drugs while taking antianxiety drugs.
- Teach patients to take benzodiazepines exactly as prescribed to decrease the risk of developing dependence on these drugs.
- Teach patients that the signs of dependence on benzodiazepines include:
  - Strong desire or need to continue taking the drug
  - Need to increase the dose to feel the effects of the drug
  - Withdrawal effects after the drug is stopped (e.g., irritability, nervousness, trouble sleeping, abdominal cramps, trembling, or shaking)
- Teach patients taking a benzodiazepine to take the drug 1 hour before or 2 hours after an antacid.
- Teach patients who take alprazolam, diazepam, midazolam, triazolam, or buspirone to avoid drinking grapefruit juice.
- Benzodiazepines should not be used during pregnancy because the fetus can become dependent on these drugs and experience withdrawal symptoms after birth.
- Teach family members to watch for and report changes in cognition or decreased mental alertness in older adults taking antianxiety drugs.
- Psychotic disorder symptoms include delusions, illusions, and hallucinations.

- A person experiencing a psychotic disorder may be unaware that anything is wrong and unable to ask for help.
- It may take up to 8 weeks for improvement of depression symptoms after an antidepressant drug is prescribed.
- Be sure to ask a patient with a mental disorder about suicidal thoughts or plans and report these immediately to the prescriber because hospitalization with suicide precautions may be necessary.
- Most antipsychotic drugs work by causing CNS depression.
- Antipsychotic drugs should never be used to restrain patients who wander, have insomnia, or are uncooperative.
- Encourage patients taking antipsychotic drugs to drink extra fluids to prevent constipation.
- Instruct patients not to stop taking these drugs without talking with their prescriber.
- Assess a patient with an anxiety disorder for physical signs such as changes in blood pressure, heart rate, and respiratory rate.
- Tell patients taking prochlorperazine (Compazine, Compro) that it may turn their urine pink or reddish-brown.
- Instruct patients taking quetiapine (Seroquel) to avoid temperature extremes because this drug impairs body temperature regulation.
- Instruct patients taking lithium carbonate to have a blood level drawn 4 to 7 days after beginning to take the drug, and once a month thereafter.
- Teach patients taking benzodiazepines to take the drugs exactly as prescribed to decrease the risk of developing drug dependence.
- To prevent falls, teach older adults to change positions slowly while taking chlorpromazine (Thorazine) because it can cause a rapid drop in blood pressure.

Additional Learning Resources

Be sure to visit your Evolve website (http://evolve.elsevier.com/Workman/pharmacology/) for additional online resources.

SG Go to your Study Guide for additional learning activities to help you master this chapter content.

Review Questions

See *Answers to In-Text Review Questions* in the back of the book for answers to these questions.

1. Which statement about depression is true?
   A. Depression does not affect the way a person interacts with others.
   B. Men are twice as likely to experience depression as women.
   C. Many older adults with depression are undiagnosed and untreated.
   D. Women are less likely than men to seek treatment for depression.

2. Which characteristic is typical of bipolar disorder?
   A. Severe highs and severe lows
   B. Increased risk for suicide
   C. Persistently low moods
   D. Lack of pleasure in life

3. A patient who was prescribed citalopram 1 week ago for depression reports feeling no different now from 1 week ago and wants to stop taking the drug. What is the nurse's best response?
   A. "Treatment for depression is highly individual and this may not be the right drug for you."
   B. "Most drugs for depression take at least 2 weeks to start making you feel better."
   C. "Are you certain that you are taking the drug exactly the way it was prescribed?"
   D. "Be sure to stop smoking because cigarette smoking inactivates this drug."

4. A patient is prescribed bupropion (Wellbutrin SR) 100 mg twice daily. It is time for the second dose today, and the drug sent from the pharmacy is Wellbutrin 100 XL. What is the nurse's **best** action?
   A. Administering the Wellbutrin XL tablet in place of the Wellbutrin SR tablet

B. Cutting the Wellbutrin XL tablet in half and then giving the dose

C. Calling the pharmacy and obtaining a Wellbutrin SR 100 mg tablet

D. Holding the dose and notifying the prescriber immediately

5. A patient who has been prescribed prochlorperazine calls the clinic and reports pink-tinged urine. What is the nurse's **best** action?

A. Asking the patient whether grapefruit or grapefruit juice has been ingested within the last 24 hours.

B. Reminding the patient to drink more water to prevent this drug from damaging the kidneys.

C. Reassuring the patient that this is an expected side effect of the drug and needs no action.

D. Instructing the patient to hold the next drug dose and notify the prescriber immediately.

6. Which assessment is **most important** for the nurse to measure or perform before administering the first dose of amitriptyline to a patient?

A. Heart rate and rhythm

B. Core body temperature

C. Level of consciousness

D. Blood pressure in the sitting position

7. The parents of a 12-year-old who was prescribed fluoxetine inform the nurse that their child is having trouble sleeping. What is the nurse's **best** response?

A. "This is a normal expected side effect of fluoxetine."

B. "We may need to ask the prescriber to order something to help your child sleep."

C. "Children are more sensitive to the effects of this drug and may need a lower dose."

D. "Before bedtime be sure that your child does not eat or drink anything with caffeine."

8. Although serotonin reuptake inhibitors (SSRIs) are used more commonly now to treat anxiety disorders than are benzodiazepines, for which patient situation does the nurse expect a benzodiazepine to be prescribed instead of an SSRI?

A. The patient is 18 years old.

B. Anxiety has been present daily for 6 months.

C. The patient has compulsive repetitive actions.

D. The anxiety attack is severe with hallucinations.

9. What is the advantage of treating a patient with anxiety with a benzodiazepine drug rather than a selective serotonin reuptake inhibitor (SSRI)?

A. Benzodiazepines are not likely to cause patient dependence when used for an extended period of time.

B. Benzodiazepines have milder side effects and almost no adverse effects when compared with SSRIs.

C. Benzodiazepines control anxiety and allow patients to live a relatively normal lifestyle.

D. Benzodiazepines act to treat anxiety within 20 minutes and can be given on an as-needed basis.

10. A patient asks the nurse why the prescriber is changing his anxiety medication from lorazepam to sertraline. What is the nurse's **best response?**

A. "Sertraline is a stronger drug and will do a better job of controlling your anxiety."

B. "Sertraline has milder side effects and a decreased risk for drug dependence."

C. "Sertraline acts much faster to get the symptoms of your anxiety under control."

D. "Sertraline can be taken only when needed to control symptoms of anxiety."

11. How do the major antipsychotic drugs exert their effects to reduce psychotic episodes?

A. Blocking dopamine receptors and reducing neuronal impulse transmission

B. Redirecting nerve impulses away from excitatory areas of the brain and into brain inhibitory areas

C. Enhancing the breakdown of excitatory neurotransmitter chemicals so that impulse transmission is slower

D. Blocking the reuptake of neurotransmitters so that the concentration of these chemicals is increased in the brain

12. Four hours after receiving risperidone, the patient on the psychiatric unit has a temperature elevation of 2°F. What is the nurse's **best** action?

A. Administering the next dose of the drug as prescribed

B. Assessing the patient for other signs and symptoms of infection

C. Holding the next drug dose and notifying the prescriber immediately

D. Attempting to arouse the patient from sleep by gently shaking his or her arm

Clinical Judgment

1. A patient with anxiety is prescribed oxazepam. What safety measures must the nurse include in this patient's plan of care? **Select all that apply.**

A. Call for help when getting out of bed.

B. Use a walker for ambulation.

C. Assess gait for steadiness.

D. Limit fluid intake to 1.5 L/day.

E. Have the patient report any side effects to the prescriber.

F. Change positions slowly.

G. Consult with physical therapy to measure for a cane.

H. Take two tablets whenever a dose is missed.

I. Teach about signs of dependency.

2. The nurse is providing care for a 38-year-old patient who is a fireman. He states that he often thinks about his experiences on the job and also has nightmares about burning buildings and being unable to save victims of fires. He describes feelings of irritability on the job and at home with his family. He tells the nurse that he often has difficulty concentrating, and also has difficulty falling asleep at night. He has experienced these symptoms for the past 3 years, and his health care provider diagnosed him with posttraumatic stress distress (PTDS) and prescribed paroxetine. His past medical history includes hypertension for which he is prescribed metoprolol, 100 mg orally once a day. **Place an X in the box to indicate whether each nursing action is Appropriate or Not Appropriate for this patient at this time.**

NURSING ACTION	APPROPRIATE	NOT APPROPRIATE
Suggesting that a better choice for long-term treatment would be a benzodiazepine drug such as diazepam		
Discussing the benefits of cognitive behavioral therapy (CBT) with the patient		
Recommending relaxation techniques such as meditation, deep breathing, massage, or yoga		
Asking the patient if he believes he can cope with his PTSD at home		
Discussing proper nutrition and diet with the patient because taking paroxetine can lead to weight gain		
Reminding the patient that his prescriber will want to follow him closely while he is taking this drug		

Drug Therapy for Insomnia

Learning Objectives

The content presented in this chapter should help you to:

1. Describe the names, actions, usual adult dosages, possible side effects, and adverse effects of drugs for insomnia.
2. Discuss the priority actions to take *before* and *after* giving drugs for insomnia.
3. Prioritize essential information to teach patients taking drugs for insomnia.
4. Discuss life span considerations for drugs for insomnia.

Key Terms

barbiturates (bär-BĬ-chŭrets) (p. 484) A class of drugs formed from barbituric acid that induce a general depression over all central nervous system functions and induce sedation.

benzodiazepine receptor agonists (běn-zō-dī-ĂZ-ĕ-pēnz rē SĔP-tŭrz ĂG-ō-nĭsts) (p. 484) A class of non-benzodiazepine sedative-hypnotics that interact with the same receptor site that benzodiazepine drugs do, turning on the receptors to induce sleep.

benzodiazepines (běn-zō-dī-ĂZ-ĕ-pēnz) (p. 484) A class of drugs that depress the central nervous system by binding to gamma-aminobutyric acid (GABA) receptors, resulting in hypnotic and sedating effects. They are used mainly to control symptoms of anxiety or stress.

sedatives (SĔD-ĕ-t«êvz) (p. 484) Drugs that promote sleep by targeting signals in the brain to produce calm and ease agitation.

REVIEW OF RELATED PHYSIOLOGY AND PATHOPHYSIOLOGY OF INSOMNIA

Insomnia is the inability to go to sleep or remain asleep throughout the night. It is the most common sleep problem. Most people experience acute, short-term insomnia at some time during their lives. It may occur in people at any age. Insomnia is considered to be chronic if a person has trouble falling asleep or staying asleep at least three nights a week for 3 months or longer.

Sleep is a natural and necessary periodic state of rest for the mind and body. When sleep occurs, the body rests and restores energy levels. Sleep helps a person recover from illness, cope with stress, and solve problems. During sleep, consciousness is partially or completely lost, the eyes close, body movements decrease, metabolism slows, and responsiveness to external stimuli declines. Normal sleep and wake states are generated by a complex neuronal network in the brain and are regulated by homeostatic and circadian mechanisms. Sleep may be divided into two main stages: rapid eye movement (REM) and non-REM (NREM) sleep.

Insomnia is considered to be a disorder of excessive activation of the arousal systems of the brain (e.g., hyperarousal). Hyperarousal in the physiologic, emotional, or cognitive networks is believed to prevent sleep regulatory processes from naturally occurring in people with insomnia. The neurotransmitter associated with insomnia is gamma-aminobutyric acid (GABA). GABA is the most common *inhibitory* transmitter in the brain. It is sometimes called the brain's "brake fluid." GABA decreases or stops the transmission of nerve impulses, allowing for sleep. A research study showed that GABA levels were reduced by 30% in adults with chronic insomnia. Symptoms of insomnia include difficulty falling asleep, waking often during the night or early morning, and not feeling rested after sleep.

Failing to get enough sleep because of insomnia causes *sleep deprivation*, which is a shortage of quality, undisturbed sleep that reduces physical and mental well-being. Coordination, judgment, reaction time, and social function are all impaired by lack of sleep. Drowsiness interferes with the ability of the brain to concentrate, learn, and

 Memory Jogger

Sleep is divided into two main stages—rapid eye movement (REM) and non–rapid eye movement (non-REM).

remember. Simple tasks seem more difficult to perform, and complex tasks may seem impossible to complete. People become anxious, moody, and impatient and have increased difficulty interacting with others.

Signs of sleep deprivation include falling asleep at the wheel while driving, watching television, or reading a book; sleeping for extra-long periods; difficulty waking in the morning; irritability during the day; and falling asleep during quiet times of the day. Sleep deprivation may be short term or long term.

Common causes of insomnia include stress, an irregular sleep schedule, poor sleeping habits, mental health disorders like anxiety and depression, physical illnesses and pain, medications, neurological problems, and specific sleep disorders (Figure 26.1). Treatment of insomnia includes cognitive therapy and drugs. Box 26.1 lists tips for coping with insomnia. Cognitive behavioral therapy for insomnia can help to control or eliminate negative thoughts and actions that keep a person awake and is generally recommended as the first line of treatment for people with insomnia.

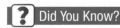 **Did You Know?**

Sleep deprivation decreases immune function and increases the risk for infection.

Long-distance travel

Heavy meals

Alcohol, smoking, or caffeine

Uncomfortable bed or pillow

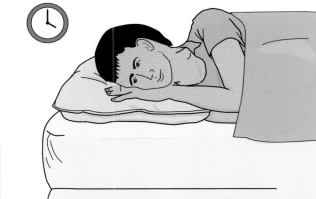

Blue light (e.g., TVs, smartphones)

Medications

Stress

Environmental factors

FIG. 26.1 Causes of insomnia.

| Box **26.1** | **Techniques for Coping with Insomnia** |

1. Wake up and go to bed at the same time, even on weekends.
2. Make your bedroom into a dark, quiet, cool sanctuary
3. Be physically active with regular exercise.
4. Avoid using stimulants (e.g., caffeine) at night.
5. Avoid taking frequent naps during the day.
6. Reserve your bed for sleep and sex.
7. Avoid blue light (e.g., shut off television, smartphones) 30 min before bedtime.
8. Avoid eating large meals close to bedtime.
9. Learn to relax by practicing yoga or meditation, listening to soothing music, or reading a good book.
10. Perform deep breathing.
11. Consider cognitive or massage therapy.
12. Release daily worries before sleeping.

TYPES OF DRUGS FOR INSOMNIA

HOW DRUGS FOR INSOMNIA WORK

The most commonly prescribed sleep drugs are sedatives, a broad group of drugs that promote sleep by decreasing signals in the central nervous system (CNS), which then produces calm and eases agitation. Sedatives include benzodiazepine receptor agonists, benzodiazepines, antihistamines, sedating antidepressants, and skeletal muscle relaxants. Melatonin, a natural hormone that helps with sleep, can also be taken as a supplement for insomnia.

Benzodiazepine receptor agonists, also called non-benzodiazepine sedative-hypnotics or Z-drugs (because many generic names start with the letter z), are a class of drugs that interact with the same receptor site as benzodiazepine drugs, turning on the receptors to induce sleep. Drugs from this class are now the first-line sleep aids to treat insomnia. They are less likely to be addictive but must be carefully monitored by the prescriber because of the possibility of misuse. These drugs have a very rapid onset of action (15 to 30 minutes).

Benzodiazepines are drugs that depress the central nervous system (CNS) by binding to gamma aminobutyric acid (GABA) receptors, resulting in hypnotic and sedating effects. GABA is an inhibitory rather than an excitatory neurotransmitter in the brain. When increased amounts of GABA are present or GABA receptors are stimulated, CNS activity is reduced. Although benzodiazepines are mainly used to treat anxiety or stress, a few are used as a short-term treatment of insomnia. They can be habit forming when used for prolonged periods of time (more than 2 to 4 weeks) and are no longer the first-line drugs for insomnia.

Older drugs rarely, but occasionally still used to treat insomnia for short time periods are the barbiturate-based drugs. Barbiturates are drugs formed from barbituric acid that induce a general depression over all CNS functions along with inducing sedation. Both motor and sensory functions are inhibited, and the seizure threshold is elevated. Barbiturates may be prescribed short-term when other drugs for insomnia have not been successful. If they are used regularly (e.g., every day) for insomnia, they are usually not effective for longer than 2 weeks. Most barbiturates, including those used for sleep, are categorized as Schedule II controlled substances with a high potential for abuse and dependence. In addition, because all CNS functions are depressed, overdoses with the barbiturates are serious and can lead to death. These drugs are more commonly used to induce sedation and reduce anxiety before surgery. Some are used as part of seizure control management with epilepsy.

Antihistamines are drugs used to treat allergies and allergic reactions. Some, such as diphenhydramine (Benadryl), have sedating effects and are available over the counter. See Chapter 10 for a complete discussion of the actions and uses of antihistamine drugs, as well as the responsibilities.

Sedating antidepressants also have some effect on insomnia, especially trazodone, amitriptyline, and doxepin. When used for insomnia, antidepressant drug doses are lower than those used to treat depression. See Chapter 25 for a complete discussion of the action and uses of antidepressants as well as the responsibilities.

Skeletal muscle relaxants are another group of drugs that are used at times for insomnia. The most common ones used for this purpose are the carbamates and the cyclobenzaprines. Both of these drug groups work by depressing the CNS and producing significant sedation. A more complete discussion of the actions, dosages, responsibilities, and side effects of these drugs is presented in Chapter 9.

Melatonin is a naturally occurring hormone in the body that helps promote **sleep.** Because of its calming and sedating effects, it is also called the "sleep hormone." It regulates the sleep-wake cycle by chemically causing drowsiness and lowering the body temperature. As an over-the-counter supplement, it is often used for the short-term treatment of insomnia.

Generic names, brand names, and adult dosages of the most commonly prescribed drugs for insomnia are listed in the following table. Be sure to consult a reliable drug resource for information about less commonly prescribed drugs for insomnia.

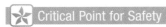 **Critical Point for Safety**

The barbiturate drugs (pentobarbital and secobarbital) are rarely used for insomnia because they are classified as Schedule II controlled substances with a high potential for abuse and addiction.

QSEN: Safety

Dosages for Commonly Used Drugs for Insomnia

Drug Class	Drug	Dosage
Benzodiazepine Receptor Agonists (Z-Drugs)	eszopiclone (Lunesta)	1 mg orally immediately before bedtime, and with at least 7–8 hr remaining before the planned time of awakening. May increase to 2–3 mg if needed. Max: 3 mg/day
	zaleplon (Sonata)	10 mg orally at bedtime. May take either at bedtime or after an attempt to fall asleep without medication, provided at least 4 or more hours of sleep time remain. Max: 20 mg/day For short-term use: 7–10 days
	zolpidem (Ambien, Edluar)	Female: 5 mg orally immediately before bedtime and with at least 7–8 hr remaining before the planned time of awakening Male: 5–10 mg orally immediately before bedtime with 7–8 hr before planned time of awakening. Sublingual dose (Edluar) same as oral dosage. Max: 10 mg/day
	zopiclone (Imovane)	3.75–7.5 mg orally before bedtime. It takes about 1 hr to work ***Special considerations:* Use of this drug is controversial because of potential for abuse and addiction. Use is short term**
Benzodiazepines	estazolam (ProSom)	1 mg orally at bedtime. Max: 2 mg/day. Used for insomnia in adults and with generalized anxiety disorder (GAD)
	flurazepam (Dalmane)	15–30 mg orally at bedtime. Max: 30 mg at bedtime. Has been demonstrated to be effective for 28 consecutive nights
	quazepam (Doral)	7.5–15 mg orally once daily at bedtime. Max: 15 mg/day
	temazepam (Restoril)	Usual dose: 15 mg orally once daily 30 min before bedtime, may increase to 30 mg. Max: 30 mg/day
	triazolam (Halcion)	0.25 mg orally at bedtime is the usual dose. May decrease to 0.125 mg. Max: 0.5 mg/day With 0.5-mg dose, there is increased risk of adverse reactions
Antihistamines	diphenhydramine (Benadryl)	12.5–50 mg orally at bedtime as needed
Herbal Supplement	melatonin	0.3–12 mg orally 30 min to 1 hr before bedtime as needed. Max: 12 mg/day 0.5–12 mg sublingually 30 min to 1 hr before bedtime

 Do Not Confuse

Benadryl *with* **benazepril**

An order for Benadryl may be confused with benazepril. Benadryl is an antihistamine used to relieve symptoms of allergy, hay fever, and the common cold or insomnia, whereas benazepril is an angiotensin-converting enzyme (ACE) inhibitor used to treat high blood pressure.

QSEN: Safety

 Do Not Confuse

zolpidem *with* **Zyloprim**

An order for zolpidem may be confused with Zyloprim. Zolpidem is a benzodiazepine receptor agonist used to treat insomnia, whereas Zyloprim is a xanthine oxidase inhibitor used to treat gout and certain types of kidney stones.

QSEN: Safety

Do Not Confuse

Restoril *with* **Risperdal**

An order for Restoril may be confused with Risperdal. Restoril is a benzodiazepine used to treat insomnia, whereas Risperdal is an atypical antipsychotic used to treat schizophrenia and bipolar disorder.

QSEN: Safety

INTENDED RESPONSES OF DRUGS FOR INSOMNIA

- Insomnia is relieved, and sleep is improved.
- Person is sedated, and sleep is induced.
- Length of time to fall asleep is decreased.
- Sleep duration is increased.

COMMON SIDE EFFECTS OF DRUGS FOR INSOMNIA

Benzodiazepine receptor agonists can cause amnesia, daytime drowsiness, dizziness, and a feeling of "being drugged." Additional side effects of zaleplon (Sonata) include hallucinations, impaired memory, and impaired psychomotor functions for a brief period of time after the drug dose.

Common Side Effects
Drugs for Insomnia

Dizziness   Confusion   Drowsiness, Lethargy

Headache   Nausea/Vomiting, Diarrhea, Constipation

Blurred vision   Dry mouth

Benzodiazepines may cause confusion, daytime drowsiness, decreased ability to concentrate, dizziness, headache, and lethargy. These drugs can also cause blurred vision, constipation, diarrhea, nausea, and vomiting.

Diphenhydramine can also cause dry mouth, nose, and throat, as well as chest congestion. *Melatonin* can lead to daytime drowsiness and may increase the risk of bleeding from anticoagulant medications such as warfarin (Coumadin).

POSSIBLE ADVERSE EFFECTS OF DRUGS FOR INSOMNIA

Drugs for insomnia are metabolized by the liver and excreted by the kidney. When liver or kidney function is reduced, drug levels can become very high, with more side effects and adverse effects. A serious adverse effect of the benzodiazepine receptor agonists is *somnambulism* or sleepwalking. Some people taking these drugs experience *parasomnia*, a disruptive sleep disorder that can cause dangerous behaviors while asleep. They may have episodes of talking in their sleep, sleep-eating, or sleep-driving without any recollection of these actions when they wake. The person may appear alert, but the brain is not fully alert and judgement is frequently impaired.

Benzodiazepines are potentially addictive. Psychologic and physical dependence can develop within a few weeks or months of regular or repeated use. In addition, overdose is possible. The reversal agent for a benzodiazepine overdose is *flumazenil* (Romazicon). When given intravenously, it can reverse the sedation effects of a benzodiazepine overdose. Its duration of action is not as long as any of the benzodiazepines. This means that more than one dose may be needed. It does not reverse the depressed respiratory functions associated with benzodiazepine overdose, and the patient may still need mechanical ventilation. Flumazenil can lower the seizure threshold, especially in a person who has used benzodiazepines for a long time.

⭐ PRIORITY ACTIONS TO TAKE *BEFORE* GIVING DRUGS FOR INSOMNIA

In addition to the general actions to take listed in Chapter 2 before giving any drug for insomnia to a patient for the first time, ask the patient about usual sleep patterns and his or her specific difficulty with sleeping. In addition, ask about a history of depression, confusion, falls, and pain. Assess the patient's current mental status. Ask patients about a history of kidney or liver disease because these drugs are eliminated through the kidneys and liver, and if a patient has these problems, they are more slowly eliminated, resulting in an increased risk for overdose.

⭐ PRIORITY ACTIONS TO TAKE *AFTER* GIVING DRUGS FOR INSOMNIA

For patients in an acute care or residential setting who are taking a drug for insomnia for the first time, check the patient's vital signs and reassess the level of consciousness. Watch for and report changes in heart rate, blood pressure, and level of consciousness. Check for orthostatic hypotension, and excessive sedation or confusion, especially in older adults.

Instruct patients to call for help when getting out of bed and ensure that the call light is within easy reach because these drugs can cause drowsiness and dizziness. Remind patients to get up or change positions slowly.

⭐ TEACHING PRIORITIES FOR PATIENTS TAKING DRUGS FOR INSOMNIA

Use these teaching points and precautions:
- Take these drugs exactly as directed by your prescriber.
- Take drugs for insomnia only for a short period of time (1 to 4 weeks) and only when needed.
- If you are prescribed a benzodiazepine drug, you may become dependent if it is taken for an extended period of time.
- Do not take drugs for insomnia unless you have adequate time to sleep (4 to 8 hours, depending on the sleep drug).
- The amnesia side effect of drugs for insomnia can be reduced or avoided if you are able to get 4 or more hours of sleep after taking the drug.
- If you are prescribed a benzodiazepine receptor agonist, you should have another person with you for the first night you take the drug to determine whether somnambulism (sleepwalking) will be a problem.

- You should go to bed immediately after taking a drug for insomnia because its rapid onset of action will cause drowsiness and dizziness.
- Do not take these drugs on overnight airplane flights of less than 7 to 8 hours because you may experience transient memory loss called *traveler's amnesia*.
- Because drugs for insomnia can cause drowsiness and blurred vision, avoid driving, operating heavy or complicated equipment, or performing any activities that require alertness.
- Avoid drinking alcohol while taking drugs for insomnia to avoid intensifying the sedating effects.
- Keep follow-up appointments to monitor the progress of your treatment.
- Never take a double dose of these drugs.
- Report side effects and adverse effects to your prescriber immediately.

LIFE SPAN CONSIDERATIONS FOR DRUGS FOR INSOMNIA

Pediatric Considerations

Watch children receiving any sedating drug for unusual or paradoxical responses. A paradoxical response is one that is the opposite of what is expected. Antihistamines (e.g., diphenhydramine) are the most commonly used drugs for treating sleep disorders for children.

Considerations for Pregnancy and Lactation

Benzodiazepines have a high likelihood of increasing the risk for birth defects or fetal harm and should not be taken during pregnancy. Most benzodiazepine receptor agonists have a moderate likelihood of increasing the risk for birth defects or fetal harm and are generally considered safe for use during pregnancy, but only if the benefits outweigh the possible side effects. Most drugs for insomnia cross the placenta and enter breast milk and can have sedating effects on the fetus or infant.

Considerations for Older Adults

Older adults should be given lower doses of drugs for insomnia because they are more sensitive to the effects of these drugs and more likely to experience side effects. In addition, older adults are at increased risk for falls while taking these drugs.

 Critical Point for Safety

Teach patients prescribed a *benzodiazepine receptor agonist* to have another person with them during the first night of taking the drug at home, to determine whether somnambulism (sleepwalking) will be a problem.

QSEN: Safety

 Drug Alert

Teaching Alert

Teach patients to be sure that there is adequate time (4–8 hr) for sleep before taking a drug for insomnia.

QSEN: Safety

 Drug Alert

Teaching Alert

Teach patients taking an insomnia drug to avoid alcohol and other CNS-depressing substances because of the risk for oversedation.

QSEN: Safety

 Critical Point for Safety

Most drugs for insomnia should not be taken during pregnancy or breastfeeding because they are passed from the mother to the fetus or infant.

QSEN: Safety

Get Ready for the NCLEX® Examination!

Key Points

- Insomnia is the inability to go to sleep or remain asleep throughout the night.
- Sleep deprivation decreases immune function and increases the risk for infection.
- All drugs to relieve insomnia cause some degree of central nervous system depression.
- Psychologic and physical dependence can develop within a few weeks or months of regular or repeated use of many drugs for insomnia, especially benzodiazepines.
- The barbiturate drugs (pentobarbital and secobarbital) are rarely used for insomnia because they are classified as Schedule II controlled substances with a high potential for abuse and addiction.
- A serious adverse effect of the benzodiazepine receptor agonists is the development of parasomnia, with possible actions such as sleepwalking (somnambulism), sleep-eating, and sleep-driving with the patient having no recollection of these actions.

- If a patient is prescribed warfarin and also taking melatonin, report this immediately to the prescriber because of the increased risk for bleeding when the two are taken together.
- Do **not** give flumazenil (Romazicon), which is the reversal agent for benzodiazepines, to anyone who has a seizure disorder, because it can lower the seizure threshold.
- To better monitor for effectiveness and for side effects, assess the level of consciousness before and after giving a drug for insomnia.
- Teach patients taking drugs for insomnia to be sure that there is adequate time for sleep (4 to 8 hr depending on the drug) before taking these drugs.
- Teach patients taking any insomnia drug to avoid alcohol and other CNS-depressing substances because of the risk for oversedation.
- A family member should be taught to watch the patient taking a benzodiazepine receptor agonist for sleepwalking.
- Warn patients to avoid operating any heavy equipment, driving a car, or making critical decisions while under the influence of any CNS depressant drug.

- Most drugs for insomnia should not be taken during pregnancy or breastfeeding because they are passed from the mother to the fetus or infant.

Additional Learning Resources

🌐 Be sure to visit your Evolve website (http://evolve.elsevier.com/Workman/pharmacology/) for additional online resources.

SG Go to your Study Guide for additional learning activities to help you master this chapter content.

Review Questions

See *Answers to In-Text Review Questions* in the back of the book for answers to these questions.

1. What is the **most important** precaution to teach a patient who is prescribed a drug for insomnia?

   A. "Avoid drinking fluids with caffeine before bedtime."
   B. "Rinse your mouth frequently with water or saline."
   C. "Avoid driving within 8 hours of taking this drug."
   D. "Do not take this drug for more than 1 week."

2. A patient who has been taking flurazepam for insomnia is now prescribed zolpidem instead. The patient asks why the prescription was changed. What is the nurse's **best** response?

   A. "Zolpidem is a first-line drug for the treatment of insomnia."
   B. "Flurazepam is a benzodiazepine drug that can become habit-forming."
   C. "Zolpidem is also used to treat any anxiety or stress that may contribute to your insomnia."
   D. "Flurazepam has both hypnotic and sedative effects that are less effective in the treatment of insomnia."

3. How do benzodiazepines depress the central nervous system and induce sleep?

   A. Raising the seizure threshold
   B. Reducing the number of neurotransmitter receptors in the brain
   C. Decreasing the amount of excitatory neurotransmitters in the brain
   D. Increasing the amount of gamma amino butyric acid present in the brain

4. What adjustment does the nurse expect will be made for an 82-year-old patient who is newly prescribed zopiclone for insomnia?

   A. Seizure precautions will be implemented.
   B. The first dose will be given with a meal or a substantial snack.
   C. The initial dose will be lower than that for a younger adult.
   D. The patient will have continuous telemetry monitoring.

5. A patient is scheduled for a procedure to test mental function at 6 a.m. At 3 a.m. the patient requests something for sleep. What is the nurse's **best** response?

   A. "I'll call your prescriber and request an order for something to help you sleep."
   B. "Your prescriber has ordered temazepam. I will give you a dose now."

   C. "I'm sorry, but there is not enough time for sleep now before your procedure."
   D. "I'm sorry, but you already received a dose of temazepam last evening at 9."

6. An adult patient is prescribed 0.5 mg of triazolam as a one-time order. The available drug is triazolam 0.125 mg per tablet. How many tablets will the nurse give for this dose?

   A. 2 tablets
   B. 3 tablets
   C. 4 tablets
   D. 5 tablets

7. Which drug, when prescribed for a patient, will the nurse be sure to question after discovering that the patient has a history of seizures?

   A. pentobarbital
   B. flumazenil
   C. secobarbital
   D. triazolam

8. A patient with insomnia tells the nurse that she has been reading about Z drugs and asks if a Z drug might help her to sleep. What is the nurse's **best** response?

   A. "These drugs are currently second-line sleep aids to treating insomnia."
   B. "Z-drugs are called that because most of their generic names start with the letter Z."
   C. "These drugs are more likely to be misused and become addictive."
   D. "Z-drugs are another name for benzodiazepine receptor agonists which are first-line for treatment of insomnia."

9. A patient with insomnia has been prescribed eszopiclone 1 mg orally per day. Which points will the nurse include in a teaching plan about this drug? **Select all that apply.**

   A. Be sure you have 7 to 8 hr to sleep before you must get up.
   B. Taking this drug for a long period increases the risk of addiction.
   C. Have someone stay with you the first night that you take this drug at home.
   D. This drug is an antihistamine and will cause you to have a very dry mouth.
   E. Take your eszopiclone 2 hr before you go to bed to give it time to work.
   F. Be sure to let your prescriber know if you have liver or kidney problems.

10. A patient who is prescribed warfarin is admitted to the patient care unit. Which information from the patient's initial assessment will the nurse report **immediately** to the health care prescriber?

   A. Takes over-the-counter melatonin
   B. Has a medical history of type 2 diabetes
   C. Has been dieting and lost 15 pounds
   D. Patient's mother struggled with insomnia for 15 years

Clinical Judgment

1. Which symptoms will the nurse expect to assess in a patient with insomnia? **Select all that apply.**

   A. Difficulty falling asleep
   B. Sleeping too much
   C. Waking often during the night
   D. Feeling unrested after sleep
   E. Uncontrollable urge to sleep
   F. Sleepwalking at least once per week
   G. Nightmares most of the nights
   H. Daytime tiredness and sleepiness
   I. Avoiding naps during the day
   J. Difficulty focusing on tasks

2. The nurse has given the 76-year-old patient with insomnia a dose of zolpidem 5 mg at bedtime for sleep. The patient was admitted to the patient care unit with a diagnosis of coronary artery disease and is to have a cardiac catheterization in the morning. Which priority actions will the nurse take before and after giving this drug? **Place an X in the boxes to indicate which nursing actions are Appropriate and which are Not Appropriate.**

NURSING ACTION	APPROPRIATE	NOT APPROPRIATE
Ensuring that the patient will have 7–8 hr to sleep before awakening		
Questioning the prescriber about giving this drug because the patient has coronary artery disease		
Asking the patient about a history of confusion, dizziness, or falls		
Assessing the patient's current mental status before giving the drug		
Before and after giving the drug, checking the patient's vital signs and assessing the level of consciousness		
Teaching the patient to go to bed within 2 hr after receiving this drug for insomnia		
Instructing the patient to have someone stay with him or her during the first night of taking this drug at home		
Telling the patient that he or she can get up to the bathroom independently		

27

Drug Therapy for Eye Problems

http://evolve.elsevier.com/Workman/pharmacology/

Learning Objectives

The content presented in this chapter should help you to:

1. Describe the proper technique to administer eye drops and eye ointments.
2. Describe the names, actions, usual adult dosages, possible side effects, and adverse effects of drugs for glaucoma.
3. Discuss the priority actions to take before and after giving drugs for glaucoma.
4. Prioritize essential information to teach patients taking drugs for glaucoma.
5. Discuss life span considerations for drugs for glaucoma.
6. Discuss intravitreal injection for macular degeneration.

Key Terms

alpha-adrenergic agonists (ăd-rĕn-ĔRJ-ĭk ĂG-ō-nĭsts) (p. 498) Drugs that bind to receptor sites in the eye that also bind to naturally occurring adrenalin, which "turns on" the receptor and reduces the amount of aqueous humor produced.

beta-adrenergic blocking agents (BĔ-tă ăd-rĕn-ĔRJ-ĭk blŏk-ēng Ā-jĕntz) (p. 497) Drugs that bind to adrenergic receptor sites and act as antagonists, which prevents naturally occurring adrenalin from binding to the receptors.

carbonic anhydrase inhibitors (CAIs) (kăr-BŎN-ĭk ăn-HĪ-drāz ĭn-HĪB-ĭ-tŏrz) (p. 502) A type of diuretic that also can lower intraocular pressure by reducing the production of aqueous humor by as much as 60%.

cholinergic agents (kō-lĭn-ĔRJ-ĭk Ā-jĕntz) (p. 500) Drugs that increase the response that occurs when the naturally produced substance (acetylcholine) binds to its receptor and activates it. In the eye, less aqueous humor is produced, and its flow is improved.

glaucoma (glŏ-KŌ-mă) (p. 492) A condition in which the aqueous humor does not drain normally out of the eye, causing a rise in intraocular pressure to levels that may damage the optic nerve.

intraocular pressure (IOP) (ĭn-trŭ-ŎK-yū-lŭr PRĔSH-ŭr) (p. 491) The fluid pressure inside the eyeball that helps to maintain the correct shape of the eye. The normal range for intraocular pressure is 10 to 20 mm Hg.

intravitreal injection (ĭn-trŭ-VĪT-rē-«îl ĭn-JĔK-shŭn) (p. 503) Intravitreal injection is a route of drug administration in which the drug is injected into the vitreous humor of the eye.

prostaglandin agonists (prŏ-stă-GLĂN-dĭn ĂG-ō-nĭsts) (p. 496) Drugs that bind to prostaglandin receptor sites in the eye and cause eye blood vessel smooth muscles to relax, which allows these blood vessels to dilate and drain more aqueous humor.

Rho kinase inhibitors (RŌ KĪ-nāz ĭn-HĪB-ĭ-tŭrz) (p. 499) Drugs that help lower intraocular pressure (IOP) by increasing aqueous humor (AH) fluid, reducing AH production, and decreasing epis-cleral venous pressure (an important determinant of intraocular pressure [IOP]).

OVERVIEW

 The eye, working with the brain, is the organ that allows sight (vision) (Animation 27.1). The most common problems affecting the eye that can be treated or controlled by drug therapy are inflammation, infection, and glaucoma. These disorders are most often treated with drugs delivered as eye drops and eye ointments. General issues for ophthalmic therapy are discussed on pp. 492–495 in this chapter. Chapter 10 discusses various types of antiinflammatory drugs, nearly all of which have an ophthalmic form. Chapters 6, 7, and 8 discuss the drug therapy for bacterial infections, viral infections, and fungal infections. Many anti-infective drugs have an ophthalmic form. This chapter focuses on drug therapy to manage glaucoma, which can be controlled if found and treated early, allowing the patient to continue to have effective vision. Also included is a section discussing intravitreal injection for the treatment of macular degeneration.

REVIEW OF RELATED PHYSIOLOGY AND PATHOPHYSIOLOGY

NORMAL EYE FUNCTION

The eyes are sense organs that react to light and help create vision. They change light to nerve impulses which are sent to the brain where images are created. Figure 27.1 shows the features of the eye from the front, looking at a person's face. Eyes sit in bony cavities called orbits. They are hollow balls made up of several layers. The *cornea*, the clear portion of the sclera that covers the front section over the eye and allows light to enter, sits at the front of the eye. The *iris* is the ring of color that surrounds the pupil. The *pupil* is a round opening in the center of the iris that lets light into the eye. It dilates to increase in size, letting more light into the eye, and constricts to decrease in size, letting less light into the eye. *Miosis* is constriction of the pupil, making the opening smaller and letting less light into the eye. *Mydriasis* is the dilation of the pupil, making the opening larger and letting more light into the eye (Figure 27.2).

The hollow eyeball is filled with clear substances that allow light to bend and penetrate all the way from the front of the eye to the retina on the back wall of the eye. The *retina* is the lining of the back part of the eye, opposite the pupil, that contains light-sensitive photoreceptors. *Photoreceptors,* the true sense organs for vision, are special smaller nerve endings of the large optic nerve. Photoreceptors react to light and change it into electrical impulses that are transmitted to the brain, where they are perceived as images. Figure 27.3 shows a cutaway side view of the eye. The optic nerve connects the photoreceptors in the retina to the brain and sends impulses that are changed to images in the brain.

The eye is divided into two segments, the posterior segment and the anterior segment (see Figure 27.3). The *posterior segment* is the entire back part of the eye from the lens to the area of the sclera where the optic nerve leaves the eye. It contains the *vitreous body (vitreous humor),* which is the gel-like filling of the eye. The *anterior segment* is the front of the eye that extends from the lens to the cornea and contains both the anterior and posterior chambers. It is filled with a small amount of clear fluid known as *aqueous humor (AH).* Because the eye is hollow and needs to retain a ball shape for vision, the gel in the posterior segment (vitreous body) and the fluid in the anterior segment (aqueous humor) must be present in set amounts that apply pressure inside the eye to keep it round. This pressure is known as **intraocular pressure (IOP)**, and it

Memory Jogger

Constriction of the pupil is miosis (small word, small pupil size). Dilation of the pupil is mydriasis (larger word, larger pupil size).

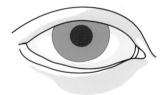

A   Normal pupil slightly dilated for moderate light.

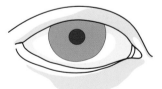

B   Miosis—pupil constricted when exposed to increased light or close work, such as reading. (Smaller word, smaller opening.)

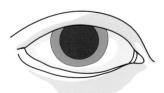

C   Mydriasis—pupil dilated when exposed to reduced light or when looking at a distance. (Larger word, larger opening.)

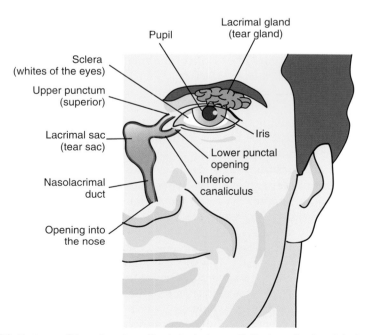

Pupil

Lacrimal gland (tear gland)

Sclera (whites of the eyes)

Upper punctum (superior)

Lacrimal sac (tear sac)

Iris

Lower punctal opening

Nasolacrimal duct

Inferior canaliculus

Opening into the nose

FIG. 27.1 Features of the external eye (front view) along with the tear gland and duct system.

FIG. 27.2 Miosis and mydriasis.

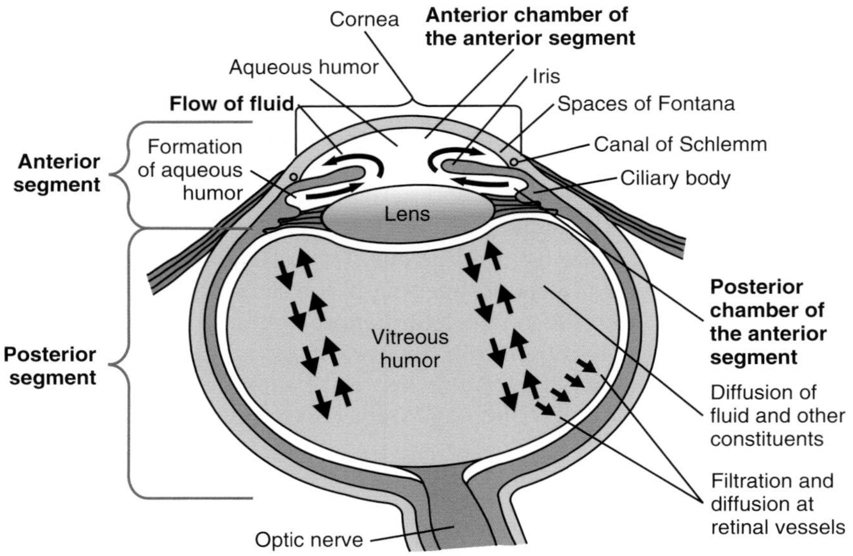

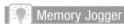

FIG. 27.3 Side view (cutaway) of the internal features of the eye and flow of aqueous humor.

has to be just right. If the pressure is too low, the eyeball is soft and collapses, preventing light from striking the photoreceptors in the back of the eye. If the pressure is too high, it compresses blood vessels in the eye, reducing blood flow and oxygen delivery to the photoreceptors. Without enough oxygen, the photoreceptors and the optic nerve die, and sight is lost permanently.

Aqueous humor is the clear fluid made continuously by the ciliary body. This fluid circulates from the posterior chamber through the pupil and into the anterior chamber, where it drains (see Figure 27.3). At the outer edges of the iris, beneath the cornea, there are blood vessels (the *trabecular network*) that collect this fluid and drain it through the canal of Schlemm, returning it to the blood. About 1 mL of aqueous humor is always present in each eye, but it is continuously made and reabsorbed. When fluid is made at the same rate that it is reabsorbed, the pressure inside the eye remains within the normal range (10 to 20 mm Hg). When fluid is reabsorbed too slowly, the amount in the eye increases, and so does the IOP.

GLAUCOMA

Glaucoma is a condition of increased IOP caused by an increase in the amount of AH fluid. Both eyes can have the problem, or it may affect only one eye. There are many types and causes of glaucoma. The most common type is a chronic condition related to aging called *primary open-angle glaucoma (POAG)*, which affects both eyes. Although we usually think of glaucoma as a disorder of older adults, children can also have it. In children, the problem most often is caused by eye trauma that blocks the canal of Schlemm and usually only affects the eye that was injured.

POAG occurs when aqueous humor is made at the normal rate but reabsorption is reduced, leading to an increase in the amount of fluid and pressure inside the eye. This type of glaucoma is painless and has no early symptoms. The damage occurs so slowly that the patient may not even be aware that sight is being lost. Usually, side vision (also known as *peripheral vision*) is lost first. Once photoreceptors die, they cannot be replaced. Without treatment, glaucoma leads to blindness.

GENERAL ISSUES FOR LOCAL EYE DRUG THERAPY

Drugs placed directly into the eye are *local* eye drug therapy. Eye drops are thin, sterile, liquid drugs that are squeezed as a small drop or drops from a small container. Eye ointments are thick, greasy drugs that stay in contact with the eye surface longer than drops. They can deliver a high concentration of drug and blur vision for minutes to hours after instillation.

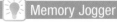

Memory Jogger

Keeping the IOP within the normal range (10–20 mm Hg) is important to maintain vision.

Memory Jogger

Drug therapy for glaucoma does not cure the problem; it only controls it.

Although drugs for eye problems can be taken orally or by another systemic method, they most often are administered as eye drops or eye ointments. Other routes include eye injections and placing drug disks on or in the eye. The following section discusses information about the correct use of eye drops and eye ointments, regardless of their specific actions or why they are prescribed.

Many different drug types can be delivered as eye drops or eye ointments. Each type has different actions and effects, along with some common actions and effects. General responsibilities for the common effects of eye drops and eye ointments are listed in the following paragraphs. Any specific responsibilities are listed with the discussion of each individual drug class.

INTENDED RESPONSES FOR ALL DRUG THERAPIES FOR GLAUCOMA

- IOP is reduced to the normal range.
- There is no further loss of sight.

★ PRIORITY ACTIONS TO TAKE *BEFORE* GIVING EYE DRUGS AND OINTMENTS

Check the order to see which eye is to receive the drug. A problem may affect only one eye, and the drug should be applied only to that eye. To avoid confusion, issues related to the right eye are indicated by writing "right eye" rather than using the Latin abbreviation "OD" (*oculus dexter*). Issues related to the left eye are indicated as "left eye" rather than "OS" (*oculus sinister*). Issues related to both eyes are indicated as either "both eyes" or "left and right eyes" rather than "OU" (*oculus uterque*). When eye drugs are ordered, the prescriber will indicate which eye or eyes are to be treated, and the pharmacist or pharmacy technician indicates this information on the drug containers. If the eye drop bottle or eye ointment tube is not labeled with this information, the health care professional labels it to correspond to the eye or eyes being treated.

Always wash your hands. Although the eye is not sterile, aseptic technique is used when touching the eye or placing drugs into the eye because it is not well protected by the immune system and can be infected easily.

Many eye drugs come in different strengths. Always check the strength prescribed with that of the drug you have on hand to be sure that you are giving the correct dose.

Check to be sure that a tube of ointment is for ophthalmic (eye) use. Some drugs for the eye are also available as regular topical ointments, but these contain larger particles that should not be placed in the eye.

Check to see whether any other eye drops are to be administered. If so, wait at least 5–10 minutes after instilling the first set and before instilling the second set of eye drops. If more than two drugs are to be instilled, wait at least 5–10 minutes between each set.

If a patient wears contact lenses, ask him or her to remove them before instilling the drop into the eye. For some drugs, the contact lens can be replaced 15 minutes after the drug is instilled. For other drugs, especially ointments, contact lenses should not be worn until drug therapy is complete. Inspect the eye for redness, drainage, or open areas. If open areas are present, check to determine whether the drug can be instilled. Some drugs should not be instilled into an eye with open areas because the drug is rapidly absorbed into systemic circulation when applied to an open area, and the side effects are widespread. For other drugs, this is not a problem.

For ointments, after removing the cap from the ointment tube, squeeze a small amount out onto a tissue (without touching the tip of the tube or letting it come into contact with the tissue) and discard this ointment. This action reduces the chance of instilling contaminated ointment into the patient's eye.

Follow the steps in Box 27.1 for placing eye drops or ointments into another person's eye. Figure 27.4 shows a common technique for instilling eye drops or ointments.

★ PRIORITY ACTIONS TO TAKE *AFTER* GIVING EYE DRUGS AND OINTMENTS

For any eye drop that can have systemic side effects, apply gentle pressure to the punctum in the corner of the eye nearest the nose for about 1 minute (Figure 27.5).

Critical Point for Safety

For clarity, **avoid** the use of the Latin terms for right eye (OD), left eye (OS), and both eyes (OU). These older abbreviations can be confused easily and, when handwritten, may not be readily distinguished. Instead, use right eye, left eye, or both eyes written out.

QSEN: Safety

Drug Alert

Interaction Alert

Always wait at least 5–10 min between instilling different eye drops to prevent a drug interaction or dilution of drug concentration.

QSEN: Safety

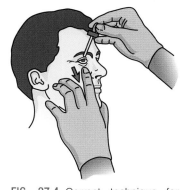

FIG. 27.4 Correct technique for instilling eye drops.

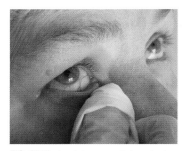

FIG. 27.5 Applying punctal occlusion to prevent systemic absorption.

| Box 27.1 | **How to Instill Eye Drops or Ointments** |

SELF-ADMINISTRATION

1. Check the name, strength, expiration date, color, and clarity of the eye drops to be instilled. If the drug is an ointment, be sure that it is an ophthalmic (eye) preparation and not a general topical ointment.
2. Check to see whether only one eye is to have the drug or if both eyes are to receive the drug.
3. If both eyes are to receive the same drug and one eye is infected, use two separate bottles or tubes and carefully label each with "right" or "left" for the correct eye.
4. Wash your hands.
5. Remove the cap from the bottle or tube, keeping the cap upright to prevent contaminating it.
6. Tilt your head backward, open your eyes, and look up at the ceiling.
7. Using your nondominant hand, gently pull the lower lid down against your cheek, forming a small pocket.
8. Hold the eye drop bottle or ointment tube (with the cap off) like a pencil with the tip pointing down with your dominant hand.
9. For ointment, squeeze a small amount out onto a tissue (without touching the tip to the tissue) and discard this ointment.
10. Rest the wrist that is holding the bottle or tube against your mouth or upper lip.
11. For eye drops, gently squeeze the bottle and release the prescribed number of drops into the pocket that you have made with your lower lid. Do not touch any part of the eye or lid with the tip of the bottle. For ointment, gently squeeze the tube and release a small amount of ointment into the pocket that you have made with your lower lid. Do not touch any part of the eye or lid with the tip of the tube.
12. Gently release the lower lid.
13. Close the eye gently (without squeezing the lids tightly) and roll your eye under the lid to spread the drug across the eye.

14. For eye drops, gently press and hold the corner of the eye nearest the nose to close off the punctum and prevent the drug from being absorbed systemically.
15. Without pressing on the lid, gently blot or wipe away any excess drug or tears with a tissue.
16. Gently release the lower lid.
17. Keep the eye closed for about 1 minute.
18. Place the cap back on the bottle or tube.
19. Wash your hands again.
20. Do not drive or operate heavy machinery while your vision is blurry.

ADMINISTERING DRUGS TO ANOTHER PERSON

1. Follow self-administration steps 1 through 5.
2. Put on gloves if secretions are present in or around the eye.
3. Explain the procedure to the patient.
4. Have the patient sit in a chair and the person applying the drug stand behind the patient (or alternatively stand in front of the patient who is sitting in a chair or over the patient who is lying in bed).
5. Ask the patient to tilt the head backward, with the back of the head resting against the body of the person applying the drug (or against the back of the chair) and looking up at the ceiling.
6. Gently pull the lower lid down against the patient's cheek, forming a small pocket.
7. Hold the eye-drop bottle or ointment tube (with the cap off) like a pencil, with the tip pointing down.
8. For ointment, squeeze out and discard a small amount of ointment as described in step
9. Follow steps 11 through 16.
10. Tell the patient to keep his or her eyes closed for a minute.
11. Remove your gloves.
12. Place the cap back on the bottle or tube.
13. Wash your hands again.
14. Remind the patient not to drive or operate heavy machinery while his or her vision is blurry.

| ⚠ Drug Alert |

Teaching Alert

Teach patients the steps in Box 27.1 for correctly instilling drops into one or both eyes. Using saline eye drops for practice, demonstrate the steps to patients and have patients demonstrate them back to you. If a patient has physical problems or is confused and cannot instill the eye drops, teach a family member, friend, or neighbor how to do this correctly.

Teach patients how to use punctal occlusion by applying pressure over the punctum immediately after instilling the drops. This action keeps the drug on the eye longer and helps to prevent systemic effects.

The *punctum* is the opening of the tube at the inner corner of the eye that drains tears into the nose and mouth (see Figure 27.1). This area is also called the *inner canthus* and can be blocked by lightly pressing on it. Applying pressure to this area immediately after drops are instilled lets the drug coat the entire eye before any of it leaves the area. This action is called *punctal occlusion* and reduces systemic absorption of the drug.

Instruct patients to keep the eye closed for about 1 minute after instilling the drug to ensure that it spreads evenly across the eye.

⊛ TEACHING PRIORITIES FOR PATIENTS TAKING EYE DRUGS AND OINTMENTS

- Use the exact number of drops that have been prescribed to prevent complications with this drug, including having systemic effects and too strong an effect on your eye.
- Administering eye drugs to an infant or child can be difficult. Sudden head movement can cause the tip of the bottle or tube to scratch the eye.

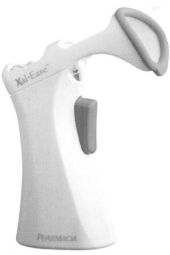

FIG. 27.6 The Xal-Ease adaptive device for self-administering eye drops. (From Pfizer, Inc., New York.)

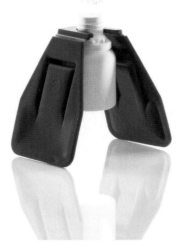

FIG. 27.7 Autosqueeze device attached to eye-drop bottle neck. (Courtesy Owen Mumford, Marietta, GA.)

- If you have difficulty giving yourself eye drops, adaptive devices are available that hold the bottle of eye drops and help keep the eyelids open. When the device is placed around the eye, the tip of the bottle lines up directly over the center of your eye (Figure 27.6). You then only have to trigger the right number of drops. Although this method does not place the drops in a lid pocket, it is acceptable. Another useful device is an Autosqueeze eye-drop bottle squeezer (Figure 27.7). Remove the cap from the eye-drop bottle and slide the Autosqueeze around the neck of the bottle then apply the eye drops by gently squeezing.
- Do not share the eye drops or ointment with anyone else to prevent spreading eye infections from one person to another.
- Remember not to drive or use heavy equipment while the drug is in your eye and your vision is blurred.
- Report any new symptoms (general or specific to the eye) to your prescriber as soon as possible.
- Call their prescriber or go to the emergency department immediately if you have a sudden loss or reduction of vision.

LIFE SPAN CONSIDERATIONS FOR DRUGS USED TO TREAT GLAUCOMA

Pediatric Considerations
The safety and effectiveness of these drugs have not been established in children. However, glaucoma can occur in children and must be treated to preserve sight. Teaching the child, the parent, or any other caregiver how to instill eye drops safely is critical (see Box 27.1). It is also important to stress that if only one eye is affected, which is common when glaucoma is the result of trauma, the drugs must only be placed in the affected eye.

Considerations for Pregnancy and Lactation
Most drugs for glaucoma therapy have a moderate likelihood of increasing the risk for birth defects or fetal harm. Unless the risk for sight loss is severe, these drugs should be avoided during the first trimester of pregnancy and used with caution during the later 6 months of pregnancy. Breastfeeding is not recommended during glaucoma therapy.

Considerations for Older Adults
Focus on the correct technique for administering eye drops. Teach older adults with physical limitations how to use adaptive devices for eye-drop administration.

 Drug Alert

Teaching Alert

Ensure that the patient understands the importance of taking only the correct dose of the drug and occluding the punctum immediately after placing the drops in his or her eye.

QSEN: Safety

 Drug Alert

Teaching Alert

If infants or young children need eye drugs, demonstrate drug instillation to the parent or guardian and teach them to obtain the assistance of another adult.

QSEN: Safety

 Drug Alert

Teaching Alert

Teach patients using eye drugs for any eye problem to immediately call their prescriber or go to the emergency department if a sudden reduction or loss of vision occurs.

QSEN: Safety

TYPES OF DRUGS FOR GLAUCOMA

Drugs for glaucoma improve the reabsorption of aqueous humor and/or reduce the amount that is made. These actions restore good blood flow inside the eye and keep the remaining photoreceptors of the optic nerve healthy. Most glaucoma drugs are administered as eye drops. For sudden-onset glaucoma (acute closed-angle glaucoma), systemic drugs may be used.

PROSTAGLANDIN AGONISTS

How Prostaglandin Agonists Work

Prostaglandin agonists bind to prostaglandin receptor sites in the eye and relax eye blood vessel smooth muscles, which allows these blood vessels to dilate and drain more aqueous humor. This allows the fluid to leave the eye more quickly and lowers the IOP. The prostaglandin agonists are very effective, are used only once a day, and seem to have fewer systemic side effects than other drugs. Generic names, trade names, and usual dosages of these drugs are listed in the following table. Be sure to consult a reliable drug reference for specific information about glaucoma drugs.

Adult Dosages for Commonly Prescribed Prostaglandin Agonists

Drug Name	Usual Maintenance Dose
bimatoprost (Lumigan)	1 drop of a 0.01% solution or a 0.03% solution in affected eye(s) daily in the evening
latanoprost (Xalatan)	1 drop (1.5 mcg) in affected eye(s) daily in the evening
tafluprost (Zioptan)	1 drop (0.0015%) in the conjunctival sac of the affected eye(s) once daily in the evening
travoprost (Travatan)	1 drop (0.004% solution) in affected eye(s) daily in the evening

Common Side Effects of Prostaglandin Agonists

The most common side effects of prostaglandin agonists are eye itching, eye redness, a permanent change in the iris color from lighter colors to brown (Figure 27.8), thickening and lengthening of the eyelashes, and darkening of the skin on the eyelids.

Possible Adverse Effects of Prostaglandin Agonists

Adverse effects related to systemic absorption of prostaglandin agonists are rare. These include muscle weakness, hypotension, elevated liver enzymes, and an increase in body hair.

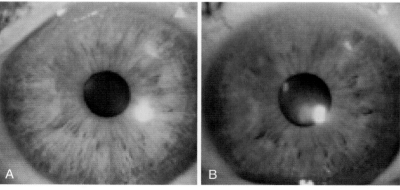

FIG. 27.8 Changes in iris color associated with prostaglandin agonist drug therapy for glaucoma. (A) Before treatment. (B) After treatment. (From Yanoff, M., & Duker, J. [2009]. *Ophthalmology* [3rd ed.]. St. Louis: Mosby.)

Priority Actions to Take *Before* and *After* Giving Prostaglandins Agonists

In addition to the general responsibilities related to eye drug therapy (pp. 493–494), inspect the eye for any corneal abrasions or other signs of trauma. These drugs should not be used if the surface of the eye is not intact.

Teaching Priorities for Patients Taking Prostaglandin Agonists

In addition to teaching the patient about the general care needs and precautions related to eye drugs (pp. 494–495), include these teaching points and precautions:

* Take these drugs exactly as prescribed. Remember that using higher doses than prescribed can reduce the effectiveness of the drug in controlling glaucoma.
* Your eye and eyelid color can change over time and your eyelashes can become thicker and longer.
* If only one eye has glaucoma, the color and lash changes will occur only in that eye. Do *not* use these drugs in the eye that does not have glaucoma.

BETA-ADRENERGIC BLOCKING AGENTS

How Beta-Adrenergic Blocking Agents Work

Beta-adrenergic blocking agents are drugs that bind to adrenergic receptor sites and act as antagonists in the ciliary body, which prevents naturally occurring adrenalin from binding to the receptors. This response in the eye causes less aqueous humor to be produced and also causes the fluid to be absorbed slightly. Generic names, trade names, and common dosages of these drugs are listed in the following table. Be sure to consult a reliable drug reference for specific information about glaucoma drugs.

Adult Dosages for Commonly Prescribed Beta-Adrenergic Blocking Agents

Drug Name	Usual Maintenance Dose
betaxolol hydrochloride (Betoptic, Kerlone)	1–2 drops (0.5% solution) in affected eye(s) every 12 hr (intraocular pressure lowering effects may require a few weeks to stabilize)
carteolol (Cartrol, Ocupress)	1 drop (1% solution) in affected eye(s) every 12 hr
levobetaxolol (Betaxon)	1 drop (0.5% ophthalmic suspension) in affected eye(s) every 12 hr (intraocular pressure lowering effects may require a few weeks to stabilize)
levobunolol (AK-Beta, Betagan)	1–2 drops (0.25% solution) in affected eye(s) every 12 hr; or 1 drop (0.5% solution) in affected eye(s) once daily
metipranolol (OptiPranolol)	1 drop (0.3% solution) in affected eye(s) every 12 hr
timolol ❶ (Betimol, Istalol, Timoptic)	1 drop (0.25% solution or 0.5% solution) in affected eye(s) twice daily
timolol GFS ❶ (gel-forming solution) (Timoptic-XE, timolol-GFS)	1 drop (0.25% solution or 0.5% solution) in affected eye(s) once daily

❶ High-alert drug.

Common Side Effects of Beta-Adrenergic Blocking Agents

Common side effects for beta blockers used in the eye include tearing, blurred vision, and a mild burning sensation within the first few minutes after the drug is instilled. Later tear production is reduced; and the eyes are dry, itchy, and red. The pupil is constricted *(miosis)*. The eyelids can become inflamed and crusty.

Possible Adverse Effects of Beta-Adrenergic Blocking Agents

Long-term use of beta blockers can increase the risk of cataracts. The most serious adverse effects occur when these drugs are absorbed systemically. They can block beta receptors in the heart, slowing the heart rate, and may even lead to heart failure. In the lungs beta blockers can make the airways narrower, making asthma and bronchitis worse.

Drug Alert

Administration Alert

Do not instill prostaglandin agonists into an eye that does not have an intact surface.

QSEN: Safety

Drug Alert

Teaching Alert

Remind patients using a prostaglandin agonist for glaucoma in only one eye **not** to place the drops in the unaffected eye even though their eye colors may now be different.

QSEN: Safety

Common Side Effects

Beta-Adrenergic Blocking Agents

Miosis, Itchiness, Redness

Blurred vision

Increased tearing

Drug Alert

Action/Intervention Alert

When beta-blocking eye drops are absorbed systemically, they can worsen asthma and heart failure. Be sure to apply *punctal occlusion* to reduce systemic absorption of these drugs.

QSEN: Safety

⭐ **Priority Actions to Take *Before* Giving Beta-Adrenergic Blocking Agents**

In addition to the general responsibilities related to eye drug therapy (p. 493), assess the patient's vital signs (especially blood pressure, heart rate, respiratory rate, and pulse oximetry). Use these data as a baseline to determine whether an adverse reaction occurs.

Check to see whether the patient is also taking an oral beta blocker to control blood pressure or heart rhythm problems. An oral drug taken along with beta-blocking eye drops could make the adverse effects more severe.

Check the patient's record to determine whether the patient has asthma, chronic obstructive pulmonary disease (COPD), or heart failure. Beta blockers should be used cautiously in patients with any of these problems.

⭐ **Priority Actions to Take *After* Giving Beta-Adrenergic Blocking Agents**

In addition to the general responsibilities related to eye drug therapy (pp. 493–494), tell the patient to call immediately if wheezing develops or if dizziness is present. Assess his or her blood pressure, heart rate, respiratory rate, and pulse oximetry at least every 4 hours for the presence of an adverse effect. Notify the prescriber if the heart rate drops below 60 beats per minute, wheezes develop, or the pulse oximetry reading drops below 92%.

⭐ **Teaching Priorities for Patients Taking Beta-Adrenergic Blocking Agents**

In addition to teaching the patient about the general care needs and precautions related to eye drugs (pp. 494–495), include these teaching points and precautions:

*   Excessive use of these drugs increases the risk for heart and breathing problems.
*   Use good light when reading and be careful in darker rooms. The pupil of your eye will not open farther to let in more light, and it may be harder to see objects in dim light. This problem can increase your risk for falls.
*   If you have diabetes, drugs from this class can mask the symptoms of hypoglycemia if the drug is absorbed systemically. Be sure to check your glucose level more often.

Life Span Considerations for Beta-Adrenergic Blocking Agents

Considerations for older adults. Focus on preventing severe systemic side effects. With high doses, systemic absorption is possible, and the effects on the cardiac and respiratory systems can be severe. Heart failure and bronchospasms can become worse. The risk for hypoglycemia increases among patients with diabetes. Thus, these drugs should either not be used or used cautiously in older adults who have heart failure, asthma, COPD, other respiratory problems, or diabetes. If they are used, stress the importance of using the right dose and the need to occlude the punctum after administration.

ALPHA-ADRENERGIC AGONISTS

How Alpha-Adrenergic Agonists Work

Alpha-adrenergic agonists are drugs that bind to alpha-adrenergic receptor sites that bind to naturally occurring adrenalin, which "turns on" the receptor and reduces the amount of aqueous humor produced in the eye. They also dilate the pupil and improve fluid flow through it. These actions reduce the amount of fluid in the eye, lowering the IOP.

When used as eye drops, the effects of these drugs should be present only in the eye. They are normally used for short-term therapy to prevent or reduce pressure after eye surgery. Generic names, trade names, and common dosages of these drugs are listed in the following table. Be sure to consult a reliable drug reference for specific information about glaucoma drugs.

Adult Dosages for Commonly Prescribed Alpha-Adrenergic Agonists

Drug Name	Usual Maintenance Dose
apraclonidine (Iopidine)	1–2 drops (0.5% solution) in affected eye(s) every 8 hr Wait 5 minutes before or after using apraclonidine to instill other glaucoma agents
brimonidine (Alphagan, Lumify)	1 drop (0.1%, 0.15%, 0.2%) in the affected eye(s) 3 times daily, approximately every 8 hr
dipivefrin (AK-Pro, Propine)	1 drop (0.1% solution) in affected eye(s) every 12 hr

Drug Alert

Action/Intervention Alert

Notify the prescriber immediately if heart rate drops, difficulty breathing develops, or pulse oximetry readings drop below 92% after a beta blocker has been instilled in the eye.

QSEN: Safety

Common Side Effects of Alpha-Adrenergic Agonists

Common side effects are tearing and blurred vision for a few minutes after instilling the drug. The pupil dilates (*mydriasis*) and remains dilated, even when there is plenty of light. The sclera may also be red and itchy. Less common side effects include eyelid crusting, eye discharge, and nasal dryness.

Possible Adverse Effects of Alpha-Adrenergic Agonists

If the drug is absorbed systemically, the patient may become drowsy. Blood pressure can decrease, and the heart rate can become slow and irregular. Usually, these symptoms occur only when the drug is overused.

⭐ Priority Actions to Take *Before* Giving Alpha-Adrenergic Agonists

In addition to the general responsibilities related to eye drug therapy (p. 493), assess the patient's vital signs, especially blood pressure and heart rate. Use this information as a baseline to determine whether an adverse reaction is occurring.

Check to find out whether a patient is also taking a monoamine oxidase (MAO) inhibitor drug. Alpha-adrenergic agonists are contraindicated for use in these patients. Taking MAO inhibitors with alpha-adrenergic agonists may cause a serious (possibly fatal) drug interaction. Patients should not take MAO inhibitors (e.g., isocarboxazid, linezolid, methylene blue, moclobemide, phenelzine, procarbazine, rasagiline, safinamide, selegiline, tranylcypromine) during treatment with these medications. MAO inhibitors should also not be taken for 2 weeks before treatment with alpha-adrenergic agonists.

⭐ Priority Actions to Take *After* Giving Alpha-Adrenergic Agonists

In addition to the general responsibilities related to eye drug therapy (pp. 493–494), assess the patient's vital signs at least once per shift to determine whether the drug is having an effect on blood pressure or heart rate.

Most alpha-adrenergic agonists should be protected from light and heat. The container is a solid color that does not allow light to enter. Refrigerate these drugs, but do not allow them to freeze.

⭐ Teaching Priorities for Patients Taking Alpha-Adrenergic Agonists

In addition to teaching the patient about the general care needs and precautions related to eye drugs (pp. 494–495), include these teaching points and precautions:

- Store the drug properly and protect it from light.
- Refrigerate but do not freeze the drug.
- Because your pupil is dilated, you will experience increased sensitivity to light. Wear sunglasses when in the sunlight or in other bright light conditions.
- If you have been prescribed to use the drug for a limited time such as 1 week, remember to not continue using the drug beyond that time period.
- The action of these drugs does not only lower elevated IOP, but they can also lower normal IOP, which can cause problems with your eyes. So, only use the exact number of drops prescribed.

RHO KINASE INHIBITORS

How Rho Kinase Inhibitors Work

Rho kinase inhibitors are a newer type of glaucoma treatment. They help lower intraocular pressure (IOP) by increasing aqueous humor (AH) outflow, reducing AH production, and decreasing episcleral venous pressure (EVP). This is thought to slow the progression of glaucoma optic neuropathy not only by lowering IOP and by working directly on optic nerve blood vessels. Generic names, trade names, and common dosages of these drugs are listed in the following table. Be sure to consult a reliable drug reference for specific information about glaucoma drugs.

Common Side Effects

Alpha-Adrenergic Agonists

Eye itchiness,
Eye redness,
Mydriasis

Blurred vision

Increased tearing

 Drug Alert

Interaction Alert

Alpha-adrenergic agonist eye drops for glaucoma should **not** be administered to anyone who is taking a monoamine oxidase (MAO) inhibitor or who has taken a drug from this class within the past 14 days because this may cause a serious (possibly fatal) drug interaction.

QSEN: Safety

 Drug Alert

Teaching Alert

Remind patients using alpha-adrenergic agonists to wear sunglasses when in bright light conditions.

QSEN: Safety

Drug Alert

Teaching Alert

Remind patients to remove contact lenses prior to using netarsudil ophthalmic solution because the solution contains the preservative benzalkonium chloride, which may be absorbed by soft contact lenses.

QSEN: Safety

❓ Did You Know?

Cholinergic drugs are named after acetylcholine.

Adult Dosages for Commonly Prescribed Rho Kinase Inhibitors

Drug Name	Usual Maintenance Dose
netarsudil (Rhopressa)	1 drop into affected eye(s) once daily in the evening

Common Side Effects of Rho Kinase Inhibitors

Side effects are generally very mild. Common side effects of these drugs include eye redness, blurred vision, tearing, and sometimes pain after using the eyedrops.

Possible Adverse Effects of Rho Kinase Inhibitors

An allergic reaction may occur with symptoms including hives; difficulty breathing; and swelling of the face, lips, tongue, or throat. Additional adverse reactions include small deposits on the cornea and broken blood vessels on the white of the eye. Reduced visual acuity has been reported in 5% to 10% of patients.

⭐ Priority Actions to Take *Before* Giving Rho Kinase Inhibitors

In addition to the general responsibilities related to eye drug therapy (p. 493), remove contact lenses prior to giving netarsudil ophthalmic solution because the solution contains the preservative benzalkonium chloride, which may be absorbed by soft contact lenses.

⭐ Priority Actions to Take *After* Giving Rho Kinase Inhibitors

In addition to the general responsibilities related to eye drug therapy (pp. 493–494), contact lenses may be replaced 15 minutes after giving netarsudil.

⭐ Teaching Priorities for Patients Taking Rho Kinase Inhibitors

In addition to teaching the patient about the general care needs and precautions related to eye drugs (pp. 494–495), include these teaching points and precautions:
- If you wear contact lenses, be sure to remove them before taking netarsudil.
- You may reinsert your contact lenses 15 minutes after taking your netarsudil drop.

CHOLINERGIC DRUGS

How Cholinergic Drugs Work

Cholinergic agents increase the response that occurs when the naturally produced substance (acetylcholine) binds to its receptor and activates it. One type of cholinergic drug is an acetylcholine agonist and acts just like acetylcholine. The other type of cholinergic drug works on the enzyme that destroys acetylcholine. The result of this action causes there to be more natural acetylcholine around to bind to the acetylcholine receptor.

By either acting like acetylcholine, or allowing it to remain in higher concentrations, the cholinergic drugs lower IOP by decreasing the amount of aqueous humor produced and improving its flow. These drugs make the pupil smaller (miosis) but at the same time make more room between the iris and the lens, allowing the fluid to flow better through the pupil even though it is smaller. Generic names, trade names, and dosages of the common cholinergic drugs are listed in the following table. Be sure to consult a reliable drug reference for specific information about less common drugs in this class.

Adult Dosages for Commonly Prescribed Cholinergic Drugs

Drug Name	Usual Maintenance Dose
carbachol (Carboptic, Carbastat, Isopto Carbachol)	2 drops (1.5% solution or 3% solution) in affected eye(s) up to 3 times/day
echothiophate (Phospholine Iodide)	1 drop (0.125% solution) in affected eye once or twice daily in the morning and at bedtime. May consider reducing the dose to 1 drop per day or every other day if needed

Drug Name	Usual Maintenance Dose
pilocarpine (Adsorbocarpine, Akarpine, Isopto Carpine, Ocu-Carpine, Ocusert, Piloptic, Pilopine, Pilostat)	1 drop (1% solution or 2% solution) in affected eye up to 4 times/day Ophthalmic gel: Apply a one-half inch ribbon in the lower conjunctival sac of the affected eye(s) once daily at bedtime

Common Side Effects of Cholinergic Drugs

The local side effects of cholinergic drugs for the eye include miosis, tearing, a mild burning sensation, blurred vision, and eye redness. These drugs are absorbed easily through the mucous membranes of the eyelids and can cause systemic effects such as headache, flushing, increased saliva, and sweating.

Possible Adverse Effects of Cholinergic Drugs

When larger amounts of the drug are absorbed into the blood, systemic adverse effects are possible. These include hypotension, heart rhythm problems, diarrhea, and urinary incontinence.

⭐ Priority Actions to Take *Before* and *After* Giving Cholinergic Drugs

In addition to the general responsibilities related to eye drug therapy (pp. 493–494), assess the patient's vital signs, especially blood pressure, heart rate, respiratory rate, and pulse oximetry. Use these data as a baseline to determine whether an adverse reaction is occurring.

Check to see whether the patient is also taking an oral cholinergic drug for other health problems (such as urinary retention or myasthenia gravis). An oral drug taken along with the eye-drop form of a cholinergic drug could make adverse effects more severe.

Check the patient's record to determine whether he or she has asthma, COPD, or heart failure. Cholinergic drugs should be used cautiously in patients with any of these problems because the drugs can make them worse.

If excess drug is present on the patient's skin, wipe it off immediately to prevent systemic side effects (these drugs can be absorbed through the skin).

Check the patient's blood pressure, heart rate, respiratory rate, and pulse oximetry at least every 4 hours for the presence of an adverse effect. Notify the prescriber if the heart rate drops below 60 beats per minute, wheezes develop, or the pulse oximetry reading drops below 92%.

Tell the patient to call you immediately if he or she develops wheezing or notes an increase in drooling or sweating or if dizziness is present.

Remind the patient that the pupils will not open as wide when light is low. He or she may need more light to read and see easily.

⭐ Teaching Priorities for Patients Taking Cholinergic Drugs

In addition to teaching patients about the general care needs and precautions related to eye drugs (pp. 494–495), include these teaching points and precautions:

- Use good light when reading and be careful in darker rooms. The pupil of the eye will not open wider to let in more light, and it may be harder to see objects in dim light. This problem can increase your risk for falls.
- Report an increase in drooling or sweating to your prescriber immediately because these are often the symptoms of a drug overdose.

COMBINATION GLAUCOMA EYE DROPS

Combination of glaucoma eye drops can lead to better control of intraocular pressure (IOP) through increased compliance and efficiency, although they should only be used when single eye drop therapy does not work. Some of these drugs are given as 1 drop to each affected eye once a day, reducing the number of drugs used and the frequency of eye drop administration, which according to research shows improved patient compliance with the use of these drugs. Always shake the drug container before using and apply punctal occlusion to decrease systemic absorption.

Common Side Effects
Cholinergic Drugs

Eye redness, Miosis

Blurred vision

Increased tearing

! Drug Alert
Action/Intervention Alert

Wipe any excess cholinergic drug from the patient's skin to prevent systemic side effects.

QSEN: Safety

! Drug Alert
Action/Intervention Alert

Notify the prescriber immediately if the heart rate drops below 60, if breathing problems develop, or pulse oximetry drops below 92% after a cholinergic drug has been administered.

QSEN: Safety

! Drug Alert
Administration Alert

Always apply punctal occlusion to decrease systemic absorption of combination glaucoma eye drops.

QSEN: Safety

Be sure to consult a reliable drug reference for specific information about combination glaucoma drugs. Also, refer to the information in this chapter on each of the elements of these combination drugs for additional information.

Adult Dosages for Commonly Prescribed Combination Drug Eye Drops for Glaucoma

Drug Name	Usual Maintenance Dose
Combigan (brimonidine tartrate and timolol maleate)	1 drop in the affected eye(s) twice daily approximately 12 hr apart
Cosopt (dorzolamide HCL and timolol maleate)	1 drop in the affected eye(s) 2 times per day. Remove contact lenses before applying eye drop and wait 15 minutes after before reinserting contact lenses
Rocklatan (netarsudil and xalatan)	1 drop in the affected eye(s) once daily in the evening
Simbrinza (brinzolamide and brimonidine tartrate)	1 drop in the affected eye(s) 3 times daily
Xalacom (latanoprost and timolol maleate)	1 drop in the affected eye(s) once daily in the evening, at the same time each day

CARBONIC ANHYDRASE INHIBITORS

How Carbonic Anhydrase Inhibitors Work

Carbonic anhydrase inhibitors (CAIs) are a type of diuretic that also can lower IOP by reducing the production of aqueous humor by as much as 60%. They can be taken orally and as eye drops to control glaucoma. Generic names, trade names, and dosages of common CAIs are listed in the following table. Be sure to consult a reliable drug reference for specific information about less common CAIs.

Adult Dosages for Commonly Prescribed Carbonic Anhydrase Inhibitors

Drug Name	Usual Maintenance Dose
acetazolamide (Diamox)	Tablets: 250 mg orally 1–4 times daily. Extended-release capsules: 500 mg orally twice daily. 500 mg IV over 1 min; may repeat the dose in 2–4 hr
brinzolamide (Azopt)	1 drop (1% solution) in affected eye every 8 hr
dorzolamide (Trusopt)	1 drop (2% solution) in affected eye every 8 hr
methazolamide (Neptazane)	50–100 mg orally every 8–12 hr

Common Side Effects of Carbonic Anhydrase Inhibitors

When carbonic anhydrase inhibitors are used as eye drops, the most common side effect is blurred vision briefly after instilling the drug. The sclera may also become red and itchy.

When these drugs are given systemically, there are many more side effects such as changes in blood glucose levels (up or down), headache, fever, nausea, vomiting, and diarrhea.

Possible Adverse Effects of Carbonic Anhydrase Inhibitors

Carbonic anhydrase inhibitors are related to sulfonamide antibacterial drugs ("sulfa" drugs). If a patient has an allergy to sulfonamides, he or she may also have an allergy to carbonic anhydrase inhibitors, even when they are used as eye drops.

When taken systemically, these drugs can cause acidosis; severe skin reactions; electrolyte imbalances; dizziness; confusion; and numbness of the hands, feet, and face. Carbonic anhydrase inhibitors also interact with many drugs. Be sure to check a reliable drug resource or the package insert before administering any of these drugs by mouth or as an injection.

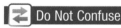

Do Not Confuse

acetaZOLAMIDE with **acetoHEXAMIDE**

An order for acetaZOLAMIDE can be confused with acetoHEXAMIDE. AcetaZOLAMIDE is a drug to treat glaucoma, whereas acetoHEXAMIDE is a drug for type 2 diabetes.

QSEN: Safety

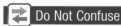

Do Not Confuse

Diamox with **Diabinese**

An order for Diamox can be confused with Diabinese. Diamox is a diuretic drug to treat glaucoma, whereas Diabinese is an older drug used for type 2 diabetes.

QSEN: Safety

Common Side Effects

Carbonic Anhydrase Inhibitors

Blurred vision

Eye redness, Eye itchiness

⭐ **Priority Actions to Take *Before* Giving Carbonic Anhydrase Inhibitors**

In addition to the general responsibilities related to eye drug therapy (p. 493), ask the patient whether he or she is allergic to sulfonamide antibacterial drugs. Because carbonic anhydrase inhibitors are a type of sulfonamide, the patient may also have an allergy to these drugs. If he or she has a known allergy to sulfonamides, report this to the prescriber before administering the eye drops because of the possibility of an allergic reaction.

⭐ **Priority Actions to Take *After* Giving Carbonic Anhydrase Inhibitors**

In addition to the general responsibilities related to eye drug therapy (pp. 493–494), after giving the first dose of a drug from this class, check the patient's vital signs every hour for the first 2 hours. Also ask the patient whether any shortness of breath, dizziness, or general skin itchiness is occurring. These are all symptoms of an allergic reaction.

⭐ **Teaching Priorities for Patients Taking Carbonic Anhydrase Inhibitors**

In addition to teaching patients about the general care needs and precautions related to eye drugs (pp. 494–495), include these teaching points and precautions:
- Take this drug exactly as directed by your prescriber.
- Report any signs of an allergic reaction (e.g., shortness of breath, dizziness, itching skin) immediately to your prescriber.

Life Span Considerations for Carbonic Anhydrase Inhibitors

Pediatric considerations. Carbonic anhydrase inhibitors are not used in children with glaucoma because these drugs slow growth when used long term.

Considerations for pregnancy and lactation. Carbonic anhydrase inhibitors are known to cause birth defects in animals. Unless the risk for sight loss is severe, these drugs should be avoided during pregnancy. Carbonic anhydrase inhibitors are not recommended during breastfeeding.

Considerations for older adults. The use of carbonic anhydrase inhibitors can increase the risk for acidosis. The risk for acidosis is low when the patient is taking the drug in eye-drop form. However, misuse or overuse of the drug can lead to acidosis and other systemic problems.

INTRAVITREAL INJECTIONS FOR MACULAR DEGENERATION

Macular degeneration is a disease that leads to loss of vision when damage occurs to the macula, which is the part of the retina that facilitates sharp central vision (needed for reading, driving, and recognition of faces). In dry macular degeneration, the center of the retina deteriorates. With wet macular degeneration, leaky blood vessels grow under the retina (Figure 27.9). **Intravitreal injections** (Figure 27.10) are a treatment for wet macular degeneration. Vascular endothelial growth factor (VEGF) is a protein that promotes the growth of blood vessels when the body needs them. With macular degeneration, growing new blood vessels is not healthy for the eyes because they tend to be weak and grow in places that harm the eye, which in turn can help curb fluid leakage in the retina. There are four main kinds of anti-VEGF treatments which are biologics (see Chapter 9) given by intravitreal injections:

Adult Dosages for Commonly Prescribed Anti-VEGF Treatments

Drug Name	Usual Maintenance Dose
aflibercept (Eylea)	2 mg (0.05 mL) via intravitreal injection into the affected eye(s) every 4 weeks (approximately every 28 days, monthly) for the first 12 weeks (3 months), followed by 2 mg (0.05 mL) once every 8 weeks (2 months)
bevacizumab (Avastin)	1.25 mg (0.05 mL) once a month by intravitreal injection into affected eye(s)

 Drug Alert

Administration Alert

Do not administer a carbonic anhydrase inhibitor to a patient who has a "sulfa drug" allergy.

QSEN: Safety

 Drug Alert

Administration Alert

Do **not** give carbonic anhydrase inhibitors to children, or women who are pregnant or breastfeeding.

QSEN: Safety

Drug Name	Usual Maintenance Dose
brolucizumab (Beovu)	6 mg (0.05 mL) via intravitreal injection into the affected eye(s) once monthly (approximately every 25–31 days) for the first 3 doses; then give 6 mg (0.05 mL) intravitreally every 8–12 weeks
ranibizumab (Lucentis)	0.5 mg by intravitreal injection to affected eye once a month (approximately every 28 days) 2 mg (0.02 mL of 100 mg/mL solution) continuously delivered via an ocular implant

Common Side Effects

Anti-VEGF Treatments

Bleeding, Infection/ Inflammation

Headache

Blurred vision

Common Side Effects of Anti-VEGF Treatments

The main side effect risks are infection or inflammation in the eye, and bleeding into a gel inside the eye called the vitreous gel. Other side effects may include headaches and blurred vision for a day.

Possible Adverse Effects of Anti-VEGF Treatments

Retinal detachment can occur with these treatments.

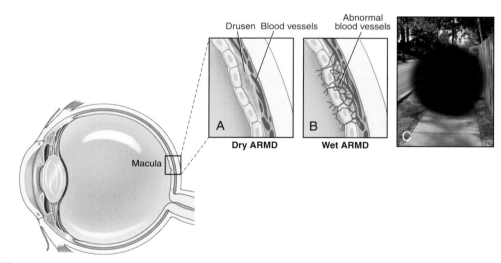

FIG. 27.9 Macular degeneration. (A) Dry macular degeneration, (B) Wet macular degeneration, (C) Lost central vision. (From LaFleur Brooks, M., & LaFleur Brooks, D. [2018]. *Exploring medical language: A student-directed approach* (10th ed.). St. Louis: Elsevier.)

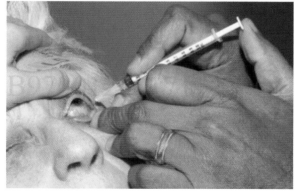

FIG. 27.10 Intravitreal injection of anti-VEGF agent. (Courtesy Jack Scully, Wills Eye Hospital.)

⊛ **Priority Actions to Take *Before* and *After* Receiving Anti-VEGF Treatments**

In addition to the general responsibilities related to eye drug therapy (pp. 493–494), remind patients that improvement in wet macular degeneration symptoms may be seen within a week of the injection. The patient may experience soreness in the eye for a few days following the injection, and their vision may be a little foggy. Over-the-counter pain relievers such as acetaminophen or ibuprofen can be taken to help with the discomfort. Also, applying a cool washcloth to the eyes for about 10 minutes every half-hour may also help relieve the soreness. If the needle hit a blood vessel in the eye there may be some redness in the sclera for up to 2 weeks. This is a harmless side effect as long as it is not accompanied by pain or vision difficulty.

⊛ **Teaching Priorities for Patients Receiving Anti-VEGF Treatments**

In addition to teaching patients about the general care needs and precautions related to eye drugs (pp. 494–495), include these teaching points and precautions:

- Report any of these occurrences to your prescriber: eye pain, sensitivity to light, vision changes, increased eye pressure, and "floaters" in your vision.
- Report pain, sensitivity to light, and vision changes to your prescriber because they may be signs of an infection.
- Do not rub your injected eye.
- You should not wash your face and hair or shower for 48 hours after the injection.
- Avoid swimming for a week after the injection.
- Keep your follow-up appointments which will be 4 to 8 weeks after the injection or course of injections.
- The beneficial effects of consistent treatment extend out to 10 years.

Get Ready for the NCLEX® Examination!

Key Points

- Use aseptic technique when instilling eye drugs because the eye can easily become infected.
- Apply only ointments that are labeled "for ophthalmic use" in the eye.
- Place eye drops or eye ointments only in the affected eye(s).
- If both eyes are to be treated and one eye is infected, use a separate bottle or tube for each eye.
- Place the drops or ointment into a pocket created by gently pulling the lower lid downward.
- Never touch any part of the patient's eye with the tip of the bottle or tube.
- Drugs administered as eye drops can enter the blood and cause systemic effects.
- When instilling eye drops that can have systemic effects, apply gentle pressure to the corner of the eye nearest the nose (the inner canthus where the drainage ducts are located) for 1 to 2 minutes after instilling the drops (punctal occlusion).
- Teach the patient to use eye drops or ointments exactly as directed and never to use more drug than prescribed.
- Glaucoma can occur at any age and can affect one or both eyes.
- Untreated glaucoma leads to blindness.
- The goal of glaucoma therapy is to keep the IOP within the normal range (10 to 20 mmHg) and prevent the loss of photoreceptors.
- Constriction of the pupil is miosis (small word, small pupil size). Dilation of the pupil is mydriasis (larger word, larger pupil size).

- Most drugs for glaucoma come in different strengths; be sure to check the strength of the drug that you have on hand with that of the prescription to prevent overdosing or underdosing.
- Adrenergic agonists cause the pupils to dilate and the eye to be more sensitive to light. Urge patients to wear dark glasses or a hat with a brim in bright conditions.
- Beta blockers and cholinergic drugs make the pupil smaller even in low-light conditions. Teach patients to be more cautious in dim lighting to avoid falls and to use more light to read or do close work.
- Beta blockers and cholinergic drugs, if absorbed systemically, can slow the heart rate, lower blood pressure, and cause asthma. Be sure to warn patients about these side effects and tell them to notify their prescriber if symptoms appear or worsen.
- Warn patients with diabetes that beta blockers can mask the symptoms of hypoglycemia. Blood glucose levels may need to be checked more often.
- Over time the prostaglandin agonist eye drops change the color of the iris to brown, darken the eyelids, and increase the number and length of eyelashes.
- Teach patients using eye drugs for any eye problem to immediately call their prescriber or go to the emergency department if a sudden reduction or loss of vision occurs.
- Alpha-adrenergic agonist eye drops for glaucoma should not be administered to anyone who is taking a monoamine oxidase inhibitor or who has taken a drug from this class within the past 14 days.
- Remind patients to remove contact lenses prior to using netarsudil ophthalmic solution because the solution contains the

preservative benzalkonium chloride, which may be absorbed by soft contact lenses.
- Notify the prescriber immediately if the heart rate drops below 60 or if breathing problems develop after a cholinergic drug has been administered.
- Do not administer a carbonic anhydrase inhibitor to a patient who has a "sulfa drug" allergy.
- Do not give carbonic anhydrase inhibitors to children or women who are pregnant or breastfeeding.
- Teach patients what to expect when an intravitreal injection is given.

- After an intravitreal injection, instruct patients to report any of these occurrences to the prescriber: eye pain, sensitivity to light, vision changes, increased eye pressure, and "floaters" in their vision.

Additional Learning Resources

🌐 Be sure to visit your Evolve website (http://evolve.elsevier.com/Workman/pharmacology/) for additional online resources.

SG Go to your Study Guide for additional learning activities to help you master this chapter content.

Review Questions

See *Answers to In-Text Review Questions* in the back of the book for answers to these questions.

1. **Which statement regarding primary open-angle glaucoma (POAG) is true?**

   A. It is most common in children.
   B. The major cause is trauma to the eye.
   C. The problem usually affects both eyes.
   D. The first symptom is chronic eye pain.

2. **How does untreated elevated intraocular pressure (IOP) eventually lead to visual impairment?**

   A. It compresses blood vessels and causes hypoxia of the photoreceptors.
   B. It clouds the lens and prevents light from striking the photoreceptors.
   C. It constricts the pupil and prevents light from entering the posterior chamber.
   D. It pushes the cornea forward and distorts the placement of the image on the retina.

3. **Which safety precaution will the nurse teach a patient who is prescribed eye drops or eye ointment?**

   A. "Check your blood pressure before and after applying the drug."
   B. "Allow at least 15 minutes between taking different types of drops or ointments."
   C. "Avoid drinking alcoholic beverages while taking this drug."
   D. "Do not drive or use heavy equipment while your vision is blurred."

4. **Which assessment is *most important* for the nurse to perform before instilling latanoprost into a patient's eyes?**

   A. Measuring the patient's temperature
   B. Measuring the patient's intraocular pressure
   C. Checking the cornea for abrasions or open areas
   D. Assessing heart rate and rhythm for 1 full minute

5. **A patient has been taking bimatoprost for the last 2 months. Which statement by the patient indicates to the nurse a correct understanding of this drug therapy?**

   A. "When my eyes are red or itchy, I should wait until the next day to use my glaucoma medicine."
   B. "Even though my intraocular pressure is now normal, I will continue to take the drug once daily."

   C. "One indication that I have used too much of this drug is when my vision becomes blurry or fuzzy."
   D. "If I forget to take the eye drops one day, I should apply them as soon as I remember them the next day and also take the regular dose for that day."

6. **Which problem indicates to the nurse that a patient may be over-using apraclonidine eye drops for glaucoma?**

   A. Anorexia
   B. Blurred vision
   C. Conjunctival itching
   D. Drowsiness

7. **A patient who has been using travoprost eye drops for glaucoma reports that the eyelashes seem longer and thicker. What is the nurse's *best* action?**

   A. Teaching the patient that the drug is absorbed by the blood vessels of the eye and has no effect on other eye or lid structures
   B. Instructing the patient to apply only the number of drops prescribed and to blot the area with a tissue after each dose
   C. Reminding the patient that eye drops are liquid and that wet lashes appear both longer and thicker
   D. Reassuring the patient that this is an expected side effect of the drug and no action is needed

8. **Which drugs for glaucoma cause marked mydriasis? *Select all that apply.***

   A. apraclonidine
   B. bimatoprost
   C. brimonidine
   D. carbachol
   E. carteolol
   F. dipivefrin
   G. levobunolol

9. **How do beta-adrenergic blocking agents (antagonists) lower intraocular pressure?**

   A. They increase the rate that the vitreous humor is reabsorbed.
   B. They slow the production of aqueous humor inside the eye.
   C. They reduce systemic blood pressure, which results in lower intraocular pressure.
   D. They increase the movement of aqueous humor from the posterior chamber into the anterior chamber.

10. What is the **most important** action for the nurse to perform after administering eye drops to a patient who is prescribed pilocarpine?

    A. Placing the patient in the supine position
    B. Wiping the excess drug from the patient's skin
    C. Instructing the patient to keep the eyes closed for 2 minutes
    D. Checking pupillary responses by shining a penlight into each eye

11. **A patient is prescribed methazolamide 75 mg orally. The drug available is methazolamide 25 mg per tablet. How many tablets should be administered to the patient for each dose?**

    A. 1 tablet
    B. 2 tablets
    C. 3 tablets
    D. 4 tablets

12. Which action is **most important** for the nurse to take when giving a patient a combination eye drop drug for glaucoma?

    A. Asking the patient to blink his or her eyes several times
    B. Applying punctal occlusion to the affected eye(s)
    C. Wiping away any residual fluid from around the eye(s)
    D. Instructing the patient to keep his or her eyes closed for 10 minutes

---

Clinical Judgment

1. Which important teaching points will the nurse include when preparing a patient for what to expect when an intravitreal injection is given by the physician? **Select all that apply.**

    A. "First, your eye will be numbed with numbing eye drops."
    B. "Second, your eye will be cleaned with a hydrogen peroxide solution."
    C. "A small device may be placed in the eye to hold the top and bottom eyelid out of the way."
    D. "The needle used to give the injection is very small and thin."
    E. "The injection is to be given very slowly, over about 1 minute."
    F. "The physician may ask you to look up as the needle is placed into the sclera of your eye."
    G. "The procedure usually causes some pain but you must be very still during the injection."
    H. "As the anti-VEGF drug mixes with the fluid in the middle of the eye, you may see wavy lines."
    I. "When the needle is removed the prescriber will put a sterile cotton tip over the injection site for about 10 seconds to put pressure on it and keep fluid from escaping."
    J. "Finally, your eye will be flushed with a solution to lubricate it and keep it from getting irritated."

2. The patient is a 78-year-old man newly diagnosed with primary open-angle glaucoma (POAG) in both eyes. He has never used eyedrops for any reason. The nurse has completed teaching the patient about his prescribed Xalacom (latanoprost and timolol maleate) eye drops. **Use an X to indicate which patient statement about issues related to this therapy is either Understood or Requires Further Teaching.**

PATIENT STATEMENT	UNDERSTOOD TEACHING	REQUIRES FURTHER TEACHING
"My combination glaucoma eye drops can cause better control of my eye pressure."		
"I will be sure to shake my bottle of eye drops every day after I use it."		
"I will only have to put the drops in my eyes once a day."		
"After I use my eye drops, I will put pressure on the inner corner of my eyelids."		
"These eye drops are less likely to cause systemic side effects."		
"I will be sure to use my eye drops at the same time every day."		

28

Drug Therapy for Male Reproductive Problems

http://evolve.elsevier.com/Workman/pharmacology/

Learning Objectives

The content presented in this chapter should help you to:

1. Describe the common names, actions, usual adult dosages, possible side effects, and adverse effects of drugs for benign prostatic hyperplasia (BPH).
2. Discuss the priority actions to take *before* and *after* giving drugs for benign prostatic hyperplasia.
3. Prioritize essential information to teach patients taking drugs for benign prostatic hyperplasia.
4. Discuss life span considerations for drugs for benign prostatic hyperplasia.

5. Describe the common names, actions, usual adult dosages, possible side effects, and adverse effects of drugs for male hormone replacement therapy and erectile dysfunction.
6. Discuss the priority actions to take *before* and *after* giving drugs for male hormone replacement therapy and erectile dysfunction.
7. Prioritize essential information to teach patients taking drugs for male hormone replacement therapy and erectile dysfunction.
8. Discuss life span considerations for drugs for male hormone replacement therapy and erectile dysfunction.

Key Terms

androgens (ĂN-drō-jĕnz) (p. 508) The group of male sex hormones that include testosterone.

dihydrotestosterone (DTH) inhibitors (dī-hī-drō-tĕs-TŎS-tĕ-rōn ĭn-HĬB-ĭ-tŭrz) (p. 509) A class of drugs with effects that are used primarily in the treatment of benign prostatic hyperplasia. These drugs are designed to stop the growth of the prostate or even shrink its size. by lowering the production of the hormone DHT.

phosphodiesterase-5 (PDE-5) inhibitor drugs (F«ëS-fō-dī-ĔST-ĕr-ās-FĪV ĭn-HĬB-ĭ-tŭr DRŬGZ) (p. 515) Drugs that relax

smooth muscle and allow the penis to fill with blood, used to treat erectile dysfunction.

selective alpha-1 blockers (sŭ-LĔK-tĭv ĂL-fă-WŬN BLŎ-kŭrz) (p. 509) Drugs that help to relax the muscles in the bladder and prostate, allowing urine to flow more freely.

testosterone (tĕs-TŎS-tĕ-rōn) (p. 512) A hormone (sex hormone) produced in the testes that is responsible for the development and maintenance of male sexual characteristics.

REVIEW OF RELATED PHYSIOLOGY AND PATHOPHYSIOLOGY FOR BENIGN PROSTATIC HYPERPLASIA

The *prostate gland* is a walnut-sized male sex gland that surrounds the upper part of the urethra and secretes a milky white mix of simple sugars, enzymes, and alkaline chemicals into seminal fluid. It is located between the bladder and the penis (Fig. 28.1). Secretions (LLC2) from the prostate gland improve the chance of pregnancy with intercourse by increasing the amount of seminal fluid, improving sperm movement, and reducing acidity in the vagina. Both the activity and size of the prostate gland depend on the presence of *testosterone*, the main androgen secreted by the testes and adrenal glands. **Androgens** are a group of male sex hormones that include testosterone, dihydrotestosterone (DHT), and androstenedione. The prostate gland has testosterone receptors in the nucleus of each cell that bind circulating testosterone. When bound, these receptors trigger the genes for prostate cell growth and activity.

Many men over age 50 have *benign prostatic hyperplasia (BPH)*, an enlargement of the prostate gland as a result of increased numbers of cells in the gland. Although the amount of circulating testosterone decreases with age, the number of testosterone receptors in the prostate gland *increases*. Because of this, even small amounts of testosterone, especially DHT, are more likely to bind with receptors and eventually cause the prostate gland to enlarge.

The symptoms of prostate enlargement are uncomfortable and can interfere with adequate sleep and rest. Often urine stays in the bladder much longer than normal,

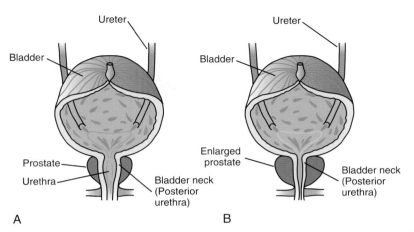

FIG. 28.1 (A) Normal prostate gland. (B) Enlarged prostate gland showing the narrowing of the urethra, decreasing urine flow.

leading to an increased risk for urinary tract infections. With rapid or severe prostate enlargement, the bladder can become completely blocked, causing urine to back up into the ureters and kidneys, and leading to kidney damage or failure. With severe blockages, surgery is needed. When symptoms are mild to moderate, drug therapy can reduce prostate pressure and improve urine flow.

TYPES OF DRUGS FOR BENIGN PROSTATIC HYPERPLASIA

DHT Inhibitors and Selective Alpha-1 Blockers

Selective alpha-1 blockers and DHT inhibitors are the two main categories of drugs used to treat prostate enlargement. Because the actions of these two drug types differ, they can be used alone or together to improve urine flow.

How drugs for BPH work. **Selective alpha-1 blockers** act to relax the smooth muscle tissue in the prostate gland, the neck of the bladder, and the urethra. These smooth muscles contain alpha-1 adrenergic receptors. When the receptors are activated, the smooth muscle constricts, tightening the prostate, which increases the pressure and squeezes the urethra. Smooth muscle in the bladder neck and urethra also contract and make the urethra narrower. When these receptors are bound with selective alpha-1 blockers, the smooth muscle relaxes, placing less pressure on the urethra and improving urine flow.

Dihydrotestosterone (DTH) inhibitors work directly on the prostate gland. They are a "counterfeit" drug that looks like testosterone and binds to the enzyme that normally converts testosterone to DHT, its most powerful form. This counterfeit drug cannot be converted to DHT, and although it is bound to the enzyme, the enzyme is not available to convert the real testosterone to DHT. With much less DHT in the prostate, the cells in the prostate gland do not receive the signal to grow. As a result, the gland shrinks and puts less pressure on the urethra, allowing better urine flow.

Generic names, brand names, and adult dosages of the most commonly prescribed drugs for BPH are listed in the following table. Be sure to consult a reliable drug resource for information about less commonly prescribed drugs for BPH.

Adult Dosages for Commonly Prescribed Drugs for Benign Prostatic Hyperplasia

Drug Category	Drug Name	Usual Maintenance Dose
DHT Inhibitors	dutasteride (Avodart)	0.5 mg orally once daily
	finasteride (Propecia, Proscar)	5 mg orally once daily ***Special Considerations:*** **A minimum of 6 months of therapy may be necessary to assess response, with up to 12 months necessary in some patients**

 Memory Jogger

As men age, testosterone levels *decrease* but the number of testosterone receptors in the prostate *increases*.

Because of its location, when the prostate enlarges, it squeezes the urethra, narrowing it and decreasing urine flow from the bladder (see Fig. 28.1).

Symptoms of BPH are:
- Increased frequency of urination
- *Nocturia* (increased urination at night)
- Difficulty in starting (hesitancy) and continuing urination
- Reduced force and size of the urine stream
- The feeling of incomplete bladder emptying
- Dribbling after urinating

 Critical Point for Safety

Because the signs and symptoms of BPH and prostate cancer are the same, urge any man with symptoms of BPH to be seen by his health care provider to rule out prostate cancer.

QSEN: Safety

 Memory Jogger

The two main groups of drugs used to treat BPH are DHT inhibitors and selective alpha-1 blockers.

Do Not Confuse

finasteride *with* furosemide

An order for finasteride may be confused with furosemide. Finasteride is a DTH inhibitor used for BPH. Furosemide is a loop diuretic used to treat pulmonary edema, hypertension, and conditions with excess fluid in the body.

QSEN: Safety

 Do Not Confuse

Flomax *with* Fosamax

An order for Flomax may be confused with Fosamax. Flomax is a selective alpha-1 blocker used to treat BPH. Fosamax is a bone-resorption inhibitor used for the prevention of osteoporosis.

QSEN: Safety

Common Side Effects

Drugs for Constipation

Decreased libido   Hypotension

Dizziness

Drug Alert

Interaction Alert

The patient who has an allergy to sulfa drugs may also have an allergy to tamsulosin.

QSEN: Safety

Drug Category	Drug Name	Usual Maintenance Dose
Selective Alpha-1 Blockers	alfuzosin (Uroxatral)	10 mg orally once daily with food, with the same meal each day
	doxazosin (Cardura, Cardura XL)	1–8 mg orally once daily. Max: 8 mg/day XR: 4-8 mg orally once daily with breakfast *Special Considerations:* **May be given in combination with finasteride for better results**
	silodosin (Rapaflo)	8 mg orally once daily with a meal at about the same time every day.
	tamsulosin (Flomax)	0.4–0.8 mg orally once daily 30 min after a meal *Special Considerations:* **Give at approximately the same time each day**
	terazosin (Hytrin)	1 mg orally once daily at bedtime. Doses are increased to 2 mg, 5 mg, then 10 mg once daily based on improvement of symptoms and urine flow rates. Maintenance doses of 5–10 mg/day have been used. Max: 20 mg/day, given in 2 divided doses every 12 hr

Intended responses of drugs for BPH
- Pressure on the urethra is decreased.
- Urine flow from the bladder through the urethra is improved.
- BPH symptoms (frequency, difficulty starting or stopping the urine stream, dribbling, excessive nighttime urination, feeling of incomplete bladder emptying) are decreased.

Common side effects of drugs for BPH. The most common side effect of drugs for BPH is a decreased interest in sexual activity (decreased libido).

Side effects of DHT inhibitors also include erectile dysfunction, decreased seminal fluid, and reduced fertility. Other side effects for some men are a slowing of hair loss from the scalp and, in some cases, scalp hair regrowth.

Selective alpha-1 blockers also relax the vascular smooth muscle to some degree. As a result, they may lower blood pressure, especially when changing positions (orthostatic hypotension), causing dizziness or light-headedness. Other side effects may include back pain and runny or stuffy nose.

Possible adverse effects of drugs for BPH. Drugs for BPH are metabolized by the liver. If the patient's liver is impaired, the drug is excreted more slowly, and higher blood levels could result. Higher blood levels lead to more severe side effects. Patients with liver impairment should be prescribed lower dosages of these drugs.

DHT inhibitors can adversely affect other hormones or sex tissues. Breast changes such as enlargement, lumps, pain, or fluids leaking from the nipple can occur. Any of these changes or pain in the testicles are reasons to consult a physician, who will likely stop the drug.

DHT inhibitors can cause birth defects when taken or handled by a pregnant woman. Women who are pregnant or who may become pregnant should avoid handling the tablets or capsules, especially if they are crushed or broken. Because these drugs enter the seminal fluid of men who take them, men should wear a condom when having sex with a woman who is pregnant or may become pregnant.

Alpha-1 blockers are excreted by the kidneys. Patients who have renal impairment retain the drug longer and have more severe hypotension. Although these drugs are not toxic to the kidney (*nephrotoxic*), they should not be taken by patients who have severe renal impairment or kidney failure.

Tamsulosin is made from a sulfonamide and may cause an allergic reaction in patients who are allergic to sulfa drugs.

All of the alpha-1 blockers can interact with many other drugs and herbal supplements, especially antihypertensives, cardiac drugs, and drugs for erectile dysfunction. The interactions can be complex and serious.

Alpha-1 blockers have been associated with a problem called *floppy iris syndrome* during cataract surgery. With this problem, the iris does not respond as expected to drugs that dilate or constrict it and can collapse toward the surgical site. Although this is not a reason to stop the drug, the surgeon performing cataract surgery must take special steps to prevent a floppy iris from causing complications.

 Priority actions to take before giving drugs for BPH. The signs and symptoms of BPH are the same as for prostate cancer. Before a drug for BPH is taken, the patient should have a digital rectal examination by his prescriber and have his blood tested for prostate-specific antigen (PSA) levels to rule out prostate cancer.

Because liver impairment can increase the blood level of the drugs for BPH, make sure that the patient does not have a liver problem before starting these drugs. Check the patient's most recent laboratory values for liver problems (elevated liver enzymes). (See Table 1.3 in Chapter 1 for a listing of normal values.)

Because alpha-1 blockers may cause orthostatic hypotension, take the patient's blood pressure in the lying, sitting, and standing positions.

If a patient will be taking tamsulosin, ask whether he has ever had an allergic reaction to sulfa drugs. If he has had such a reaction, report this to the prescriber.

 Priority actions to take after giving drugs for BPH. Assess the patient for orthostatic (postural) hypotension and related problems (dizziness, light-headedness), especially after the first dose. Remind the patient to call for assistance when getting out of bed.

 Teaching priorities for patients taking drugs for BPH. Use these teaching points and precautions:
- Be sure to continue your annual prevention and early detection practices for prostate cancer. These include a digital rectal examination and blood PSA levels.
- If you are taking a DHT inhibitor drug, be sure that women who are or may become pregnant do not come into contact with the drug or handle it. Methods for men to reduce exposure to women include wearing a condom during sexual intercourse and avoiding blood donation which could be given to a pregnant woman.
- Remember that some common herbal preparations have an action similar to that of DHT inhibitors (e.g., saw palmetto [*Serenoa repens*] and soy isoflavones). If you take a DHT inhibitor with one of these substances, a possible increase in the intended responses of the drug and side effects can occur.
- If you are taking an alpha-1 blocker drug, change positions slowly, especially when rising to a standing position, because a rapid drop in blood pressure can cause dizziness. Although this problem is more likely to occur when you first start taking an alpha-1 blocker, it can occur at any time, especially if you are dehydrated or taking drugs for hypertension, erectile dysfunction drugs, or cardiac drugs such as beta blockers or calcium channel blockers.
- Avoid driving or operating dangerous equipment, as well as any activities requiring mental alertness, until you know how your prescribed drug will affect you.
- If you are taking an alpha-1 blocker, be sure to tell all other health care providers because of the potential for drug interactions.
- Do **not** take over-the-counter drugs without checking with their prescriber.
- If you are taking an alpha-1 blocker, be sure to inform your surgeon when cataract surgery is being planned.

Life span considerations for drugs for BPH

Considerations for pregnancy and lactation. DHT inhibitors have a very high likelihood of increasing the risk for birth defects or fetal harm. They are teratogens and can cause birth defects, especially in male fetuses. Women who are pregnant, may become pregnant, or are breastfeeding should not take these drugs or handle them if

Memory Jogger

Testosterone levels begin to decrease around age 30 and continue to decrease for the rest of a man's life.

Symptoms of insufficient testosterone include (Fig. 28.2):
- Decreased interest in sex
- Decreased sense of well-being
- Depression, irritability
- Difficulty concentrating and remembering
- Erectile dysfunction
- Decreased muscle and increased body fat
- Anemia with fatigue and decreased energy
- Decreased bone density
- Decreased body hair

the tablet or capsule is crushed or broken. Although selective alpha-1 blockers have a low likelihood of increasing the risk for birth defects or fetal harm, they are used only to treat BPH in men and are not indicated for women, regardless of pregnancy or breastfeeding status.

Considerations for older adults. Drugs for BPH are more commonly prescribed for older men. Prostate cancer is much more common in this age group. Ensure that older men taking drugs for BPH understand the need to have annual prostate cancer screening.

The risk for orthostatic (postural) hypotension is higher in older patients taking alpha-1 blockers than in younger adults, especially with the first dose. Monitor older adults carefully for severe hypotension.

REVIEW OF RELATED PHYSIOLOGY AND PATHOPHYSIOLOGY FOR MALE HORMONE REPLACEMENT THERAPY

Testosterone is a hormone (sex hormone), produced in the testes, and is responsible for the development and maintenance of male sex characteristics. It is also important for maintaining muscle mass, adequate levels of red blood cells (RBCs), bone density, sense of well-being, and sexual and reproduction functions. As men age, the level of testosterone in their bodies decreases. This is natural, usually beginning around age 30 and continuing through the remainder of life. Low blood testosterone level, also called hypogonadism, occurs in many men over age 45. There are also several other potential causes of low testosterone (Box 28.1).

TYPES OF DRUGS FOR MALE HORMONE REPLACEMENT THERAPY

Testosterone

How drugs for testosterone replacement therapy work. Testosterone replacement therapy drugs promote the growth and development of men's sexual organs, as well as help maintain secondary sexual characteristics. Box 28.2 lists methods of testosterone replacement. Testosterone is a schedule III drug (with moderate to low potential for physical and psychological dependence). Oral testosterone tablets are available but are generally not used because of the danger of liver damage. Be sure to consult a reliable drug reference for additional information on testosterone drugs.

Box 28.1　Causes of Low Testosterone Levels

- Injury, infection, or loss of the testicles
- Chemotherapy or radiation treatment for cancer
- Genetic abnormalities such as Klinefelter syndrome (extra X chromosome)
- Hemochromatosis (too much iron in the body)
- Dysfunction of the pituitary gland (a gland in the brain that produces many important hormones)
- Inflammatory diseases such as sarcoidosis (a condition that causes inflammation of the lungs)
- Medications, especially hormones used to treat prostate cancer and corticosteroid drugs
- Chronic illness
- Chronic kidney failure
- Liver cirrhosis
- Stress
- Alcoholism
- Obesity (especially abdominal)

Box 28.2　Methods of Testosterone Replacement

- Intramuscular injections, given anywhere from 2 to 10 weeks apart
- Testosterone patch worn either on the body or on the scrotum (the sac that contains the testicles)
- Testosterone gel applied to the skin or inside the nose
- Mucoadhesive material applied above the teeth twice a day
- Oral tablets
- Long-acting subcutaneous implant
- Testosterone stick (apply like underarm deodorant)

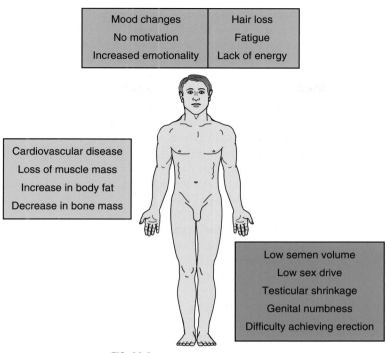

FIG. 28.2 Signs of low testosterone.

Adult Dosages for Commonly Prescribed Drugs for Male Hormone Replacement

Drug Category	Drug Name	Usual Maintenance Dose
Testosterone Replacement Drugs	testosterone undecanoate injection (Aveed)	Initially, 750 mg IM. After 4 weeks, give a repeat dose of 750 mg IM, then 750 mg IM every 10 weeks thereafter
	testosterone cypionate or testosterone enanthate	50 to 400 mg intramuscularly once every 2 to 4 weeks
	testosterone (Xyosted)	75 mg subcutaneously in the abdominal region once weekly
	testosterone patch (Androderm)	Transdermal patch: 4 mg/day patch applied to arm or upper body once daily at night
	testosterone gel (AndroGel, Testim)	5 g of 1% gel (containing 50 mg of testosterone and delivering 5 mg of testosterone systemically) applied once daily (preferably in the morning) to clean, dry, intact skin of the upper arms and/or abdomen
	testosterone (Natesto)	11 mg gel (2 pump actuations; 1 actuation per nostril) intranasally 3 times daily for a total of 33 mg/day [morning, afternoon, and evening (6–8 hr apart, preferably at the same times each day)
	testosterone (Tland)	*Tland:* 225 mg (taken as two 112.5 mg capsules) orally twice daily, once in the morning and once in the evening; give with food
	testosterone (Jatenzo)	*Jatenzo:* 237 mg orally twice daily initially, once in the morning and once in the evening; give with food
	testosterone pellets (Testopel)	150–450 mg (2–6 pellets) inserted subcutaneously by a health care professional every 3–6 months

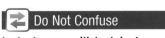 **Do Not Confuse**

testosterone *with* testolactone

An order for testosterone can be mistaken for testolactone. Testosterone is used for hormone replacement. Testolactone is used to treat advanced stage breast cancer.

QSEN: Safety

Common Side Effects

Drugs for Testosterone Replacement Therapy

Itchiness   Difficulty urinating   Sleep apnea

Male breast enlargement   Injection site reaction

Intended responses of drugs for testosterone replacement therapy
- *Increased anabolic effects* (e.g., increased muscle mass and bone density)
- *Increased androgenic effects* (e.g., maturation of sex organs, development of secondary sex characteristics such as deepened voice and growth of pubic and axillary hair)
- Relief of symptoms
- Increased interest in sex

Common side effects of drugs for testosterone replacement therapy. Side effects of testosterone are uncommon. Some side effects include acne or oily skin, mild fluid retention, increased size of the prostate with difficulty urinating, breast enlargement, sleep apnea, and decreased testicle size. Pain or inflammation may occur at intramuscular (IM) injection sites, and pruritus (itching), erythema (redness), or skin irritation may occur with transdermal patches.

Possible adverse effects of drugs for testosterone replacement therapy. Liver damage, including peliosis hepatitis, neoplasms, and hepatocellular carcinoma, are adverse effects of these drugs. Increases in the incidence of heart attacks and strokes have been reported and are a major concern.

⭐ ***Priority actions to take*** *before* ***giving drugs for testosterone replacement therapy.*** Ask men about history of prostate or breast cancer because if this is present, they should not receive testosterone replacement therapy. Before this therapy, all men should have prostate cancer screening including a rectal exam and PSA blood test.

Also check for a history of diabetes, kidney, liver, or cardiovascular disease. Testosterone can cause decreased blood glucose levels.

Get a baseline weight and blood pressure. Check laboratory tests including complete blood count (CBC) with hemoglobin and hematocrit, liver function tests, electrolytes, and cholesterol.

⭐ ***Priority actions to take*** *after* ***giving drugs for testosterone replacement therapy.*** Check weight every day to assess for fluid retention, and report weight gain of 5 or more pounds to the prescriber. Assess blood pressure at least twice a day. Monitor laboratory tests including electrolytes, liver function tests, hemoglobin/hematocrit, and cholesterol.

Assess injection sites for redness, swelling, or pain. Ask the patient about his sleep pattern. In collaboration with nutrition services, ensure that the patient's diet contains adequate protein and calories.

⭐ ***Teaching priorities for patients taking drugs for testosterone replacement therapy.*** Use these teaching points and precautions:
- Check your weight daily (same time, scale, and amount of clothes), keep a record of your weights, and report a weight gain of 5 pounds or more per week to your prescriber.
- Report frequent erections, difficulty with urination, or breast enlargement to your prescriber.
- Be sure to include high protein sources in your diet.
- If you experience gastrointestinal discomfort, eat smaller, more frequent meals.
- Consult with your prescriber before taking any other drugs while receiving testosterone replacement therapy.
- Keep regular follow-up visits with your prescriber and have laboratory tests done as directed by your prescriber.
- If you are prescribed testosterone gels or patches, remind family members and significant others (especially women and children) to avoid touching your skin, or any linen, or clothing that has been in contact with the drug.

Life span considerations for testosterone replacement drugs

Pediatric considerations. Safe use has not been established. Testosterone replacement must be used with caution in children.

Considerations for pregnancy and lactation. Testosterone has a very high likelihood of increasing the risk for birth defects or fetal harm and should not be used during pregnancy or breastfeeding.

Considerations for older adults. Older males are at increased risk of prostate hyperplasia, or growth stimulation of occult prostate carcinoma. They should have more frequent digital rectal examinations performed, as well as PSA levels.

REVIEW OF RELATED PHYSIOLOGY AND PATHOPHYSIOLOGY FOR ERECTILE DYSFUNCTION

Penile erections occur as a result of a complex process involving the central nervous, peripheral nervous, hormonal, and vascular systems. An abnormality occurring in any of these systems can interfere with the ability to develop and sustain an erection or ejaculate and experience an orgasm (Animation 28.1).

Erectile dysfunction (ED) is the inability of a man to achieve or maintain an erection sufficient for satisfying sexual activity. For more than 20 years, ED (also called *impotence*) has been recognized as a common problem as men age. Many men are affected by age 40, and the incidence continues to increase as men age.

Physical disorders that pose organic risk factors for ED include cardiovascular disease (e.g., hypertension, atherosclerosis, hyperlipidemia), diabetes, drug side effects (e.g., antihypertensives), alcohol use, smoking, pelvic surgery or trauma, neurological disease, obesity, and radiation to the pelvis. Hormone deficiency or hypogonadism (reduction or absence of hormone secretion or other physiological activity of the gonads [testes]) can also cause ED. Psychological (sometimes called "functional) ED, which is not associated with an organic or physical problem, may be caused by depression, anxiety, or stress.

ED is diagnosed by a thorough history and a complete physical examination. Signs and symptoms of ED include:
- Difficulty getting an erection
- Difficulty keeping an erection
- Decreased sexual desire

Treatment may include penile pumps, implants, surgery, psychological counseling, or drugs. Phosphodiesterase-5 (PDE-5) inhibitor drugs have been very successful in treating ED in many men.

DRUGS FOR ERECTILE DYSFUNCTION

Phosphodiesterase-5 (PDE-5) Inhibitor Drugs
How drugs for erectile dysfunction work. When a man develops an erection, blood fills tissue in the penis, which causes it to become enlarged and stiff. **Phosphodiesterase-5 (PDE-5) inhibitor drugs** relax smooth muscle and allow the penis to fill with blood (Fig. 28.3). Each of these drugs requires sexual stimulation to cause an erection. They begin working within 15 or 30 minutes to an hour. The effects of sildenafil and vardenafil last for up to 4 hours, whereas the effects of tadalafil can last up to 36 hours.

In addition to treating ED, some of these drugs are prescribed to increase blood flow in the lungs of people who have pulmonary vascular problems such as pulmonary arterial hypertension and some forms of pulmonary fibrosis (see Chapter 18). Be sure to consult a reliable drug reference for additional information about a specific ED drug.

Memory Jogger

ED may be caused by physical problems (organic) or psychological (functional) factors.

Memory Jogger

Drugs for erectile dysfunction require sexual stimulation to cause an erection.

Adult Dosages for Commonly Drugs for Erectile Dysfunction

Drug Category	Drug Name	Usual Maintenance Dose
Phosphodiesterase-5 (PDE-5) Inhibitor Drugs	avanafil (Stendra)	100–200 mg orally 15 min before sexual activity once daily, or decreased to 50 mg orally, approximately 30 min before sexual activity
	sildenafil (Revatio, Viagra)	50 mg orally once daily, 30 min to 1 hr before sexual activity

Drug Category	Drug Name	Usual Maintenance Dose
	tadalafil (Adcirca, Cialis)	10 mg orally once daily, taken prior to anticipated sexual activity. The dose may be increased to 20 mg or decreased to 5 mg, based on individual efficacy and tolerability **For use once daily for ED without regard to timing of sexual activity:** 2.5–5 mg orally once daily at about the same time each day
	vardenafil (Levitra, Staxyn)	10 mg orally once daily, 1 hr before sexual activity. For males 65 years of age or older, consider a lower starting dose of 5 mg

Do Not Confuse

sildenafil *with* **avanafil, tadalafil, or vardenafil**

All four of these drugs are used to treat ED. Be sure to double-check that you are giving the prescribed drug.

QSEN: Safety

Common Side Effects

Drugs for Erectile Dysfunction

Headache

Abdominal discomfort

Muscle aches

Nasal congestion

Flushing

Postural hypotension

Critical Point for Safety

PDE-5 drugs for ED should not be taken at the same time as nitrate drugs because of the danger of extremely low blood pressure. Angina (chest pain) or heart attack (myocardial infarction) can occur.

QSEN: Safety

Intended responses of drugs for ED
- Ability to have an erection
- Ability to maintain an erection
- Increased interest in sexual intercourse

Common side effects of drugs for erectile dysfunction. Common side effects of PDE-5 drugs include acid reflux, heartburn, indigestion, diarrhea, nasal congestion, flushing of the skin, bloody nose, headache, and muscle aches. Patients may experience changes in vision, hearing, or postural hypotension, but these are not common.

Use of avanafil may also cause stuffy or runny nose, sore throat, or back pain.

Possible adverse effects of drugs for erectile dysfunction. PDE-5 drugs may cause prolonged erections lasting more than 4 hours. *Priapism* (painful erections lasting more than 6 hours) can occur but is rare. Tadalafil may cause nephrotoxicity, neurotoxicity, or pleural effusions. If these drugs are taken with nitrate drugs, angina (chest pain) or heart attack (MI) can occur. These drugs are not recommended for use when male patients have underlying cardiovascular conditions, or for men for whom sexual activity is inadvisable due to cardiovascular issues (e.g., heart attack, stroke, life-threatening dysrhythmias, heart failure, hypotension [blood pressure less than 90/50 mm Hg], hypertension [blood pressure greater than 170/100 mm Hg]).

⭐ *Priority actions to take* before *giving drugs for erectile dysfunction.* Ask patients about cardiovascular problems, including angina, and about BPH. Check laboratory

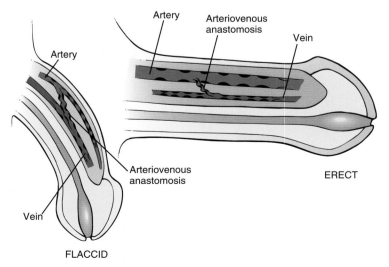

FIG. 28.3 The normal erection process. (From Swartz, M. [2015]. *Textbook of physical diagnoses: History and examination.* St. Louis: Elsevier.)

test results for kidney and liver function. Contact the prescriber if the patient is taking a nitrate drug because giving the two drugs together may result in severe hypotension.

Check baseline heart rate, blood pressure, and oxygen saturation. Assess cardiovascular status. Ask about current medications (these drugs are contraindicated for patients using any form of nitrate drug because extreme low blood pressure can occur) and herbal preparation use (St. John's wort may decrease the concentration of the drugs). Patients taking alpha-adrenergic blockers with these drugs may also experience hypotension.

⭐ *Priority actions to take after giving drugs for erectile dysfunction.* Continue to monitor patients' heart rate, blood pressure, and oxygen saturation. Ask patients about any vision or hearing changes. Assess patients for intended or side effects such as headache, flushing, and gastrointestinal upset. Instruct them to report prolonged or painful erections.

Give acetaminophen (if ordered) for headache relief.

⭐ *Teaching priorities for patients taking drugs for erectile dysfunction.* Use these teaching points and precautions:

- Remember that these drugs have no effect without sexual stimulation.
- Notify your prescriber immediately for an erection that lasts longer than 4 hours or if you experience priapism (prolonged painful erections).
- Report any sudden loss of vision or hearing to the prescriber.
- Take the drugs 15 minutes to an hour before anticipated sexual activity. The action of avanofil, sildenafil, and tadalafil lasts about 4 hours, and the action of tadalafil lasts up to 36 hours.
- Avoid the use of nitrate drugs while taking these drugs because this combination of drugs may cause severe hypotension.
- Using correct techniques, monitor your blood pressure and heart rate daily and keep a record of the results.
- Avoid alcohol while taking these drugs because it increases the risk of orthostatic hypotension.
- Avoid using the herbal preparation St. John's wort because it can decrease the concentration and effect of these drugs.
- If you are overweight, consider a weight loss program because being overweight can worsen ED.
- Include exercise in your daily routine because it will help with weight loss, increasing blood flow, and decreasing stress.
- Avoid grapefruit and grapefruit juice because it may increase the concentration of the drugs and cause toxicity.
- Remember that high-fat meals may delay the maximum effectiveness of these drugs.
- Get up slowly when rising from a lying or sitting position because of side effects such as dizziness, light-headedness, or hypotension.

Drug Alert

Administration Alert

Patients prescribed a drug for erectile dysfunction should not take the herbal preparation St. John's wort because it can decrease the concentration and effect of these drugs.

QSEN: Safety

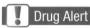

Drug Alert

Teaching Alert

Teach patients to report prolonged or painful erections to the prescriber.

QSEN: Safety

Drug Alert

Teaching Alert

Teach patients to take drugs for erectile dysfunction 15 min to an hour before anticipated sexual activity.

QSEN: Safety

Drug Alert

Teaching Alert

Teach patients to avoid alcohol while taking drugs for ED because of increased risk for orthostatic hypotension.

QSEN: Safety

Get Ready for the NCLEX® Examination!

Key Points

- As men age, testosterone levels decrease but the number of testosterone receptors in the prostate increases.
- An enlarged prostate squeezes the urethra, narrowing it and decreasing urine flow from the bladder.
- Because BPH and prostate cancer have similar symptoms, all men being treated for BPH should be screened for prostate cancer annually.
- Women who are pregnant, may become pregnant, or are breastfeeding should neither take DHT inhibitors nor handle these drugs if the tablet or capsule is crushed or broken.

- Orthostatic hypotension may occur with selective alpha-1 blocker therapy, especially with the first dose.
- A patient who has an allergy to sulfa drugs may also have an allergy to tamsulosin.
- Alpha-1 blockers interact with many drugs and herbal supplements. Before giving an alpha-1 blocker, ask the patient about all other drugs or supplements he takes and then check with the pharmacist to avoid a possible drug interaction.
- Remind men taking DHT inhibitors that it may take 3 to 6 months of therapy before the prostate shrinks and symptoms improve.

- Instruct patients who take a DHT inhibitor with saw palmetto (*Serenoa repens*) or soy isoflavones to notify the prescriber if any unusual side effects occur.
- Testosterone replacement methods include IM, subcutaneous, patch, and gel.
- Teach patients prescribed drugs for BPH to schedule annual prostate cancer screening.
- Be sure that patients receive prostate cancer screening before beginning testosterone replacement therapy.
- Men with a history of prostate or breast cancer should not receive testosterone replacement therapy.
- Report weight gain of 5 pounds or more in a week with testosterone replacement because this indicates fluid retention.
- Family members should avoid touching skin, clothing, or linens that have been in contact with testosterone preparations.
- Drugs for erectile dysfunction require sexual stimulation to work.
- Report any prolonged or painful erections to the prescriber immediately.
- Drugs for erectile dysfunction should not be taken with nitrate drugs or alcohol because of the increased risk for severe hypotension.

- Patients prescribed a drug for erectile dysfunction should not take the herbal preparation St. John's wort because it can decrease the concentration and effect of these drugs.
- Drugs for erectile dysfunction also may be used to treat pulmonary artery hypertension and some forms of pulmonary fibrosis.
- Teach patients to take drugs for erectile dysfunction 15–30 minutes to an hour before anticipated sexual activity and teach them that achieving an erection requires sexual stimulation.
- Teach patients to report erections that last longer than 4 hr or are painful to their prescriber.

Additional Learning Resources

Be sure to visit your Evolve website (http://evolve.elsevier.com/Workman/pharmacology/) for additional online resources.

SG Go to your Study Guide for additional learning activities to help you master this chapter content.

Review Questions

See *Answers to In-Text Review Questions* in the back of the book for answers to these questions.

1. **How do DHT inhibitors work to reduce benign prostatic hyperplasia?**

   A. Relaxing the muscles of the bladder
   B. Increasing urine production
   C. Shrinking the prostate gland
   D. Relaxing prostate smooth muscle

2. **When a patient with benign prostatic hyperplasia (BPH) is prescribed a selective alpha-1 blocker drug, for which side effect will the nurse monitor to prevent harm?**

   A. Low blood pressure
   B. Male-pattern baldness
   C. Erectile dysfunction
   D. Urinary retention

3. **An 82-year-old-man is prescribed a dihydrotestosterone (DHT) inhibitor to treat benign prostatic hyperplasia (BPH). Which health promotion activity is most important for the nurse to teach this patient to prevent harm?**

   A. Have vision and glaucoma checks yearly.
   B. Participate in yearly prostate cancer screening.
   C. Avoid both alcohol and caffeine while on the drug.
   D. Avoid donating blood when taking the drug and for at least 6 months after drug therapy.

4. **A patient taking tamsulosin asks how the drug works. What is the nurse's best response?**

   A. "This drug works on your prostate gland to decrease its size."
   B. "This drug signals the cells in your prostate gland not to grow."
   C. "This drug works by relaxing the detrusor muscle of your bladder."

   D. "This drug relaxes the muscle around your urethra to improve urine flow."

5. **For which intended response will the nurse assess when a patient is prescribed 5 mg orally or finasteride each day?**

   A. Urine is less concentrated
   B. Urine flow from urethra improves
   C. Nocturia increases
   D. Bladder empties incompletely

6. **For which patient will the nurse question an order for the dutasteride 0.5 mg orally once daily?**

   A. 55-year-old male with chronic obstructive pulmonary disease (COPD)
   B. 63-year-old male with gastroesophageal reflux disease (GERD)
   C. 71-year-old male with liver disease (hepatotoxicity)
   D. 82-year-old male with kidney disease (nephrotoxicity)

7. **A patient is prescribed the testosterone patch 4 mg/day applied to the upper body once daily at night. Which side effect(s) will the nurse teach the patient may occur?**

   A. Itching and redness at the application site
   B. Acne and dry skin in the genital region
   C. Increased ease with starting urine stream
   D. Increased testicular size

8. **A 58-year-old male prescribed testosterone replacement is married to a 34-year-old woman who is expecting their first child. What safety measure would the nurse teach the patient and his wife to prevent harm?**

   A. "Avoid having sex with your wife any time during the pregnancy."
   B. "Do not touch linens that have been in contact with your husband's testosterone gel."

C. "Never enter the bathroom while your husband is applying the testosterone gel."

D. "Avoid high protein containing foods because they can interact with the testosterone gel."

9. The patient prescribed sildenafil tells the nurse that he has a painful erection that has lasted almost 7 hours. What is the nurse's best action?

A. Instructing the patient to think of a quiet, peaceful place so the erection will subside.

B. Telling the patient to get up and take a cool shower until the erection subsides.

C. Contacting the pharmacy to send an antidote for this drug.

D. Notifying the prescriber about the length of time and the pain associated with the erection.

10. A patient is prescribed testosterone 100 mg IM every 4 weeks. What finding will the nurse teach the patient to report to the prescriber **immediately**?

A. Blood pressure decrease of 10 mm Hg systolic

B. Urine output increase of 200 mL/day

C. Weight gain of 5 pounds

D. Increased penile size

11. Which patient will the nurse caution to avoid handling a DHT inhibitor drug?

A. 55-year-old woman who is postmenopausal

B. 25-year-old woman who is 3 months pregnant

C. 35-year-old man whose sister is 5 months pregnant

D. 45-year-old man who has diabetes and hypertension

12. A patient is prescribed testosterone 250 mg IM every 3 weeks. Testosterone is available as 100 mg/1 mL. How many mL will the nurse give with each dose?

A. 1.5 mL

B. 2.0 mL

C. 2.5 mL

D. 3.0 mL

Clinical Judgment

1. Which signs and symptoms will the nurse assess for when a patient is diagnosed with benign prostatic hyperplasia (BPH)? **Select all that apply.**

A. Burning with urination

B. Frequency of urination

C. Decreased urination at night

D. Difficulty starting and continuing urination

E. Increased force and size of urine stream

F. Dribbling after urination

G. Feeling of incomplete bladder emptying

H. Pale yellow color of urine

I. Inadequate sleep and rest

J. Increased thirst

2. The patient is a 44-year-old married male who visits his primary health care provider's office reporting decreased sexual desire as well as difficulty achieving and maintaining an erection. His health history includes hypertension, obesity, and type 2 diabetes. The health care provider diagnoses erectile dysfunction (ED) and after discussion with the patient, prescribes sildenafil, 50 mg. The nurse prepares a teaching plan for the patient. Use an X to indicate which instructions are Relevant, Not Relevant, or Potentially Harmful for this patient.

INSTRUCTION	RELEVANT	NOT RELEVANT	POTENTIALLY HARMFUL
Take your sildenafil at least 2 hours before anticipated sexual activity.			
If you are prescribed a nitrate drug, be sure to have at least 2 hours between taking sildenafil and your nitrate.			
The drug will not work without sexual stimulation.			
Priapism is an expected side effect of sildenafil.			
Notify your prescriber if you experience an erection that lasts longer than 4 hours.			
A side effect while taking sildenafil is weight loss.			
Report any sudden loss of vision or hearing to the prescriber.			
Get up slowly when rising from a lying or sitting position.			
The action of sildenafil will last up to 36 hours.			
Be sure to eat grapefruit or drink grapefruit juice at least twice a week while taking sildenafil.			

Learning Objectives

The content presented in this chapter should help you to:

1. Explain the names, actions, usual dosages, possible side effects, and adverse effects of drugs for perimenopausal hormone replacement and hormonal contraceptives.
2. Prioritize essential information to teach patients taking perimenopausal hormone replacement drugs and hormonal contraceptives.
3. Explain the names, actions, usual dosages, possible side effects, and adverse effects of drugs for osteoporosis.

4. Explain priority actions to take before and after giving drugs for osteoporosis.
5. Prioritize essential information to teach patients taking drugs for osteoporosis.
6. Describe appropriate life span considerations of drugs for perimenopausal hormone replacement drugs, hormonal contraception, and osteoporosis.

Key Terms

bisphosphonates (BĬ-ō-FŌS-fō-nătz) (p. 528) A class of drugs known as calcium-modifying drugs that both prevent bones from losing calcium and increase bone density.

estrogen (ĔS-trō-jĕn) (p. 520) The main female sex hormone secreted by the ovaries and adrenal glands.

estrogen agonists/antagonists (ĔS-trō-jĕn ĂG-ŏ-nĭsts/ăn-TĂG-ŏ-nĭsts) (p. 530) Hormone receptor drugs that selectively bind to and activate estrogen receptors in some tissues and bind to and block estrogen receptors in other tissues.

follicle-stimulating hormone (FŎL-ĭ-kŭl STĬM-yū-lā-tĭng HŌR-mōn) (p. 521) A hormone secreted by the pituitary gland that

causes the ovary to secrete estrogen and allows one ovum each month to complete maturation.

hormonal contraception (hŏr-MŌN-ŭl kŏn-tră-SĔP-shŭn) (p. 525) The use of hormone-based drugs that suppress ovulation and prevent pregnancy.

progesterone (prō-JĔS-tŭr-ōn) (p. 521) The female hormone that supports pregnancy by maintaining the thickened uterine lining.

sclerostin antagonists (skle-ROS-tĕn ăn-TĂG-ŏ-nĭsts) (p. 530) Drugs composed of antibodies directed against immature osteoclasts.

REVIEW OF RELATED PHYSIOLOGY FOR FEMALE HORMONE FUNCTION

The secretion of female hormones changes during adolescence and continues throughout a woman's menstruating years to promote conception and pregnancy. Conception occurs when a mature egg (*ovum*) is released from a woman's ovary and is fertilized by a sperm (*spermatozoon*) during sexual intercourse. When the fertilized egg then successfully implants in the uterus, the condition of pregnancy results, and an infant may be born 9 months later. The maturation of an egg and proper preparation of the uterine lining to support pregnancy depend on the presence and timing of specific hormones.

MENARCHE

Menarche is the beginning of the years of menstruation in an adolescent female. *Menstruation* is the periodic shedding of the uterine lining that occurs as a result of the cyclic changes in hormone levels in females after menarche (Animation 29.1). The onset of menarche occurs as a result of the secretion of *gonadotropin-releasing hormone (GnRH)* in the brain. This hormone starts to be secreted in both females and males at the beginning of puberty so that sex hormone secretion can occur and cause the physical changes leading to an interest in sexual activity (*libido*) and the ability to perform sexual intercourse. **Estrogen** is the main female sex hormone secreted by the ovaries and adrenal glands.

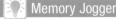
Memory Jogger

GnRH is secreted by the hypothalamus of both males and females to start the hormone changes needed for puberty. In females, this hormone is secreted cyclically throughout the menstruating years.

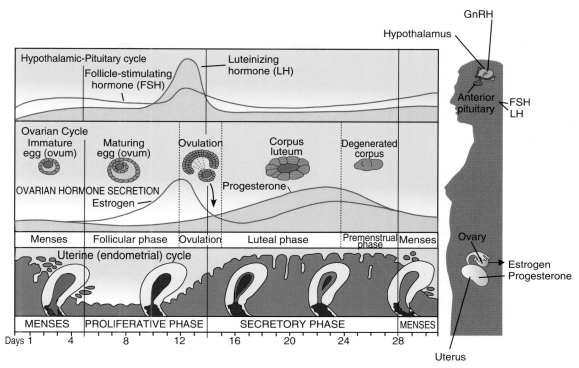

FIG. 29.1 Hormone interactions for ovulation and menstruation. GnRH, Gonadotropin-releasing hormone.

In females, the secretion of GnRH stimulates the release of two hormones from the pituitary gland: *follicle-stimulating hormone* and *luteinizing hormone* (Fig. 29.1). (The role of GnRH in males is discussed in Chapter 28.) **Follicle-stimulating hormone (FSH)** causes the ovary to secrete estrogen and allows one ovum in the ovary to complete maturation each month. As estrogen levels rise in the blood, the lining of the uterus grows and thickens (see Fig. 29.1). After about 14 days of lining growth, it is thick enough to support the implantation of a fertilized egg. At this optimal midcycle time, GnRH triggers the pituitary gland to release *luteinizing hormone (LH)*, which causes secretion of progesterone by the ovary and allows *ovulation*, the release of a mature ovum. The outer covering (*corpus luteum*) from the released ovum also secretes progesterone.

Progesterone supports any pregnancy that occurs by maintaining the thickened uterine lining and allowing it to secrete nutrients needed by the early embryo. If fertilization and pregnancy do not occur, the outer covering from the released ovum degenerates in about 12 days, and circulating levels of estrogen and progesterone drop. Decreased secretion of these hormones allows the lining of the uterus to stop growing and to shed as menstruation. Fig. 29.2 shows the feedback loops controlling the secretion of estrogen and progesterone.

When the mature ovum is fertilized by a sperm, the outer covering from the released ovum continues to grow and secrete both estrogen and progesterone. Together these hormones keep the uterine lining thickened and secreting nutrients to support a pregnancy until the placenta takes over these functions for the rest of the pregnancy. So, pregnancy depends first on conception, in which a mature ovum is released from the ovary and fertilized by a sperm. Then, within 5 to 8 days, the fertilized ovum must implant itself into the prepared uterine lining.

MENOPAUSE

Menopause is the cessation of menstrual periods and ovulation. Natural menopause occurs as a result of age-related changes in the ovary in which glandular cells shrink and become nonfunctional, a process called *involution*. The ovaries become smaller

 Memory Jogger

Estrogen causes the uterine lining to thicken during the first half of the menstrual cycle. Progesterone maintains the lining and causes it to secrete nutrients during the second half of the cycle. The drop in the level of these hormones allows menstruation to occur.

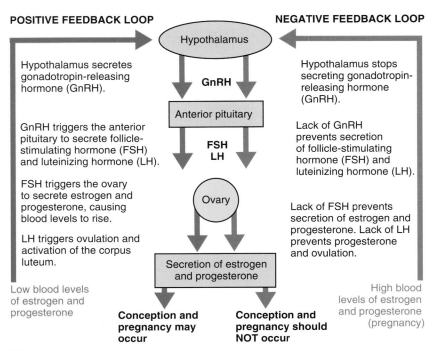

POSITIVE FEEDBACK LOOP

Hypothalamus secretes gonadotropin-releasing hormone (GnRH).

GnRH triggers the anterior pituitary to secrete follicle-stimulating hormone (FSH) and luteinizing hormone (LH).

FSH triggers the ovary to secrete estrogen and progesterone, causing blood levels to rise.

LH triggers ovulation and activation of the corpus luteum.

Low blood levels of estrogen and progesterone

Conception and pregnancy may occur

NEGATIVE FEEDBACK LOOP

Hypothalamus stops secreting gonadotropin-releasing hormone (GnRH).

Lack of GnRH prevents secretion of follicle-stimulating hormone (FSH) and luteinizing hormone (LH).

Lack of FSH prevents secretion of estrogen and progesterone. Lack of LH prevents progesterone and ovulation.

High blood levels of estrogen and progesterone (pregnancy)

Conception and pregnancy should NOT occur

Hypothalamus — GnRH — Anterior pituitary — FSH LH — Ovary — Secretion of estrogen and progesterone

FIG. 29.2 Positive and negative feedback control over estrogen and progesterone secretion.

and can no longer respond to the hypothalamic and pituitary hormones by secreting estrogen and releasing mature eggs. Natural menopause occurs gradually, over months to years. (Menopause caused by surgery or drug therapy can be sudden.)

Perimenopause is the transition in a woman from having regular hormone cycles with menstrual periods to the time when menstrual periods have stopped for a full year. During this time, hormone levels change, causing the woman to have a variety of uncomfortable but usually minor symptoms.

When the glandular cells of the ovary shrink, they no longer produce normal levels of estrogen. The decreased blood levels of estrogen trigger the brain to secrete GnRH, which then triggers the pituitary gland to secrete FSH (see Fig. 29.2). Before menopause, the FSH acts on the ovary and causes ovarian cells to secret estrogen, which then inhibits the pathway through negative feedback. With nonfunctional ovarian cells unable to respond to FSH by increasing estrogen secretion, this pathway is disrupted. For a time, the continued low blood levels of estrogen constantly stimulate the hypothalamus to secret GnRH in large amounts, resulting in the secretion of very large amounts of FSH (Fig. 29.3). This extra FSH is useless because the ovary cannot respond to it, and it has effects on other body tissues. Box 29.1 lists the symptoms associated with decreased estrogen levels and increased FSH levels.

High levels of FSH act on blood vessels, making them dilate suddenly, resulting in the woman experiencing sudden whole-body flushes and radiant heat. These are commonly called *hot flashes* or *hot flushes*. At night, these flushes are often followed by excessive sweating that leaves nightclothes and bedding wet.

Perimenopausal Hormone Replacement Therapy (HRT)

Hormone replacement therapy (HRT) is the replacement of naturally secreted estrogen and progesterone with exogenous forms of these hormones during the perimenopausal period. HRT is used by some women to relieve the intensity of perimenopausal symptoms and reduce the risk for health problems associated with low or absent hormone levels. It is not the intention of this therapy to prevent or "fix" menopause. There are several natural estrogens used in HRT, including conjugated estrogen and estradiol. Both natural progesterone and synthetic forms (progestin) may be used alone for HRT or in combination with estrogens. In addition, a variety

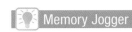

Memory Jogger

Menopause symptoms are caused by *low* levels of estrogen and *high* levels of FSH.

Positive but ineffective feedback loop

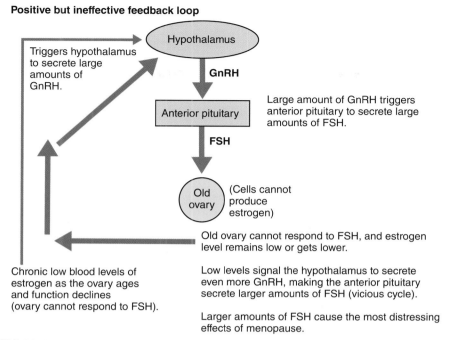

FIG. 29.3 Mechanism for hot flushes and night sweats associated with menopause. FSH, Follicle-stimulating hormone; GnRH, gonadotropin-releasing hormone.

of non-hormone drugs may be used to assist the patient to feel better during this time, such as antidepressants, gabapentin, and oxybutynin, among others. This chapter focuses on drugs for hormone replacement therapy.

For women who have a uterus, either an estrogen and progesterone combination or a progesterone-only drug is usually prescribed to avoid excessive build-up of the uterine lining and excessive uterine bleeding. For women who have had a hysterectomy, estrogen-alone drugs are often prescribed because there is no risk for excessive bleeding.

Replacement hormones are available as tablets or capsules, injections, patches, gels, transdermal sprays, skin creams, and vaginal creams. The type and amount of HRT drugs used depend on the degree of patient discomfort with perimenopausal symptoms, whether or not the woman still has her uterus, and overall patient health and health risks. (Remember, menopause is a normal physiologic state and not all women choose to participate in HRT.) The table below lists common oral HRT drugs. Dosages and schedules vary from person to person. Consult a reliable drug reference source for dosing and scheduling information.

Common Drugs for Oral Perimenopausal Hormone Replacement Therapy

Hormone Contents	Drug Names
Estrogen-only	conjugated estrogens (Cenestin, Enjuvia, Premarin) estradiol (Estrace) estradiol acetate (Femtrace) esterified estrogen (Menset) estropipate (Ortho-Est)
Progestin-only	medroxyprogesterone (Provera) micronized progesterone (Prometrium)
Combination estrogen/ progesterone	drospirenone/estradiol (Angeliq) estradiol/norethindrone (Activella, Femhrt) estradiol/norgestimate (Prefest) estradiol/progesterone (Bijuva) conjugated estrogen/medroxyprogesterone (Prempro)

Box **29.1** Common Perimenopausal Symptoms

Symptoms from Low Estrogen Levels	Symptoms from High FSH Levels
Atrophy of vaginal tissue	Decreased mental concentration
Dry skin	Hot flushes
Increased rate of osteoporosis	Night sweats
Painful intercourse	Sleep difficulties
Reduced cervical mucus	

How perimenopausal HRT works. HRT replaces naturally secreted estrogen and progesterone with exogenous hormones. Providing low doses of estrogen increases blood estrogen levels, which helps with perimenopausal symptoms in two ways. First, it relieves the direct problems of low estrogen levels (see Box 29.1). Second, it also inhibits the feedback system and lowers the levels of FSH. This reduces the side effects of high FSH levels (see Box 29.1).

Intended responses of perimenopausal HRT
- The number and severity of hot flushes and night sweats are reduced.
- Vaginal dryness is reduced.
- Patient's quality of sleep is increased.

Common side effects of perimenopausal HRT. Common side effects of perimenopausal HRT include breast tenderness, breakthrough bleeding, fluid retention, weight gain, and acne. These occur with conjugated estrogen alone and when estrogen is combined with progesterone.

Possible adverse effects of perimenopausal HRT. Recent studies indicate that women taking estrogen-based HRT have a slightly higher incidence of myocardial infarction (heart attack). For this reason, estrogen-based HRT is not recommended for long-term therapy, just to help reduce symptoms during the first year of perimenopause.

Drugs for perimenopausal HRT increase blood clotting, placing the patient at risk for thrombosis and emboli. Cigarette smoking and nicotine vaping worsen this risk. Results of increased clot formation include increased risks for heart attack, stroke, pulmonary embolism, and deep vein thrombosis.

The hormones in perimenopausal HRT can increase the growth of cancers that are hormone sensitive such as cervical, breast, ovarian, and uterine cancers. These drugs should not be used in women who have a history of these types of cancer. These hormones are metabolized by the liver and increase the risk for liver impairment, gallbladder disease, and pancreatitis.

HRT drugs that contain drospirenone as the progestin can increase the serum potassium level (normal levels 3.5 to 5.0 mEq/L or mmol/L), leading to hyperkalemia. When severe, it can cause complete heart block and other life-threatening irregular heart rhythms. This drug combination should be avoided in women who have kidney, liver, or adrenal disease and in those who are taking other drugs that increase potassium levels (e.g., angiotensin-converting enzyme [ACE] inhibitors for hypertension, potassium-sparing diuretics).

⭐ *Teaching priorities for women taking perimenopausal HRT*
- Take your prescribed perimenopausal HRT drugs exactly as prescribed with regard to dosage and timing, because taking them more often than prescribed or not following instructions for timing increases the risk for excessive uterine bleeding.
- Avoid using nicotine in any form, including smoking, vaping, nicotine patches, or gum. Nicotine increases your risk for blood clot formation leading to serious health problems such as stroke and heart attack.
- Check yourself weekly for any yellowing of your skin, the roof of your mouth, and the whites of your eyes. These are symptoms of possible liver problems and HRT can increase the risk for liver problems.

Common Side Effects
Perimenopausal HRT

Breast tenderness

Fluid retention

Weight gain

Acne

✦ Critical Point for Safety

Perimenopausal HRT increases the risk for blood clot formation leading to pulmonary embolism, heart attacks, strokes, and other problems. Nicotine use in **any** form, including vaping, increases this risk. Emphasize to patients prescribed HRT to avoid nicotine in any form.

QSEN: Safety

- If you develop chest pain, difficulty breathing, facial drooping, garbled speech, or any symptom of a stroke, call 911 immediately.
- If you develop swelling in one leg, notify your prescriber immediately.
- If you think you have become pregnant while using HRT, contact your prescriber immediately. Hormones can adversely affect pregnancy.

CONTRACEPTION

In the United States, the age when females begin menarche (start menstruating) and can become pregnant may be as young as 9 years. Although sexual maturity is often early, social maturity is considerably later. Many people prefer to delay or prevent pregnancy while still engaging in sexual intercourse.

Contraception is the intentional prevention of pregnancy. Many methods are used to prevent pregnancy. The most reliable method is completely abstaining from sexual intercourse, which is not a reasonable choice for many people. Other forms of contraception include surgery, barrier methods, spermicidal foams and gels, and intrauterine devices. Specific hormone-based drugs can be highly effective at preventing conception and pregnancy.

Types of Drugs for Hormonal Contraception

Hormonal contraception is the use of hormones that suppress ovulation and prevent pregnancy. It is highly effective when used correctly. The hormones that prevent conception and pregnancy can be taken orally; used as topical applications in the form of transdermal patches, uterine rings, and some intrauterine devices; implanted under the skin; and injected parenterally as a slow-absorbing drug form. The most commonly used form of hormonal contraception is the oral contraceptive. *Oral contraceptives* (OCs) (often called birth control pills or BCPs) are hormone-based drugs taken orally that are generally effective in preventing pregnancy. Regardless of the form of hormonal contraception used, the mechanism of action and side effects are the same.

 Memory Jogger

Regardless of how hormonal contraception drugs are delivered, the mechanism of action and side effects are the same.

How hormonal contraceptives work. As described earlier in the chapter, the control of natural estrogen and progesterone secretion is through a "feedback" system of the hormone pathway that includes the hypothalamus, the pituitary gland, and the ovary (see Figure 29.2). Oral contraceptives interfere with the body's natural production of estrogen and progesterone by "turning off" the tissues in the pathway through negative feedback (see Figure 29.2). The most effective oral contraceptives contain two types of hormones, synthetic estrogen and a synthetic type of progesterone known as progestin. When a woman consistently takes this hormone combination, the blood levels of estrogen and progesterone are high, which sends signals to the hypothalamus that secretion of these hormones is not needed. Thus, GnRH secretion is inhibited. Without GnRH, the anterior pituitary does not secrete FSH and LH. Without FSH and LH, the ovary does not produce more estrogen or progesterone. Without this influence, ovulation does not occur, and the lining of the uterus stays thin, unable to support a pregnancy. In a sense, oral contraceptives fool the endocrine system by mimicking pregnancy hormones. This "feeds back" to the hypothalamus, signaling that further hormone production is not needed.

 Memory Jogger

Hormonal contraceptives fool the endocrine system into not secreting estrogen and progesterone by mimicking pregnancy hormones.

Some oral contraceptives contain only progestin rather than a combination of estrogen and progestin. These are known as "mini-pills" and raise blood levels of progesterone, causing the hormone pathway to be turned off through negative feedback. The exact mechanism by which the surge of LH and ovulation are prevented is not known. However, in addition to suppressing ovulation, other changes occur that prevent pregnancy. These changes include thickening of the cervical mucus, which prevents movement of sperm into the uterus, and changing of the endometrium so that a pregnancy is not supported. These progestin-only oral contraceptives are usually taken daily and continuously. The specific drugs in combination and their dosages vary, as does the dosing schedule. Be sure to consult a drug handbook for specific dosages and scheduling of any oral contraceptive.

Intended responses of hormonal contraceptives
- Suppression of ovum maturation
- Suppression of ovulation
- No conception and pregnancy

Common side effects of hormonal contraceptives. Common side effects of oral contraceptives include breast enlargement and tenderness, nausea, fluid retention, weight gain, and breakthrough bleeding. The severity of side effects is related to the dosage of the specific hormones used for contraception. Some women have more acne while taking oral contraceptives and others have less acne.

Possible adverse effects of hormonal contraceptives. Oral contraceptives increase the risk for blood clots that can cause deep vein thrombosis, pulmonary embolism, myocardial infection, and stroke, especially among women who use nicotine in any form. This risk is greater in women older than 35 years.

Most oral contraceptives (and other hormonal contraceptives) cause some degree of fluid and sodium retention, leading to hypertension. Women with moderate to severe hypertension should not use hormonal contraceptives.

Estrogen and progestin are metabolized by the liver and can cause liver toxicity. The patient with liver toxicity has elevated liver enzymes, yellowing of the skin and whites of the eyes, tiredness, dark urine, pale or clay-colored stools, and nausea. Women with known liver problems should not use hormonal contraceptives.

The synthetic hormones in oral contraceptives and other hormonal contraceptives can increase the growth rate of cancer cells sensitive to the presence of hormones. Such cancers include cervical, breast, uterine, and ovarian cancers. Hormonal contraceptives should not be used by women who have or who have had any of these cancers.

The oral contraceptives that use drospirenone as the progestin can increase the serum potassium level (normal levels 3.5 to 5.0 mEq/L or mmol/L), leading to hyperkalemia. When severe, it can cause complete heart block and other life-threatening irregular heart rhythms. This drug combination should be avoided in women who have kidney, liver, or adrenal disease and in those who are taking other drugs that increase potassium levels (e.g., angiotensin-converting enzyme [ACE] inhibitors for hypertension, potassium-sparing diuretics).

⭐ **Teaching priorities for women taking normonal contraceptives**
- Be sure to use an additional method of contraception during the first cycle of oral contraceptives because they require a full cycle before they are effective.
- Check the recommended scheduling of the specific contraceptive you have been prescribed. The scheduling is important for best effectiveness. Take the drugs according to the recommended schedule to prevent an unplanned pregnancy.
- Take your prescribed oral contraceptive with food once daily. The drug works best for contraception if you take it at the same time each day.
- Do not take more than one dose per day.
- These drugs increase your risk for developing blood clots that could lead to stroke, heart attack, and other serious health problems, especially among women who use nicotine-containing products. It is critical to avoid using nicotine in any form, including smoking, vaping, and using nicotine gum or patches.
- If one dose is missed within the cycle, the drug should still be effective in preventing pregnancy. However, if more than one dose is missed within a cycle, especially if two doses in a row are missed, continue to use it for the rest of the cycle and also use another method of contraception for the rest of the cycle.
- Be sure to tell all your health care providers that you are using hormonal contraceptives because of the possibility for drug interactions. Also, do not take any over-the-counter drug without checking with your health care provider who prescribed the contraceptive.
- If you develop yellowing of the skin or eyes, darkening of the urine, or lightening of the stools, notify your prescriber immediately because these problems are signs of liver toxicity, a serious complication of hormonal contraceptives.

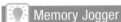

Common Side Effects
Hormonal Contraceptives

Nausea   Weight gain   Breast tenderness

💡 **Memory Jogger**

The most serious adverse effect of hormonal contraceptives is the formation of blood clots that could lead to deep vein thrombosis, myocardial infarction, pulmonary embolism, and stroke.

❗ **Drug Alert**
Interaction Alert

Oral contraceptives interact with many drugs and herbal supplements. Ask the patient about all other drugs she takes, including prescribed drugs and over-the-counter drugs or supplements. Check with the pharmacist to avoid a possible drug interaction or a reduction of contraceptive effectiveness.

QSEN: Safety

❗ **Drug Alert**
Teaching Alert

Remind women that oral contraceptives are only effective at preventing pregnancy when taken exactly as prescribed.

QSEN: Safety

- If you think you have become pregnant while using a hormonal contraceptive, contact your prescriber immediately. Hormones can adversely affect pregnancy.
- Remember that although hormonal contraceptives protect against pregnancy, they provide no protection against HIV and other sexually transmitted diseases. Condom use is needed to protect against contracting these infections.

REVIEW OF RELATED PHYSIOLOGY AND PATHOPHYSIOLOGY FOR OSTEOPOROSIS

NORMAL BONE MAINTENANCE

For good skeletal support and mobility, bones must remain strong throughout the life span by staying firm and dense. So, even though bones do not get longer after puberty and during adulthood, they do continue to grow throughout the life span. Bone formation with the removal of old bone cells (osteocytes) and replacement with new bone cells occurs throughout life. The process of old bone cell removal is *osteoclastic activity*. Osteoclastic activity also causes bones to lose minerals, especially calcium *(bone resorption of calcium)*. Replacement with new bone cells is *osteoblastic activity*.

In infancy, childhood, and adolescence, osteoblastic activity occurs at a faster rate than osteoclastic activity. This results in bones becoming longer as the person grows taller, and becoming denser to support body structures as the person grows heavier. In addition to bone cells, minerals such as calcium and phosphorus deposit and form a matrix within the bone to add density and strength. Osteoblastic activity and hormones contribute to the deposition and retention of these minerals, as does weight-bearing.

In adulthood, when osteoblastic activity and osteoclastic activity are balanced, bone does not become longer or thicker but does maintain its density. As older cells are removed, they are replaced with new cells, and minerals are retained in the matrix for bone strength.

OSTEOPOROSIS

With aging, osteoblastic activity can slow down. If osteoclastic activity then continues at a normal or faster rate, bone formation becomes unbalanced with bone cell removal occurring faster than bone cell replacement. This results in thinner, more fragile bones that can break easily even without trauma. When osteoclastic activity outstrips osteoblastic activity, bone mineral loss also reduces bone density (Animation 29.2).

Imbalanced bone metabolism is osteopenia. When *osteopenia* becomes more severe and bone density is lost, *osteoporosis* is present. All older people have some degree of osteopenia as a result of normal aging. However, osteoporosis occurs to a greater degree and at earlier ages among people who have a smaller stature (women more than men), those who have a strong family history of the problem, those who smoke, those who are taking corticosteroids on a daily basis, those who have lower levels of androgens (men) or lower levels of estrogen (women), and those who do not participate in sufficient weight-bearing activity. (Weight-bearing activity involves the direct use of the legs, such as walking, dancing, running, and performing resistance exercises of the lower body.) Along with age, body size, and gender, the risk for osteoporosis varies with race, ethnicity, and family history. Those at greatest risk for osteoporosis are Asian Americans; African Americans have the lowest risk for it.

Many health problems are associated with osteoporosis. Foremost is the greatly increased risk for bone fractures and the resulting mobility limitations. However, other problems can occur when bone density decreases unevenly. Posture changes, and the person loses height as the spine bends forward, outward, or inward (Fig. 29.4). These changes can limit lung expansion and lead to pulmonary problems.

TYPES OF DRUGS TO MANAGE OR SLOW OSTEOPOROSIS

In addition to ensuring adequate intake of vitamins and minerals, especially activated vitamin D (calciferol), calcium, and magnesium, a variety of different types of drugs are used to manage or slow the progression of osteoporosis. These include

Drug Alert

Teaching Alert

Remind women that hormonal contraceptives provide no protection against HIV or any other sexually transmitted disease.

QSEN: Safety

Memory Jogger

Osteoclastic activity reduces bone density and strength whereas osteoblastic activity improves bone density and strength.

Memory Jogger

Osteoporosis occurs with aging, but the rate of progression varies as a result of many individual patient factors.

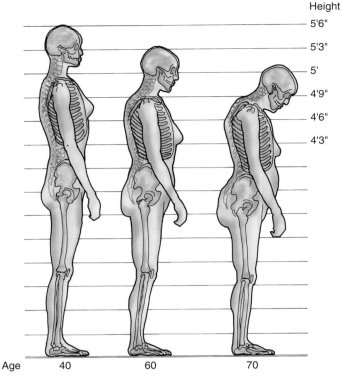

Height
- 5'6"
- 5'3"
- 5'
- 4'9"
- 4'6"
- 4'3"

Age 40   60   70

FIG. 29.4 A normal spine at age 40 years and osteoporotic changes at ages 60 and 70 years. (From Ignatavicius, D. D., & Workman, M. L. [2016]. *Medical-surgical nursing: Patient-centered collaborative care* [8th ed.]. St. Louis: Saunders.)

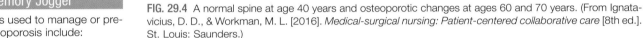

> **Memory Jogger**
>
> The drugs used to manage or prevent osteoporosis include:
> - Bisphosphonates
> - Estrogen agonists/antagonists
> - Biologics: RANKL inhibitors
> - Biologics: osteoblastic monoclonal antibodies
> - Biologics: parathyroid hormone (PTH) agonists

bisphosphonates, estrogen agonists/antagonists, and biologics, including RANKL inhibitors, osteoblastic monoclonal antibodies, and parathyroid hormone (PTH) agonists.

First-Line Therapy for Osteoporosis: Bisphosphonates

Bisphosphonates are a type of calcium-modifying drug that both prevents bones from losing calcium and increases bone density rather than just maintaining bone density. Drugs from this class are used as first-line therapy for osteoporosis. The major use of these drugs is the prevention and management of osteoporosis with a reduction of the risk for bone fractures, especially in women. They are less effective in preventing and managing osteoporosis in men.

The currently prescribed bisphosphonates are second- and third-generation drugs that contain nitrogen and are much more effective than the first-generation drugs. However, these drugs are only effective in adults who have an adequate intake of both calcium and vitamin D. For this reason, some formulations of the bisphosphonates also contain calcium and vitamin D. The following table presents adult dosages for the most commonly used bisphosphonates to prevent or treat osteoporosis. These drugs are not approved for use with children who have osteoporosis.

> **Do Not Confuse**
>
> **Fosamax** *with* **Flomax**
>
> An order for Fosamax can be confused with Flomax. Fosamax is a drug to manage or prevent osteoporosis and Flomax is a drug to improve urine flow for men with an enlarged prostate gland.
>
> QSEN: Safety

Adult Dosages of Common Bisphosphonates for Osteoporosis

Drug Name	Usual Maintenance Dosage
alendronate (Binosto, Fosamax)	10 mg orally once daily 35 mg orally once **weekly**
ibandronate (Boniva)	150 mg orally once **monthly** on the same date each month 3 mg IV (over 15–30 s) every 3 months

Drug Name	Usual Maintenance Dosage
risedronate (Actonel, Atelvia)	5 mg orally once daily or 35 mg orally once **weekly** or 150 mg orally once **monthly**
zoledronic acid (Reclast, Zometa)	5 mg IV infusion over at least 15 min, given once **yearly** for osteoporosis treatment; **every other year** for osteoporosis prophylaxis

How bisphosphonates work. Bisphosphonates all work by moving blood calcium into the bone, binding to calcium in the bone, and preventing osteoclasts from destroying bone cells and resorbing calcium. They also inhibit the activity of tumor necrosis factor (TNF) within bone, preventing certain white blood cells from damaging or destroying bone. It is not known exactly how bisphosphonates increase bone production.

Intended responses of bisphosphonates
- Progression of osteopenia to osteoporosis is slowed or stopped.
- Bones maintain density and strength.
- Blood calcium levels remain normal.
- Bone fractures do not occur.

Common side effects of bisphosphonates. The most common side effects of bisphosphonates are abdominal pain, headache, esophageal reflux, and nausea.

Possible adverse effects of bisphosphonates. The most serious adverse effect of bisphosphonates is the development of *jawbone osteonecrosis* (JON), especially with tooth extraction or other invasive dental procedures involving the jawbone in which the bone is damaged. The exact mechanism causing JON is not known but it is thought to occur because the drugs interfere with bone healing. It is more common in patients taking higher doses and with IV doses of the drugs.

The oral bisphosphonates are irritating to tissues they contact directly. This irritation is responsible for mouth ulcers, esophageal ulcers, and gastric ulcers. The tissue irritation can be reduced by taking the drugs with plenty of water and remaining in the upright position to reduce gastroesophageal reflux.

⭐ *Teaching priorities for patients taking bisphosphonates*
- For an oral bisphosphonate, take the drug early in the morning, right after breakfast, and drink a full glass of water with it to reduce the risk for irritation of your mouth, esophagus, and stomach.
- Remain in the upright position (sitting, standing, or walking) for at least 30 minutes after taking the oral drug to help ensure the drug does not remain in your esophagus and cause irritation and sores to form there.
- Be sure to inform your dentist or oral surgeon that you are taking a bisphosphonate before having a tooth extraction or any invasive dental procedure involving the jawbone.

Second-Line Drugs for Osteoporosis
A variety of newer classes of drugs are now available to prevent or manage osteoporosis. Although mechanisms of action and dosing schedules vary, all second-line drugs for osteoporosis require the patient to have adequate levels of calcium and activated vitamin D for drug effectiveness. The following table lists the adult dosages of common second-line therapy drugs for osteoporosis. These drugs are prescribed for patients whose osteoporosis is more severe, who have not shown improvement with first-line drugs, or who have not been able to tolerate first-line drugs, and for those who remain at high risk for bone fractures.

 ⇄ Do Not Confuse

Actonel *with* **Actos**

An order for Actonel (risedronate) can be confused with Actos. Actonel is a bisphosphonate drug to manage or prevent osteoporosis. Actos is an antidiabetic drug to control blood glucose.

QSEN: Safety

 Critical Point for Safety

Some bisphosphonates are taken daily; others are now given or taken on a weekly, monthly, or even yearly schedule. Ensure that you are giving and that patients are taking the proper dosage of these drugs for the prescribed schedule to prevent severe dosing errors.

QSEN: Safety

Common Side Effects

Bisphosphonates

Abdominal pain, Nausea   Headache

Adult Dosages of Second-Line Therapy for Osteoporosis

Drug Class	Drug Name	Usual Maintenance Dosage
Estrogen Agonists/Antagonists	raloxifene (Evista)	60 mg orally once daily
Biologics: RANKL Inhibitors	denosumab (Prolia, Xgeva)	Prolia: 60 mg subcutaneous injection once every 6 months
Biologics: Sclerostin Antagonists	romosozumab (Evenity)	210 mg subcutaneously once monthly for 12 months
Biologics: Parathyroid Hormone Agonists	abaloparatide (Tymlos)	80 mcg subcutaneously once daily for no more than 2 years
	teriparatide (Forteo)	20 mcg subcutaneously once daily for no more than 2 years

 Critical Point for Safety

All second-line drugs for osteoporosis require the patient to have adequate levels of calcium and activated vitamin D for drug effectiveness. These drugs have more side effects than do the first-line drugs. Unless the patient maintains adequate levels of calcium and vitamin D, these drugs have minimal effect and are not worth the risk for adverse effects.

QSEN: Safety

 Critical Point for Safety

All of the biologic drugs for osteoporosis are given subcutaneously. If the patient will be self-injecting these drugs after the first dose, teach her or him to use the techniques presented in Box 2.3 in Chapter 2 for safe administration into the abdominal area or the thigh.

QSEN: Safety

 Critical Point for Safety

Estrogen agonist/antagonist drugs increase the risk for blood clot formation leading to pulmonary embolism, heart attacks, strokes, and other problems. Nicotine use in **any** form, including vaping, increases this risk. Emphasize to patients prescribed an estrogen agonist/antagonist for osteoporosis to avoid nicotine in any form.

QSEN: Safety

How second-line drugs for osteoporosis work. Estrogen agonists/antagonists are hormone receptor drugs that selectively bind to and activate estrogen receptors in some tissues and bind to and block estrogen receptors in other tissues. When used together, these drugs selectively activate some estrogen receptors and block others, which provides a protective influence in preventing bone density loss with fewer of the problems associated with estrogen use after menopause.

RANKL inhibitors are monoclonal antibodies directed against a receptor that allows an activator (RANK) to bind with it. When RANK binds to its receptor, osteoclastic cells mature and break down bone tissue at a faster rate than osteoblastic (bone cell formation) activity occurs. Thus, RANKL inhibitors suppress osteoclastic activity, preventing excessive bone destruction.

Sclerostin antagonists are directed against sclerostin, which is a regulatory protein in bone metabolism. By inhibiting the action of *sclerostin*, osteoblastic activity and bone formation are increased at the same time that osteoclastic activity and bone resorption are decreased. As a result, overall bone mass is increased, especially in the spine.

Parathyroid hormone agonists are synthetic forms of natural parathyroid hormone (PTH). At therapeutic dosages, these agonists bind to receptors on bone cells, kidney cells, and intestinal cells in the same way that PTH does. As a result, more calcium is absorbed from the intestinal tract to be taken up by bone cells. In addition, the kidneys reabsorb more calcium back into the blood to help maintain bone density. If these drugs are taken at higher than therapeutic dosages, just like for many other hormones and receptor-based drugs, their effects are either reduced or work in the opposite way.

Common side effects of second-line drugs for osteoporosis. Estrogen agonist/antagonists often cause muscle spasms (especially severe in the lower legs), nausea, indigestion, and weight gain. Symptoms associated with perimenopause also may occur, including hot flushes and night sweats. Other common side effects include breast tenderness and peripheral edema.

Sclerostin antagonists have skin rashes and musculoskeletal pain as common side effects. Because these drugs are taken subcutaneously, injection site reactions and infections are also possible. Some people develop "flu-like" symptoms of headache, general achiness, tiredness, and low-grade fever for the first 24 to 48 hr after injection. Peripheral edema also is common.

Parathyroid hormone agonists induce nausea, gastric distress, and constipation. These effects are most likely associated with hypercalcemia. The drugs are also associated with orthostatic hypotension.

Possible adverse effects of second-line drugs for osteoporosis. Just as for the bisphosphonates, *all* the second-line drugs for osteoporosis can cause *jawbone osteonecrosis*. In addition, although bone mass may be increased, the risk for atypical fractures not usually associated with osteoporosis also is increased.

Estrogen receptor agonist/antagonists have an increased risk for clot formation, although this risk is lower than for estrogen agonists alone. Consequences of this problem include increased risk for strokes, heart attacks, and deep vein thrombosis, especially in people who use nicotine in any form. The incidence of gall bladder disease and of gall stone formation also is higher with these drugs.

Sclerostin antagonists have an increased risk for severe allergic reactions and possible anaphylaxis. The risk for severe allergic reaction increases with repeated dosages of the drug.

For *denosumab*, severe and even life-threatening low blood calcium levels *(hypocalcemia)* along with low magnesium levels have occurred, as have elevated blood cholesterol levels and pancreatitis. Shortness of breath has been frequently reported among patients receiving denosumab, although the cause of this is not known.

With *romosozumab*, the risk for atypical bone fractures appears higher than for other drugs. The bone most commonly involved is the shaft of the femur, and the fracture can be bilateral. Symptoms of this fracture include pain in the thigh, hip, and/or groin.

Biologics that are *parathyroid hormone* agonists can cause elevated blood calcium levels *(hypercalcemia)* and also increase the risks for the development of bone cancers, especially osteosarcoma. The elevated blood calcium levels also increase the risk for kidney stone formation.

<table>
<tr><td>⚠️ **Drug Alert**</td></tr>
</table>

Administration Alert

Assess the patient for an allergic reaction during and after subcutaneous injections of any of the biologics. Keep emergency equipment in the room with the patient.

QSEN: Safety

⭐ *Teaching priorities for patients taking second-line drugs for osteoporosis*

- Be sure you understand how often to take your prescribed drug. Some are taken daily, and others may be taken monthly, every 6 months, or once a year. If a drug is taken too often, serious side effects can result.
- If you are self-injecting your drug for osteoporosis, use the instructions taught to you for injecting into the abdomen or thighs.
- Check your injection sites daily for indications of infection such as warmth, redness at or around the injection site, swelling, pain, skin that is firm to the touch, or foul-smelling drainage.
- If you have any difficulty breathing, chest pain, severe dizziness, or swelling of the lips, tongue, or throat, call 911 immediately because these are signs of a severe allergic reaction.
- Observe yourself for symptoms of blood calcium levels that are either higher than normal or lower than normal. *High calcium* symptoms include a slow or irregular heart rate, muscle weakness, nausea, and constipation. *Low calcium* symptoms include sensations of tingling and numbness in the fingers, toes, lips, and nose; painful muscle cramps; abdominal cramping and diarrhea; and dizziness on standing.
- If you have new or unusual pain in the thigh, hip, or groin, notify your prescriber immediately because unusual thigh bone fractures have occurred, even without trauma.
- If you take abaloparatide or teriparatide, keep all cancer screening appointments because these drugs increase your risk for bone cancer.
- If you take raloxifene or Duavee, do not use nicotine in any form. These drugs increase your risk for blood clots that can lead to stroke and heart attack. This risk is much greater if you also smoke or use nicotine in any form.

Get Ready for the NCLEX® Examination!

Key Points

- Drugs for perimenopausal hormone replacement should be taken only short term to reduce the symptoms of menopause.
- Drugs for perimenopausal HRT, hormonal contraceptives, and estrogen agonist/antagonists for osteoporosis increase blood clot formation, increasing the risks for heart attack, stroke, pulmonary embolism, and deep vein thrombosis.
- Women on perimenopausal hormone replacement therapy or who are taking hormonal contraceptives should not smoke or use nicotine in any form.

- Whether taken orally or applied as a patch, vaginal ring, intrauterine device, or implanted into subcutaneous tissue, hormonal contraceptives have the same mechanism of action and side effects.
- The estrogen and progesterone in hormonal contraceptives disrupt the female hormone pathway by using negative feedback and mimicking pregnancy hormones.
- Hormonal contraception should not be used by women who use nicotine; have a personal history of breast, uterine, ovarian, or cervical cancer; have moderate to severe hypertension; or have other significant risk factors for stroke or myocardial infarction.

- Teach women to seek medical help immediately for any symptom associated with deep vein thrombosis, myocardial infarction, stroke, or pulmonary embolism.
- Hormonal contraceptives do not protect against sexually transmitted infections.
- Osteoclastic activity reduces bone density and strength, whereas osteoblastic activity increases bone density and strength.
- Osteoporosis occurs with aging, but the rate of progression varies as a result of many individual patient factors, including gender, race, ethnicity, body size, general health, use of other drugs, and level of weight-bearing activity.
- Instruct patients taking oral bisphosphonates to drink a full glass of water with each dose and to remain in the upright position for at least 30 minutes after taking the drug to prevent esophageal reflux and irritation.
- Any drug for osteoporosis can cause jawbone osteonecrosis after tooth extraction or oral surgery. Remind patients to inform their dental health practitioners that they take these drugs.

- Remind patients taking estrogen agonists/antagonists not to use nicotine in any form to reduce the risk for thrombotic events.
- Biologic monoclonal antibodies have a greater incidence of severe hypersensitivity reactions than any other drug class for osteoporosis.
- Patients taking second-line drugs for osteoporosis have an increased risk for developing atypical bone fractures with or without trauma, particularly of the femur shaft. Teach them to report any new or unusual pain in the thigh, hip, or groin to their prescriber immediately.

Additional Learning Resources

Be sure to visit your Evolve website (http://evolve.elsevier.com/Workman/pharmacology/) for additional online resources.

SG Go to your Study Guide for additional learning activities to help you master this chapter content.

Review Questions

See *Answers to In-Text Review Questions* in the back of the book for answers to these questions.

1. **Which hormone is responsible for initiating sex hormone production and secretion at the beginning of puberty in both males and females?**

   A. Estrogen
   B. Luteinizing hormone
   C. Follicle-stimulating hormone
   D. Gonadotropin-releasing hormone

2. **Which side effect is most important for the nurse to teach a patient who has never had surgery and who is now prescribed an estrogen-only hormone replacement therapy (HRT) drug to relieve perimenopausal symptoms?**

   A. New onset migraine headaches
   B. Increased breast tenderness
   C. Excessive uterine bleeding
   D. Weight gain

3. **For which patient will the nurse question a prescription of drospirenone/estradiol for hormone replacement therapy (HRT)?**

   A. 45-year-old who still has a uterus
   B. 48-year-old who recently had gall bladder surgery
   C. 50-year-old who takes an angiotensin-converting enzyme (ACE) inhibitor for blood pressure control
   D. 55-year-old who takes a sodium-glucose cotransport inhibitor for control of type 2 diabetes

4. **A 22-year-old patient who started taking an oral hormonal contraceptive 1 month ago calls to report that her breasts are now enlarged and tender. What is the nurse's best action?**

   A. Reassuring her that this is an expected and normal side effect of the drug
   B. Asking her whether there is any possibility that she may be pregnant
   C. Instructing the patient to wear a tighter bra
   D. Notifying the prescriber immediately

5. **How do "mini pills" prevent pregnancy?**

   A. Suppressing secretion of gonadotrophin-releasing hormone and follicle-stimulating hormone
   B. Thickening the endometrium to prevent movement of a fertilized egg into the uterus
   C. Suppressing ovulation and thickening cervical mucous
   D. Decreasing the patient's interest in having sex (libido)

6. **Which two supplements will the nurse suggest to a patient at risk for osteoporosis to reduce or delay its onset?**

   A. Calcium and vitamin C
   B. Calcium and vitamin D
   C. Phosphorous and Vitamin C
   D. Phosphorous and Vitamin D

7. **For which patient will the nurse question a prescription for oral risedronate?**

   A. 40-year-old with gastroesophageal reflux disease
   B. 40-year-old with type 2 diabetes mellitus
   C. 50-year-old with metastatic breast cancer
   D. 50-year-old with chronic obstructive respiratory disease

8. **What dosing schedule will the nurse tell a patient who is prescribed to take oral alendronate 35 mg for prevention of osteoporosis to use for best effect?**

   A. Once daily with breakfast
   B. Once weekly with breakfast
   C. Once monthly on the same day each month
   D. Once yearly in the same month every year

9. **Which patient does the nurse identify as at increased risk for osteoporosis as a result of drug therapy for another health problem?**

   A. Woman who uses oral hormonal contraceptives
   B. Woman who takes acetaminophen daily for arthritic pain
   C. Man who takes an oral anticoagulant daily for heart failure
   D. Man who takes an oral corticosteroid for a chronic respiratory problem

Clinical Judgment

1. Which drugs for osteoporosis treatment or prevention will the nurse prepare to administer to a patient by intravenous infusion? **Select all that apply.**

   A. Abaloparatide
   B. Alendronate
   C. Denosumab
   D. Ibandronate
   E. Raloxifene
   F. Risedronate
   G. Teriparatide
   H. Zoledronic acid

2. The patient is a 48-year-old woman who works as a teacher's aide. She has two teenaged children and began having perimenopausal symptoms about 4 months ago. She says that she feels her symptoms are "taking over her life." Her women's health care provider has prescribed a drospirenone/estradiol combination of 1 tablet orally daily to relieve her perimenopausal symptoms. The nurse has prepared and delivered a teaching plan for this patient. **For each patient statement, use an X to indicate whether the statement demonstrates Correct Understanding or demonstrates that More Teaching Is Needed.**

PATIENT STATEMENT	CORRECT UNDERSTANDING	MORE TEACHING IS NEEDED
"My friends tell me that I shouldn't smoke when taking drugs for menopause, so I have switched to vaping instead."		
"It's a good thing my husband has had a vasectomy because estrogen will increase my risk for getting pregnant."		
"I will make certain to have a mammogram every year."		
"If I forget a dose one day, I will take two doses the next day."		
"I will take the drug for a year and see what happens when I stop taking it."		
"If my skin or eyes start to get yellow, I will contact my prescriber immediately."		

CHAPTER 1

1. C

Although some non–health-care-related people consider drugs to be illicit and medication to be helpful, they are interchangeable terms and both have the same meaning. Remember that another name for "pharmacy" is drug store.

2. B

Not only do schedule I drugs have the highest potential for abuse, they currently have no accepted medical use in treatment in the United States. As a schedule II drug, morphine is an opioid that is frequently prescribed to help manage some types of severe pain. It may or may not be combined with another agent and is carefully regulated because it does have a relatively high risk for dependency and addiction.

3. A

Lasix and Furocot are two brand names for the same actual drug (furosemide), produced by different manufacturers. Both brands must be 97% identical to the generic drug and can be interchanged without causing problems.

4. D

When two drugs have the same or a similar chemical structure and one of them is known to cause an adverse reaction, the use of the nearly identical drug is contraindicated because of the high risk for cross-reactivity. Such a problem would greatly increase the patient's risk for having an adverse reaction to a drug with a similar chemical composition.

5. C

St. John's wort can somewhat increase the time required for blood to clot and increase the risk for bleeding. Often, St. John's wort makes bleeding risk greater when a patient is also taking some anticoagulants. The best option is to check with the pharmacist who would know for certain whether or not St. John's wort can be taken safely along with the newly prescribed anticoagulant so that the nurse can provide the patient with accurate information.

6. A

When naturally occurring adrenaline binds with its receptor, a specific action results. An antagonist is an extrinsic drug that blocks the receptor site of a cell, which prevents the naturally occurring body substance from binding to the receptor and decreases the cell's expected response.

7. A, E

Shortness of breath and chest pain are indicators of an adverse reaction that could be life threatening and must be managed immediately. The other changes are considered side effects and are not serious.

8. C

With increased metabolic enzyme activity and more rapid elimination, drugs will leave the body more quickly and have less time to exert their intended actions. In order to have a therapeutic response, this patient may need higher drug doses or more frequent dosing (or both).

9. A

A paradoxical response to a drug is one in which the drug induces the opposite response from its intended action. A sedative is used to induce sleep and rest. When the person has increased insomnia or alertness rather than sleepiness, the response is a paradoxical reaction.

10. D

The drug is being administered intravenously because it is poorly absorbed from the stomach. Even if the drug enters breast milk, the infant will not absorb it or be harmed by it.

CHAPTER 2

1. B

A prescriber's drug order should be in written form and include all the minimal information required by the U.S. government. Verbal orders should only be accepted in emergency situations. As soon as the emergency is resolved, verbal orders must be written and signed. For safety, when a nurse contacts a prescriber or follows a verbal order, the nurse should be sure to write the order, read it back, and ask for confirmation that what was written is correct.

2. D

A patient has the right to refuse to take any drug. Although it is important that the patient understand why the drug has been prescribed and the consequences of refusing to take it, the nurse should investigate why the patient prefers not to take a drug. For example, if a patient is having diarrhea and understands the action of docusate, refusing the drug is not only the patient's right but is also the right action to take.

3. B

Drug errors can occur any time while a drug is in the control of the health care professional or the patient. Because nurses give most drugs to patients, nurses are the final defense for detecting and preventing drug errors. To prevent drug errors, nurses must always follow the "eight rights."

4. C

Omeprazole comes in time-released capsules, which should not be opened to prevent rapid absorption of the drug and consequent side effects or adverse effects. Mixing the drug with applesauce and asking the patient to swallow it when the patient has difficulty swallowing puts the patient at high risk for aspiration.

5. A

The intravenous route is used when a drug needs to enter the bloodstream rapidly or a large dose of a drug must be given. The rates of absorption and action are very rapid with this route, and this route is best for a patient with severe postoperative pain.

6. A

When giving ear drops to a child younger than 3 years of age, pulling the earlobe down and back straightens the ear canal. This helps the nurse to place the ear drops where they are needed to be effective.

7. D

The patient should be taught to remain lying down for 10 to 15 minutes after receiving a vaginal drug to keep the drug in place and ensure that it is fully absorbed.

8. C

STAT drugs are prescribed to correct or help an immediate problem; they are given as soon as they are available. If the drug is not available on the unit, the nurse must call the pharmacy for an immediate drug dose. PRN drugs may be important but are given at the patient's indication of a need for the drug. The diphenhydramine order is written as a standing order and does not indicate an immediate need. Although cyanocobalamin is written as a single-dose drug order, there is no indication for immediate administration.

9. B

These symptoms indicate there has been IV infiltration and the needle is no longer in the vein. No further drugs can be delivered through this IV setup, even if they are well diluted. IV administration of the drug must be discontinued. The prescriber should be notified before restarting IV administration of the drug. The prescriber may change the drug to a different form or prescribe a different drug. A new IV must be started at another site.

10. A, D, E, F

Diarrhea may make the rectal route of drug administration undesirable because the patient may be unable to hold the drug in the rectum long enough to be absorbed. Disposable gloves are used, but they do **not** need to be sterile. The suppository is inserted pointed end first, not blunt end. The modified left lateral recumbent position (with the patient turned to the side and one leg bent over the other) is the best position for giving a rectal suppository. The suppository is pushed into the rectum about 1 inch for better absorption. Be sure to instruct the patient about how long the suppository should be held in the rectum.

11. B, C, F

Because of the rich blood supply in the muscles, IM drugs are absorbed much faster than subcutaneous drugs. IM injections can also be much larger than subcutaneous injections. They require needles that are longer (1 to 1.5 inches) and larger (22 to 20 gauge) and tend to be more painful. IM

injections are deeper (into the muscle) than subcutaneous. Both subcutaneous and intramuscular injections require rotation of injection sites to prevent tissue damage.

12. A

All of these questions are important to know when giving a new drug. The information that is most critical, however, is whether the patient has an allergy to this drug or any other drug. A drug allergy can result in life-threatening effects.

CHAPTER 3

1. D

The bottom number of a fraction is the denominator. The top number is the numerator.

2. C

An improper fraction is one in which the numerator is larger than the denominator. As a result, the answer to an improper fraction is always greater than 1.

3. A

When 16 is divided by 1, the answer is the whole number 16. If 16 is divided by 16, the answer would be the whole number 1. When 1 is divided by 16, the answer is a fraction and not a whole number. When 16 is divided by 2, the answer is the whole number 8.

4. A

When 9 is divided by 2, the correct answer is the whole number 4 and the fraction ½.

5. B

The fraction $17/29$ cannot be reduced further. The fraction $5/25$ can be reduced to $1/5$ by dividing the numerator and the denominator both evenly by 5. The fraction $2/8$ can be reduced to ¼th by dividing the numerator and the denominator evenly by 2. The fraction $12/16$ can be reduced to ¾ by dividing the numerator and the denominator evenly by 4.

6. C

The lowest number that the denominators for these three fractions can share is 20. The denominator 5 cannot divide 12 evenly. The denominator 4 cannot divide 15 evenly nor can it divide 30 evenly.

7. A

The fractions in this series can only be added when they are expressed as their lowest common denominator. ¾ = $15/20$, ¼ = $5/20$, 3/5 = $12/20$. $15 + 5 + 12 = 32/20$, reduced to 1 and $3/5$.

8. C

To divide $1/3$ by ½, the fraction ½ is inverted (flipped) to $2/1$. Then the numerators are cross-multiplied with $1 \times 2 = 2$, and the denominators are cross-multiplied with $3 \times 1 = 3$. The result is $2/3$.

9. C

The divisor is the number the dividend is divided by (or that is divided into the dividend).

10. B

The answer to a division problem. When 26.4 is divided by 16.22, the initial answer is 1.62762. Rounding to the 10th place involves changing the .627 to 0628 because the 6 next to the 7 is greater than 5. The final answer is 1.628.

11. A

To express $5/8$ as a decimal, 5 is divided by 8. The answer is 0.625.

12. B

To get 18% of 52, 52 is multiplied by 0.18, which equals 9.36.

13. C

The dose of the drug on hand is 3 mg/tablet. This dose is much less than the 20 mg dose prescribed and multiple tables will need to be given to ensure the correct dose.

14. D

The dose on hand (have) is 250 mg/tablet. The dose wanted is 1000 mg. 1000 divided by 250 = 4. Thus 4 tablets are needed to equal a 1000 mg dose.

15. D

A proportion is an equal mathematic relationship between two numbers or two sets of numbers. Thus, if 50 mL of morphine contains 500 mg of morphine, then to keep the same proportion 1 mL would contain 10 mg of morphine (not 5). The only set of numbers that retains the same proportion as 50 mL containing 500 mg of morphine is 15 mg containing 150 mg.

16. 2.4 mL

Set up as a want versus have problem. Have 25 mg/1 mL; want 60 mg. 60 mg divided by 25 mg = 2.4 mL.

CHAPTER 4

1. A

There are 3 teaspoons in a tablespoon. 60 × 3 = 180 for 1 tablespoon × 2 = 360 in 2 tablespoons.

2. D

1 ounce = 30 mL. 150 mL divided by 30 mL = 5 ounces

3. 3 Tbs

1 Tbs contains 3 teaspoons. 3 teaspoons × 5 mL = 15 mg/Tbs. 45 mg divided by 15 mg = 3 Tbs.

4. C

1 mcg is equal to 1/1000 of a mg; or 1/1,000,000 of a gram; or 1/1,000,000,000 of a kg.

5. 250 mL

1 L = 1000 mL. 0.25 × 1000 = 250 mL

6. 79.5 kg

1 kg = 2.2 lb; 175 divided by 2.2 = 79.54 kg, round down to 79.5

7. 1.5 mL

10 mg/mL = 1 mg/0.1 mL 15 × 0.1 mL = 1.5 mL

8. 0.6 mL

20,000 units/mL concentration = 2000/0.1 mL; 12,000 divided by 2000 = 6; 6 × 0.1 mL = 0.6 mL

CHAPTER 5

1. C

The drop factor is the number of drops (gtt) needed to make 1 mL of IV fluid. The larger the drop, the fewer drops needed to make 1 mL.

2. A

At 10 gtts/mL × 31 gtts/min = ~3 mL/min, 180 mL/hr, infusion complete in about 6 hours
At 15 gtts/mL × 31 gtts/min = ~2 mL/min, 120 mL/hr, infusion complete in about 8 hours
At 20 gtts/mL × 31 gtts/min = ~1.5 mL/min, 90 mL/hr, infusion complete in about 11 hours
At 60 gtts/mL × 31 gtts/min = ~ 0.5 mL/min, 30 mL/hr, infusion complete in about 31 to 33 hours

3. C, D, F, G

A valid prescription for IV therapy must include the specific drug or IV solution to be infused, the dosage or volume, the duration, and the rate of infusion. The drip rate (of gtts/min) must be calculated by the nurse based on the drop factor of the specific IV administration set used.

4. B

Infiltration is a condition that occurs when an IV needle or catheter pulls from the vein and begins to leak the fluids into the surrounding tissue, causing tissue swelling. When the fluid or drug that infiltrates is irritating and leads to tissue damage or loss, the condition is termed extravasation. Although checking the site frequently does not prevent *infiltration*, if the problem is discovered quickly, *extravasation* with tissue damage is avoided or reduced.

5. A

The amount infused is equal to the starting amount (1000 mL) minus the volume to be infused (VBTI or the amount remaining in the IV bag) of 250 mL. 1000 − 250 = 750 mL have infused.

6. D

At 125 mL/hr, the patient should receive 2 mL/min (125 mL/60 min). With a drop factor of 10 gtts/mL, the total number of drops per minute should be 20. The 15-second drop rate should be 5 (20 gtts/min/4).

7. 21 gtts/min

1000 mL divided by 8 hours = 125 mL/hr, divided by 60 minutes = 2.08 mL/min
2.08 mL × 10 gtts/mL = 20.8 gtts/min, round to 21 gtts/min

8. 30 gtts/min

When using microdrip tubing, the drop factor of 60 drops/mL is the same as the number of minutes in 1 hour (60) and, as in the formula below, the two 60s cancel each other out. *This is why the flow rate for microdrip tubing always equals the drop rate.*

$$\frac{30}{60} \times \frac{60}{1}(\text{drop factor}) = \frac{30}{1} = 30 \text{ microdrops/minute}$$

CHAPTER 6

1. A

Resistant bacteria are difficult to control and the infection may not be cured, leading to increased sepsis and death. Opportunistic infections are caused by normal flora and only occur in people whose immune function is reduced. Even though bacteria become more resistant, people will not be more susceptible, but when an infection does develop it will be more serious.

2. C

Bactericidal drugs directly kill bacteria; bacteriostatic drugs only stop bacteria from reproducing while the immune system kills the bacteria.

3. C

For all antibacterial therapy, it is important to keep the blood level high enough to affect the bacteria causing the infection. Therefore, teach the patient to take the drug evenly throughout a 24-hour day. If the drug is to be taken four times daily, teach the patient to take it every 6 hours. Doubling the dose every 12 hours does not increase the drug's half-life or keep the blood level even.

4. A

Infusing the drug slowly allows more blood to flow in the vein at the same time and reduces irritation. Cooling the drug does not change its irritating quality. Using less diluent would concentrate the drug and increase its irritation effect. Keeping the patient's IV site above the level of the heart would only increase the rate of blood return to the heart and would not reduce the risk for vein irritation.

5. C

The most important action is to prevent the patient from receiving any more of the drug causing this life-threatening reaction. Although discontinuing the IV would accomplish this, one of the major problems with anaphylaxis is circulatory collapse leading to shock (and death). The patient will still need the IV access. Slowing the infusion while assessing the patient is not sufficient to prevent more of the harmful drug to enter and will only delay life-saving interventions. Notifying the prescriber is the least important action, although calling a code or the rapid response team would be the second most important action to take.

6. D

Cephalosporins lower the seizure threshold and should not be given to a patient who has a seizure disorder. If the infection is only sensitive to cephalosporins, special precautions must be taken to prevent seizures from occurring.

7. B

Penicillin has no particular risk for embryonic or fetal harm in early pregnancy and does not need to be changed. If taken while breastfeeding, the baby may have an increased risk for a penicillin allergy and is highly likely to develop diarrhea. If the patient stops taking the drug after only 6 days, her strep throat will be inadequately treated and may recur. Also, this increases the chance for bacteria to become drug resistant.

8. A

Amikacin is not penicillin and is not structurally similar to penicillin. An allergy to penicillin does not predispose a patient to an allergy to an aminoglycoside antibiotic like amikacin. Continuing with the infusion after reassuring the patient that it is safe is the appropriate action. The nurse does need to document the patient report of a penicillin allergy to ensure all health care providers are aware of this patient fact.

9. D

Warfarin is an anticoagulant. Macrolides change the metabolism of warfarin and it stays in the body longer, greatly increasing the risk for bleeding. Both drugs are important for this patient. The dosage of the macrolide cannot be decreased because the infection is serious. The atrial fibrillation still requires the use of warfarin; however, the dosage can be lowered.

10. B

Sulfonamides can crystalize in the kidneys, causing obstruction and kidney impairment. It is critically important that the patient increases fluid intake to ensure good urine flow through the kidneys. For this drug, skin rashes are a common side effect and not an allergic response. There is no evidence that this drug reduces the effectiveness of oral contraceptives. Although hyperkalemia is possible with trimethoprim, sodium levels are not changed.

11. C

Ciprofloxacin is a fluoroquinolone drug that concentrates in the urine, making the urine irritating to surrounding tissues. The patient may experience pain or burning of the urethra and nearby tissues during urination. An incontinent patient may have skin irritation over the entire perineal area. To avoid this, teach the patient to drink a full glass of water with each dose and to drink more fluids throughout the day.

12. 3 mL

Want 1,800,000 units/*X* mL; have 2,400,000 units/4 mL or 600,000/1 mL. 1,800,000/600,000 = 3 mL

CLINICAL JUDGMENT

1. A, C, D, F, G, I

Vancomycin is a powerful glycopeptide cell wall synthesis inhibitor that can cause a histamine release with vasodilation if given too fast. This dilation results in an appearance known as "red man syndrome" with flushing of the face, neck, chest, back, and arms. Although not a true allergic reaction, it can result in hypotension and cardiac dysrhythmias. The first action is to stop the IV infusion while asking whether breathing is impaired (to rule out anaphylaxis). After determining that the patient is not having an allergic reaction, the nurse would allow the infusion to continue at a slower rate. Then the nurse would reassure the patient and family that this is a common response and that appropriate actions are being taken. The nurse would also document the occurrence, the nurse's actions, and the patient's response to slowing the infusion. Under these circumstances would the nurse **not** discontinue

the IV access. Calling the Rapid Response Team for this patient response is not necessary. The drug does not have a side effect or adverse effect that would cause urine to be bloody.

2.

INSTRUCTION/PRECAUTION	MOST RELEVANT	NOT RELEVANT	POTENTIALLY HARMFUL
Take this drug with food or milk to prevent stomach problems.			X
Drink a full glass of water with each capsule and increase your overall daily water intake.	X		
Avoid pickled food, red wine, soy-containing food or drinks, and sauerkraut while taking this drug.		X	
Whenever you golf or are outdoors, wear a hat, long sleeves, and sunscreen because you will sunburn much more easily on this drug.	X		
Avoid taking any vitamin supplements that contain vitamin K because they will reduce this drug's effectiveness.		X	
Brush your teeth and tongue thoroughly followed by rinsing with mouthwash at least three times daily to prevent an oral infection.	X		
If you notice darkening or a yellow-gray discoloration of your teeth, notify your prescriber immediately.		X	
If you should become pregnant while on this drug, stop taking it.	X		
Keep the tablets in the container that came from the pharmacy rather than using a daily pill organizer.		X	

Tetracycline's absorption and, therefore, its effectiveness is inhibited by milk and other dairy products. It should be taken on an empty stomach. Drinking a full glass of water with each dose and increasing fluid intake throughout the day is important because this drug can irritate the esophagus. The drug does not interact with tyramine and it is not necessary to avoid food containing it. Tetracyclines increase sun sensitivity (photosensitivity), and severe burns are possible. This is especially important for this patient, who is a golfer. No vitamins interfere with this drug's action, nor does it increase vitamin excretion. Yeast infections of the mouth and vagina are common with tetracycline therapy, especially when it is taken long term. Good oral hygiene can help prevent or reduce this problem. Although the drug can cause darkening or a yellow-gray appearance when developing teeth are exposed to it (during pregnancy and in childhood), mature teeth are not affected by it. The drug does not have to be protected from light.

CHAPTER 7

1. C

Antiviral drugs do not kill the virus. Their main action is interfering with viral replication/reproduction enough to slow their growth and spread so that the immune system actions can eliminate or neutralize them.

2. B

Antiviral drugs suppress viral replication and reduce the severity and length of the infection but do not confer immunity. It is not the same as receiving a vaccination to prevent an infection.

3. A

Peramivir is an IV antiviral drug given as a one-time dose. It does not increase the risk for seizures and can be used during pregnancy and lactation.

4. C

For all antimicrobial therapy, including antiviral drugs, it is important to keep the blood level high enough to affect the virus causing the infection. Therefore, teach the patient to take the drug evenly throughout a 24-hour day. If the drug is to be taken three times daily, teach the patient to take it every 8 hours.

5. D

Acyclovir can interfere with the effectiveness of live-virus vaccines and immunity may not be conferred. This drug is not known to cause photosensitivity or fetal harm. It is not necessary to avoid caffeine or alcohol while taking this drug.

6. C

Ribavirin is a dangerous drug and should not be inhaled by anyone except the patient. When it is aerosolized it can permeate to other areas. Standard procedure is for the nurse to wear personal protective equipment while administering the drug and keep the door to the room closed to reduce the chances of exposure to others.

7. D

HCV infection seldom has an acute phase, but the virus remains within the person. This virus is able to evade immune action because it constantly mutates within the infected person, so as soon as the person begins to make antibodies against it, the virus mutates its genetic material and those previously made antibodies are no longer effective, although the patient is **not** immunocompromised. Without an acute illness phase, the person is often unaware that he or she has been infected with HCV. However, over the course of 20 to 30 years, about 85% of people infected with HCV eventually develop chronic disease with liver cirrhosis and failure. This progression does not occur any more rapidly because the patient is unaware of his or her condition and it does not directly infect the kidneys.

8. D

The changes in the patient's urine in stool colors strongly suggest liver toxicity. The prescriber must be notified immediately and the drug therapy stopped before liver damage is irreparable.

9. A

Interferon and peginterferon can cause depression and worsen existing depression. Its use in patients with mental health problems, especially depression and suicide ideation, is contraindicated.

10. C

Antacids interfere with the absorption of Dovato and must not be taken within 2 hours of a Dovato dose. Caffeine restriction is not indicated, and the therapy is life-long. Dovato can be taken with or without food. It is not known to induce drowsiness.

11. B

The most important factor in the development of drug resistance to combination ART is missing drug doses. When doses are missed, the blood concentrations become lower than that needed to inhibit viral replication, allowing the virus to replicate and produce new viruses that may be resistant to the drugs being used. Although having multiple sex partners increases the risk for becoming infected with a drug resistant HIV strain, the practice does not contribute to the development of drug resistance.

12. D

Integrase strand transfer inhibitors bind to the active site of the viral enzyme integrase, preventing it from inserting the newly formed viral DNA strand into the host cell's DNA. Without this insertion, the host cell cannot be used to reproduce viruses.

13. 0.25 mL

Want 90 mcg; have 180 mcg/0.5 mL. 180 mcg ÷ 90 mcg = 2. 0.5 mL ÷ 2 = 0.25 mL; 0.50 mL − 0.25 mL = 0.25 to be discarded for a remaining volume of 0.25 mL containing 90 mcg.

CLINICAL JUDGMENT

1. A, B, C, D, E, F, G, H

Ribavirin can have toxic effects on many organs and causes birth defects. Before giving ribavirin, determine whether the patient is pregnant. Assess the patient's heart rate, rhythm, and pulse quality. Evaluate lung function by assessing the rate and depth of respiratory effort, breath sounds, pulse oximetry, color of skin and mucous membranes, and level of consciousness. Assess kidney function by checking the

most recent 24-hour intake and output and comparing the amount of urine excreted with the amount of fluids consumed. Assess liver function by examining for jaundice of the skin, palate, or whites of the eyes and by checking liver function tests. Because ribavirin often suppresses the growth of blood cells in the bone marrow, review the patient's most recent WBC and RBC counts before drug therapy begins. Assess the patient's vital signs (including temperature and mental status) before starting ribavirin.

2.

PATIENT STATEMENT	CORRECT UNDERSTANDING	MORE INSTRUCTION NEEDED
"If I forget a dose on one day, I will take two doses the next day."		X
"In addition to avoiding alcohol during this treatment phase, I will do my liver a favor and quit drinking altogether."	X	
"To prevent a drug interaction, I will stop my blood pressure drug just until this therapy is over."		X
"When my therapy is completed, I will be immune to being infected with this virus again."		X
"I will avoid sexual intercourse until 1 month after this therapy is completed."		X
"If I take this drug at night, I can be sure my stomach is empty."		X

Doubling the dose of the drug because of a missed dose is never to be done. Usually, the person with chronic HCV infection has some degree of liver impairment and must avoid alcohol and other liver-damaging substances during therapy. It would be best to avoid these substances forever. Hypertension must continue to be treated, although if metabolic changes occur, some dosing adjustments may be needed. The therapy suppresses viral replication and allows the immune system to eradicate or neutralize the virus. It does not confer immunity and the patient would be susceptible to becoming infected again with HCV upon exposure, especially to a virus with a different genotype. The drug can cause birth defects when taken during pregnancy. It is not necessary for male patients to avoid intercourse while on Mavyret. Mavyret is supposed to be taken with a meal and not on an empty stomach.

CHAPTER 8

1. B

When *Mycobacterium tuberculosis* is inhaled into the lungs, the bacteria multiply and form a primary TB lesion, which is a small, inflamed pocket of bacteria, white blood cells (WBCs), and exudate. The lesion is surrounded by more WBCs that cause a response known as *pneumonitis*. During this time, people who have an intact immune system develop immunity to the TB organism, and further growth of bacteria is controlled by confining it to the primary lesions.

2. C

A positive reaction to a TB indicates exposure to TB or the presence of inactive (dormant) disease, not active disease. Additional testing is needed to rule out or confirm active TB for which treatment is needed.

3. C

Most often without treatment, active tuberculosis continues to progress with destruction ("consumption") of large areas of lung tissue, interfering with gas exchange. The patient either becomes too hypoxic to support life or the tissue destruction erodes a large blood vessel in the lungs leading to a fatal hemorrhage.

4. A

If the patient does not adhere to the schedule, the infection can become worse and lead to death. Also, taking the drugs inconsistently leads to the development of drug-resistant organisms. Anyone who is cognitively impaired or living in a situation in which drug management is difficult would be best served by DOT. Only the 25-year-old homeless man who is addicted to opioids (and would have periods of reduced cognition) meets the criteria for DOT.

5. B

All the first-line drugs for TB are liver toxic and can cause liver damage. Drinking alcohol compounds this damage and should be ingested only in small quantities, if at all. Fluids are recommended to be increased, not decreased. Although some patients have nausea and taking the drugs at bedtime can help them to be less uncomfortable with this side effect, nausea does not cause harm. Grapefruit does not affect the absorption or metabolism of these drugs.

6. D

Ethambutol can cause serious eye problems that may lead to blindness in people of any age. Its use is avoided in children because they may not recognize vision changes caused by the drug soon enough to avoid permanent vision changes or blindness.

7. D

Reduced TB symptoms are indicators of therapy effectiveness. TB increases metabolism and patients lose much weight. A weight gain is a positive outcome indicator that the drug therapy is effective at this time (a negative sputum culture would be the best indicator). The TB skin test does not revert to negative with therapy. Neither hypertension nor hypotension are associated with TB. WBC counts do not reliably indicate the status of TB infection.

8. A

Two of the three drugs in this combination therapy, *bediquiline* and *linezolid*, often induce cardiac changes including a prolonged QT interval on electrocardiogram (ECG) even after the drug is stopped. This particular dysrhythmia can be fatal. Although respiratory assessment and skin assessment are important in patients receiving this therapy, cardiac assessment is most important.

9. B

These drugs can be absorbed through the skin and only the person for whom the drug was prescribed should be exposed to the drug. Anyone else applying the drug is taught to wear disposable gloves to avoid coming into direct contact with the cream or lotion.

10. D

Systemic antifungal drugs have many common side effects, including loss of taste or changes in how food tastes. Unless this problem interferes with the patient's nutritional status, it is of no consequence. The patient should be reassured that the taste changes are an expected side effect and that normal taste sensation will return after the drug has been stopped after several days or a week.

11. C

The drug can affect how the kidney reabsorbs or excretes potassium. A serum potassium level of 2.2 is very low and could lead to serious cardiac conduction and skeletal muscle problems. The low potassium level is likely to cause greater problems in an older adult.

12. A

500 mL/6 = 83.3 mL/hr. 83.3 mL/60 min = 1.38 mL/min. Round up to 1.4 mL/min.

CLINICAL JUDGMENT

1. B, D, E

Sexual intercourse should be avoided for several reasons: the drug can make holes in a condom or diaphragm and increase the risk for an unplanned pregnancy; in addition, the infection can be spread to a sexual partner. The applicator should be washed regularly with soap and water after each use. Although hands should be washed before and after applying the drug, the vagina is not a sterile body cavity, so it is not necessary to wear gloves during the application. There are no bathing restrictions while using the drug. Vaginal application of the drug does not affect pregnancy (however, a vaginal infection can have adverse effects on the pregnancy). To ensure eradication of the infection and prevent the development of resistant organisms, the drug should be used for as long as prescribed even after symptoms are no longer present. The cream will leak from the vagina even when the patient is not in the upright position. Wearing panties or pants is not contraindicated during this treatment.

2.

INSTRUCTION/PRECAUTION	MOST RELEVANT	NOT RELEVANT	POTENTIALLY HARMFUL
With a family history of TB and the fact that English is not your first language, you will need to be enrolled in a directly observed therapy program.		X	
Drink a full glass of water with each days' doses and increase your overall daily water intake.	X		
Fortunately, there is no need to modify your dietary or alcohol consumption habits with this drug therapy.			X
Try to take the drugs at the same time every day so that you do not forget any doses.	X		
You will need to eat more carbohydrates daily and decrease the dosage of your antidiabetic drug because these drugs increase the risk for hypoglycemia.			X
Do not worry about a change in urine color to a reddish orange; this is a harmless side effect.	X		
If you notice any numbness or tingling in your hands or feet, notify your prescriber immediately.	X		
Even if your symptoms go away after a month or so, it is critical that you continue taking the drugs.	X		
Keep the tablets in the container that came from the pharmacy rather than using a daily pill organizer.		X	
Keep all appointments for laboratory tests and follow-ups because these drugs can have harmful effects on your liver, kidneys, and eyes, and close monitoring is important.	X		

The patient has no characteristic that could be considered a risk for nonadherence to the daily drug therapy and does not require directly observed therapy. Increased fluid intake is important to reduce the risk of kidney damage. All four drugs for first-line therapy are liver toxic, and alcohol must be avoided to prevent even greater toxicity. Anything the patient can do to help remember to take the drugs daily is important. The risk for hyperglycemia as a side effect of this drug therapy is much more common than hypoglycemia. The patient is taught to check blood glucose levels more frequently and adjust both diet and antidiabetic therapy to prevent going out of the target range. Rifampin causes the urine to become reddish-orange and is a harmless side effect. Isoniazid can cause peripheral neuropathy. This patient is more at risk for peripheral neuropathy because he also has diabetes. Numbness and tingling in the hands and feet are often the first indications of peripheral neuropathy. TB is slow-growing and therapy is usually required for 6 months or longer. Not only can the disease progress and cause death if therapy is stopped too soon, but such action can also cause the organism to become drug-resistant. The first-line drugs are not particularly light-sensitive and can be kept in a pill organizer. Continuing follow-up with laboratory tests and other assessments is critical to identifying potential adverse reactions quickly before permanent harm occurs.

CHAPTER 9

1. C

Drug tolerance is a normal physiologic adjustment of the body to long-term opioid agonist use that increases the rate at which a drug is eliminated and reduces the main effects (pain relief) and side effects of the drug. It is an expected response and occurs fairly quickly with opioid agonist therapy that lasts a week or longer. Addiction is the psychologic need or craving for the "high" feeling that results from using opioid agonists when pain is either not present or minimally present.

2. C

The most common side effect of opioid agonists is constipation because these drugs slow intestinal movement. Most patients who are on opioid agonists for 2 or more days experience constipation. Assess patients who are prescribed opioid agonists for constipation and the need for stool softeners or laxatives.

3. A

The most reliable indicator of pain relief is the patient's self-report of reduced pain. Being drowsy or actually sleeping does not mean that pain is absent. Tolerating a dressing change without grimacing may only indicate that the dressing change manipulation is not the source of the pain. Although anxiety may increase pain perception, receiving an antianxiety medication does not indicate pain reduction.

4. C

Have 5 mg in 1 mL; want 3 mg in X mL. 1×3 divided by $5 = 0.6$ mL

5. A

Acetaminophen can cause severe liver damage and even liver failure when taken at high doses or too often. This adverse reaction is much more likely to occur in people who drink alcoholic beverages while on acetaminophen therapy. Drowsiness or sleepiness is an expected side effect of this drug and notifying the prescriber is not necessary. Ingesting caffeine is not contraindicated with this drug. Although codeine with or without acetaminophen can induce constipation, this is not the most important precaution for the prevention of harm caused by the drug.

6. C

Gabapentin is an anti-epilepsy drug that works on nerves and neurotransmitters to reduce seizure activity. It also reduces neuropathic pain, which is characterized by burning and tingling sensations in the affected areas.

7. B

Ubrogepant is a monoclonal antibody biologic agent that prevents CGRP from binding to its receptors in the trigeminovascular system of the head and neck. When CGRP binds to its receptors, it causes complete and prolonged vasodilation that causes the severe throbbing of migraine pain. This drug stops the cause of the pain, not the patient's perception of it.

8. C

The main effect of ergotamine is strong vasoconstriction. This effect is systemic and increases blood pressure, greatly increasing the risk for heart attacks and strokes. Preexisting hypertension is a contraindication for ergotamine therapy.

9. A

The inclusion of the mouth and lips in the area of reduced muscle response is most likely as a result of the spread of the drug from the injected areas. It may continue to spread and cause more problems. This patient needs to be evaluated immediately for changes in muscle responses in other areas.

10. D

Although most of these drugs can lower blood pressure to some extent, they all interact with more than 100 other drugs, which can result in severe or dangerous adverse effects. The main effect of these drugs is to stop the source of the pain, the muscle spasms, not directly relieve the pain. These drugs can result in temporary muscle weakness and reduced deep tendon reflexes, but assessing these parameters is not the most important action to take.

11. B

Methocarbamol usually causes some facial flushing. This problem does not indicate any type of allergic response and does not require either stopping the drug or implementing an intervention.

12. A

Discontinuing tizanidine abruptly can cause dangerous rebound hypertension. The drug is not related to any naturally occurring hormone. It does lower the seizure threshold, which means that the risk for seizures is increased while the patient takes the drug, not when the drug is discontinued.

CLINICAL JUDGMENT

1. A, E, F

Acute pain is a stressor that causes a client to have a sympathetic nervous system reaction similar to the "fight or flight" responses. These responses include diaphoresis, increased heart rate and blood pressure, dilated pupils, and increased respiratory rate.

2.

PATIENT STATEMENTS	CORRECT UNDERSTANDING	MORE INSTRUCTION NEEDED
If I develop a migraine on a day when I have already taken a dose for prevention, I will wait 2 hours to repeat the dose.		X
If I lose more than 2 lb in a week, I will notify my prescriber.		X
Even though I love grapefruit juice, I will not take it on the days I take the drug.	X	
If I have nausea and am unable to keep an oral dose of the drug down, I will go to the prescriber to get an injection of the drug.		X
I will test my facial muscles daily, especially around my eyes, to make sure they are not weaker or won't work.		X
I will drink plenty of water and take a stool softener daily to prevent constipation.	X	

This drug can only be taken once on any given day as a single dose. The patient must be taught not to repeat the dose if a migraine develops after already having taken the prevention dose. Some people do lose weight on these drugs but 2 lb in a week is not a cause for concern or to notify the prescriber. None of the oral CGRP monoclonal antibodies should be taken with grapefruit juice. This drink slows the elimination of the drug, intensifying the side effects and increasing the risk for dangerous adverse reactions. Rimegepant is available only as an oral agent. The drug with the ability to spread the effect of reducing muscle responses beyond the trigeminovascular system is onobotulinumtoxinA given by local subcutaneous injection. This is not a side effect or adverse effect of rimegepant. All of the CGRP monoclonal antibodies cause constipation as a side effect. The patient is taught to be proactive in preventing constipation.

CHAPTER 10

1. C

Inflammatory responses start tissue actions that cause visible and uncomfortable symptoms. Despite the discomfort, these actions are important in ridding the body of harmful organisms and helping repair damaged tissue. The response can occur in any tissue or organ, not just those of the immune system. Although infection most often is accompanied by inflammation, inflammation also occurs in response to noninfectious triggers.

2. B

After corticosteroid therapy is stopped, many side effects resolve, although this can take months to years. The sleep disturbance, weight gain, and moon-shaped face do go away over time. The stretch marks are permanent because they result from actual structural changes and skin damage, although they usually change from reddish-purple to silver over time so that they are less noticeable.

3. C

Histamines cause capillary leak syndrome by increasing the size of the capillary pores, which causes fluid to leave the capillaries and collect in the interstitial space with edema and swelling.

4. A

Corticosteroid drugs closely resemble cortisol. When a person is taking corticosteroids, the blood levels of the drug are high and the adrenal glands atrophy and stop or greatly reduce their production of cortisol. The atrophied adrenal glands become a problem if the person suddenly stops taking corticosteroids and when stress or illness are present. The unresponding adrenal glands cannot provide the extra cortisol needed, and adrenal insufficiency can result. Because more cortisol is needed during periods of stress or illness and the adrenal gland may not be able to release more, most patients will require a higher daily dose during these times.

5. D

Prednisolone and prednisone are not interchangeable because the strength of the cortisol in each is different. Although an equivalent dose of prednisolone can be calculated, it is not the nurse's role to do this. The best first course of action is to have the pharmacy send the correct drug and dose. The drug is to be administered quickly. There is no guarantee that the prescriber can be notified soon enough, and this should only be done if the pharmacy has no prednisone.

6. B

All NSAIDs are antiinflammatory drugs that are not similar to cortisol but prevent or limit the tissue and blood vessel general responses to injury or invasion by slowing the production of one or more inflammatory mediators. Most NSAIDs are nonselective and suppress both the COX-1 and COX-2 forms of the enzyme, so production of the helpful housekeeping mediators along with the inflammatory mediators is slowed. This means that these drugs cause side effects that are related to a reduction in the housekeeping mediators. Selective NSAIDs primarily suppress the COX-2 form of the enzyme and have fewer side effects from reducing the "housekeeping" mediators.

7. A

Celecoxib, as a selective COX-2 inhibitor, can increase clot formation in the small arteries of the heart and brain, especially when these arteries are narrowed by atherosclerosis or cigarette smoking. This drug should be avoided by any patient who has angina, smokes, or has undergone coronary artery bypass graft surgery (CABG).

8. A

An allergic asthma attack is the result of excessive release of histamine. However, during an asthma attack, the bronchioles are constricted and moving air in and out of the airways becomes more difficult. Extra conscious effort is needed by the patient to work the skeletal muscles of inhalation and exhalation. If the patient is given diphenhydramine, he or she can become too sleepy to put forth the extra muscle effort needed to breathe. This is the reason why the drug is only used during an asthma attack if the patient is also being mechanically ventilated.

9. D

Want 2.5 mg; have 5 mg/5 mL. 5 mg divided by 5 mL = 1 mg/mL
2.5 mg divided by 1 mg/mL = 2.5 mg in 2.5 mL

10. C

Naproxen's mechanism of action only interferes with blood clotting fairly briefly. Blood clotting returns to normal within 24 to 48 hours after stopping the drug. Aspirin, on the other hand, interferes with blood clotting for up to 7 days after the last dose.

11. C

Although questions A and B are important for the nurse to ask a patient who is to start taking sulfasalazine, C is the most important. This drug has a sulfa component. Any patient with an allergy to a sulfonamide drug is likely to have an allergy to sulfasalazine.

12. D

An adverse effect of hydroxychloroquine is the development of ocular toxicities and retinal damage. If the drug is not stopped when vision changes, particularly blurred vision, are first noticed, the damage can result in permanent vision loss. This drug is taken daily, not weekly, and is more likely to cause weight loss rather than weight gain. Although all general disease-modifying antirheumatic drugs (DMARDs) do cause some degree of immunosuppression and an increased risk for infection, the most important precaution is to prevent vision loss.

CLINICAL JUDGMENT

1. A, D, F, G, H

Patients on long-term therapy with corticosteroids lose bone density and muscle mass, and the skin becomes thinner and fragile. These patients are at high risk for falls, fractures with minimal trauma, and skin breakdown, especially pressure injuries. The sodium and fluid retention caused by corticosteroids can lead to fluid overload with pulmonary edema, and peripheral edema (also increasing the risk for skin breakdown). In addition to padding bony areas (heels and elbows), weighing the patient daily, and keeping track of intake and output, AP are instructed to handle the patient gently and move her using a lift sheet to avoid grasping the patient and causing fragile fractures and to assist the patient to ambulate using a gait belt to prevent falls and possible fractures.

2.

PATIENT STATEMENT	CORRECT UNDERSTANDING	MORE INSTRUCTION NEEDED	NEITHER CORRECT NOR INCORRECT
I have watched nurses give a lot of injections and am sure I can learn to give them to myself.		X	
My husband had a vasectomy 3 years ago, so I don't have to worry about getting pregnant while taking this drug.	X		
I understand that I should see my dentist and ophthalmologist regularly while I am taking this drug.	X		
I plan to take the methotrexate at the same time daily so I won't forget to take it.		X	
My daughter gave me a large hat to protect me when I am out in the sun.			X
Wearing gloves when I prepare my dose of methotrexate will protect me from absorbing it.		X	
Luckily, I am not allergic to sulfa types of antibiotics.			X
Last month I took my "flu shot" so I won't need another one until next year.	X		

Methotrexate as a general DMARD is an oral drug, not an injectable one. Methotrexate is a known teratogen and patients taking the drug must avoid getting pregnant. If her husband is now sterile from a vasectomy, the patient does not need to use two reliable forms of contraception. The drug can cause ocular toxicities that may lead to permanent blindness. Being checked regularly by an ophthalmologist is important while taking this drug. Methotrexate is only taken once per week, not daily. It is critically important to ensure the patient understands this dosing schedule to prevent a dangerous overdose. Although methotrexate is not known to have the side effect of increased photosensitivity, wearing sun protection is not harmful. Methotrexate is a high-alert drug that can be absorbed through the skin. It should not be handled directly by anyone except the patient. Because the patient will be absorbing the drug (through the intestinal tract), it is not necessary for her to avoid skin contact with it. This drug does not have a sulfa component and does not cause an allergic reaction in a patient who also has a sulfonamide allergy. All of the general DMARDs, including methotrexate, reduce immunity and increase the risk for infection. Getting a yearly flu shot is part of self-protection.

CHAPTER 11

1. **A**

   Sensitized B-cells, in response to initial recognition of a specific antigen, such as a virus, learn to secrete immunoglobulins (antibodies) directed against that antigen (invading virus). Although this response does not always prevent the person from becoming ill as a result of the exposure, it does limit the duration of illness and provides protection against future illness if the person is ever invaded by the same virus.

2. **D**

   A vaccine used to generate immunity is artificial rather than natural because it is purposefully placed in the patient's body with the intent of triggering immunity. Because it is a vaccine rather than preformed antibodies, the person's own immune system must take an active part in generating sufficient antibodies to provide full immunity.

3. **D**

   All immunosuppressant drugs reduce immune function to some degree and increase the risk for the person to develop an infection.

4. **B**

   RhoGAM is an agent that is composed of many anti-Rh antibodies. The purpose of giving an Rh-negative mother RhoGAM after she has given birth to an Rh-positive infant is to bind to and remove any Rh-positive red blood cells that may have been transferred into the mother's blood during labor and delivery. By removing these cells from the mother's blood, she will not begin to make any anti-Rh antibodies that may harm the red blood cells of an Rh-positive fetus she may become pregnant with in the future.

5. **C**

   Autoimmune disorders represent a failure of the immune system to recognize a person's normal cells as "self" and attack these cells as if they were foreign invaders. These inappropriate immune actions are progressive and destructive. The total white blood cell count is not affected by the autoimmune disorder, only by the drugs used to manage it.

6. **A**

   Use of direct-acting monoclonal antibodies suppresses the immune system and permits reactivation of organisms that a patient may have been previously infected with, especially tuberculosis and any viral hepatitis. These are contraindications for this therapy. These drugs are given parenterally and, therefore, are not affected by grapefruit or grapefruit juice. Although a patient can be taught how to self-inject the subcutaneous form of these drugs, that is not a critical piece of information to gather before the first injection. These drugs are not cross-reactive to sulfa.

7. D

The JAK inhibitors are associated with a risk for bowel perforation. This risk is greatly increased among people who have diverticulosis or diverticulitis. These drugs are prescribed to manage rheumatoid arthritis. Neither low blood pressure nor diabetes are contraindications to JAK inhibitor therapy.

8. A

A recipient with a normally functioning immune system will recognize a transplanted donor organ from anyone who is not an identical sibling as foreign tissue and take immunologic steps to destroy it. This is the normal job of the immune system. It does not know that the transplanted organ is beneficial to the recipient. Thus, in order to prevent rejection of a transplanted organ, certain components of the recipient's immune response must be suppressed.

9. B

Gingival hyperplasia is a side effect of cyclosporine. Although it changes appearance, it is harmless as long as the patient continues to keep his mouth very clean.

10. C

Want 520 mg/*X* mL; have 50 mg/1 mL. 520 mg divided by 50 mg = 10.4 mL

CLINICAL JUDGMENT

1. A, C, D, F, H

The information required to be documented in the patient's medical record or permanent log for vaccination includes the age and name of the patient; name of the vaccine; manufacturer, lot number, and expiration date of the vaccine; dosage of the vaccine; site of the vaccination; and condition of the site.

2.

INSTRUCTION/PRECAUTION	MOST RELEVANT	NOT RELEVANT	POTENTIALLY HARMFUL
Use two reliable forms of birth control because this drug is known to cause birth defects and fetal death.		X	
The weeks you take this drug, stop taking your other drugs for rheumatoid arthritis to avoid any possible serious drug interactions.			X
Wear nonsterile gloves when preparing your dose of adalimumab to prevent absorbing it through the skin.		X	
Rotate the sites so that you do not inject within 8 inches of the most recently used site.	X		
Pull back on the plunger after placing the needle in the skin and check to see if blood enters the syringe. If it does, do not inject that dose and prepare another dose to be injected at a different site.	X		
If you develop swelling of the face, lips, or tongue after injecting the drug, apply cold packs to the sites to reduce the swelling and avoid drinking anything until your lips can comfortably form a seal around a straw.			X

At age 60, this woman is not at risk for becoming pregnant regardless of how frequently she has sexual intercourse. Adalimumab is used with the other drugs to control her RA, not as monotherapy. The other drugs need to be taken as prescribed even in the same weeks she takes the adalimumab for the best effect. In addition, prednisone should never be stopped suddenly to prevent acute adrenal insufficiency. Wearing gloves to prepare the dose is not important (although using sterile technique is). She is self-injecting the drug and will experience maximum exposure to it. All of the direct-acting monoclonal antibodies injected subcutaneously require that the sites be rotated to prevent scar tissue formation and other tissue injuries. Subcutaneous preparations must not be injected intravenously. Thus, aspiration is very important to perform to avoid injecting the drug into a blood vessel. Swelling of the face, lips, or tongue after an injection are indicators of a severe allergic reaction. The patient is at risk for having her airway blocked. She needs to be instructed to call 911 for immediate medical attention and not attempt to use cold packs to reduce the swelling.

CHAPTER 12

1. D

Any type of diuretic increases water loss through urination. This water loss can cause dehydration if a patient's fluid intake does not keep pace with his or her urine output.

2. A

Diuretic drugs cause water loss and are often prescribed for edema. One liter of water weighs 2.2 lb. In helping the patient rid the body of excess water, the patient is expected to lose weight.

3. C

Too much time has passed to take both yesterday's dose and today's dose. Additional dosing would amount to doubling the dose, which could lead to more side effects and possible complications.

4. A

Diuretics do not cure high blood pressure (hypertension), they only control the problem. If the patient stops taking the diuretic, blood pressure will increase

5. B

Normal blood levels of potassium range between 3.5 and 5.0 mEq/L. This value, 2.6 mEq/L, is low (hypokalemia) and can weaken the skeletal muscles of respiration. Most likely, the diuretic therapy caused the kidneys to excrete too much potassium. Although the blood urea nitrogen level also is lower than normal, it does not pose an immediate health threat.

6. A

Furosemide is ototoxic (can reduce hearing). This effect is more likely to occur when the drug is administered intravenously at a rapid rate (faster than 10 mg/min).

7. A

Most salt substitutes are made by replacing sodium with potassium. Use of salt substitutes at the same time as potassium-sparing diuretics such as spironolactone increases the patient's risk of a high potassium level (hyperkalemia).

8. C

Extended-release tablets or capsules are meant to release a drug at a relatively even dose throughout the day. Chewing or crushing the drug ruins the timed-release feature and allows most of the drug dose to be absorbed at once. This can cause more side effects and limits how long the drug will be effective.

9. B

Tolterodine is an anticholinergic drug that can close the angle of the iris of the eye and decrease the outflow of aqueous fluid in the eye. For people who have closed-angle glaucoma, the intraocular pressure can become even higher and the risk for blindness increases.

CLINICAL JUDGMENT

1. A, B, D, H, I, J

Removing the old patch before applying the new patch to a different site helps maintain skin integrity. Any redness, itchiness, or irritation is reported to the prescriber. Transdermal patches are usually changed every 3 to 4 days. Before applying a new patch, clean and dry the selected site, and remove the adhesive backing. When the patch is placed, apply firm pressure for at least 15 seconds. Side effects of this drug include dry mouth and eyes. The expected actions of oxybutynin are decreases in urinary frequency and urgency, along with decreased urinary incontinence.

2.

PATIENT STATEMENT	UNDERSTOOD TEACHING	REQUIRES FURTHER TEACHING
"While I'm taking this drug my urine will be lighter in color and the amount will increase."	X	
"I will avoid foods like bananas and broccoli."		X
"I will sit on the side of the bed for 1–2 min before standing up."	X	
"If my blood pressure is 120/70 mmHg, I will report it to my doctor immediately."		X
"I will check my heart rate daily and report any irregular rhythms to my prescriber."	X	
"If I miss taking my morning dose, I will take two pills the next day."		X
"I will get my blood potassium tested as ordered by my doctor."	X	

Expected actions of thiazide diuretics include increased urine output, lighter colored urine, and lowered blood pressure. Thiazide drugs also result in a decrease in potassium, so increased intake of foods high in potassium (e.g., bananas, broccoli) is often encouraged. Decreased blood pressure can cause dizziness or lightheadedness, and the nurse will teach the patient to rise from bed slowly. A blood pressure of 120/70 is normal and does not need to be reported. Irregular heart rhythms can occur when the blood potassium is low and must be reported. The nurse teaches a patient never to take a double dose the next day when a dose is missed. The nurse teaches the patient to have blood drawn to check potassium levels as ordered by the prescriber.

CHAPTER 13

1. C

There are four classifications of hypertension (see Table 13.1 in the text). This patient's blood pressure is consistently within the range for stage 1 high blood pressure.

2. A, B, E, F

Health problems that can result from untreated hypertension include arteriosclerosis, heart attack, stroke, enlarged heart, kidney damage, and blindness. High blood pressure can affect the ability of the kidneys to remove waste from the blood by hardening, thickening, and narrowing the arteries to the kidneys. About 25% of patients who are on kidney dialysis have kidney failure that was caused by hypertension.

3. A

Antihypertensive drugs do not cure high blood pressure, they only control it. The patient must continue to take the drug to keep blood pressure at target levels unless the factors that are increasing the blood pressure are changed or eliminated. For example, sometimes blood pressure becomes normal again when the person is no longer overweight. In addition, if another drug is causing the hypertension, like corticosteroids, and the patient no longer needs to take that drug, blood pressure can become normal again.

4. B

Drugs that lower blood pressure can make a normal pressure too low and can make a low blood pressure worse. Checking the patient's blood pressure before giving a drug ensures that the patient is not hypotensive at the time he or she receives the drug. Some drugs can change the body's electrolyte concentration so much that an irregular heart rate can occur; however, **all** antihypertensive drugs can lower blood pressure.

5. D

This patient's blood pressure is quite low. If the patient is receiving this drug because he or she has hypertension, another dose of the drug right now could make the patient's blood pressure dangerously low. Sometimes a patient may be prescribed an antihypertensive drug for another reason. The nurse holds the drug and checks with the prescriber before administering this antihypertensive drug dose.

6. A

After taking the first dose of any antihypertensive drug, a patient may develop dizziness, light-headedness, or hypotension.

The patient should be given the call light and instructed to call for help getting up out of bed. The patient should also be instructed to change positions slowly.

7. D

Atenolol is a beta blocker that blocks the action of epinephrine on the heart. This results in a decreased heart rate and force of contraction, which leads to decreased blood pressure. Thus, the heart does not work as hard and requires less oxygen.

8. C

About 15% of patients taking an angiotensin-converting enzyme (ACE) inhibitor, such as lisinopril, develop allergies to the drug with the first symptom of angioedema (swelling) of the face, lips, tongue, and neck. The swelling can become severe enough to block the patient's airway, although this reaction is not usually as immediately life threatening.

9. B

Salt substitutes are mostly composed of potassium. Losartan is an angiotensin receptor blocker (ARB), a class of drugs that causes the kidneys to retain potassium. Taking in more potassium along with this drug could lead to high blood potassium levels (hyperkalemia), which has severe effects on heart contractility.

10. C

Carvedilol is an alpha-beta blocker drug. These drugs can cause elevated blood glucose levels, so the nurse should monitor blood glucose levels regularly in patients with diabetes.

CLINICAL JUDGMENT

1. A, F, G, H, J

Prazosin is an alpha blocker antihypertensive drug. Priority teaching points for this patient include: Do not drive or use machines for at least 24 hours after taking the first dose of an alpha blocker because a sudden drop in blood pressure can cause dizziness or confusion; get up slowly, especially during the middle of the night; the first dose is given at bedtime and the patient is instructed to rise slowly because of the potential for orthostatic hypotension; weigh yourself twice a week and check for ankle swelling because weight gain and swelling are signs that the body is holding on to extra fluid and must be reported to the prescriber; and a woman who is pregnant or planning to become pregnant should inform their prescriber because alpha blockers have a moderate likelihood of increasing the risk for birth defects or fetal harm.

2.

PATIENT STATEMENT	UNDERSTOOD TEACHING	REQUIRES FURTHER TEACHING
"While I'm taking this drug my urine will be darker and the amount will decrease."		X
"I will check and keep a record of my blood pressure every day."	X	
"I will get up slowly from bed or from the chair."	X	
"If my blood pressure is 120/70 mmHg, I will report it to my doctor immediately."		X
"I will get to the emergency department if I notice any swelling in my face or throat."	X	
"When I'm working outside, I will be sure to wear protective clothing."	X	
"If my heart rate is 90 beats a minute, I will increase the dosage of my beta blocker."		X
"I will be sure to let my prescriber know if I notice any weight gain or ankle swelling."	X	

Expected actions of thiazide diuretics include lighter colored and increased urine output. Any patient prescribed drugs for hypertension control must check and keep track of blood pressure. Because of the hypotensive effects of antihypertensive drugs, patients must be taught to rise from a bed or chair slowly. Swelling of the face or throat are indicators of angioedema which must be treated rapidly to prevent airway blockage. A side effect of beta blockers is sun sensitivity. A patient should not increase the dosage of any drug without consulting the prescriber. Weight gain and ankle swelling are signs of fluid retention and possible heart failure. A blood pressure of 120/70 mmHg is a normal finding and does not need to be reported.

CHAPTER 14

1. D

When the left ventricle fails, less blood is pumped out to the body and backs up into the pulmonary system causing signs of pulmonary congestion such as crackles and wheezes. Weight gain, peripheral swelling, and jugular vein distention are all signs of right ventricular failure.

2. C

Ankle swelling is associated with heart failure, although other conditions also can cause it. If this is a new symptom or is occurring even when the patient is not spending a lot of time sitting or standing, the nurse should assess the patient for other symptoms of heart failure. Although the blood pressure is not high, the pulse pressure is wide, which does not indicate failure. A pounding headache is most associated with elevated blood pressure. Foul-smelling urine is associated with urinary tract infection.

3. D

Some drugs for heart failure also slow the heart rate. If the heart rate is slow before taking the drug, the drug can slow the heart rate so much that the patient cannot adequately perfuse and oxygenate his or her vital organs. Usually, if the heart rate is less than 60 beats per minute, the prescriber is notified. The next dose may be held until the pulse rate returns to normal.

4. C

Heart failure can be improved with drug therapy, but the underlying condition remains. When heart failure is a result of damage, it is **not** cured. Drug dosage needs may change to control heart failure, but usually, the dosages only increase as time goes on.

5. B, C, E, F

Lifestyle changes that are important in treating heart failure include weight loss, smoking cessation, and a low-salt and low-fat diet. A fluid restriction of 1000 mL is not appropriate because it can result in decreased perfusion of the kidneys. Patients with heart failure may not be able to tolerate an aerobic exercise program. Alcohol can raise a patient's blood pressure and risk of heart problems. It should be kept to less than one to two drinks a day for a man or one drink for a woman.

6. C

Beta blockers and ACE inhibitors are often used together to treat heart failure. Beta blockers block the effects of epinephrine on the heart resulting in decreased heart rate and force of contraction, thus decreased blood pressure. A heart rate of 68 per minute is a normal finding. The nurse would notify the prescriber if the heart rate is less than 60 per minute.

7. D

Common side effects of nitroglycerin ointment include hypotension and headaches. When a nurse is administering this drug, if his or her skin comes into contact with this drug as it is squeezed onto the special lined paper, these side effects may develop. Wearing gloves prevents skin contact with the drug and decreases the risk of side effects.

8. A, C, E, F

Nesiritide is given by the IV route, so the nurse should always ensure that the IV line is patent. Heart and respiratory rate, as well as blood pressure, should always be assessed before giving this drug. The heart rate should be between 60 and 100 beats per minute and the respiratory rate should be between 12 and 20 breaths per minute.

9. B

Common side effects of potassium include nausea, vomiting, diarrhea, gas, and abdominal discomfort. Taking the drug with food or right after meals with a full glass of water or fruit juice will decrease or prevent these side effects. A patient should never take a double dose of any prescribed drug. Most salt substitutes are made by replacing sodium with potassium. Use of salt substitutes or eating excessive amounts of foods that are high in potassium while taking a potassium supplement increases the risk of hyperkalemia (high blood potassium).

10. A

Although all the actions are important, the most important is to ensure that the pulse rate is between 60 and 100 beats

per minute and is regular before administering digoxin or any other cardiac glycoside. For an irregular heart rate or one that is outside of this range, the dose must be held and the prescriber notified immediately.

11. A, D, E, F

Entresto lowers blood pressure by dilating blood vessels and reducing sodium levels, which improves blood flow. It lowers the risk for hospitalization when heart failure symptoms worsen and decreases the risk of death from heart failure. Kidney problems are a common side effect of this drug.

12. B

Serum potassium level affects the activity of digoxin. A value of 2.8 is low (hypokalemia). Any abnormal potassium value (high or low) requires the prescriber to change the digoxin dosage. In addition, action is needed to bring this critical electrolyte value back to its normal range. Although the other laboratory values are slightly abnormal, none are critically abnormal or likely to have an effect on digoxin activity.

CLINICAL JUDGMENT

1.

ACTION	RELEVANT	LESS RELEVANT	POTENTIALLY HARMFUL
Checking the patient's saline lock for patency and signs or infiltration or irritation	X		
Giving the potassium by the IV push route			X
Using an IV pump when infusing each dose of potassium	X		
Diluting the potassium in 20 mL of normal saline			X
Infusing each dose over a full hour	X		
Instructing the patient to report if the infusion is burning or painful	X		
Sending a blood sample for potassium after the first dose is given		X	
Checking the patient's heart monitor rhythm before and after giving each dose of potassium	X		

Before giving any IV drug, the nurse checks the IV site for patency and irritation or infiltration. If the site is not patent or shows signs of infiltration, a new IV must be placed. Potassium doses are **never** given by IV push. It is always diluted with 50 or 100 mL of normal saline and given slowly over an hour. An IV pump is always used to prevent the drug from infusing too rapidly. The nurse monitors the patient's heart rhythm before and after the infusion. A blood sample for potassium is sent to the laboratory after both doses are given to recheck the level. The nurse also instructs the patient to report any pain or discomfort at the IV site.

2. **A, C, E, F, I, J**

Dobutamine is a positive inotrope drug. Intended responses of these drugs include increased contractility, increased cardiac output, increased blood vessel dilation, decreased preload and afterload, improved heart function and contractility, decreased blood pressure, and improved circulation. While the nurse would monitor for all of these responses, decreased contractility, irregular heart rate, tachycardia, and discomfort at the IV site are not intended responses of the drug.

CHAPTER 15

1. **A**

The SA node initiates electrical impulses at a rate of 60 to 100 per minute. When the ECG shows P waves before every QRS complex with a rate between 60 and 100 per minute, the rhythm is a normal sinus rhythm which is initiated by the SA node.

2. **D**

A slow heart rate (less than 50 beats per minute) results in a decrease in cardiac output, blood pressure, and perfusion to a patient's vital organs. This leads to symptoms such as dizziness, light-headedness, syncope, and decreased peripheral pulses. While the nurse will want to notify the prescriber, the patient's blood pressure should be checked **first**.

3. **C**

A dry mouth is an expected response to atropine, which inhibits oral secretions. The nurse would also offer the patient the opportunity to brush the teeth and rinse the mouth; however, the **first** action is to relieve the patient's concerns about this side effect.

4. **A, C, D, F**

Use the acronym NAVEL to remember which drugs may be given by endotracheal tube: *N*arcan (naloxone), *a*tropine, *V*alium, epinephrine, and *l*idocaine.

5. **B**

Signs of digoxin overdose (toxicity) include nausea, vomiting, loss of appetite, diarrhea, and vision problems. Other signs include heart rate or rhythm changes, palpitations, and fainting. When these signs and symptoms occur, hold the dose, notify the prescriber, and check the patient's serum digoxin level. This drug has a very narrow therapeutic range (0.8 to 2 ng/mL), and any blood level higher than 2 ng/mL can cause serious problems or death.

6. **C**

Lidocaine can only be given by IV or by airway inhalation (ET tube). When given orally, the liver destroys most of the drug, making it ineffective.

7. **D**

With older adults, signs of confusion may indicate lidocaine toxicity. Older adults are more sensitive to the effects and side effects of this drug. Notify the prescriber immediately; the drug must be stopped and the patient started on another antidysrhythmic drug to prevent life-threatening dysrhythmias such as ventricular tachycardia. Once the drug is discontinued and metabolized, these symptoms will resolve.

8. **C**

When a patient is prescribed propafenone, the nurse always checks whether the patient has a history of bronchospasm, asthma, or COPD. This drug blocks beta-adrenergic activity and can cause bronchospasm.

9. **A**

Sotalol is a beta blocker. When a beta blocker is prescribed for a patient with kidney damage, a lower dose of the drug should be ordered. A creatinine level of 2.4 mg/dL indicates kidney damage. Whereas all of these laboratory results are abnormal and should be reported to the prescriber, the creatinine level is the **most** important.

10. **B**

Depression is a side effect associated with taking beta blockers such as propranolol. The depression may be new onset, or a patient with a history of depression may find that it gets worse while taking these drugs. The patient should be instructed to report increased depression symptoms to the prescriber. The patient also is instructed **not** to suddenly stop taking the drug. Although beta blockers often do affect sexual ability, this is not related to depression.

11. **B**

Want 1600 mg/*X* tablets; have 400 mg/1 tablet. 1600/400 = 4 tablets.

12. **D**

A male patient may experience pain or swelling in the scrotum while taking amiodarone. This problem is reported to the prescriber immediately so that the drug dosage can be decreased.

CLINICAL JUDGMENT

1. **C, E, H, J**

Intended responses of adenosine include slower impulse conduction through the AV node, decreased heart rate, elimination of SVT, and normal and regular heart rhythm. Common side effects of adenosine include facial flushing, shortness of breath, and transient dysrhythmias such as atrial fibrillation or atrial flutter.

2.

ACTION/TEACHING POINT	RELEVANT	LESS RELEVANT	NOT RELEVANT
Informing the patient of the increased risk for torsades de pointes	X		
Explaining that dofetilide is used to treat all tachydysrhythmias			X
Placing the patient on a cardiac monitor for 72 hr	X		
Documenting the patient's heart rhythm every 2 hr		X	
Inserting a urinary catheter to monitor urine output for 3 days.			X
Instructing the patient to report any chest pain	X		
Instructing the patient to drink at least 2 L of fluid daily		X	
Asking if the patient has a history of kidney problems	X		
Checking laboratory kidney function test results	X		
Inserting an IV catheter to give the drug IV			X

Dofetilide is a class III potassium channel blocker used to treat highly symptomatic atrial fibrillation or flutter. One of the adverse effects of this drug is the life-threatening ventricular dysrhythmia, torsades de pointes. Because of this risk, the patient is placed on a cardiac monitor and hospitalized for 72 hours after starting the drug. The drug is eliminated from the body by the kidneys and the drug is not given when a patient has kidney problems. Heart rate is assessed often and documented, but this does not need to be done every hour. ECGs may be ordered but not every 4 hours. A urinary catheter is not necessary and would increase the risk of infection. The drug is given orally; however, a saline lock may be placed in case of the need for emergency drugs.

CHAPTER 16

1. **D**

People who do not show lipid profile improvement after following a low-fat diet for 3 months often have a genetic factor that leads to familial hyperlipidemia. This tends to run in families and requires antilipidemic drugs to lower blood lipid levels. Telling the patient that a drug is definitely required may be correct in this case, but it does not address the patient's question.

2. **A**

All lipid-lowering drugs reduce high blood lipid levels, but they do not cure the problem. Treatment is long term, and these drugs need to be taken even after blood fat levels are normal.

3. **C**

The total cholesterol, triglyceride, and HDL levels are all within the normal range. The LDL level is high and should be reported to the prescriber because a high level increases the patient's risk for atherosclerosis.

4. **A, B, D**

Chronic hyperlipidemia contributes to the development of narrowed arteries. It can cause health problems including atherosclerosis, coronary artery disease (angina, heart attack), hypertension, pancreatitis, peripheral vascular disease, stroke, and xanthomas (skin atheromas or abnormal fat deposits).

5. **B**

Atorvastatin is a statin drug and can cause the adverse reaction of rhabdomyolysis, which is the destruction of skeletal muscle. The symptoms of this problem include muscle aches, pain, and weakness, as well as vomiting, stomach pain, and dark urine. When a patient develops this problem, the drug should be stopped and a different type of antilipidemic drug prescribed.

6. **C**

Renal failure can occur if rhabdomyolysis (muscle breakdown) occurs as an adverse effect of statin drugs. The proteins released from broken-down muscle can block urine flow through the kidneys leading to decreased urine output. Telling the patient that intake and output measurement is an important assessment of kidney function is essentially correct, but it does not fully address the patient's question.

7. **B**

Bile acid sequestrants are taken by mouth and work directly on dietary fats in the intestinal tract. They bind with cholesterol in the intestine, preventing fats from being absorbed into the blood. This action then eliminates the cholesterol from the body through the stool and also is likely to change the general activity of the intestinal tract, leading to intestinal side effects.

8. **D**

Colestipol can change the action of the anticoagulant warfarin in two ways. It can decrease the absorption of vitamin K, which would intensify the effects of warfarin and increase the risk for bleeding (as evidenced by a high INR). Bile acid sequestrants can also directly bind warfarin in the intestinal tract and cause its rapid elimination. This action would inactivate warfarin activity and increase the risk for clot formation (as evidenced by an INR level that is lower than the therapeutic range). Although all of the above laboratory blood values can help diagnose a bleeding problem, the most sensitive test is the INR.

9. **C**

Swelling under the skin, usually around the eyes, nose, and lips, is a symptom of angioedema, a rare adverse effect of ezetimibe. It is caused by blood vessel dilation and may be life threatening when it affects the airways.

10. A

Niacin causes a mild systemic inflammatory response with vasodilation that can result in the sensation of itching. This is not an allergy but can be very distressing to the patient. Often, taking aspirin reduces the inflammatory response and eliminates the itchiness. If the patient has no other health problems that would be worsened by aspirin, this should be tried first.

11. C

Niaspan is an extended-release form of niacin that is taken once a day. Niacor is an immediate release form of niacin. Immediate-release niacin should not be substituted for extended-release niacin. Additionally, extended-release niacin should be swallowed whole and never crushed or chewed because this causes immediate release of the entire drug dose and could lead to overdose symptoms.

12. D

Although all of these actions are important for a patient taking gemfibrozil, the priority action is to check the patient for signs of bleeding. Fibrate drugs such as gemfibrozil increase the effectiveness of warfarin by causing a prolonged prothrombin time, which can lead to excessive bleeding and become life threatening.

CLINICAL JUDGMENT

1. A, D, E, G, H, J

Excessive LDL cholesterol levels cause plaques to form in blood vessels and narrow the area where blood flows through these vessels. This results in reduced blood flow, and vital organs may not be well oxygenated. As a result, the risk for angina and stroke is increased. The same narrowing of blood vessels increases the resistance in the arterial system and raises blood pressure, leading to hypertension. With hypertension, the heart has to work much harder and may have less blood feeding the heart from the coronary arteries. These two conditions increase the risk for a heart attack. Other decreased risks with controlled normal levels of LDL include peripheral vascular disease and pancreatitis. High LDL levels are not associated with an increased risk for asthma, colitis, cystitis, or Parkinson disease.

2.

PATIENT STATEMENT	UNDERSTOOD TEACHING	REQUIRES FURTHER TEACHING
"Simvastatin will help my body eliminate cholesterol through my bowels."		X
"I will take my simvastatin once a day in the evening before I go to bed."	X	
"I will immediately get in touch with my prescriber if I start having pain in my leg muscles."	X	
"When my prescriber sends me to the laboratory for a lipid profile, I will have it done right after breakfast."		X
"I will continue to watch what I eat and get some exercise while taking this drug."	X	
"Once my cholesterol is back to normal, I will no longer need to take the simvastatin."		X
"If I get an upset stomach with gas and abdominal pain or cramps, I will stop taking this medicine."		X
"If I notice any yellowing or my eyes or skin, I will contact my prescriber right away."	X	

Simvastatin is a short-acting statin that helps lower blood lipids. It works by controlling the amount of cholesterol produced in the body. It works best when taken in the evening because the liver enzyme that creates cholesterol is more active at night. The prescriber must be notified of adverse effects such as rhabdomyolysis (symptoms include general muscle soreness and pain) and decreased liver function (symptoms include yellowing of skin and whites of the eyes). A person with familial hypercholesterolemia is not cured by statin drugs and will need to take them long-term. Stomach upset and other gastrointestinal symptoms are common side effects that usually disappear when the body adjusts to the drug. Continuing to follow a low-fat diet and exercise will help with normalizing blood lipids.

CHAPTER 17

1. B

Both thrombolytics and anticoagulants disrupt steps in clot formation. However, anticoagulants have no effect on clots that have already formed. Only thrombolytics can dissolve an existing clot. Neither drug causes a "thinning" of the blood. Blood viscosity (thickness or specific gravity) remains the same when a person receives either class of drug.

2. D

Aspirin is an over-the-counter drug with antiplatelet activity. However, it is not a high-alert drug.

3. C

Not all antibiotics can be administered intravenously. Although it is best to avoid IM injections, when it is necessary to use this route, firm pressure is applied to the site for at least 5 minutes after the injection.

4. C

Too much time has passed to receive an additional dose by any route. The dose of these drugs is never doubled. The nurse instructs the patient to take the usual evening dose now and just begin again with the prescribed doses and timing tomorrow. Patients taking an anticoagulant are taught to avoid aspirin.

5. D

The bolus dose of IV heparin is based on the patient's weight. Thus, obtaining the most accurate weight is the most important of these assessments.

6. C

With HIT, the platelets (thrombocytes) are consumed by microclot formation and the overall circulating number is way below normal. Other blood cells are unaffected. The INR is not influenced by heparin.

7. B

Ginkgo biloba interferes with blood clotting and must be avoided when taking either an anticoagulant or a thrombolytic agent. Taking it at a different time of day is not sufficient to prevent increased bleeding risk. Only warfarin-induced excessive bleeding can be helped with vitamin K, and it should be given parenterally for best effect.

8. A

When an ischemic stroke occurs, there is an existing clot in an artery in the brain. To resolve this problem early after symptoms develop, a thrombolytic drug (clot buster) is prescribed. These drugs must be administered within 3 hours of the onset of symptoms of stroke. Thrombin inhibitors and clotting factor synthesis inhibitors prevent new clots from forming and existing clots from getting larger. Antiplatelet drugs prevent platelets from clumping together (aggregating).

9. C

The only anticoagulant approved for use to manage DVT during the first and second trimesters of pregnancy is heparin. Aspirin alone would not provide sufficient anticoagulation for a DVT.

10. B

Vorapaxar is a relatively new drug. For best effectiveness, it is always prescribed with another antiplatelet drug, most commonly aspirin, although sometimes clopidogrel is prescribed instead.

11. D

Oprelvekin is a thrombocyte (platelet) stimulating agent. It is used to help a patient achieve a platelet count of at least 50,000/mm^3.

12. 0.5 mL

Want 10,000 units/X mL; have 20,000 units/1 mL. 10,000/20,000 = 0.5 mL

CLINICAL JUDGMENT

1. D, E, G

The drug is meant to be given as a deep subcutaneous (never as an intradermal injection) injection with the skinfold pinched up and the needle inserted at a 90-degree angle. Both aspiration before the injection and massaging the site after the injection are no longer recommended for most subcutaneous injections. The area for a 2-inch radius around the umbilicus is avoided for subcutaneous injections. The thigh may be used for subcutaneous injections, especially if the patient does not also use that site to self-administer any other subcutaneous drugs.

2.

INSTRUCTION/PRECAUTION	MOST RELEVANT	NOT RELEVANT	POTENTIALLY HARMFUL
If you lose an additional 10 lb or more, report this to your prescriber because the dose will need to be reduced.		X	
Try to take the drug at the same time every day as close as possible to 12 hr apart.	X		
If you forget one dose, double the next dose.			X
Switch to an electric shaver to shave your legs and other body hair.	X		
Do not take aspirin or NSAIDs while on this drug.	X		
If you develop swelling of the lips, tongue, and face, put ice on the swollen areas.			X
Make and keep weekly laboratory appointments to have your INR measured.		X	
Keep the tablets in the container that came from the pharmacy rather than using a daily pill organizer.	X		
Avoid eating grapefruit or drinking grapefruit juice while on this drug.	X		
If you fall and hit your head or spine, contact your prescriber immediately.	X		

The dosage of apixaban is not weight-based and no adjustments are needed for weight loss or weight gain. Maintaining a good blood level of any drug is important for its effectiveness. Thus, a drug prescribed for twice daily would have the best blood level when the two doses are taken as close as possible to 12 hours apart. Taking a double dose of any anti-coagulant is very dangerous and can lead to life-threatening excessive bleeding. Any anticoagulant increases the risk for excessive bleeding, even in response to a relatively minor injury. Patients are instructed to avoid actions and activities that have a high risk for skin injuries, such as shaving with a safety razor or straight razor instead of an electric shaver. Aspirin and NSAIDs are platelet inhibitors and should be avoided while taking a direct-acting thrombin inhibitor because they increase the risk for uncontrolled excessive bleeding. Swelling of the lips, face, and tongue are indications of a serious allergic reaction that will not respond to ice therapy. Patients are instructed to call 911 or go to the nearest emergency department if these symptoms appear. The effectiveness of direct-acting thrombin inhibitors is not measured using the INR and regular monitoring is not needed. The direct-acting thrombin inhibitors are light-sensitive and lose potency quickly when exposed to light. They should be kept in the non-light pene-trating container supplied by the pharmacy. Grapefruit and grapefruit juice alter the metabolism of these drugs. The direct-acting thrombin inhibitors increase the risk for internal bleeding when an injury occurs. Bleeding in the brain can be fatal and bleeding in the spine can lead to paralysis.

CHAPTER 18

1. D

Mast cell stabilizers work by preventing the membranes of mast cells from degranulating and releasing histamine and leukotriene. They do not stop the synthesis of these media-tors but keep them confined inside the mast cell where they do not induce tissue inflammation.

2. A, C, E

All drugs commonly used for asthma control and relief are also used for COPD. An additional drug category often prescribed daily for COPD management is the mucolytics, some of which are delivered by nebulizer daily. The focus for COPD manage-ment is on long-term control therapy with longer-acting drugs in two- and three-drug combinations. These are not recom-mended (and some are contraindicated) for asthma manage-ment. Although cholinergic antagonists are used more com-monly for COPD, they are also prescribed for asthma control. Interleukin 5 antagonists are not prescribed for COPD because disease symptoms do not appear to be caused by eosinophils.

3. C

Beta$_2$-adrenergic agonists are reliever or rescue drugs and are not taken on a regular schedule for COPD management. Instead, they are to be used whenever breathlessness is increased. These drugs do not alter mucus consistency.

4. B, C, E

Tiotropium is a cholinergic antagonist and can cause specific side effects if it reaches the bloodstream. These effects in-clude urinary retention, blurred vision, eye pain, nausea, constipation, dry mouth, and headache.

5. C

The mist contains slow-moving heavy particles that move down respiratory passages rather than up and out through the nose. Because these particles are slow-moving, the pa-tient has more time to breathe them in with an inhalation.

6. A

The drug works best when released and absorbed over time at a continuous rate. Chewing or crushing the tablet ruins this property and results in uneven blood drug levels.

7. B

Most inhalers require a significant degree of fine muscle co-ordination and strength. A person with severe arthritis of the hands may have an easier time preparing and taking doses by nebulizer than by inhaler.

8. B

The symptoms are those of an allergic reaction that can be life threatening. To prevent further harm, the infusion must be stopped immediately while maintaining IV access. Then the prescriber is notified and further assessment is made.

9. D

Endothelin receptor antagonists cause vasodilation of sys-temic as well as pulmonary blood vessels, which can lead to severe hypotension. These oral drugs do not increase clot formation or lead to sepsis. Urine output is only affected when hypotension becomes profound.

10. C

At 45 mcg/puff, two puffs are needed per dose for 90 mcg. A drug taken every 4 hours should be taken a total of six times in 24 hours. $6 \times 2 = 12$ puffs.

CLINICAL JUDGMENT

1.

PATIENT STATEMENT	UNDERSTOOD	REQUIRES FURTHER TEACHING
"I am lucky that I have the eosino-philic type of asthma for this drug to work."	X	
"My wife is willing to learn how to give me those subcutaneous in-jections."	X	
"It will be great to take asthma drugs only once every 8 weeks instead of daily."		X
"If I have a fever or any sign of infec-tion I will call my health care pro-vider immediately."	X	
"I will use a condom whenever my wife and I have sex to limit her ex-posure to this drug."		X
"If the injection site becomes red or sore, I will go to the emergency department immediately."		X

Benralizumab is a biologic specific for eosinophilic asthma and does not benefit patients with other types of asthma. This drug is administered as a subcutaneous injection. Although adverse reactions are always possible, selected patients or their family members can be taught to give the injections at home. Drugs in this class are "add-on" drugs taken in addition to traditional daily prescribed controller drugs for asthma, not in place of them. The patient must still take his traditional asthma controller drugs daily as prescribed and should use his rescue inhaler when needed. Although benralizumab is most specific for suppressing eosinophil activity, it does cause some general immunosuppression and increases the risk for the patient to develop an infection. He needs to know the signs and symptoms of an infection and report them immediately to the prescriber. Benralizumab does not pose a health risk from seminal fluid exposure. The patient may want to wear a condom for a variety of personal reasons, but limiting exposure of this drug to his partner is not needed. Soreness or redness at the injection site of benralizumab is an expected side effect, not an adverse reaction, and does not require emergency medical attention.

2. **A, B, C, E, G, I**

Short-acting beta$_2$-adrenergic agonists are rescue inhalers and are taken when needed, not on a regular basis. The drug reaches the lower airways best when it is inhaled slowly and deeply using a spacer and holding the breath in the lungs for at least 10 seconds. Because an attack can occur at any time, the patient must keep the inhaler with him or her at all times. Cleaning the inhaler at least once daily helps prevent an oral infection. Using the drug before participating in activities that are known to induce an attack for a specific patient can help prevent the attack or reduce its severity. The effectiveness of the drug is not affected by meals. The drug is not harmful to an embryo or fetus.

CHAPTER 19

1. **D**

Normal bowel function varies from person to person, from several times a day to several times a week. Consistency is more important than frequency. Stool should be soft enough to pass easily from the bowel, but not liquid. Bowel movements are a complex process involving several muscles and nerves located on the pelvic floor.

2. **A**

To prevent constipation, a patient should be taught to consume a diet that is high in fiber, drink plenty of fluids, and be physically active. Misuse of laxatives can cause constipation because the body becomes dependent on these drugs, needing higher and higher doses until the bowel no longer works.

3. **B**

While drinking bottled water is good, ice cubes may be made with tap water, which in some countries may contain bacteria that can cause diarrhea. Washing hands before and after handling raw meat or poultry is important, but it is not necessary to wear gloves. The patient should continue drinking adequate fluids while having diarrhea to prevent dehydration. Washing hands after using the bathroom or changing diapers can prevent the spread of diarrhea.

4. **A**

Ondansetron is an antinausea drug that is given 30 minutes before meals and at bedtime to prevent the nausea

that is associated with chemotherapy. Metoclopramide increases peristalsis to help move food through the GI tract. Antihistamines prevent the nausea and vomiting caused by opiate drugs such as morphine. If the drug were given after meals, its purpose would not be met because nausea and vomiting could occur before the drug is present to exert its effects.

5. **A**

Metoclopramide increases stomach and small intestine contractions (peristalsis), which help move food through the GI system. Increased peristalsis causes increased and sometimes loud bowel sounds (gurgling). The patient should be instructed that this is an expected action of the drug.

6. **C**

Promethazine, a phenothiazine-based drug, induces sedation and confusion in addition to having antiemetic effects. Some patients have reduced memory about events occurring within a few hours after receiving the drug. This is an expected, temporary side effect and does not indicate any permanent reduced cognition. Both the patient and the spouse should be aware of this effect so that the patient is not at risk for injury. Driving, cooking, or operating dangerous equipment should not be performed until the drug's effects have worn off.

7. **A**

Cyclizine is an antiemetic drug. Most of these drugs cause drowsiness as a side effect. The nurse instructs the patient to call for help when getting out of bed and makes sure that the call light is within easy reach. This is especially important because this is the patient's first dose of the drug, and its effects on this patient are unknown.

8. **B**

Laxative drugs are not meant for long-term use and should not be used for longer than one week unless following a prescriber's advice. The use of laxatives long-term can cause other health problems and can result in worse constipation.

9. **D**

Psyllium is a bulk-forming laxative and can be used once a day to help prevent constipation. Bulk-forming laxatives are the one exception to the rule that laxatives should not be used long-term. This drug is not absorbed from the intestines into the body and is safe for long-term use.

10. **B**

A common side effect of bisacodyl is hypokalemia (low blood potassium). The nurse monitors the potassium level when a patient is prescribed this drug and reports decreased values to the prescriber.

11. **D**

Scopolamine is an anticholinergic drug that can cause urinary retention. Older men often have some degree of prostate enlargement that may be undiagnosed and results in some urinary retention. Scopolamine makes this problem worse and can cause kidney damage. Comparing urine output to fluid intake is important for this patient to determine whether severe urinary retention is occurring.

12. C

Prochlorperazine can trigger neuroleptic malignant syndrome, a rare and life-threatening adverse effect in which dangerously high body temperatures can occur. Without prompt and expert treatment, this condition can be fatal in as many as 20% of those who develop it. One of the first warning signs is increasing body temperature. At this point, steps must be taken quickly to prevent this adverse reaction from becoming worse.

13. A, C, D

Adequate fluid intake (1500 to 2000 mL), bulk foods in the diet, and regular daily exercise are important strategies to prevent constipation. Patients should be taught to use the bathroom right away when the urge to have a bowel movement occurs. At least 8 ounces of fluid should be given with oral laxatives so that they can be safe and effective. Polyethylene glycol is an osmotic laxative and should work within 2 to 3 days.

14. D

Antidiarrheal drugs should not be taken for more than two days unless instructed by a prescriber. When a patient's diarrhea is not relieved after two days, the prescriber should be contacted.

CLINICAL JUDGMENT

1. A, C, E, F, G, I

When teaching patients about antiemetic drugs, the nurse includes getting up slowly from a bed or a chair because of hypotension and dizziness; using sunscreen, wearing protective clothing, and avoiding tanning beds because of sun sensitivity; drinking enough fluids to prevent constipation; taking antiemetic drugs before events that usually cause nausea; consulting with the prescriber before taking OTC drugs; using a mild analgesic such as acetaminophen for relief from headaches; and using frequent mouth rinses and oral care to manage dry mouth. If long-term use of these drugs is planned, seeing the dentist regularly (**not** every 2 months) to prevent dental disorders is recommended. Never take a double dose of any drug because of toxicity risks. CNS depressants including sleeping drugs are avoided because with many antiemetics there is increased CNS depression.

2.

INSTRUCTION	RELEVANT	LESS RELEVANT	NOT RELEVANT
Weighing the patient every morning	X		
Inserting a urinary catheter for accurate intake and output			X
Giving each loperamide dose with a meal or snack			X
Listening for active bowel sounds every shift	X		
Checking the patient's skin turgor for tenting on the back of the hand			X
Preparing a full glass of water to give with each dose of loperamide		X	
Placing call light within easy patient reach	X		
Assisting the patient up to the bathroom	X		
Sending a stool sample for bacteria and parasites	X		
Monitoring for changes in skin and mucous membranes	X		
Checking for signs of constipation		X	

Because the patient has diarrhea with dehydration, checking baseline and daily weights is helpful in monitoring the progress of the treatment. Loperamide is an antimotility drug used to treat diarrhea. Common side effects include dizziness and drowsiness, so the nurse would be sure to instruct the patient to use his or her call light and ask for help when getting out of bed. A stool sample is sent to the laboratory to help determine the cause of the diarrhea. Essential assessments for this patient include monitoring for active bowel sounds and abdominal distention. The nurse would also monitor for skin breakdown and check the condition of mucous membranes in relation to the dry mouth side effects of the drug. Adequate fluid intake is important, but the patient is also receiving IV fluids. Constipation is a possible side effect but is not the primary concern at this time. A urinary catheter is not essential and increases the risk of infection. Loperamide is not necessarily given with food. This patient is an older adult, and the places to check for "tenting" as an indicator of dehydration are the sternum and forehead.

CHAPTER 20

1. B

The stomach is the site where protein digestion begins. Acid is secreted in the stomach to enhance this process. Because the acids can damage the stomach lining, the stomach secretes a thick, gel-like mucus to protect it. Neither the esophagus nor the duodenum has this protection. Stomach contents that reflux up into the esophagus are highly acidic and cause inflammatory damage with ulcer formation to the lining.

2. D

The most common symptom of peptic ulcer is burning, gnawing pain caused by stomach acid coming into contact with an open wound (ulcer). The pain usually occurs somewhere between the navel and breastbone and may last from a few minutes to many hours. Even though foods and antacids may relieve the pain, the fact that this is new onset pain indicates that the nurse should notify the prescriber immediately.

3. D

Sucralfate is a cryoprotective drug. These drugs form a thick coating that covers an ulcer to protect the open sore from further damage and allow healing to occur. Histamine blockers decrease the secretion of gastric acids. Proton pump inhibitors block the secretion of gastric acids. Antibiotics are used to treat H. pylori infections.

4. C

Ulcers do not heal in an acidic environment. Histamine increases acid production by stimulating the stomach's parietal cells to secrete hydrochloric acid. Histamine (H_2) blockers reduce the amount of histamine that is present, which then results in less stimulation of the parietal cells.

5. A

Famotidine is a histamine H_2 blocker. The most common side effect of these drugs is confusion. You must teach the patient's family to monitor for changes in the level of consciousness and confusion and to notify the prescriber if this occurs.

6. B

Famotidine is a histamine H_2 blocker. This class of drugs can cause anemia. The patient's red blood cell count is more than 50% below normal.

7. A, C, D, E

When a patient has peptic ulcer disease, not smoking is highly recommended because smoking slows ulcer healing; is related to ulcer recurrence; increases acid secretion; reduces prostaglandin, mucus, and bicarbonate production; and decreases mucosal blood flow.

8. B, C, E, F

Risk factors for the development of GERD are listed in Box 20.3 in the text. Risk factors for GERD include being overweight or pregnant, certain diseases (e.g., diabetes, asthma, peptic ulcers), certain drugs (e.g., NSAIDs), drinking alcohol or caffeinated beverages, eating foods high in acid (e.g., tomatoes, orange juice), eating fatty or spicy foods, lying down too soon after meals, and smoking.

9. B

The change in the acidity of stomach contents reduces the absorption of calcium through the intestinal tract. As calcium is lost from bones, it is not replaced and the bones become more fragile. More bone density is lost from the hip, making hip fractures more likely, even without a fall or other trauma.

10. C

Aluminum hydroxide is an aluminum-based antacid. The most common side effect of these drugs is constipation. Patients should be taught to consume a diet rich in fiber-containing foods to prevent this side effect.

11. A

When a patient is prescribed an immunomodulator drug for IBD, the nurse assesses for signs of liver toxicity such as dark urine, jaundice, itching, and light-colored stools.

12. B

Possible adverse effects of biologics include increased risk for infection because of their effects on the immune system. The nurse monitors patients with previous infections such as tuberculosis or hepatitis B carefully because they may experience reactivation of these conditions when they start on biologic therapy.

CLINICAL JUDGMENT

1. A, B, E, F, H, J

Alcohol, caffeine, and spicy foods irritate an existing ulcer and promote inflammation. Smoking slows cell division and can delay healing. In addition, smoking promotes acid secretion. NSAIDs inhibit prostaglandin synthesis, which reduces the amount of gel-like mucus in the stomach and increases the likelihood that ulcers will continue to form. Stress is a risk factor for the development of PUD. Neither dairy products nor exercise promote ulcer formation or delay or reduce healing.

2.

PATIENT STATEMENT	UNDERSTOOD TEACHING	REQUIRES FURTHER TEACHING
"After I've been taking the rabeprazole for a couple of weeks my ulcer will be cured and I can stop taking it."		X
"I will be sure to report any black and tarry looking bowel movements as well as diarrhea to my doctor."	X	
"I will be sure to take some time to sit in the sun whenever I can."		X
"I will be careful not to drive until I know how this drug affects me because it can cause dizziness."	X	
"My doctor prescribed the rabeprazole because it will decrease the acid in my stomach so my ulcer can heal."	X	
"Once my prescription runs out, I will buy rabeprazole over-the-counter and take it so my ulcer doesn't come back."		X

Antacids do not cure an ulcer, but they change the GI environment so that healing is more likely to occur. Also, the patient should take the drug exactly as prescribed for as long as it is prescribed. Patients should report any black, tarry stools, diarrhea, or abdominal pain to their prescriber because these are signs of bleeding and possible hypovolemia. Rabeprazole can cause increased sun sensitivity, and the patient is taught to apply sunscreen and wear protective clothing when exposed to the sun. Patients prescribed rabeprazole (also lansoprazole and omeprazole) are cautioned not to drive or engage in activities that require increased alertness because these drugs can cause dizziness. The patient should not continue using the drug unless instructed to do so by the prescriber. Also, the patient must consult with the prescriber before taking any over-the-counter drug.

CHAPTER 21

1. C

When insulin binds to insulin receptors on cells, the cells' membranes become more open (permeable) to glucose, and glucose transport proteins in the cell membranes become more active. The overall result is the movement of glucose into the cells, which lowers blood glucose levels.

2. A

Noninsulin antidiabetic drugs are not insulin and only make the patient's insulin secretion and use more effective. Patients with type 1 diabetes have such destruction of pancreatic beta cells that they no longer produce any insulin.

3. A

Glyburide is a second-generation sulfonylurea that contains a "sulfa" compound. A patient who has an allergy to any other sulfa drug, including sulfonamide antibiotics, is likely to be allergic to a sulfonylurea and should not take glyburide.

4. C

Metformin is an oral antidiabetic drug that works in two ways to lower blood glucose levels. It decreases the conversion of glycogen into glucose within the liver and increases the sensitivity of the insulin receptor to binding insulin. The sulfonylureas and the meglitinide analogues force beta cells to release more insulin. None of the drugs inactivate the enzyme that breaks down insulin, nor do they increase the person's need for glucose.

5. A

Miglitol is an oral alpha-glucosidase inhibitor. It exerts its effects in the intestinal tract to prevent the conversion of starches into glucose. If it is not taken with the first bite of every meal, it has no effect on blood glucose levels.

6. D

Rosiglitazone is an antidiabetic drug used to help manage type 2 diabetes. It can cause heart failure and worsens existing heart failure. This drug has a black box warning that moderate to severe heart failure is a contraindication for prescribing this drug.

7. A

Semaglutide is a long-acting GLP-1 agonist given only once weekly and comes only as a self-injection pen. It does not have to be administered by a health care professional. It is not associated with any vision changes.

8. C

The abdominal site has the fastest and most consistent rate of absorption because of the blood vessels in the area and not because of its proximity to the pancreas. The other statements demonstrate a correct understanding about injection site selection and rotation.

9. B

The patient is very thin. Using either a longer needle or injecting the insulin at a 90-degree angle increases the likelihood of performing an intramuscular injection instead of a subcutaneous one, which would affect insulin absorption. Selecting a shorter needle and injecting at a 45-degree angle prevents an intramuscular injection into this patient.

10. D

The character of NPH insulin is uniformly cloudy. If the expiration date has not passed it can be safely used. Insulin should never be warmed by placing the vial in water.

CLINICAL JUDGMENT

1. B, D, E, F, G, H, I

The drug classes or groups that can lead to serious hypoglycemia when used alone are insulin, sulfonylureas, meglitinides, GLP-1 agonists, amylin analogs, DPP-4 inhibitors, and the sodium-glucose cotransport inhibitors. The alpha-glucosidase inhibitors, biguanides, and thiazolidinediones are only associated with serious hypoglycemia episodes when used with other blood glucose-lowering agents.

2.

ASSESSMENT FINDINGS	EFFECTIVE	INEFFECTIVE	UNRELATED
Weighs 10 lb (4.5 kg) less than 1 month ago	X		
Fasting blood glucose 132 mg/dL		X	
Serum sodium level 139 mEq/L			X
A1C = 5.9%	X		
Reports drinking one 12-ounce beer daily with supper	X		
Eats a full meal within 30 minutes of injecting exenatide	X		
Reports using sunscreen of SPF 40 or wearing a hat when outdoors			X
Walks at a moderate pace for 2 miles 5 days each week	X		

The weight loss is associated with a positive change in diet and exercise. The fasting blood glucose level is out of the target range, although this patient's overall glucose control is quite good as indicated by the A1C of 5.9%. This may represent a bad adherence day on the day before the test, not fasting the day of the test, or could mean improvement because no data were supplied to indicate what this value was 1 month ago before plan implementation. The serum sodium level, although within the normal range, is not directly related to this patient's management plan except to indicate that he is not dehydrated. Keeping his alcohol consumption to just one drink daily and taken with a meal is acceptable for controlling diabetes and preventing hypoglycemia. The patient is taking his prescribed drug at an appropriate time with regard to his food intake. Using sunscreen is a good action but not one that is required by this diabetes management plan. The patient's level of exercise with walking is appropriate for this stage of his diabetes care and does indicate the plan is effective.

CHAPTER 22

1. C

When thyroid hormones leave the thyroid gland and enter other body cells, they bind to receptors inside the cell and activate the genes for metabolism and energy use of every cell, tissue, and organ. This regulates the function and amount of work performed in the entire body. When thyroid hormone levels are abnormal, the symptoms are widespread because all tissues and organs are affected.

2. B

Autoimmune disease-causing Hashimoto thyroiditis results in a permanent loss of thyroid function. Without continuous thyroid replacement drugs, the patient's metabolism would eventually stop and death would occur. Antibiotics do not help this condition.

3. A

The side effects and adverse effects of thyroid hormone replacement drugs increase metabolic rate and cardiac activity. Checking heart rate and rhythm before giving the drug provides a baseline to determine whether or not the drug is working correctly or is causing an overdose effect. Although changes in core body temperature and bowel sounds will eventually indicate responses to the prescribed therapy, the most critical to assess are those related to cardiac function.

4. D

Although changes in dosages may eventually be prescribed, when starting thyroid hormone agonists, the patient must take the drug exactly as prescribed. Taking a lower dose does not improve the hypothyroidism, which has serious consequences on body function. Increasing the dose can lead to dangerous cardiac and central nervous system toxicities.

5. A

Although methimazole is not as toxic to the liver as propylthiouracil is, it can worsen damage associated with existing liver problems. If the drug is used temporarily before the patient can have surgery for hyperthyroidism, he or she will need to be monitored more closely for worsening liver problems.

6. C

Thyroid hormones should be taken on an empty stomach, at least 2 to 3 hours before or 3 hours after a meal, because the dose is so small and almost any other substances interfere with its absorption. Drinking a full glass of water with the drug can help its absorption.

7. B

Methimazole enters the thyroid gland and combines with the enzyme responsible for connecting iodine (iodide) with tyrosine to make active T_3 and T_4. However, the drug does not affect the hormones already formed and stored in the thyroid gland, so it may take as long as 3 or 4 weeks for a person to use all of the thyroid hormones made and stored before the drug was started.

8. C

Fludrocortisone increases the reabsorption of sodium and water. This response can cause heart failure or worsen existing heart failure. Continuous shortness of breath is a major symptom of heart failure. Although edema may also indicate heart failure, it has many other causes.

9. B

With adrenal hypofunction, reduced levels of cortisol and aldosterone decrease serum sodium levels below normal (hyponatremia) and increase serum potassium levels above normal (hyperkalemia). Adequate drug therapy with hormone replacement is expected to return these electrolytes back to their normal ranges (sodium = 135 to 145 mEq/L [mmol/L]; potassium = 3.5 to 5.0 mEq/L [mmol/L]). Response A indicates hypernatremia and hyperkalemia. Response C indicates hyponatremia and hypokalemia. Response D indicates severe hyponatremia and hyperkalemia.

10. C

Electrical conduction through the heart is reduced with any degree of hyperkalemia, and the condition can lead to heart block or lethal dysrhythmias. It is the most important assessment to perform for a client with an elevated serum potassium level. Respiratory rate and depth are more affected by hypokalemia because of the accompanying muscle weakness. The reduction then affects oxygen saturation. Although deep tendon reflexes may be increased with hyperkalemia, cardiac changes are more critical.

CLINICAL JUDGMENT

1. A, B, C, D, E, F, G

All precautions are a priority. The hormone replacement therapy reduces inflammation and Immunity, increasing the risk for infection. A pathologic problem with adrenal hypofunction and reduced aldosterone is increased serum potassium levels that cause cardiac dysrhythmias. Adrenal hypofunction causes low sodium levels, and the client needs to ensure an adequate intake of this mineral. The disorder is associated with hypotension and postural hypotension. Another common problem is hypoglycemia. The client should always have a concentrated oral glucose source on hand and eat it whenever symptoms of hypoglycemia are present. Skipping hormone replacement therapy increases the likelihood that serious and potentially life-threatening complications can occur quickly. Blood hormone levels need to be relatively constant. These drugs increase the risk for gastric problems and GI bleeding. Taking the drugs with food can help prevent these effects.

2.

INSTRUCTION/PRECAUTION	MOST RELEVANT	NOT RELEVANT	POTENTIALLY HARMFUL
Without a family history of hypothyroidism, your disease is probably milder and you may be able to stop the therapy once the symptoms have gone away.			X
Drink a full glass of water with each days' dose and increase your overall daily water intake.		X	
If you forget a day's dose, be sure to take a double dose the next day.			X
Try to take the drug at the same time every day so that you do not forget to take it.	X		
You do not need to change your usual food choices but be sure to take this drug at least 2–3 hours before or 3 hours after eating a meal or taking a fiber supplement.	X		
As your metabolism increases, you should recover your usual mental alertness and cognition.	X		
If you have any chest pain, call 911 or go the nearest emergency department immediately.	X		
Do not increase or decrease the dose of the drug unless your prescriber tells you to do so.	X		
Keep the tablets in the container that came from the pharmacy rather than using a daily pill organizer.		X	

Hypothyroidism, unless caused by drugs, is not a temporary problem no matter how mild the symptoms are when it is diagnosed. The thyroid hormone agonists must be taken for the rest of the patient's life. Drinking a full glass of water, although overall a good action, is not essential with this drug therapy. Doubling the next day's dose is NOT appropriate. If possible, the patient takes the missed dose as soon as it is remembered the same day and then takes the next day's dose as usual. Taking the drug at the same time each day helps the patient remember to take it. The dose of the drug is so low that it must be taken either 2 to 3 hours before or 3 hours after a meal so that substances in the GI tract do not interfere with its absorption. Although telling patient that their mental awareness will improve is not always a priority, this patient was concerned about it. When hypothyroidism is corrected too quickly, it can increase cardiac activity and cause chest pain (or even a heart attack). This is an emergency that must be investigated. The dosing of thyroid hormone agonists requires initially low doses that are *gradually* increased. Increasing the drug too quickly can lead to adverse effects such as a heart attack or seizures. Decreasing the drug (without prescriber input) reduces its effectiveness. The drug is not particularly sensitive to light. It can be safely kept in a daily pill organizer, especially if this helps the patient remember to take it.

CHAPTER 23

1. **B**

A person with a seizure disorder is more likely to have a seizure during times of increased emotional or physical stress (such as training for a marathon). While watching the diet and pacing the exercise program are important, they are not related to the patient's seizure disorder. Most antiseizure drugs do not require the patient to avoid exercise.

2. **A**

Before a seizure, some people experience an aura, which is a strange sensation. It can be an odor, sound, taste, or visual sensation such as bright spots or flashes. It is a common occurrence and not an indicator of tumors or pressure in the brain. Confusion, lethargy, and an inability to respond are common for the postictal phase of a seizure, but asking about these symptoms does not address the patient's question.

3. **C**

Absence (petit mal) seizures are more common in children. They involve a brief (few seconds) loss of consciousness and blank staring. A child may appear to be daydreaming. After the seizure, the child returns to normal immediately.

4. **C**

A common side effect of phenytoin is gingival hyperplasia (excessive growth of gum tissue). The change does not cause physical problems or endanger the teeth. Some patients choose to change drug therapy to avoid this effect, but this is a choice and not a requirement.

5. **A**

Carbamazepine can suppress bone marrow activity and decrease the number of WBCs. This patient's WBC count is much lower than normal (normal range is 5000 to 10,000/mm^3), greatly increasing his or her risk for infection. The drug must be discontinued as soon as possible (but not abruptly). The blood sodium level is slightly low as well, but it is not an immediate problem.

6. **D**

Female patients of childbearing age should be taught that birth control pills may not work effectively while taking this drug. To prevent pregnancy, patients should be taught to use another form of contraception.

7. D

It is important to try to keep to the dosing schedule to maintain blood levels of antiseizure drugs and prevent seizures. However, it has now been 10 hours since the missed dose. Taking it now and also taking the regularly scheduled second dose could cause blood levels to be too high. The missed dose should not be taken at all. The second dose can be taken now or at its regularly scheduled time and back to the regular schedule the next day.

8. C

Among the most common side effects of ethosuximide are GI symptoms such as nausea, vomiting, and indigestion. The nurse should give this drug with food or a snack to minimize or prevent these symptoms.

9. B

Lamisil is **not** a brand of lamotrigine; it is an antifungal drug. This drug is easily confused with the Lamictal brand of lamotrigine. The drug should not be given. The pharmacy needs to be informed about the confusion and asked to send the correct drug.

10. A

When a patient is prescribed morphine at the same time as gabapentin, the blood level of gabapentin is increased. The nurse should expect that the ordered dose of gabapentin will be decreased.

11. B

With an atonic seizure, typically there is a sudden loss of muscle tone for a few seconds, followed by postictal (after the seizure) confusion.

12. C

Ratio and proportion: 340 mg/X mL is equal to 500 mg/5 mL; $1700X/500 = 3.4$ mL.

CLINICAL JUDGMENT

1. A, C, H, I, J

The single most common cause of seizures is not known. However, for adults, the most common causes of seizures include head injury, stroke, and tumors. When a patient has a seizure disorder, seizures are more likely to occur during periods of increased emotional or physical stress.

2.

TEACHING POINT	SHOULD BE INCLUDED	SHOULD NOT BE INCLUDED	MAY CAUSE HARM IF INCLUDED
Valproic acid has a high likelihood of increasing the risk for birth defects or fetal damage.	X		
Breastfeeding while taking AEDs is safe and recommended.			X
A woman taking lamotrigine should take folic acid supplements throughout the pregnancy.	X		
If you are taking phenobarbital, you can use birth control pills to prevent pregnancy.		X	
Primidone had been reported to cause bleeding problems in newborn infants.	X		
Fetal hydantoin syndrome is a rare disorder that is caused by exposure of a fetus to gabapentin.		X	
If you are prescribed primidone or lamotrigine, you may consume only 1–2 alcoholic drinks per day.			X
Valproic acid during pregnancy has been associated with developmental defects, low IQ, birth defects, congenital anomalies, and damage to the infant's liver.	X		

Valproic acid has a high likelihood of increasing the risk for birth defects or fetal damage. Many of these drugs pass into breast milk and should not be taken by a woman who is breastfeeding because they may cause unwanted side effects in infants. Lamotrigine limits the body's production of folic acid. Folic acid deficiency during pregnancy is associated with a variety of birth defects. To prevent deficiency during pregnancy, a woman taking lamotrigine should take folic acid supplements throughout the pregnancy. Phenobarbital interferes with the actions of birth control pills. If you are a woman taking this drug you should use another form of contraception to prevent pregnancy. Primidone may cause increased birth defects, and there have been reports of newborns with bleeding problems. Fetal hydantoin syndrome is a rare disorder that is caused by exposure of a fetus to phenytoin. The symptoms of this disorder may include abnormalities of the skull and facial features, growth deficiencies, underdeveloped nails of the fingers and toes, and/or mild developmental delays. If you are prescribed primidone or lamotrigine you should avoid alcohol because it adds to the drowsiness that these drugs may cause. Valproic acid during pregnancy has been associated with developmental defects, low IQ, birth defects, congenital anomalies, and damage to the infant's liver.

CHAPTER 24

1. C

Alzheimer's disease is a form of dementia. Parkinson's disease is a neurodegenerative disease. Both illnesses involve interrupted nerve impulse transmissions.

2. C

Alzheimer's disease symptoms begin very slowly. In the early stage, the first symptom is mild forgetfulness, which is sometimes confused with age-related memory changes.

3. D

Age is the greatest risk factor for development of Alzheimer's disease. A patient with Down syndrome has an increased risk by age 50 to 60 years. Whiplash and head injuries, hypertension, smoking, and high cholesterol all increase the risk for Alzheimer's disease.

4. A

Because patients with Alzheimer's disease have difficulty with memory and cognition, the person or persons providing care in the home should be included when doing any teaching about the disease, including drugs and dosages.

5. B

Both rivastigmine and galantamine (Reminyl) commonly cause the side effect of GI upset. The nurse should give these drugs with food twice a day to minimize this side effect.

6. A

As for any drug delivered by transdermal patch, the old patch should be removed before applying the new one to prevent a drug overdose. The patches can irritate the skin and should not be replaced in the same position as the previous patch. Rotating sites prevents skin irritation and breakdown. Applying the patch closer to the brain does not increase brain absorption of the drug.

7. D

Entacapone is a COMT inhibitor. These drugs can cause the adverse effect of rhabdomyolysis, a serious and potentially fatal effect involving the destruction or degeneration of skeletal muscle. Signs and symptoms of rhabdomyolysis include muscle aches, muscle weakness, and dark cola-colored urine. The nurse must hold the drug and notify the prescriber immediately.

8. C

Carbidopa-levodopa can suppress bone marrow activity and reduce the circulating levels of WBCs (neutropenia), greatly increasing the risk for infection. More patients with Parkinson's disease are older adults and may already have some age-related decrease in immune function. Neutropenia and infection are more likely when the patient's WBC count is low before treatment with the drug is started.

9. D

An adverse effect of ropinirole, a dopaminergic/dopamine antagonist drug, is episodes of falling asleep suddenly (narcolepsy). Neuroleptic malignant syndrome is an adverse effect of COMT inhibitors. Depression with suicidal tendencies is an adverse effect of carbidopa-levodopa. Central nervous system depression is an adverse effect of apomorphine and can include respiratory depression, coma, and cardiac arrest.

10. A

Entacapone may discolor a patient's urine brownish-orange. This is an expected side effect and is not harmful.

11. B, C, D

The four major symptoms of Parkinson's disease are tremors at rest, rigidity, bradykinesia (slow movements and difficulty starting movements), and abnormal gait. Lack of facial expression is a symptom of this illness, but not a major symptom. Sleeplessness or insomnia is more characteristic of Alzheimer's disease.

12. B

Have 100 mg/1 tablet; want 200 mg/X tablets. 200/100 = 2 tablets.

CLINICAL JUDGMENT

1. B, C, E, G, H, J

Rasagiline is an MAO-B inhibitor. Patients must be taught to avoid foods with tyramine, an amino acid that can cause a hypertensive crisis when patients are taking these drugs. Examples of such foods are aged cheeses, sour cream, liver, yogurt, salami, and soy sauce (see Box 24.2 for additional examples of food to avoid).

2.

HOME CARE PROVIDER STATEMENT	CORRECT UNDERSTANDING	MORE INSTRUCTION NEEDED
"Now that the patient is taking istradefylline, she will no longer need to take her carbidopa/levodopa."		X
"Istradefylline is given for "off" times when the usual drugs wear off and PD symptoms reappear."	X	
"The istradefylline can be given up to five times a day to control PD symptoms."		X
"Pimavanserin is a drug used for treatment of the patient's hallucinations."	X	
"When the patient has difficulty swallowing capsules, I can open the pimavanserin and mix it with a teaspoon of applesauce."	X	
"Because of her age, the patient has no additional risk while taking pimavanserin."		X

Drugs for PD that are used as needed for "off" episodes in adults with Parkinson's disease who are treated with regular carbidopa/levodopa medicine. They do **not** replace regular carbidopa/levodopa. Istradefylline is given once a day. Inhaled levodopa is given as the contents of 2 capsules (42 mg per capsule for a total of 84 mg) via oral inhalation with the provided inhaler as needed for 'off' symptoms up to five times daily. Pimavanserin is a newer drug used for the treatment of hallucinations and delusions in patients with PD. The pimavanserin capsule can be opened and mixed with a tablespoon (15 mL) of applesauce, yogurt, pudding, or a nutritional supplement if a patient has difficulty swallowing pills or cap-sules. Pimavanserin has a safety warning because this drug can increase the risk of death in older patients with dementia-related psychosis.

CHAPTER 25

1. C

Because depression is often mistaken for a normal part of aging, many older adults with depression may be undiag-nosed and untreated. Depression affects the way people feel about themselves and how they interact with others. Women are twice as likely as men to experience depression and women are also more likely than men to seek treatment.

2. A

Bipolar disorder, also called manic-depression, is character-ized by cycling moods from severe highs (mania) and severe lows (depression). Increased risk for suicide and lack of plea-sure in life are characteristics of major depression. Persis-tently low moods are characteristic of both major depression and dysthymia.

3. B

Citalopram is a selective serotonin reuptake inhibitor (SSRI). SSRIs work by increasing the amount of serotonin in the brain by inhibiting reuptake. This drug begins inhibiting the reuptake of serotonin immediately, but the patient's symp-toms often do not respond for 2 to 8 weeks. In order to know whether this is an effective drug for a particular patient, he or she needs to take the drug daily for at least 8 weeks.

4. C

An order for Wellbutrin SR can be confused with Wellbutrin XL. Both drugs are norepinephrine and dopamine reuptake inhibitors used to treat depression. But Wellbutrin SR is a slow-release form of the drug given twice a day, whereas Wellbutrin XL is an extended-release form of the drug given once a day. Because of their absorption and differences in onset of action, these drugs are not interchangeable.

5. C

Prochlorperazine usually changes urine color to pink or reddish-brown. It is not an indication of bleeding or of any kidney problem. No action needs to be taken other than reassuring the patient about this change.

6. A

Amitriptyline is a tricyclic antidepressant that can cause un-stable ventricular dysrhythmias. Therefore, heart rate and rhythm are **most** important to assess to establish a baseline and determine possible adverse effects of this drug. Al-though the drug can also lower blood pressure and increase drowsiness, changes in heart rhythm can be life threatening.

7. C

Because children are more sensitive to the effects of fluox-etine, the drug may cause unusual excitement, restlessness, irritability, or trouble sleeping. The prescriber should be notified

if these side effects occur because a lower dose or a differ-ent drug may be needed to control the child's depression symptoms.

8. D

Benzodiazepines, even when given orally, act within 30 minutes of administration. SSRIs need to build up to a certain blood level and may take as long as 3 to 5 weeks to reduce anxiety. When an anxiety attack is sudden or severe, a benzodiazepine may be most helpful, even if it is just given once.

9. D

Benzodiazepines have stronger side effects than SSRIs and are more likely to cause dependence in a patient who uses them for an extended period of time. Both benzodiaz-epines and SSRI drugs control anxiety and allow patients to live nearly normal lives. The major benefit of benzodiaz-epines is that they act within 20 to 30 minutes and can be taken as needed.

10. B

Sertraline is a selective serotonin reuptake inhibitor (SSRI). This class of drugs has milder side effects and a much lower likelihood of developing drug dependence than benzodiaze-pines such as lorazepam. However, it takes 3 to 5 weeks for symptoms of anxiety to improve, and it must be taken on a daily basis.

11. A

All antipsychotic drugs tend to block dopamine receptors in the dopamine pathways in the brain. The normal effect of releasing the neurotransmitter dopamine is decreased. Transmission of impulses is decreased which in turn de-creases the symptoms of hallucinations, illusions, and delu-sions.

12. C

A rapid temperature elevation is often the first sign of an adverse reaction called *neuroleptic malignant syndrome.* This reaction involves the autonomic nervous system and is po-tentially life threatening. Until the cause of the temperature elevation is identified, further drug dosages should be with-held.

CLINICAL JUDGMENT

1. A, C, G, I

Oxazepam is a benzodiazepine. Common side effects of these drugs include sedation, sleepiness, depression, light-headedness, ataxia, and unsteadiness. The patient's gait must always be assessed for steadiness when these drugs are prescribed. Patients may need assistance getting out of bed, changing positions, or walking, but do not necessarily need a walker or cane. Patients should be taught not to take double doses of any drug because this could cause drug overdose with severe side effects or adverse effects. Patients taking benzodiazepine drugs are at risk for the development of dependency.

2.

NURSING ACTION	APPROPRIATE	NOT APPROPRIATE
Suggesting that a better choice for long-term treatment would be a benzodiazepine drug such as diazepam		X
Discussing the benefits of cognitive behavioral therapy (CBT) with the patient	X	
Recommending relaxation techniques such as meditation, deep breathing, massage, or yoga	X	
Asking the patient if he believes he can cope with his PTSD at home		X
Discussing proper nutrition and diet with the patient because taking paroxetine can lead to weight gain	X	
Reminding the patient that his prescriber will want to follow him closely while he is taking this drug	X	

Paroxetine is an SSRI drug used to treat anxiety while diazepam is a benzodiazepine. SSTIs have milder side effects and patients are less likely to become dependent on them. CBT is a type of psychotherapy that has consistently been found to be the most effective treatment of PTSD both in the short term and the long term. Relaxation techniques such as meditation, deep breathing, massage, or yoga can activate the body's relaxation response and ease symptoms of PTSD. The patient has experienced these symptoms for the past 3 years so asking him to self-treat is not appropriate. Paroxetine can cause weight gain, as can other SSRI antidepressant medications. In its class, Paxil causes the most weight gain, perhaps because it can be sedating, which tends to limit physical activity. The health care provider will want to see the patient often while they are taking paroxetine, especially at the beginning of treatment to monitor progress and check for side effects or adverse effects.

CHAPTER 26

1. C

Driving or operating dangerous equipment within 6 to 8 hours after taking any of these drugs can result in an accident or injury. Tasks that require mental alertness also should be delayed until these effects have subsided. All drugs for insomnia produce drowsiness and blurred vision and can impair judgment.

2. B

Flurazepam is a benzodiazepine with hypnotic and sedative effects, used mostly to treat anxiety or stress. Benzodiazepines are schedule IV drugs, which means that abuse of these drugs or their long-term use may lead to limited physical

dependence or psychological dependence. These drugs can be habit-forming when used for prolonged periods (2 to 4 weeks) and are no longer first-line drugs for the treatment of insomnia. Zolpidem is a benzodiazepine receptor agonist and is less likely to be addictive.

3. D

Benzodiazepines are drugs that depress the CNS by increasing the amount of GABA (gamma amino butyric acid) in the brain. GABA is an inhibitory neurotransmitter that results in hypnotic and sedating effects. Although these drugs are mainly used to treat anxiety or stress, a few are used as a short-term treatment of insomnia.

4. C

Older adults should be given lower doses of drugs for insomnia because they are more sensitive to the effects of these drugs and more likely to experience side effects. This is especially true for the first dose of a newly prescribed drug until the patient learns how the drug will affect him or her.

5. C

Drugs for insomnia should not be taken unless there is adequate time to sleep (4 to 8 hours depending on the prescribed drug). Inadequate time for sleep can cause side effects including drowsiness or adverse effects such as amnesia. This is especially important when the patient needs to be alert as for a mental function test.

6. C

Want triazolam 0.5 mg/X tablets; have triazolam 0.125 mg/tablet. $0.5/0.125 = 4$ tablets

7. B

Flumazenil is a reversal agent for a benzodiazepine overdose and can lower the seizure threshold in a person who has epilepsy. Pentobarbital and secobarbital are barbiturates that can raise the seizure threshold and prevent seizures. Triazolam is a benzodiazepine that can reduce seizures.

8. D

Benzodiazepine receptor agonists, also called non-benzodiazepine sedative-hypnotics or Z-drugs because many generic names start with the letter z, are a class of drugs that interact with the same receptor site that benzodiazepine drugs do, by turning on the receptor sites to induce sleep. Drugs from this class are now the first-line sleep aids for the treatment of insomnia. They are less likely to be addictive but must be carefully monitored by the prescriber because of the possibility of misuse.

9. A, C, F

Eszopiclone is a benzodiazepine receptor agonist. It should be taken as 1 mg orally immediately before going to bed, with at least 7 to 8 hours remaining before the planned time of awakening. A serious adverse effect of the benzodiazepine receptor agonists is *somnambulism*, or sleepwalking. If a patient is prescribed a benzodiazepine receptor agonist, they should have another person with them for the first night they take the drug at home to determine whether somnambulism will be a problem.

10. A

When a patient is prescribed warfarin, the nurse immediately reports if the patient is taking over-the-counter melatonin because taking the two together may increase the risk of bleeding from anticoagulant medications such as warfarin.

CLINICAL JUDGMENT

1. A, C, D, H, J

Typical symptoms of insomnia include difficulty falling asleep, waking often during the night or early morning, difficulty focusing on tasks, and not feeling rested after sleep during the day. Uncontrollable urges to sleep are typical of narcolepsy.

2.

NURSING ACTION	APPROPRIATE	NOT APPROPRIATE
Ensuring that the patient will have 7–8 hr to sleep before awakening	X	
Questioning the prescriber about giving this drug because the patient has coronary artery disease		X
Asking the patient about a history of confusion, dizziness, or falls	X	
Assessing the patient's current mental status before giving the drug	X	
Before and after giving the drug, checking the patient's vital signs and assessing the level of consciousness	X	
Teaching the patient to go to bed within 2 hr after receiving this drug for insomnia		X
Instructing the patient to have someone stay with him or her during the first night of taking this drug at home	X	
Telling the patient that he or she can get up to the bathroom independently		X

It is important to ensure that a patient has 7 to 8 hours to sleep before giving a benzodiazepine receptor agonist such as zolpidem. Ask patients about a history of kidney or liver disease because drugs are eliminated through the kidneys and liver, and if a patient has these problems, they will be more slowly eliminated, resulting in an increased level of the drug and increased risk for overdose. Before giving this drug, ask about a history of depression, confusion, falls, and pain and assess the patient's current mental status. Teach patients to go to bed immediately after taking drugs for insomnia because of the rapid onset of the sedation effects of drowsiness and dizziness. Instruct the patient to call for help when getting out of bed and ensure that the call light is within easy reach because these drugs can cause drowsiness and dizziness. Remind the patient to get up or change positions slowly.

CHAPTER 27

1. C

POAG is the most common form of glaucoma and is much more common in older adults. It does not occur as a result of trauma and usually affects both eyes, although one eye may be affected to a greater degree than the other.

2. A

The photoreceptors of the retina are the part of the sensory nerve that respond to light and enable vision. These receptors require a constant supply of oxygen. Higher than normal intraocular pressure compresses retinal vessels and limits or prevents blood flow to these receptors. As a result of this lack of oxygen, the receptors die and are not replaced. Loss of any photoreceptors reduces vision. Loss of them all causes total blindness.

3. D

Both eye drops and eye ointments can blur vision immediately after instillation. Vision may remain blurry with eye ointments until the ointment is removed. Patients must not drive, operate heavy equipment, or perform any skill requiring precision (e.g., drawing up an insulin dose) until vision is clear.

4. C

Latanoprost is a prostaglandin agonist. These drugs should not be applied unless the cornea is completely intact. Measuring intraocular pressure is not necessary when a diagnosis of glaucoma has been established. Prostaglandin agonists, even if systemically absorbed, do not affect body temperature, or heart rate and rhythm.

5. B

Primary open-angle glaucoma is not cured by drugs and the eye drops must be used as prescribed continually for control of intraocular pressure. Prostaglandin agonists are applied just once daily. If one day's dose is forgotten, the patient should not take it along with the next day's dose. Overusing drugs from this class reduces their effectiveness. Eye redness and itchiness are expected as temporary local responses to eye drugs. They are not a reason to withhold the drug.

6. D

Apraclonidine is an alpha-adrenergic agonist that is generally prescribed for short-term therapy. When used excessively, it can cause drowsiness as a systemic side effect. When used as prescribed, systemic effects should not occur.

7. D

An expected side effect of prostaglandin agonists is longer and thicker eyelashes on the side in which eye drops are applied. In fact, there is now a special formulation of the drug to be applied just to the lashes to increase length and thickness. In addition, the lashes, iris, and eyelid may become darker. Other than reassurance, no action is needed.

8. A, C, F

Apraclonidine, brimonidine, and dipivefrin are adrenergic agonists that cause pupillary dilation (mydriasis). This action allows aqueous humor to flow more freely through the pupil and be absorbed. The others either do not affect pupillary size to any degree or cause pupillary constriction.

9. **B**

Beta-adrenergic blocking agents, more commonly known as *beta blockers*, bind to adrenergic receptor sites and act as antagonists. They block the receptor and prevent the naturally occurring adrenalin from binding to the receptor. Selectively blocking beta-adrenergic receptors in the eye causes less aqueous humor to be produced by the ciliary bodies. These drugs also cause the fluid to be absorbed slightly better so that less remains in the eye to contribute to intraocular pressure.

10. **B**

Pilocarpine is a cholinergic drug that can be absorbed through the skin and cause many systemic effects, including headache, flushing, increased saliva, and sweating. If excessive amounts are absorbed, the patient can develop more severe problems such as asthma, hypotension, heart block and other rhythm problems, abdominal cramps, diarrhea, urinary incontinence, vomiting, and dizziness. The usual dosage is two drops per eye, which increases the chances that some drug will overflow onto the skin. Wiping any drug that falls on the skin prevents these severe problems.

11. **C**

Want 75 mg in X tablets; have 25 mg in 1 tablet. $75/25 = 3 \times 1$ tablet = 3 tablets

12. **B**

Always apply punctal occlusion to decrease systemic absorption of combination glaucoma drugs because systemic absorption of these drugs can cause systemic side effects on the body. Blinking the eyes several times should be avoided because this can lead to loss of the eye drop fluid. Wiping excess fluid from the eyes should be done but is not as important. Instructing that the eyes be closed for 10 minutes is not necessary.

CLINICAL JUDGMENT

1. A, C, D, F, H, I, J

The nurse teaches patients what to expect when an intravitreal injection is given: first, the patient's eye is numbed with eye drops. Next the eye is cleaned with yellow iodine solution. To keep the patient from blinking during the injection, a small device may be placed in the eye to hold the top and bottom eyelid out of the way, or the prescriber and an assistant may place their fingers on the eyelids to prevent blinking. The needle used to give the injection is very small and thin, and the injection happens very quickly, in less than a second. The physician asks the patient to look up as he or she places the needle into the sclera (white part of the eye) as far as the vitreous humor (jelly-like substance in the middle of the eye) where the anti-VEGF drug is injected. This is usually painless, although some patients experience some pressure or discomfort. As the anti-VEGF mixes with the fluid in the middle of the eye, the patient may see wavy lines. Once the needle is out, the prescriber will put a sterile cotton tip over the injection site for about 10 seconds to put pressure

on it and keep fluid from escaping. Finally, the eye will be flushed with a solution to lubricate it and keep it from getting irritated.

2.

PATIENT STATEMENT	UNDERSTOOD TEACHING	REQUIRES FURTHER TEACHING
"My combination glaucoma eye drops can cause better control of my eye pressure"	X	
"I will be sure to shake my bottle of eye drops every day after I use it."		X
"I will only have to put the drops in my eyes once a day."	X	
"After I use my eye drops, I will put pressure on the inner corner of my eyelids."	X	
"These eye drops are less likely to cause systemic side effects."		X
"I will be sure to use my eye drops at the same time every day."	X	

Combination glaucoma eye drops can lead to better control of intraocular pressure (IOP) through increased compliance and efficiency, although they should only be used when single eye drop therapy does not work. Some of these drugs are given as 1 drop to each affected eye once a day, reducing the number of drugs used and the frequency of eye drop administration, which according to research shows improved patient compliance with the use of these drugs. Always shake the drug container before (not after) using and apply punctal occlusion to decrease systemic absorption. Xalcom (latanoprost and timolol maleate) eye drops are 1 drop in the affected eye(s) once daily, at the same time each day.

CHAPTER 28

1. C

DHT inhibitors work directly on the prostate gland. They are a "counterfeit" drug that looks like testosterone and binds to the enzyme that normally converts testosterone to DHT, its most powerful form. This counterfeit drug cannot be converted to DHT; and, while it is bound to the enzyme, the enzyme is not available to convert the real testosterone to DHT. With much less DHT in the prostate, the cells in the prostate gland do not receive the signal to grow. As a result, the gland shrinks and puts less pressure on the urethra, allowing better urine flow.

2. A

Selective alpha-1 blockers can lower blood pressure, especially when changing positions (orthostatic hypotension), causing dizziness or light-headedness and increasing the risk for falls.

3. B

The symptoms of BPH and prostate cancer are the same. Prostate cancer is the most common cancer type in older men. DHT inhibitors improve the symptoms of obstruction, which can mask the presence of prostate cancer. Although younger men should be cautioned not to donate blood during therapy and for 6 months after therapy (because the drug in the blood could cause birth defects if a pregnant woman received the blood), most blood centers do not permit people older than 75 years to donate blood.

4. D

Tamsulosin is a selective alpha-1 blocker that acts to relax smooth muscle tissue in the prostate gland, the neck of the bladder, and in the urethra. When these receptors are bound with selective alpha-1 blockers, the smooth muscle relaxes, placing less pressure on the urethra and improving urine flow.

5. B

The intended responses for drugs used to treat BPH include pressure is decreased, urine flow from the bladder through the urethra is improved, and BPH symptoms (frequency, difficulty starting or stopping the urine stream, dribbling, excessive nighttime urination, feeling of incomplete bladder emptying) are decreased.

6. C

Drugs for BPH are metabolized by the liver. If the patient's liver is impaired, the drug is excreted more slowly, and higher blood levels could result. Higher blood levels lead to more severe side effects. Patients with liver impairment should be prescribed *lower* dosages of these drugs (0.5 mg daily is the normal dose for this drug).

7. A

While side effects of testosterone are uncommon, some side effects that may occur including acne or oily skin, mild fluid retention, increased size of prostate with difficulty urinating, breast enlargement, sleep apnea, and decreased size of testicles. Pain or inflammation may occur at IM injection sites, while pruritus (itching), erythema (redness), or skin irritation may occur with transdermal patches.

8. B

Testosterone can cause virilization in children and women following secondary exposure. Warn them to avoid touching skin, clothing, or linens that have come into contact with testosterone preparations. Additionally, testosterone preparations have a high likelihood of increasing the risk for birth defects or fetal damage and should be avoided during pregnancy or breastfeeding.

9. D

PDE-5 drugs may cause prolonged erections lasting over 4 hours. Priapism (painful erections lasting over 6 hours) can occur but is rare. Notify the prescriber and teach patients to notify the prescriber when this happens.

10. C

Teach patients to check weight every day to assess for fluid retention, and report weight gain of 5 or more pounds (indicating significant fluid retention) to the prescriber.

11. B

DHT inhibitors are teratogens and can cause birth defects, especially in male fetuses. Women who are pregnant, may

become pregnant, or are breastfeeding should not take these drugs or handle them if the tablet or capsule is crushed or broken.

12. C

Want 250 mg/X mL; have 100 mg/1 mL. 250/100 = 2.5 mL

CLINICAL JUDGMENT

1. B, D, F, G, I

Symptoms of BPH include increased frequency of urination, nocturia (increased urination at night), difficulty in starting (hesitancy) and continuing urination, reduced force and size of the urine stream, feeling of incomplete bladder emptying, and dribbling after urinating. The symptoms of prostate enlargement are uncomfortable and can interfere with the patient getting adequate sleep and rest.

2.

INSTRUCTION	RELEVANT	NOT RELEVANT	POTENTIALLY HARMFUL
Take your sildenafil at least 2 hr before anticipated sexual activity.		X	
If you are prescribed a nitrate drug, be sure to have at least 2 hr between taking sildenafil and your nitrate.			X
The drug will not work without sexual stimulation.	X		
Priapism is an expected side effect of sildenafil.			X
Notify your prescriber if you experience an erection that lasts longer than 4 hr.	X		
A side effect while taking sildenafil is weight loss.		X	
Report any sudden loss of vision or hearing to the prescriber.	X		
Get up slowly when rising from a lying or sitting position.	X		
The action of sildenafil will last up to 36 hr.		X	
Be sure to eat grapefruit or drink grapefruit juice at least twice a week while taking sildenafil.			X

Sildenafil should be taken 30 minutes to an hour before sexual activity. Use of nitrate drugs is avoided while taking sildenafil because the combination of these drugs may cause severe hypotension. Sexual stimulation is required for sildenafil's action to work. Priapism is a dangerously long and painful erection and must be reported immediately to the prescriber. Any erection lasting longer than 4 hours must be reported to the prescriber. Weight loss is not a side effect of sildenafil; however, if a patient is overweight, weight loss is recommended because being overweight can make erectile dysfunction worse. Sudden loss of vision or hearing are potential though rare adverse reactions of this drug and should be immediately reported to the prescriber. Patients should be taught to get up slowly when taking this drug because side effects such as dizziness, light-headedness, or hypotension can occur. The action of sildenafil lasts about 4 hours while the effects of tadalafil can last up to 36 hours. Grapefruit products are avoided because they may increase the concentration of sildenafil and cause toxicity.

CHAPTER 29

1. D

Gonadotropin-releasing hormone (GnRH) is the stimulatory hormone secreted by the hypothalamus of both males and females to start the hormone changes needed for puberty.

2. C

In women who still have a uterus, estrogen-only HRT keeps thickening the uterine lining and leads to excessive uterine bleeding. Although all the other changes also can occur with this therapy, and with any HRT for relief of perimenopausal symptoms, excessive uterine bleeding is the most serious.

3. C

Drospirenone is a progesterone replacement drug that increases the reabsorption of potassium. It should not be taken with any other drug that also increases blood levels of potassium, such as ACE inhibitors, because blood potassium levels could become dangerously high.

4. A

Enlarged breasts that are firmer and at times tender are a common and expected side effect of the estrogen in oral hormonal contraceptives. This condition does not require any reporting beyond reassuring the patient.

5. C

The "mini-pills" contain only progesterone, which raise blood levels of progesterone, causing the hormone pathway to be turned off through negative feedback. This negative feedback suppresses the surge of LH and ovulation. In addition to suppressing ovulation, other changes occur that prevent pregnancy, such as thickening the cervical mucus, which prevents movement of sperm into the uterus, and thinning of the endometrium so that a pregnancy is not supported.

6. B

The two most important minerals and vitamins for maintaining bone health, preventing osteoporosis, and ensuring the effectiveness of drugs for osteoporosis are calcium and activated vitamin D. Without the presence of activated vitamin D, dietary calcium is minimally absorbed from the gastrointestinal tract.

7. A

Risedronate is a bisphosphonate. This class of drugs is irritating to the esophagus and other tissues they contact. Preexisting gastroesophageal reflux disease is a contraindication for this drug class because of the increased risk for esophageal ulceration.

8. B

Alendronate 5 mg is taken orally daily. The 35 mg dose is a once weekly dose, not daily, monthly, or yearly.

9. D

Corticosteroids increase bone density loss and suppress osteoblastic activity. This action of corticosteroids occurs in men as well as women. So, the patient with the greatest risk for osteoporosis resulting from drug therapy is the one who takes a corticosteroid daily.

CLINICAL JUDGMENT

1. D, H

Of all the drugs listed, only ibandronate and zoledronic acid can be given intravenously (although ibandronate can also be taken orally).

2.

PATIENT STATEMENT	CORRECT UNDERSTANDING	MORE TEACHING IS NEEDED
My friends tell me that I shouldn't smoke when taking drugs for menopause, so I have switched to vaping instead.		X
It's a good thing my husband has had a vasectomy because estrogen will increase my risk for getting pregnant.		X
I will make certain to have a mammogram every year.	X	
If I forget a dose one day, I will take two doses the next day.		X
I will take the drug for a year and see what happens when I stop taking it.	X	
If my skin or eyes start to get yellow, I will contact my prescriber immediately.	X	

Nicotine use in any form, vaping just as much as smoking, increases the risk for clot formation and must be avoided. The statement is erroneous in that these hormones do not increase the chances of pregnancy, but it is not a critical issue for this patient. Hormonal therapy with estrogen, progesterone, or estrogen/progesterone does increase the growth rates of hormonal-dependent cancers, including breast cancer, and also appears to play a role in breast cancer development. A double dose of this drug is not ever recommended even when a dose has been missed. HRT should be a short-term therapy option. Stopping the drug after a year to determine whether menopause is complete is a very reasonable approach. These drugs are metabolized by the liver and can contribute to liver impairment. Yellowing of the skin or sclera are indicators of possible liver impairment.

Bibliography

Alzheimer's Association (2121). Aducanumab approved for treatment of Alzheimer's disease. Retrieved from https://www.alz.org/alzheimers-dementia/treatments/aducanumab.

Alzheimer's Association. (2021). Medications for memory, cognition and dementia-related behaviors. Retrieved from https://www.alz.org/alzheimers-dementia/treatments/medications-for-memory#:~:text=Cholinesterase%20inhibitors%20(Aricept%C2%AE%2C%20Exelon,judgment%20and%20other%20thought%20processes.

American Diabetes Association Professional Practice Committee. (2022). Classification and diagnosis of diabetes: Standards of medical care in diabetes—2022. *Diabetes Care, 45*(Supp 1), s17–s38.

American Parkinson's Disease Association. New Parkinson's disease treatments. Retrieved from https://www.apdaparkinson.org/article/new-treatments-for-parkinsons-disease.

Anderson, P., & Townsend, T. (2015). Preventing high-alert medication errors in hospital patients. *American Nurse Today, 10*(5), 18–22.

Aschenbrenner, D. (2018). Drug Watch: Patient education on generic drugs. *American Journal of Nursing, 118*(10), 18–19.

Aschenbrenner, D. (2019). Drug Watch: Tofacitinib receives new boxed safety warning. *American Journal of Nursing, 119*(11), 20.

Aschenbrenner, D. (2020). Drug Watch: Hydrochlorothiazide associated with risk of skin cancer. *American Journal of Nursing, 120*(12), 22–23.

Aschenbrenner, D. (2020). Drug Watch: New drugs for breast cancer. *American Journal of Nursing, 120*(8), 22–23.

Aschenbrenner, D. (2020). Drug Watch: Ranitidine withdrawn from the market. *American Journal of Nursing, 120*(8), 23.

Aschenbrenner, D. (2020). Drug Watch: Remdesivir receives emergency use authorization for severely patients with COVID-19. *American Journal of Nursing, 120*(7), 26.

Baldwin, K., & Walsh, V. (2014). Independent double-checks for high-alert medications: Essential practice. *Nursing, 44*(4), 65–67.

Barbel, P. (2019). Vaccine safety in infants and children. *Nursing, 49*(12), 42–49.

Bartlett, D. (2017). Drug-induced serotonin syndrome. *Critical Care Nurse, 37*(1), 49–54.

Beery, T. A., Workman, M. L., & Eggert, J. (2018). *Genetics and genomics in nursing and health care* (2nd ed.). Philadelphia: FA Davis.

Bertschi, L. (2021). Back to basics: The complete blood count. *American Journal of Nursing, 121*(1), 38–45.

Beydoun, S. (2018). The art and science of medication administration. *American Nurse Today, 13*(9), 99–102.

Blevins, S. (2017). Immunizations for the adult patient. *MEDSIURG Nursing, 26*(2), 138–151.

Bohnenkamp, S. (2018). Immuno-oncology: Another option for treatment of cancer. *MEDSIURG Nursing, 27*(5), 336–340.

Branstetter-Hall, J., & Felicilda-Reynaldo, R. (2017). Antiviral medications, part 3: Evidence-based treatment of hepatitis B. *MEDSURG Nursing, 26*(6), 393–398.

Brien, L. (2019). Anticoagulant medicines for the prevention and treatment of thromboembolism. *AACN Advanced Critical Care, 30*(2), 126–138.

Cadet, M. (2021). Antiretroviral therapies and corticosteroids: Drug-drug interactions. *The Nurse Practitioner, 46*(12), 40–41.

Capriotti, T., & Sapp, S. (2021). Clinical update on the medical use of marijuana. *MEDSIURG Nursing, 30*(3), 175–180.

Centers for Disease Control and Prevention (CDC). (2019). *Biggest threats and data: Antibiotic/antimicrobial resistance (AR/AMR).* Retrieved from https://www.cdc.gov/drugresistance/biggest-threats.html.

Centers for Disease Control and Prevention (CDC). (2020). *Fast facts on diabetes.* Retrieved from https://www.cdc.gov/diabetes/data/statistics-report/index.html.

Cheek, D., & Howington, L. (2018). Pharmacogenetics in critical care. *AACN Advanced Critical Care, 29*(1), 36–42.

Chesebro, J., Armes, K., & Peterson, K. (2019). Focus on pharmacotherapy for depression. *Nursing, 49*(12), 32–39.

Chu, R. (2016). Simple steps to reduce medication errors. *Nursing, 46*(8), 63–65.

Cleveland Clinic. Dofetilde: A new class III antiarrythmic. Retrieved from https://my.clevelandclinic.org/health/drugs/16936-dofetilide-antiarrhythmic-medication.

Cleveland Clinic. Sleeping pills. Retrieved from https://my.clevelandclinic.org/health/drugs/15308-sleeping-pills.

Clinical Pharmacology powered by ClinicalKey®. Philadelphia: Elsevier. Retrieved from https://www.clinicalkey.com/pharmacology/.

Cohen, M. (2020). Medication errors. *Nursing, 50*(5), 72.

Connoe, J., Ahern, J., Cuccovia, B., Arnold, A., & Hickey, P. (2016). Implementing a distraction-free practice with the red zone medication safety initiative. *Dimensions of Critical Care Nursing, 35*(3), 116–124.

Cooper, C., Tupper, R., & Holm, K. (2016). Interruptions during medication administration: A descriptive study. *MEDSURG Nursing, 25*(3), 186-191.

Crohn's and Colitis Foundation. Fact Sheet News from the IBD Center: Corticosteroids. Retrieved from www.chronscolitis-foundation.org.

Crohn's and Colitis Foundation. Fact Sheet News from the IBD Center: Immunomodulators. Retrieved from www.chronscolitisfoundation.org.

Crohn's and Colitis Foundation. Fact Sheet News from the IBD Center: Aminosalicylates. Retrieved from www.chronscolitisfoundation.org.

Crohn's and Colitis UK. Information sheet: Biologic medicines. Retrieved from https://crohnsandcolitis.org.uk/info-support/information-about-crohns-and-colitis/all-information-about-crohns-and-colitis/treatments/biologic-medicines#:~:text=What%20biologic%20medicines%20are%20used,%2C%20golimumab%2C%20vedolizumab%20and%20ustekinumab.

Davis, L. (2021). Hypertension update: Implications for nursing practice. *American Nurse Journal, 16*(11), 6–10.

Dickinson, J. (2020). A broader look at insulin. *American Nurse Journal, 15*(6), 14–18.

DiGiulio, M., Loveless, T., Heider, G., Fagan, K., & Porsche, B. (2020). Bisphosphonate drug holidays: One size does not fit all. *The Nurse Practitioner, 45*(3), 50–55.

Drugs.com. Entresto. Retrieved from https://www.drugs.com/uk/entresto.html.

Drugs.com. Thiazide diuretics. Retrieved from https://www.drugs.com/drug-class/thiazide-diuretics.html#:~:text=

Thiazide%20diuretics%20are%20a%20type,functional%20 unit%20of%20a%20kidney).

Drug News. (2021). Migraines: FDA approves new intranasal treatment. *Nursing, 51*(11), 9.

Durham, M. (2020). Mindfulness for medication safety. *American Nurse Journal, 15*(7), 24–26.

Edvinsson, L., & Goadsby, P. (2019). Discovery of CGRP in relation to migraine. *Cephalagia, International Headache Society, 39*(3), 331–332.

Epilepsy Foundation. (2021). Summary of antiepileptic drugs. Retrieved from https://www.epilepsy.com/stories/summary-antiepileptic-drugs.

Felicilda-Reynaldo, R., & Inocian, E. (2020). Drugs for pulmonary arterial hypertension: Endothelin receptor antagonists. *MEDSURG Nursing, 29*(4), 259–262, 266.

Felicilda-Reynaldo, R., & Kenneally, M. (2019). First-line medications for osteoporosis. *MEDSURG Nursing, 28*(6), 381–330.

Felicilda-Reynaldo, R., & Patterson, K. (2017). Antiviral medications, part 1: Treating herpes and influenza viruses. *MEDSURG Nursing, 26*(1), 47–52.

Felicilda-Reynaldo, R., & Patterson, K. (2018). Antiviral medications, part 4: Evidence-based treatment of hepatitis C. *MEDSURG Nursing, 27*(1), 49–52.

Foust, J., & Kilbourne, G. (2015). Improving posthospital medication management for chronically ill older adults. *American Nurse Today, 10*(3), 26, 28–29.

Fredericks, T. (2018). Medication reconciliation. *MEDSURG Nursing, 27*(5), 329–330.

Fredrikson, K., & Fasoline, T. (2021). Pharmacogenetic testing: Clinical integration and application for chronic pain management. *The Nurse Practitioner, 46*(4), 12–19.

Galante, C. (2022). Asthma management updates. *Nursing, 52*(2) 25–33.

Gann, M. (2015). How informatics nurses use bar code technology to reduce medication errors. *Nursing 45*(3), 60–66.

Goetz, A., McCormick, S., Phillips, R., & Friedman, D. (2022). Diagnosing and managing migraine. *American Journal of Nursing, 122*(1), 32–43.

Good Therapy. (2021). Typical and atypical antipsychotic agents. Retrieved from https://www.goodtherapy.org/drugs/antipsychotics.html.

Hafeez, U., Gan, H., & Scott, A. (2018). Monoclonal antibodies as immunomodulatory therapy against cancer and autoimmune diseases. *Current Opinion in Pharmacology, 41*, 114–121.

Hafer, A., & McCann, L. (2021). Direct oral anticoagulant reversal: An update. *Nursing, 51*(6), 54–64.

Haugen, N. (2020). Promoting safe use of parenteral anticoagulants. *American Nurse Journal*, 37–40.

Huether, S., McCance, K., & Brashers, V. (2020). *Understanding pathophysiology* (7th ed.). St. Louis: Elsevier.

Hussar, D. (2017). New drugs 2017, part 1. *Nursing, 47*(11), 32–39.

Hussar, D. (2017). New drugs 2017, part 3: Selexipeg. *Nursing, 47*(11), 29.

Hussar, D. (2018). New drugs 2018, Part 1: Antiviral drugs for HCV. *Nursing, 46*(2), 36–44.

Hussar, D. (2019). New drugs 2019, Part 1. *Nursing, 49*(2), 28–34.

Hussar, D. (2020). New drugs 2020, Part 3. *Nursing, 50*(10), 32–41.

Ignatavicius, D., Workman, M. L., Rebar, C., & Heimgartner, N. (2021). *Medical-surgical nursing: Concepts for professional collaboration* (10th ed.). St. Louis: Elsevier.

Iliades, C. (2020). 10 Things to know about biologics for ulcerative colitis. Retrieved from https://www.everydayhealth.com/hs/ulcerative-colitis-treatment-management/ulcerative-colitis-biologics-things-to-know.

Inocian, E., Patterson, K., & Felicilda-Reynaldo, R. (2020). Direct-acting oral anticoagulants. *MEDSURG Nursing, 29*(6), 391–394.

Institute for Safe Medication Practices. ISMP's list of confused drug names. (2019). Retrieved from http://www.ismp.org/Tools/Confused-Drug-Names.aspx.

Jariwala, A., & Hamman, K. (2018). Stop the bleeding! Oral anticoagulation and options for reversal. *The Journal for Nurse Practitioners, 14*(1), 54–55.

Jarrell, L. (2021). Eosinophilic asthma and the role of monoclonal antibodies. *The Nurse Practitioner, 46*(4), 21–27.

Johnson, C., Miltner, R., & Wilson, M. (2018). Increasing nurse-driven heparin infusion administration safety: A quality improvement initiative. *MEDSURG Nursing, 27*(4), 243–246.

Karch, A. (2015). Preventing medication errors by empowering patients. *American Nurse Today, 10*(9), 18–22.

Kidd, T., Mitchell, S., Dehays, J., & Wibberley, E. (2022). Fluoroquinolones: With great power comes great risk. *Nursing, 52*(1), 24–27.

Kreider, K. (2021). Patient-centered medication selection for type 2 diabetes. *American Nurse Today, 16*(11), 33–36.

Maloy, P., Iacocca, M., & Morasco, B. (2019). Implementing guidelines for treating chronic pain with prescription opioids. *American Journal of Nursing, 119*(11), 22–29.

Marzlin, K. (2019). Implications of antiarrhythmic pharmacology. *AACN Advanced Critical Care, 30*(1), 85–91.

Marzlin, K. (2020). Atrial fibrillation and heart failure. *AACN Advanced Critical Care, 31*(4), 431–434.

Mayo Clinic (2021). Alzheimer's treatments: What's on the horizon? Retrieved from https://www.mayoclinic.org/diseases-conditions/alzheimers-disease/in-depth/alzheimers-treatments/art-20047780.

Mayo Clinic. (2021). Erectile dysfunction. Retrieved from https://www.mayoclinic.org/diseases-conditions/erectile-dysfunction/symptoms-causes/syc-20355776.

Mayo Clinic. (2021). Prescription sleeping pills: What's right for you? Retrieved from https://www.mayoclinic.org/diseases-conditions/insomnia/in-depth/sleeping-pills/art-20043959

Mayo Clinic. (2021). Seizures. Retrieved from https://www.mayoclinic.org/diseases-conditions/seizure/symptoms-causes/syc-20365711#:~:text=A%20seizure%20is%20a%20sudden,generally%20considered%20to%20be%20epilepsy.

McMahon, J. (2017). Improving medication administration safety in the clinical environment. *MEDSURG Nursing, 26*(6), 374–377, 409.

Medication Update. (2021). Higher-dose naloxone nasal spray approved. *The Nurse Practitioner, 46*(7), 56.

MedicineNet. (2022). How can I cure insomnia fast? 15 tips and techniques. Retrieved from https://www.medicinenet.com/how_can_i_cure_insomnia_fast_15_tips/article.htm.

MedlinePlus. Senna. Retrieved from https://medlineplus.gov/druginfo/natural/652.html.

Moore, D. (2020). Opioid-induced respiratory depression. *American Nurse Journal, 15*(5), 14.

Napier, K. (2021). Safe handling of oral chemotherapy. *Nursing, 51*(11), 11–12.

National Institutes of Health. (2021). HIV overview: FDA-approved HIV medicines. Retrieved from https://hivinfo.nih.gov/understanding-hiv/fact-sheets/fda-approved-hiv-medicines.

Ogbru, O., & Davis, C. (2019). Biologics (biologic drug class). Retrieved from https://www.medicinenet.com/biologics_biologic_drug_class/article.htm.

Olsen, M., LeFebvre, K., & Brassil, K. (2019). *Chemotherapy and immunotherapy guidelines and recommendations for practice.* Pittsburgh: Oncology Nursing Society.

Pattison, K. (2019). Medications for heart failure management: What nurses need to know. *American Nurse Today, 14*(2), 20–23.

Penkalski, M., Felicilda-Reynaldo, R., & Patterson, K. (2017). Antiviral medications, part 2: HIV antiretroviral therapy. *MEDSURG Nursing, 26*(5), 327–331.

Pich, J. (2019). Lamotrigine vs. carbamazepine monotherapy for epilepsy treatment. *American Journal of Nursing, 19*(11), 19.

Pickett, J. (2019). Direct oral anticoagulants in patients with non-valvular atrial fibrillation: Update and periprocedural management. *Critical Care Nurse, 39*(2), 54–66.

Plavskin, A. (2019). Fighting antimicrobial resistance with genetics and genomics. *MEDSURG Nursing, 28*(5), 297–302.

Priddy, M., & Bock, C. (2018). Acute decompensated heart failure: A pharmacotherapy approach. *AACN Advanced Critical Care, 29*(3), 233–239.

Pusey-Reid, E., Quin, L., & Foley, C. (2021). Review of COVID-19 for nurses. *MEDSURG Nursing, 30*(5), 297–302, 333.

Robichaux, C., Lewis, T., & Gros, R. (2022). Tools to enhance nursing students' confidence and skills in medication administration. *Nursing, 52*(3), 45–51,

Rogers, J. (2020). Understanding the most commonly billed diagnoses in primary care: Hypothyroidism. *The Nurse Practitioner, 45*(12), 36–42.

Rosenblum, R., & Manion, A. (2021). An update on practice guidelines for primary care treatment of pediatric migraine. *The Nurse Practitioner, 46*(11), 18–27.

Ruggiero, J., Smith, J., Copeland, J., & Boxer, B. (2015). Discharge time out: An innovative nurse-driven protocol for medication reconciliation. *MEDSURG Nursing, 24*(3), 165–172.

RxList. (2021). Anti-anxiety drugs (anxiolytics). Retrieved from https://www.rxlist.com/anti-anxiety_drugs_anxiolytics/drugs-condition.htm.

Sabella, D. (2018). Antidepressant medications. *American Journal of Nursing, 118*(9), 52–59.

Saccomano, S. (2019). Acute acetaminophen toxicity in adults. *The Nurse Practitioner, 44*(11), 42–47.

Sassatelli, E. (2022). Cause to pause: Preventing medication errors with high-risk opioids. *Nursing, 52*(6), 26-30.

Scuteri, D., Adornetto, A., Rombola, L., Naturale, M., Morrona, L., Bagetta, G., et al. (2019). New trends in migraine pharmacology: Targeting calcitonin gene-regulated peptide (CGRP) with monoclonal antibodies. *Frontiers in Pharmacology, 10*, 363. Retrieved from https://doi.org/10.3389/fphar.2019.00363.

Shirley, D., Sterrett, J., Haga, N., & Durham, C. (2020). The therapeutic versatility of antihistamines: A comprehensive review. *The Nurse Practitioner, 45*(2), 8–21.

Singer, A., & Wilson, S. (2017). Reversal strategies for newer oral anticoagulants. *AACN Advanced Critical Care, 28*(4), 322–331.

Sink, K., & Scardina, A. (2020). Pharmacogenomics: Importance to clinical practice. *MEDSURG Nursing, 29*(6), 375–380.

Sloan, A., & Dudjak, L. (2020). Bedside nurses: Champions of antimicrobial stewardship. *Critical Care Nurse, 40*(6), 16–22.

Smith, D., & Kautz, D. (2018). Protect older adults from polypharmacy hazards. *Nursing, 48*(2), 56–59.

Smith, G., Pueger, M., & Wagner, J. (2019). Evidence-based epilepsy care. *American Nurse Today, 14*(7), 6–11.

Taylor, K. (2021). Geriatric medication reconciliation in the home setting. *American Nurse Journal, 16*(7), 14–17.

Theisen, E., & Konieczny, E. (2019). Medical cannabis: What nurses need to know. *American Nurse Today, 14*(11), 6–10.

Trang, J., Nguyen, N., & Huynh, S. (2019). Guidance for transitioning among anticoagulants. *AACN Advanced Critical Care, 30*(3), 209–216.

Toney-Butler, J., & Wilcox, L. (2021). Dose calculation: Desired over have formula method. *StatPearls*. Retrieved from https://www.ncbi.nlm.nih.gov/books/NBK493162.

United States Department of Justice, Drug Enforcement Administration. (2020). Diversion Control Division: Controlled Substance Schedules. Retrieved from https://www.deadiversion.usdoj.gov/schedules.

United States Food and Drug Administration (FDA). FDA approves new add-on drug to treat off episodes in adults with Parkinson's disease. Retrieved from https://www.fda.gov/news-events/press-announcements/fda-approves-new-add-drug-treat-episodes-adults-parkinsons-disease#:~:text=Press%20Announcements-,FDA%20approves%20new%20add%2Don%20drug%20to%20treat%20off,in%20adults%20with%20Parkinson's%20disease&text=The%20U.S.%20Food%20and%20Drug,)%20experiencing%20%22off%22%20episodes.

Villaluz, I., & Grantner, G. (2020). Newly approved HIV medications. *U.S. Pharmacist, 45*(10), 17–25.

Volkert, D., & Ortelli, T. (2021). Medical and recreational marijuana. *American Journal of Nursing, 121*(11), 50–52.

Web MD. (2021) Biologics for Crohn's disease treatment. Retrieved from https://www.webmd.com/ibd-crohns-disease/crohns-disease/cm/biologics-crohns.

Web MD. (2021). Medications for Parkinson's disease. Retrieved from https://www.webmd.com/parkinsons-disease/guide/drug-treatments.

Web MD. (2021). On the frontline of epilepsy treatment. Retrieved from http://webmd.com/epilepsy/frontline-epilepsy-treatment.

Wieruszewski, E., Brown, C., Leung, J., & Wieruszewski, P. (2020). Pharmacologic management of status epilepticus. *AACN Advanced Critical Care, 31*(4) 349–356.

Wright, N. (2019). Antibiotic stewardship. *American Nurse Today, 14*(11), 46–47.

Index

Page numbers followed *f*, *t*, and *b* indicate figures, tables, and boxes, respectively.